FOURTH EDITION

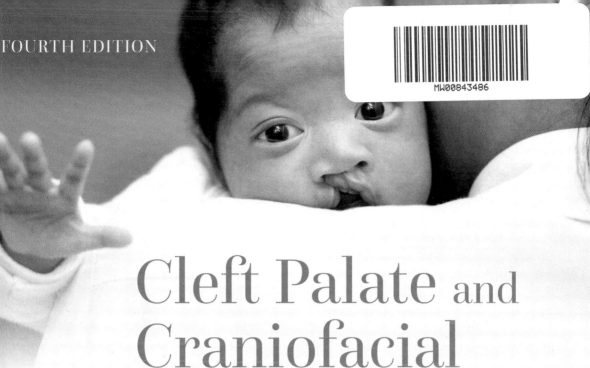

Cleft Palate and Craniofacial Conditions

A Comprehensive Guide to Clinical Management

Ann W. Kummer, PhD, CCC-SLP, FASHA

Senior Director, Division of Speech-Language Pathology (Retired)
Cincinnati Children's Hospital Medical Center
and
Professor of Clinical Pediatrics and
Professor of Otolaryngology–Head and Neck Surgery
University of Cincinnati College of Medicine
Cincinnati, Ohio

JONES & BARTLETT
L E A R N I N G

World Headquarters
Jones & Bartlett Learning
5 Wall Street
Burlington, MA 01803
978-443-5000
info@jblearning.com
www.jblearning.com

Jones & Bartlett Learning books and products are available through most bookstores and online booksellers. To contact Jones & Bartlett Learning directly, call 800-832-0034, fax 978-443-8000, or visit our website, www.jblearning.com.

Substantial discounts on bulk quantities of Jones & Bartlett Learning publications are available to corporations, professional associations, and other qualified organizations. For details and specific discount information, contact the special sales department at Jones & Bartlett Learning via the above contact information or send an email to specialsales@jblearning.com.

14972-2

Production Credits

VP, Product Management: David D. Cella
Director of Product Management: Matt Kane
Product Manager: Laura Pagluica
Product Assistant: Rebecca Feeney
Production Editor: Vanessa Richards
Senior Production Editor, Navigate: Leah Corrigan
Marketing Manager: Michael Sullivan
Product Fulfillment Manager: Wendy Kilborn

Composition: codeMantra U.S. LLC
Cover Design: Kristin E. Parker
Rights & Media Specialist: Thais Miller
Media Development Editor: Troy Liston
Cover Image (Title Page, Part Opener, Chapter Opener):
    © PeopleImages/Getty Images
Printing and Binding: LSC Communications
Cover Printing: LSC Communications

Library of Congress Cataloging-in-Publication Data

Names: Kummer, Ann W., author.
Title: Cleft palate and craniofacial conditions: a comprehensive guide to clinical management / Ann W. Kummer.
Other titles: Cleft palate and craniofacial anomalies
Description: Fourth edition. | Burlington, Massachusetts: Jones & Bartlett Learning, [2020] |
Preceded by Cleft palate and craniofacial anomalies / Ann W. Kummer. Third edition. 2014. |
Includes bibliographical references and index.
Identifiers: LCCN 2018005640 | ISBN 9781284149104 (pbk.)
Subjects: | MESH: Cleft Palate—complications | Speech Disorders—etiology |
    Cleft Palate—therapy | Speech Disorders—therapy | Craniofacial
    Abnormalities—complications | Craniofacial Abnormalities—therapy
Classification: LCC RJ496.S7 | NLM WV 440 | DDC 617.5/225—dc23
LC record available at https://lccn.loc.gov/2018005640

6048

Printed in the United States of America
22 21 20   10 9 8 7 6 5 4 3 2

DEDICATION

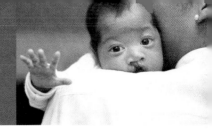

This book is dedicated to the three people who have influenced me most in my life and helped me to be the best that I can be. Without their love and support, I would never have had a career and certainly would not have had the opportunity to write this book . . . now for the fourth time.

The first dedication is to my father, who was a wonderful, caring, and talented otolaryngologist whom I always admired. I always wanted to be like my dad when I was growing up.

The next dedication is to my mother, who was the kindest, most thoughtful, and most caring person I have ever known. Once I grew up, I tried to be more like her. (I'm still trying.)

The final dedication is to my husband, who has loved me, supported me, encouraged me, and helped me to focus and succeed in my career. For that I will be eternally grateful!

Ann

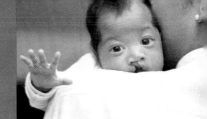

CONTENTS

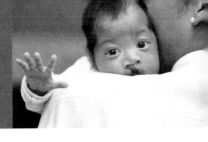

PREFACE

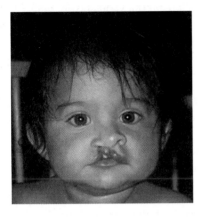

Anticipating the birth of a new baby is usually a very exciting time of life. The expectant couple does many things to prepare for the baby, including setting up a nursery, gathering baby clothes and diapers, and deciding on a name. The parents expect to have a normal baby, with 10 fingers, 10 toes, and an intact face. Usually, they are totally unprepared for the possibility of a different outcome.

Unfortunately, not all babies are born with perfect structures. When a child is born with cleft lip, cleft palate, or other craniofacial anomalies, this is a true shock, especially because it involves the face. What was expected to be a very happy and exciting time becomes a very stressful and emotional time for the parents and other family members. It may be impossible for the parents to see past the anomaly to really appreciate their newborn baby.

Cleft lip with or without cleft palate is the fourth most common birth defect and the first most common facial birth defect. In fact, about 1 in every 700 children born in the United States each year has a cleft of the lip and/or palate. About half of these children have other associated malformations. Cleft palate is a characteristic of well over 400 recognized syndromes.

Although current medical technology is not advanced enough to prevent the occurrence of these birth defects, most of the speech and functional impairments associated with craniofacial anomalies can be improved or even corrected with the help of a team of professionals. To provide the type of care that these patients require, this group of professionals must be specialists within their fields. For true quality care, they must have a thorough understanding of the current methods of evaluation and treatment of these patients.

Considering the incidence of clefts and craniofacial anomalies in the general population, however, all healthcare providers should have at least basic knowledge about the management of these patients and appropriate referrals. In particular, speech-language pathologists must be trained in the basic evaluation and treatment and appropriate referrals of individuals with these conditions, especially considering the fact that they often have a significant effect on speech. Certainly, school-based speech-language pathologists are very likely to have children on their caseloads with a history of cleft, craniofacial anomalies, or resonance disorders.

Purpose of This Text

The purpose of this text is to inform, educate, and excite students and professionals in speech-language pathology and the medical and dental professions regarding the management of individuals with clefts or craniofacial anomalies. This text is designed to be a textbook for graduate students and a sourcebook for healthcare professionals who provide services in this area. My goal in writing this text was to provide readers with a great deal of information but in a way that is both interesting and easy to read. As an active clinician myself, my intent was to make this text a very practical how-to guide as well as a source of didactic and theoretical information.

My ultimate goal with this text is to improve the knowledge of treating professionals who work with individuals who are affected by a cleft or other craniofacial conditions. It is hoped that with this knowledge, they can positively affect the quality of care provided to this population.

Organization

This text was written in a purposeful sequence so that the information from each chapter builds on the information from previous chapters.

Part 1 of this text provides basic information on the normal anatomy of the orofacial structures and the normal physiology of the velopharyngeal valve. Once the normal structures and function are described, information on genetics and patterns of inheritance is covered. The rest of Part 1 consists of information about congenital and acquired craniofacial anomalies and craniofacial syndromes. Once the reader has completed the first section, the reader should have a firm understanding of normal and abnormal facial and velopharyngeal features and the potential causes of congenital and even acquired anomalies.

Part 2 of this text includes chapters on the various functional problems associated with clefts and craniofacial conditions. In particular, this section covers the effects of these anomalies on feeding, speech and language development, psychosocial function, and speech and resonance. After completing the second section, the reader will have an understanding of the number, types, and complexity of the problems that are secondary to clefts and craniofacial conditions. It will then be apparent to the reader that there is a need for multidisciplinary management of these patients in an interdisciplinary setting.

Part 3 of this text covers the various diagnostic methods for assessing speech, resonance, and velopharyngeal function. This section includes the perceptual examination of speech and resonance and the physical examination of the oral cavity and other orofacial structures. There is an overview chapter on instrumentation that is sufficient for graduate students. There are also individual chapters on the various types of instrumental procedures. These chapters are very detailed and written to provide specific information for practicing clinicians who will be using these procedures.

Part 4 of this text covers the treatment of speech and resonance disorders secondary to clefts, craniofacial anomalies, and velopharyngeal dysfunction. This section includes surgical management, prosthetic management, and speech therapy. The speech therapy chapter includes specific therapy strategies for achieving placement. In addition, there is a section on achieving carryover using motor learning and motor memory principles.

Part 5 of this text is short but important because it emphasizes the fact that many disciplines are needed to provide care for patients affected by clefts or craniofacial anomalies. The reader will complete this section with an understanding that quality patient care requires interdisciplinary interaction and collaboration in the assessment and treatment of these patients.

Features

- **Chapter outlines:** The outline of each chapter helps readers navigate through the content and find information quickly.
- **Figures:** This text includes almost 700 figures. These photos and illustrations are meant to enhance comprehension of information and concepts discussed in the chapters.
- **Case studies:** Several chapters include patient case studies to illustrate how chapter information applies to real-life situations.
- **Speech Notes:** Chapters regarding anomalies and surgeries have boxed sections called *Speech Notes*. These sections highlight how these anomalies or surgeries affect speech and resonance.

- **For Review and Discussion:** A list of questions and topics for discussion is included at the end of each chapter. The purpose of this section is to help the reader synthesize and apply information presented in the chapter. Instructors can also use this section for class discussion, student homework, or essay exams.
- **Definitions:** Selected technical and medical terms are presented in bold and defined within the text and in the glossary.
- **Glossary:** There is a glossary of terms at the end of the text that defines all the medical and technical terms that were bold in the individual chapters. The student may find that studying the glossary is helpful for learning much of the information in the text.

Online Resources

The following resources are available for students and instructors. For more information on how to access these resources, please visit go.jblearning.com/cleftpalate.

- **Cleft Notes:** The *Cleft Notes* are basic summaries in table format provided for each chapter. There are some compare-and-contrast aspects of these tables to help students assimilate the information. There are two versions of the Cleft Notes—a blank version for students to use when taking notes or studying, and a filled-out version for instructors. By completing the Cleft Notes, the students are engaged in more active learning and have a study guide for test preparation.
- **Handouts:** There are online handouts on a variety of topics that are covered in this text. These handouts are designed primarily for parents but can also be helpful to other professionals who are not familiar with the topic area. The handouts are designed so the user can print them directly from the website.
- **Videos:** There are 295 videos/animations/audio files online. These videos illustrate different types of speech and resonance disorders. There are videos of evaluation techniques, including nasopharyngoscopy,

videofluoroscopy, and even nasometry studies. Finally, there are videos of speech therapy techniques that are effective with this population and also with other individuals with speech sound disorders. These videos are designed to help the viewer develop diagnostic and treatment skills by watching and listening to each video as many times as necessary. Because these videos are short and carefully edited, they facilitate better learning than direct observation in a clinic.

- **PowerPoint Presentations:** There are PowerPoint presentations, which include important figures and photos, for each chapter. These presentations can be used by the instructor for classroom teaching.
- **Testbank:** Assessment questions are available in a variety of different formats, including multiple choice, labeling, matching, and true/false.
- **Image Library:** The image library provides access to all the art in the textbook. This resource can be searched using keywords and subject areas.

New to This Edition

- **Photos:** Many new photos have been added, most of which are in color.
- **Drawings:** Anatomy figures have been re-rendered for consistency and improved quality.
- **Tables:** Many chapters have information summarized in tables for easy learning. There are also tables of terms for normal and abnormal craniofacial, oral, dental, and pharyngeal structures and anomalies.
- **Chapter Text:** Chapters have been heavily edited with a focus on making the information clear, concise, and easy to read.
- **Chapter Order:** The chapter order has been reorganized for better flow.
- **Research Updates:** Information within the text and the references have been updated to reflect current research and literature.

Format Notes

Service providers must be sensitive to the emotional and psychological needs of the patient. Sensitivity to the feelings of the patient is often overlooked by well-meaning service providers. It is easy to forget that we deal with real people, not just interesting cases. This lack of sensitivity is sometimes reflected in the terminology that is used in the literature and in daily use. I recall listening to a speech given by an adult who was born with a cleft palate. As he described his childhood, he pointed out that being called a "cleft palate child" evoked very negative feelings. Fortunately, this type of phrase is becoming "politically incorrect," just as the term "harelip" has in the past. Using the anomaly as an adjective to describe the individual is certainly insensitive to the feelings of the person who was born with this anomaly. Therefore, it is preferable to use "patient-first" terminology as in "child with a cleft."

The reader will note that the word "child" is frequently used throughout the text for the individual with the anomaly. This is because the speech and resonance disorders secondary to cleft lip/palate and craniofacial anomalies are usually addressed during childhood. However, it should be understood that this information also applies to adults with the same anomalies.

Acknowledgments and Thanks

There are so many people that I would like to acknowledge for their help with this edition of the text. Many thanks go to the members of our VPI/Resonance Team at Cincinnati Children's, including Jenn Marshall, Shyla Miller, Cara Werner, Margaret (Meg) Wilson, and Sarah Woodhouse. They were very helpful in providing feedback, developing the Cleft Notes, and reviewing videos. Special thanks go to Cara Werner, who proofread the entire manuscript and online content. She also provided very valuable suggestions. I would like to thank the members of the Cleft and Craniofacial Center at Cincinnati Children's for being such great colleagues, mentors, and friends! I have learned so much through our professional interactions over the years. Finally, I'm very grateful to Laura Pagluica and her entire team at Jones & Bartlett including Rebecca Feeney, Vanessa Richards, Thais Miller, and Troy Liston. It was such a great experience working with them. I have been very impressed with the entire company and the quality of their products.

Final Words

I am very grateful for the opportunity to share with you what I have learned through my clinical practice over the years. I sincerely hope that through this text you will be educated, enlightened, and inspired to provide superior clinical services for individuals with clefts or other craniofacial conditions.

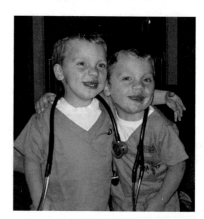

CREDITS

All photos courtesy of the Cleft and Craniofacial Center at Cincinnati Children's Hospital Medical Center.

KEY TO PHONETIC SYMBOLS

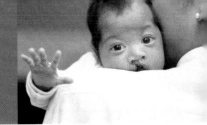

Vowels	
Symbol	**Examples**
/i/	b**ee**, s**ee**
/æ/	h**a**t, c**a**t
/ɑ/	f**a**ther, p**o**t
/ə/	teach**er**, moth**er**

Consonants		
Symbol	**Letters**	**Examples**
/ʔ/	glottal stop	bu**tt**on, mi**tt**en
/ʃ/,	sh	**sh**oe
/ʒ/	zh	mea**s**ure
/tʃ/	ch	**ch**air
/dʒ/	j	**j**ump
/θ/	th	**th**in
/ð/	th	**th**en
/ŋ/	ng	si**ng**

Note: This key includes only the phonetic symbols used in this text.

ABOUT THE AUTHOR

Ann W. Kummer, PhD, CCC-SLP, FASHA, is the former senior director of the Division of Speech-Language Pathology at Cincinnati Children's. Under her direction of over 35 years, the speech-language pathology program at Cincinnati Children's became the largest pediatric program in the nation and one of the most respected. Dr. Kummer is professor of clinical pediatrics and professor of otolaryngology at the University of Cincinnati (UC), College of Medicine.

Dr. Kummer has done hundreds of national and international lectures and seminars in the areas of cleft palate and craniofacial anomalies, resonance disorders, velopharyngeal dysfunction, and business practices in speech-language pathology. She has taught the craniofacial anomalies course for five universities. She has also written numerous professional articles and 22 book chapters in speech pathology and medical texts. In addition to this text, she is one of the authors of the text *Business Practices: A Guide for Speech-Language Pathologists*. Dr. Kummer is the co-developer of the Simplified Nasometric Assessment Procedures (SNAP) test (1996) and author of the SNAP-R (2005), which is incorporated in the Nasometer™ equipment (PENTAX Medical). She holds a patent on the nasoscope, which is marketed as the Oral & Nasal Listener™ (Super Duper, Inc.). She was one of the main developers of workflow software that won the 1995 International Beacon Award through IBM/Lotus. (Derivative software is marketed by Chart Links.)

Dr. Kummer has received numerous honors, including Honors of the Southwestern Ohio Speech-Language-Hearing Association (1995); Honors of the Ohio Speech-Language-Hearing Association (OSLHA) (1997); Distinguished Alumnus Award from the Department of Communication Sciences and Disorders, University of Cincinnati (1999); Fellow of the American Speech-Language-Hearing Association (ASHA) (2002); named one of the top 25 most influential therapists in the United States by *Therapy Times* (2006); Honors for Distinguished Service, Department of Otolaryngology–Head and Neck Surgery, University of Cincinnati (2007); named one of the 10 Most Inspiring Women in Cincinnati (2007); inducted into the National Academy of Inventors, Cincinnati Chapter (2010); Distinguished Alumnus Award, College of Allied Health, University of Cincinnati (2012), Elwood Chaney Outstanding Clinician Award from the Ohio Speech-Language-Hearing Association (OSHLA) (2012); Annie Glenn National Leadership Award, Ohio School Speech Pathology Educational Audiology Coalition (OSSPEAC) (2014); and the Media Outreach Champion award from ASHA (2014). In 2017, she received Honors of the Association from ASHA, the highest award given by the association.

CONTRIBUTORS

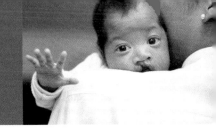

It is with great appreciation that I would like to thank the various contributors to this edition. Their expertise was essential in making the contents of many of the chapters both accurate, current, and clinically relevant. I will be forever in their debt for their contributions.

Haithem Elhadi Babiker, MD, DMD, FAAP, FACS
Assistant Professor
Plastic and Oral-Maxillofacial Surgeon
University of Cincinnati College of Medicine
Division of Plastic Surgery
Cincinnati Children's Hospital Medical Center
Cincinnati, Ohio
Chapter 17

David A. Billmire, MD
Emeritus Professor of Clinical Surgery
University of Cincinnati College of Medicine
Director of Plastic Surgery
Shriners Hospitals for Children
Cincinnati, Ohio
Chapter 17

Richard Campbell, DMD, MS
Assistant Professor
University of Cincinnati College of Medicine
Director, Orthodontics
Division of Pediatric Dentistry
Cincinnati Children's Hospital Medical Center
Cincinnati, Ohio
Chapter 6

Julia Corcoran, MD
Adjunct Associate Professor of Surgery
Feinberg School of Medicine Northwestern University
Attending Surgeon
Shriners Hospital for Children - Chicago
Chicago, Illinois
Chapter 17

Murray Dock, DDS, MSD
Associate Professor of Clinical Pediatrics
University of Cincinnati College of Medicine
Division of Pediatric Dentistry
Cincinnati Children's Hospital Medical Center
Cincinnati, Ohio
Chapter 6

Robert J. Hopkin, MD
Associate Professor of Clinical Pediatrics
University of Cincinnati College of Medicine
Division of Human Genetics
Cincinnati Children's Hospital Medical Center
Cincinnati, Ohio
Chapter 2

Deepak Krishnan, DDS, FACS
Associate Professor of Surgery & Residency Program Director
Division of Oral & Maxillofacial Surgery
University of Cincinnati Medical Center
Cincinnati, Ohio
Chapter 17

Patricia K. Marik, PsyD
Pediatric Psychologist
Psychiatry and Behavioral Medicine
Children's Hospital of Wisconsin
Assistant Clinical Professor of Psychiatry
Medical College of Wisconsin
Wauwatosa, Wisconsin
Chapter 9

Claire K. Miller, PhD, MHA
Program Director, Aerodigestive and Esophageal Center
Clinical/Research Speech-Language Pathologist
Division of Speech-Language Pathology
Cincinnati Children's Hospital Medical Center
Cincinnati, Ohio
Chapter 7

Howard M. Saal, MD
Professor of Pediatrics
University of Cincinnati College of Medicine
Director, Clinical Genetics
Division of Human Genetics
Cincinnati Children's Hospital Medical Center
Cincinnati, Ohio
Chapter 4

Janet R. Schultz, PhD
Professor
Psychology Department
Xavier University
Cincinnati, Ohio
Chapter 9

J. Paul Willging, MD
Professor
Department of Otolaryngology–Head and Neck
Surgery
University of Cincinnati College of Medicine
Cincinnati Children's Hospital Medical Center
Cincinnati, Ohio
Chapter 5

REVIEWERS

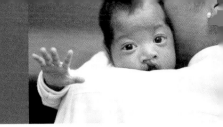

I would like to thank the reviewers who were kind enough to read through chapters and offer their advice. Their comments were greatly appreciated and most of their suggestions were incorporated in this edition.

Kate Bunton
University of Arizona

Marie E. Byrne
Mississippi University for Women

Ellen R. Cohn
University of Pittsburgh

Karen Copple
Eastern New Mexico University

Ramesh Kaipa
Oklahoma State University

Ciara Leydon
Sacred Heart University

Julie Owen Morris
University of Central Oklahoma

Amy Shollenbarger
Arkansas State University Jonesboro

Daniel Valentine
University of Motevallo

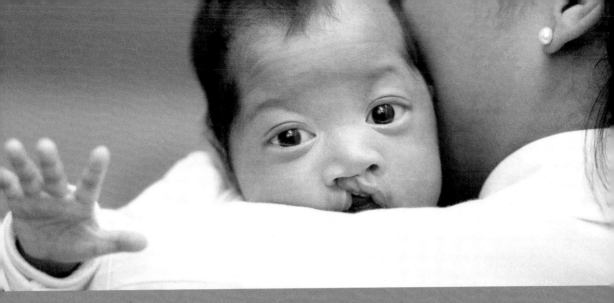

CHAPTER 1

Anatomy and Physiology

CHAPTER OUTLINE

INTRODUCTION

The nasal, oral, and pharyngeal structures are all very important for normal speech and resonance. Unfortunately, these are the structures that are commonly affected by cleft lip and palate and other craniofacial anomalies. Before the speech-language pathologist can fully understand the effects of oral and craniofacial anomalies on speech and resonance, a thorough understanding of normal structure (anatomy) and normal function (physiology) of the oral structures and the velopharyngeal valve is essential.

This chapter reviews the basic anatomy of the structures of the orofacial and velopharyngeal complex as they relate to speech production. The physiology of the subsystems of speech, including the velopharyngeal mechanism, is also described. For more detailed information on anatomy and physiology of the speech articulators, the interested reader is referred to other sources (Cassell & Elkadi, 1995; Cassell, Moon, & Elkadi, 1990; Dickson, 1972; Dickson, 1975; Dickson & Dickson, 1972; Dickson, Grant, Sicher, Dubrul, & Paltan, 1974; Dickson, Grant, Sicher, Dubrul, & Paltan, 1975; Huang, Lee, & Rajendran, 1998; Kuehn, 1979; Maue-Dickson, 1977; Maue-Dickson, 1979; Maue-Dickson & Dickson, 1980; Maue-Dickson, Dickson, & Rood, 1976; Moon & Kuehn, 1996; Moon & Kuehn, 1997; Moon & Kuehn, 2004; Perry, 2011; Seikel, King, & Drumright, 2005).

ANATOMY

Craniofacial Structures

Although the facial structures are familiar to all, some aspects of the face are important to point out for a thorough understanding of congenital anomalies and clefting. The normal facial landmarks can be seen on **FIGURE 1-1**. The reader is encouraged to identify the same structures on the photo of the normal infant face shown in Figure 1-1B.

Craniofacial Bones and Sutures

The bones of the cranium include the frontal bones, which cover the anterior portion of the brain; the parietal bones, which cover the top and sides of the cranium; the temporal bones, which form the sides and base of the skull; and finally, the occipital bone, which forms the back of the skull (**FIGURE 1-2**).

Each bone is bordered by an embryological suture line. The frontal bones are divided in midline by the metopic suture and bordered posteriorly by the coronal suture. The coronal suture is across the top of the skull horizontally (like a crown) and separates the frontal bones and parietal bones. The sagittal suture crosses the skull vertically and, therefore, divides the two parietal bones. Finally, the lambdoid suture is between the parietal, temporal, and occipital bones.

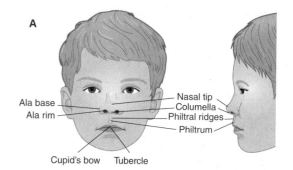

A

Ala base
Ala rim

Nasal tip
Columella
Philtral ridges
Philtrum

Cupid's bow   Tubercle

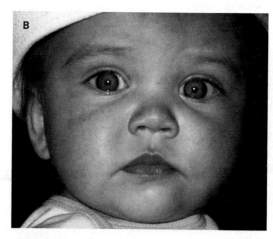

B

FIGURE 1-1 (A) Normal facial landmarks. Note the structures on the diagram. **(B)** Normal face. Try to locate the same structures on this infant's face.

Anterior

Normal skull of the newborn

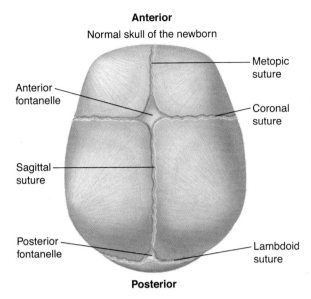

Anterior fontanelle

Sagittal suture

Posterior fontanelle

Metopic suture

Coronal suture

Lambdoid suture

Posterior

FIGURE 1-2 Cranial suture lines.

The **anterior fontanelle** ("soft spot" of an infant) is on the top of the skull at the junction of the frontal and the coronal sutures. The metopic suture closes between 3 and 9 months of age. The coronal, sagittal, and lambdoid sutures close between 22 and 39 months of age.

The facial bones include the **zygomatic bone** (also called **malar bone**), which forms the cheeks and the lateral walls of the orbits; the **maxilla**, which forms the upper jaw; and the **mandible**, which forms the lower jaw.

Ear

The ear has three distinct parts—the external ear, the middle ear, and the inner ear (**FIGURE 1-3**). A description of the anatomy of each part follows.

The **external ear** consists of the pinna and the external auditory canal. The **pinna** is the delicate cartilaginous framework of the external ear. It functions to direct sound energy into the **external auditory canal**, which is a skin-lined canal leading from the opening of the external ear to the eardrum.

The **middle ear** is a hollow space within the temporal bone. The **mastoid cavity** connects to the middle ear space posteriorly and consists of a collection of air cells within the temporal bone. Both the middle ear and mastoid cavities are lined with a **mucous membrane** (also known as **mucosa**), which consists of stratified squamous epithelium and lamina propria. (This should not be confused with **mucus**, which is the clear, viscid secretion from the mucous membranes.)

The **tympanic membrane**, also called the **eardrum**, is considered part of the middle ear. The tympanic membrane transmits sound energy through the ossicles to the inner ear. The **ossicles** are tiny bones within the middle ear and are called the malleus, incus, and stapes. The **malleus** (also known as the hammer) is firmly attached to the tympanic membrane. The **incus** (also known as the anvil) articulates with both the malleus and the stapes. The **stapes** acts as a piston to create pressure waves within the fluid-filled cochlea, which is part of the inner ear. The tympanic membrane and ossicles act to amplify the sound energy and efficiently introduce this energy into the liquid environment of the cochlea.

The **eustachian tube** (also known as the **auditory tube**) connects the middle ear with

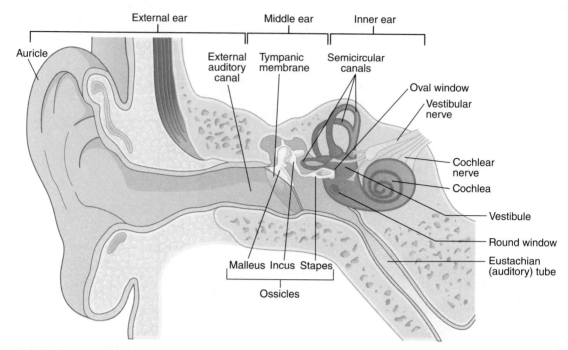

FIGURE 1-3 Ear showing external, middle, and inner ear structures and the eustachian tube.

the nasopharynx. The end of this tube, which terminates in the nasopharynx, is closed at rest but opens during swallowing. When it opens, it provides ventilation for the middle ear and mastoid cavities and results in equalization of air pressure between the middle ear and the environment (Cunsolo, Marchioni, Leo, Incorvaia, & Presutti, 2010; Licameli, 2002; Smith, Scoffings, & Tysome, 2016; Yoshida, Takahashi, Morikawa, & Kobayashi, 2007). It also allows drainage of fluids and debris from the middle ear space. (More information about the eustachian tube is noted in the Pharyngeal Structures section.)

The inner ear consists of the cochlea and semicircular canals. The cochlea is composed of a bony spiral tube that is shaped like a snail's shell. Within this bony tube are delicate membranes separating the canal into three fluid-filled spaces. The organ of Corti is the site where mechanical energy introduced into the cochlea is converted into electrical stimulation. This electrical impulse is conducted by the auditory nerves to the auditory cortex, which results in an awareness of

sound. Inner and outer hair cells (sensory cells with hair-like properties) of the cochlea may be damaged by a variety of mechanisms, leading to sensorineural hearing loss.

In addition to hearing, the inner ear is responsible for balance. The semicircular canals are the loop-shaped tubular parts of the inner ear that provide a sense of spatial orientation. They are oriented in three planes at right angles to one another. The saccule and utricle are additional sensory organs within the inner ear. Hair cells within these organs have small calcium carbonate granules that respond to gravity, motion, and acceleration.

Nose and Nasal Cavity

The nose begins at the nasal root, which is the most depressed, superior part of the nose and at the level of the eyes. The nasal bridge is the saddle-shaped area that includes the nasal root and the lateral aspects of the nose. Finally, the nasion is a midline point just superior to the nasal root and overlying the nasofrontal suture.

The nostrils are separated externally by the columella (little column). The **anterior nasal spine** of the maxilla forms a base for the columella. The columella is like a supporting column in that it provides support for the nasal tip. The columella must be long enough so that the nasal tip has an appropriate degree of projection. Ideally, the columella is straight and backed by a straight nasal septum.

The nostrils are frequently referred to as **nares**, although an individual nostril is a **naris**. The **ala nasi** (ala is Latin for "wing") is the outside curved side of the nostril. The alae (plural version of ala) are the two curved sides of each nostril. The **alar rim** is the outside curved edge that surrounds the opening to the nostril on either side, and the **alar base** is the area where the ala meets the upper lip. The **nasal sill** is the base of the nostril opening. The **nasal vestibule** is the most anterior part of the nasal cavity and is enclosed by the cartilages of the nose.

The opening to the bony inside of the nose is called the **pyriform aperture** (also spelled as "piriform," means "pear shaped"). This pear-shaped opening (thus the name) is bordered by the nasal and maxillary bones (**FIGURE 1-4**).

The **nasal septum** is located in the midline of the nose and serves to separate the nasal cavity into two nostrils (**FIGURE 1-5**). It consists of both cartilage in the anterior portion of the nose and bone in the posterior portion. The **quadrangular cartilage** forms the anterior nasal septum and projects anteriorly to the columella. The bones of the septum include the maxillary crest, the vomer, and the perpendicular plate of the ethmoid. The

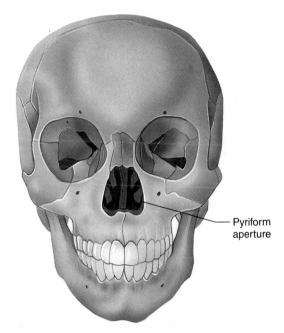

FIGURE 1-4 Pyriform aperture.

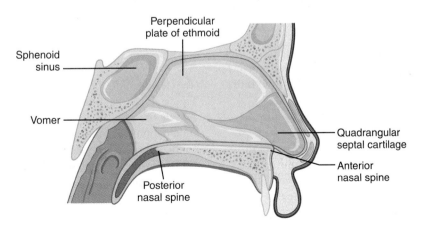

FIGURE 1-5 The nasal septum and related structures.

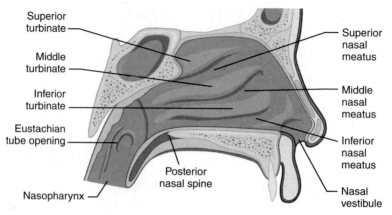

FIGURE 1-6 The lateral wall of the nose showing the turbinates.

vomer is a trapezoidal-shaped bone in the nasal septum. It is positioned perpendicular to the palate, and as such, the lower portion of the vomer fits in a groove formed by the median palatine suture line on the nasal aspect of the maxilla. The perpendicular plate of the ethmoid projects downward to join the vomer. It is not uncommon for the nasal septum to be less than perfectly straight, particularly in adults. The nasal septum is covered with mucous membrane, which is the lining tissue of the nasal cavity, oral cavity, and the pharynx.

The nasal turbinates, also called nasal conchae (concha, singular), are paired bony structures within the nose that are covered with mucosa (**FIGURE 1-6**). They are attached to the lateral walls of the nose and protrude medially into the nasal cavity. They are long, narrow, shelf-like, and curled in shape. As air flows underneath them, the curled shape helps to create turbulent airflow (thus the name "turbinate") to maximize contact of the inspired air with the nasal mucosa.

The nasal turbinates within the nose have three distinct functions. First, the mucus that covers the nasal mucosa filters inspired air of gross contaminants by trapping particulate contaminants. Second, the turbinates warm and humidify the inspired air. Finally, the turbinates deflect air superiorly in the nose in order to enhance the sense of smell.

Directly under the turbinates are the superior, middle, and inferior nasal meatuses (meatus, singular), which are the openings or passageways through which the air flows. At the back of the nasal cavity, on each side of the posterior part of the vomer, is a choana (choanae, plural), which is a funnel-shaped opening that leads to the nasopharynx.

Finally, the paranasal sinuses are air-filled spaces in the bones of the face and skull. These structures are each about the size of a walnut. There are four pairs of paranasal sinuses: frontal sinuses (in the forehead area), ethmoid sinuses (between the eyes), maxillary sinuses (under the cheeks), and sphenoid sinuses (deep in the skull). These sinuses are connected to the nose by a small opening called an ostium (ostia, plural). **FIGURE 1-7** shows the sinuses through computed tomography.

Lips

The features of the upper lip can be seen in Figure 1-1A. An examination of the upper lip reveals the philtrum, which is a long dimple or indentation that courses from the columella down to the upper lip. The philtrum is bordered by the philtral ridges on each side. These ridges are actually embryological suture lines that are formed as the segments of the upper lip fuse. The philtrum and philtral ridges course downward from the nose and terminate at the edge of the upper lip.

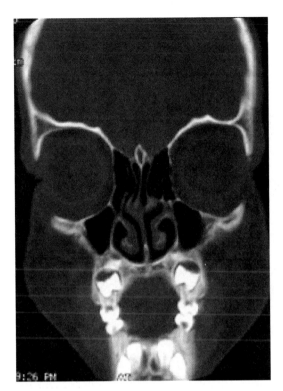

FIGURE 1-7 Radiograph of the nasal sinuses.

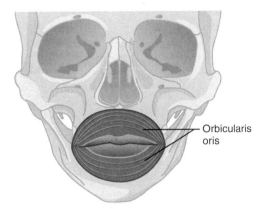

Orbicularis oris

FIGURE 1-8 Orbicularis oris muscles, which circle the mouth.

Intraoral Structures

The intraoral structures include the tongue, faucial pillars, tonsils, hard palate, soft palate, uvula, and oropharyngeal isthmus (**FIGURE 1-9**). These structures are discussed in detail as follows.

Tongue

The tongue resides within the arch of the mandible and fills the oral cavity when the mouth is closed. With the mouth closed, the slight negative pressure within the oral cavity ensures that the tongue adheres to the palate and the tip rests against the alveolar ridge. The dorsum (dorsal surface) is the superior surface of the tongue and the ventrum (ventral surface) is the inferior surface of the tongue.

Faucial Pillars, Tonsils, and Oropharyngeal Isthmus

At the back of the oral cavity on both sides are the paired curtain-like structures called the faucial pillars (Figure 1-9). Both the anterior and posterior faucial pillars contain muscles that assist with velopharyngeal movement. (See section called *Muscles of the Velopharyngeal Valve.*)

Most people think of the tonsils as the tissue in the oral cavity that can become infected,

The top of the upper lip is called the Cupid's bow because of its characteristic shape of bilateral rounded peaks with a midline indentation. On the upper lip, the inferior border of the midsection of the vermilion is referred to as the labial tubercle because it comes to a slight point and can be somewhat prominent. The lips are surrounded by border tissue, called the white roll. The skin of the lips is called the vermilion because it is redder (and darker) than the skin of the rest of the face.

In its naturally closed position, the upper lip rests over and slightly in front of the lower lip, although the inferior border of the upper lip is inverted. Movement of the lips is primarily because of the orbicularis oris muscle. The orbicularis oris muscle is actually a complex of four independent quadrant muscles in the lips that encircle the mouth (**FIGURE 1-8**). This group of muscles is responsible for pursing and puckering of the lips for kissing and whistling.

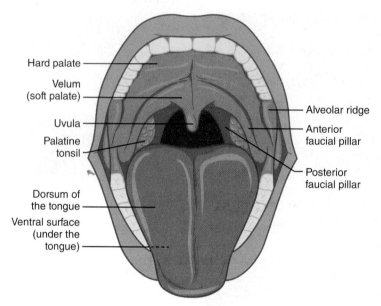

FIGURE 1-9 The structures of the oral cavity.

causing **tonsillitis**. Actually, there are three sets of tonsils, which surround the opening to the oropharynx, collectively known as **Waldeyer's ring**.

The **palatine tonsils** (usually known as just the tonsils) are located at the back of the mouth and between the anterior and posterior faucial pillars on both sides. Although the palatine tonsils are bilateral, differences in size are common, so it is not unusual for one tonsil to be larger than the other. The **lingual tonsil** is located at the base of the tongue and extends to the epiglottis (**FIGURE 1-10**). Finally, the pharyngeal tonsil, also known as the adenoids, is located in the nasopharynx. All tonsils consist of tissue similar to lymph nodes. They are covered by mucosa with various pits, called **crypts**, throughout.

Tonsillar tissue serves as part of the body's immune system by developing antibodies against infections, and therefore, this tissue is especially important during the child's first 2 years of life (Brodsky, Moore, Stanievich, & Ogra, 1988). Over time, the tonsil and adenoid tissue tends to atrophy, particularly with puberty, so that by around the age of 16, only small remnants of this

tissue remain. Fortunately, atrophy (and even surgical removal) of tonsil and/or adenoid tissue has little effect on immunity because of the redundancy in the immune system. In fact, the entire gastrointestinal tract is lined with the same type of tissue as found in the tonsils so that it also supports immunity.

The **oropharyngeal isthmus** is the opening between the oral cavity and the pharynx. It is bordered superiorly by the velum, laterally by the faucial pillars, and inferiorly by the base of the tongue.

Hard Palate

The **hard palate** is a bony structure that separates the oral cavity from the nasal cavity. It serves as both the roof of the mouth and the floor of the nose. The anterior portion of the hard palate is called the **alveolar ridge** (Figure 1-9). This ridge forms the bony support for the teeth. The rest of the hard palate forms a rounded dome on the upper part of the oral cavity, called the **palatal vault**.

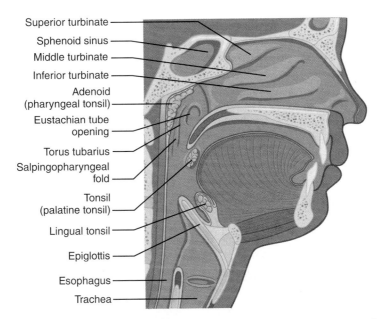

Superior turbinate
Sphenoid sinus
Middle turbinate
Inferior turbinate
Adenoid (pharyngeal tonsil)
Eustachian tube opening
Torus tubarius
Salpingopharyngeal fold
Tonsil (palatine tonsil)
Lingual tonsil
Epiglottis
Esophagus
Trachea

FIGURE 1-10 Lateral view of the nasal, oral, and pharyngeal cavities and the structures in these areas.

The hard palate is covered by a mucoperiosteum. Mucoperiosteum consists of a mucous membrane and periosteum. Mucous membrane (often called mucosa) is an epithelial tissue that lines many body cavities, in addition to the hard palate, and secretes mucus. Mucus (note the difference in spelling) is a clear and viscid (sticky) secretion. Periosteum is a thick, fibrous tissue that lies just under the mucous membrane and covers the surface of bone.

The mucosal covering of the hard palate has multiple ridges, called rugae, which run transversely. There is often a slight elevation of the mucosa in the middle of the anterior part of the hard palate, called the incisive papilla. A narrow seam-like ridge in midline (actually an embryological suture line), called the median palatine raphe (pronounced /ˈræfeɪ/), runs from the incisive papilla posteriorly over the entire length of the hard palate and velum. Bilateral midline depressions at the junction of the hard and soft palate, called the foveae palati, can often be seen. These are openings to minor salivary glands.

The bones of the hard palate include the premaxilla (a single midline bone), the palatine processes of the maxilla, and the horizontal plates of the palatine bone. These bones are separated by embryological suture lines.

The premaxilla is a triangular-shaped bone located in front of the maxillary bones (**FIGURE 1-11**). The alveolar ridge of the premaxilla contains the central and lateral maxillary incisors. The premaxilla is bordered on either side by the incisive suture lines and posteriorly by the incisive foramen. By definition, a foramen is a hole or opening in a bony structure that allows blood vessels and nerves to pass through to the area on the other side. The incisive foramen is an opening at the junction between the premaxilla and the maxillary bones. The incisive foramen also serves as a dividing point between two embryological processes. This will be discussed in the chapter *Clefts of the Lip and Palate.*

Behind the premaxilla are the paired palatine processes of the maxilla, which form the anterior three quarters of the maxilla. These bones terminate at the transverse palatine suture line

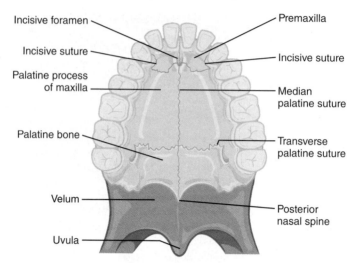

FIGURE 1-11 Bony structures of the hard palate.

(also known as the palatomaxillary suture line). Behind the transverse palatine suture line are the paired horizontal plates of the palatine bones. These bones form the posterior portion of the hard palate and end with the protrusive posterior nasal spine. The palatine processes of the maxilla and the horizontal plates of the palatine bones are both paired because they are separated in the midline by the median palatine suture line (also known as the intermaxillary suture line). This midline suture line begins at the incisive foramen and ends at the posterior nasal spine.

In some individuals, a torus palatinus, or palatine torus, can be seen as a prominent longitudinal ridge on the oral surface of the hard palate in the area of the median suture line (**FIGURE 1-12**). It can become larger with age. This finding is a normal variation, rather than an abnormality, and is most commonly seen in Caucasians of northern European descent, Native Americans, or Eskimos. It tends to occur more in females than in males (Garcia Garcia, Martinez-Gonzalez, Gomez-Font, Soto-Rivadeneira, & Oviedo-Roldan, 2010).

The sphenoid bone (an unpaired bone located at the base of the skull) and the temporal bones (located at the sides and base of the skull) provide bony attachment for the velopharyngeal musculature. The pterygoid process of the sphenoid

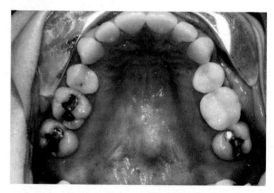

FIGURE 1-12 Small torus palatinus.

bone contains the medial pterygoid plate, the lateral pterygoid plate, and the pterygoid hamulus, which provides attachments for muscles in the velopharyngeal complex (**FIGURE 1-13**).

Velum

The velum (commonly referred to as the soft palate) is located in the back of the mouth and is attached to the posterior border of the hard palate (see Figure 1-9 and Figure 1-11). The velum consists of muscles (rather than bones), making it soft. As with the hard palate, the oral surface is covered by mucous membrane.

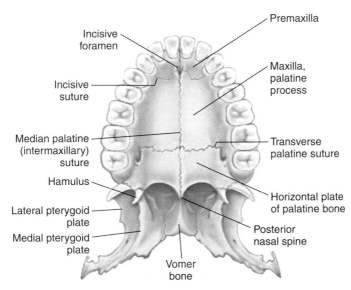

FIGURE 1-13 Inferior view of the hard palate. Note the hamulus, the lateral pterygoid plate, and the medial pterygoid plate.

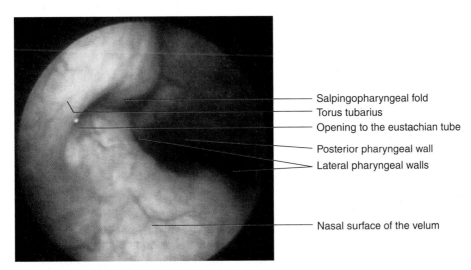

FIGURE 1-14 View of the nasal surface of the velum as seen through nasopharyngoscopy. Note the opening to the eustachian tube.

The median palatine raphe continues to course from the midline of the hard palate posteriorly through the velum to the uvula. The nasal surface of the velum (**FIGURE 1-14**) consists of pseudostratified, ciliated columnar epithelium anteriorly, and posteriorly of stratified, squamous epithelium in the area of velopharyngeal closure (Ettema & Kuehn, 1994; Kuehn & Kahane, 1990; Moon & Kuehn, 1996; Moon & Kuehn, 1997; Serrurier & Badin, 2008).

The anterior portion of the velum consists of the tensor veli palatini muscle tendon, glandular tissue, **adipose** (fat) tissue, and **palatine aponeurosis** (also called **velar aponeurosis**)

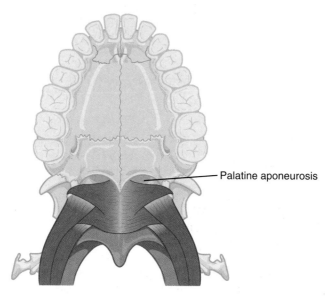

FIGURE 1-15 Position of the palatine (velar) aponeurosis. This is a sheet of fibrous tissue that is located just below the nasal surface of the velum and consists of periosteum, fibrous connective tissue, and fibers from the tensor veli palatini tendon. It provides an anchoring point for the velopharyngeal muscles and adds stiffness and velopharyngeal flexibility.

(**FIGURE 1-15**). The palatine aponeurosis consists of a sheet of fibrous connective tissue and fibers from the tensor veli palatini tendon. It attaches to the posterior border of the hard palate and courses about 1 cm posteriorly through the velum. The palatine aponeurosis provides an anchoring point for the velopharyngeal muscles and adds stiffness to that portion of the velum (Cassell & Elkadi, 1995; Ettema & Kuehn, 1994; Hwang, Kim, Huan, Han, & Hwang, 2011). The medial portion of the velum contains most of the fibers of the levator veli palatini muscles, which are described later in this chapter. The posterior portion of the velum consists of the same glandular and adipose tissue as can be found in the anterior portion.

Uvula

The uvula is a teardrop-shaped structure that is typically long and slender (see Figure 1-9 and Figure 1-11). It hangs freely from the posterior border of the velum. The uvula consists of mucosa on the surface and connective, glandular, adipose, and vascular tissue underneath. It contains no muscle fibers, however. The uvula does not contribute to velopharyngeal function and actually has no known function.

Pharyngeal Structures
Pharynx

The throat area between the nasal cavity and the esophagus is called the pharynx. The pharynx is divided into three sections, as can be seen in **FIGURE 1-16**. These sections include the nasopharynx, which is just posterior to the nasal cavity and behind the velum; the oropharynx, which is just posterior to the oral cavity; and the hypopharynx, which is below the oral cavity and extends from the epiglottis inferiorly to the esophagus. The back wall of the throat is called the posterior pharyngeal wall, and the side walls of the throat are called the lateral pharyngeal walls. The adenoids (also called the pharyngeal tonsil, adenoid pad, or just adenoid) consist of a

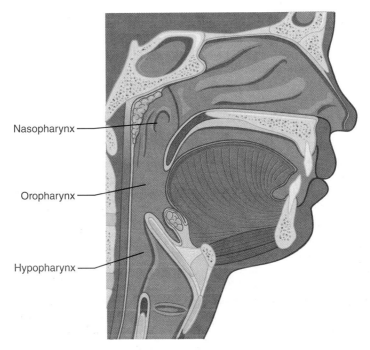

FIGURE 1-16 Sections of the pharynx. The oropharynx is at the level of the oral cavity or just posterior to the mouth. The nasopharynx is above the oral cavity, and the velum and is just posterior to the nasal cavity. The hypopharynx is below the oral cavity and extends from the epiglottis inferiorly to the esophagus.

singular mass of lymphoid tissue on the posterior pharyngeal wall, just behind the velum. Adenoids are usually present in children, but they atrophy with age. Adults have little, if any, adenoid tissue, and that which remains is relatively smooth on the surface.

Eustachian Tube

The eustachian tube is a membrane-lined tube that connects the middle ear space with the pharynx (see Figure 1-3 and Figure 1-14). The pharyngeal opening of the eustachian tube on each side is located on the lateral aspect of the nasopharynx and is slightly above the level of the velum during phonation. Bordering the posterior opening of each eustachian tube is a projection of the cartilaginous tissue, called the **torus tubarius**. Coursing down from the torus tubarius are folds of glandular and connective tissue, called the **salpingopharyngeal**

folds (Cunsolo et al., 2010; Dickson, 1975; Lukens, Dimartino, Gunther, & Krombach, 2012).

The eustachian tube is closed at rest, which helps prevent the inadvertent contamination of the middle ear by the secretions in the pharynx and back of the nose. During swallowing and yawning, however, the velum raises and the **tensor veli palatini muscles** contract to open the pharyngeal end of each of the tubes. As noted, this allows middle ear ventilation to ensure that the pressure inside the ear remains nearly the same as ambient air pressure. In addition, the opening of the tube allows drainage of fluids and debris from the middle ear space.

In the infant or toddler, the eustachian tube is essentially horizontal, and the pharyngeal opening is small. As the child grows, however, the tube changes to a downward-slanting angle from middle ear to the pharynx, and the pharyngeal opening becomes larger. As a result, the eustachian tube of an adult is at a 45° angle, and the opening is about the size of the diameter of a pencil. This gradual change in both the inclination and width of the tube during growth results in improved ventilation and drainage of the middle ear.

PHYSIOLOGY

Velopharyngeal Valve

The velopharyngeal valve consists of the velum (soft palate), lateral pharyngeal walls, and the posterior pharyngeal wall. During nasal breathing, the velopharyngeal valve remains open so that there is a patent airway between the nasal cavity and the lungs. For functions that require the nasal cavity to be separated (uncoupled) from the oral cavity, the velopharyngeal valve closes as a result of the highly coordinated movements of its component structures.

Velopharyngeal closure occurs during oral speech production as well as singing, whistling, blowing, swallowing, gagging, vomiting, and sucking (Nohara et al., 2007). In connected speech, the velopharyngeal valve must close quickly for oral sounds and open quickly for nasal sounds (Moon & Kuehn, 1996). Therefore, the velopharyngeal valve regulates and directs the transmission of sound energy and airflow into the oral and nasal cavities as appropriate.

It is important to recognize that the velopharyngeal valve is a three-dimensional structure that includes an anterior–posterior (AP) dimension, a sagittal dimension, and a vertical dimension. During closure, there must be coordinated movement of all structures in all dimensions so that the velopharyngeal valve can achieve closure like a sphincter. This can be seen in **FIGURE 1-17**, which shows an inferior view of the entire sphincter.

Velar Movement

During nasal breathing, the velum drapes down from the hard palate and rests against the base of the tongue (**FIGURE 1-18A**). This position contributes to a patent pharynx for unobstructed movement of air between the nasal cavity and lungs during nasal breathing. During velopharyngeal closure, the velum moves in a superior and posterior direction to contact the posterior pharyngeal wall or, in rare cases, the lateral pharyngeal walls (**FIGURE 1-18B**). During elevation, the velum bends at about three-quarters of the

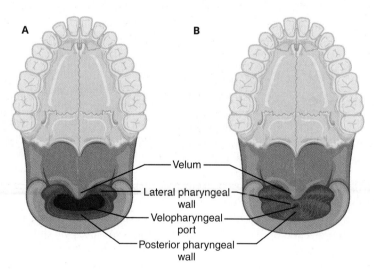

A

B

Velum

Lateral pharyngeal wall

Velopharyngeal port

Posterior pharyngeal wall

FIGURE 1-17 An inferior view of the velopharyngeal port. **(A)** The velopharyngeal port is open for nasal breathing. **(B)** The velopharyngeal port is closed for speech.

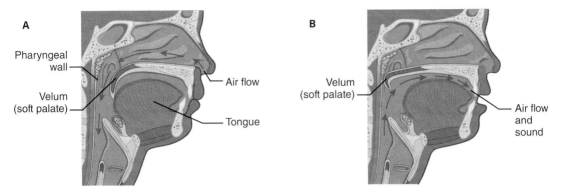

FIGURE 1-18 Lateral view of the velum and the posterior pharyngeal wall. **(A)** The velum rests against the base of the tongue during normal nasal breathing, resulting in a patent airway. **(B)** The velum elevates during speech and closes against the posterior pharyngeal wall. This allows the airflow from the lungs and the sound from the larynx to be redirected from a superior direction to an anterior direction to enter the oral cavity for speech.

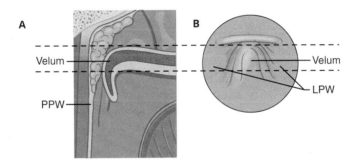

FIGURE 1-19 Lateral pharyngeal wall movement. **(A)** Lateral view of the velum as it contacts the pharyngeal wall. **(B)** Nasopharyngoscopy view of the lateral walls as the move to close against the velum.

way back from its entire length. This bending (sometimes called "knee action") results in a **velar eminence** (projection, like the knee cap, on top of the velum) on the nasal surface of the velum and a **velar dimple**, which can be seen in midline on the oral side. When a nasal phoneme is produced after an oral sound, the velum is pulled down so that sound energy can enter the nasal cavity.

As the velum elevates, it also elongates through a process called **velar stretch** (Bzoch, 1968; Mourino & Weinberg, 1975; Pruzansky & Mason, 1969; Simpson & Chin, 1981). The effective length of the velum, therefore, is the distance between the posterior border of the hard palate and the point on the posterior pharyngeal wall where there is velar contact during speech. This is measured in a line on the same plane as the hard palate (Satoh, Wada, Tachimura, & Fukuda, 2005). The amount of velar stretch and effective length of the velum vary among individuals and are dependent on the size and configuration of the pharynx.

Lateral Pharyngeal Wall Movement

The lateral pharyngeal walls contribute to velopharyngeal closure by moving medially to close against the velum or, in rare cases, to meet in midline behind the velum (**FIGURE 1-19**). Both lateral pharyngeal walls move during closure, but there is great variation among normal speakers as to the extent of movement (Lam, Hundert, & Wilkes, 2007). In addition, there is often asymmetry in movement so that one side may move significantly more than the other side. Although some lateral wall movement may be noted from an intraoral perspective, the point of greatest medial displacement occurs at the level of the hard palate (Iglesias, Kuehn, & Morris, 1980) and velar eminence (Lam et al., 2007; Shprintzen, McCall, Skolnick, & Lencione, 1975). This area is well above the area that can be seen from an intraoral inspection. In fact, at the oral cavity level, the lateral walls may actually appear to bow outward during speech (Lam et al., 2007).

Posterior Pharyngeal Wall Movement

Although there may be some anterior movement of the posterior pharyngeal wall during velopharyngeal closure, the contribution of the posterior pharyngeal wall to closure seems to be much less than that of the velum and lateral pharyngeal walls (Iglesias et al., 1980; Magen, Kang, Tiede, & Whalen, 2003).

Some speakers demonstrate a Passavant's ridge on the posterior pharyngeal wall (**FIGURE 1-20**).

Passavant's ridge

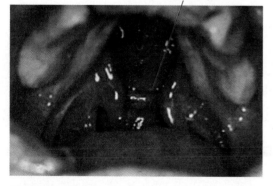

FIGURE 1-20 Passavant's ridge as noted during phonation. This patient has an open palate because of surgery for maxillary cancer. During phonation, the Passavant's ridge presents as a ridge of muscle on the posterior pharyngeal wall.

A Passavant's ridge, first described by Gustav Passavant in the 1800s, is not a permanent structure. Instead, it is a defined area on the posterior pharyngeal wall that bulges forward inconsistently during velopharyngeal movement and then disappears during nasal breathing or when velopharyngeal activity ceases (Glaser, Skolnick, McWilliams, & Shprintzen, 1979; Skolnick & Cohn, 1989). Passavant's ridge is thought to be formed by the contraction of specific fibers of the superior constrictor muscles (Dickson & Dickson, 1972; Finkelstein et al., 1993; Perry, 2011). The vertical location of the ridge is variable among individuals, but it is usually well below the site of velopharyngeal contact and, therefore, does not seem to be a factor in velopharyngeal closure (Glaser et al., 1979). Reports of the prevalence of Passavant's ridge in normal speakers range from as little as 9.5% to as high as 80% (Casey & Emrich, 1988; Finkelstein et al., 1991; Skolnick, Shprintzen, McCall, & Rakoff, 1975; Yamawaki, 2003; Yanagisawa & Weaver, 1996). In a look at the collective results of several studies, Casey and Emrich (1988) found that Passavant's ridge probably occurs in about 23% of individuals with a history of cleft and in 15% of normal speakers.

Muscles of the Velopharyngeal Valve

The velopharyngeal valve requires the coordinated action of several muscles, all of which are paired with one muscle on each side of the midline (Moon & Kuehn, 1996; Perry, 2011) (**FIGURE 1-21**). Coordinated movement of the velopharyngeal valve is very complex, requiring the interaction of not only these muscles but also that of the articulators, particularly the tongue (Kao, Soltysik, Hyde, & Gosain, 2008; Moon, Smith, Folkins, Lemke, & Gartlan, 1994; Perry, 2011; Perry & Kuehn, 2009).

Levator Veli Palatini Muscles

The levator veli palatini muscles, often referred to as the levator sling (Mehendale, 2004), are responsible for elevation of the velum during

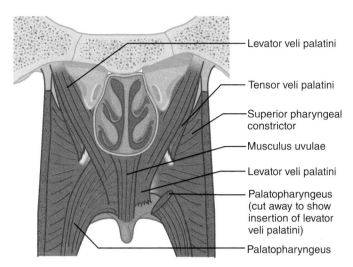

Levator veli palatini

Tensor veli palatini

Superior pharyngeal constrictor

Musculus uvulae

Levator veli palatini

Palatopharyngeus (cut away to show insertion of levator veli palatini)

Palatopharyngeus

FIGURE 1-21 The paired muscles of the velopharyngeal mechanism, as viewed from front to back. Note that the palatoglossus muscles are not shown, but would be anterior to the palatopharygeus muscles.

velopharyngeal closure. These muscles enter the velum on both sides at a 45° angle and interdigitate (blend together) in midline (Smith & Kuehn, 2007). Because of the 45° angle, the contraction of the levator muscles pulls the velum in a posterior and superior direction to close against the posterior pharyngeal wall. The point where these muscles interdigitate forms the velar dimple, which can be seen in the midline of the oral surface of the velum during phonation.

On each side of the nasopharynx, the levator veli palatini muscle originates from the apex of the petrous portion of the temporal bone at the base of the skull. The muscle then courses through an area that is anterior and medial to the carotid canal and inferior to the eustachian tube (Moon & Kuehn, 1996; Moon & Kuehn, 1997; Smith & Kuehn, 2007). The levator muscles take up the middle 40% of the entire velum and, therefore, provide its main muscle mass (Boorman & Sommerlad, 1985; Kuehn & Moon, 2005; Nohara, Tachimura, & Wada, 2006; Perry, Kuehn, & Sutton, 2011; Shimokawa et al., 2004).

Superior Constrictor Muscles

The **superior constrictor** (also called **superior pharyngeal constrictor**) muscles are responsible

for constriction of the lateral pharyngeal walls around the velum (Iglesias et al., 1980; Shprintzen et al., 1975; Skolnick, McCall, & Barnes, 1973). The paired superior constrictor muscles are located in the upper pharynx and arise from the pterygoid hamulus, pterygomandibular raphe, posterior tongue, posterior mandible, and palatine aponeurosis. They insert posteriorly in the pharyngeal raphe in the midline of the posterior pharyngeal wall.

Palatopharyngeus Muscles

The **palatopharyngeus** muscles are responsible for the medial movement of the lateral pharyngeal walls to bring them against the velum (Cassell & Elkadi, 1995; Cheng & Zhang, 2004; Sumida, Yamashita, & Kitamura, 2012). The palatopharyngeus muscles are contained within the posterior faucial pillars. They originate from the palatine aponeurosis in the anterior portion of the velum and posterior border of the hard palate. They then course down through the posterior pillars to the pharynx.

Palatoglossus Muscles

The **palatoglossus** muscles are responsible for the rapid downward movement of the velum for production of nasal consonants that follow an oral sound (Kuehn & Azzam, 1978; Moon & Kuehn, 1996). Given the speed at which the velum must be lowered for nasal phonemes and then raised for oral phonemes, gravity alone would not be effective (Cheng, Zhao, & Qi, 2006; Lam et al., 2007). The palatoglossus muscles are contained within the anterior faucial pillars. They arise from the palatine aponeurosis and then course down through the anterior pillars to insert into the posterior lateral aspect of the tongue.

Salpingopharyngeus Muscles

The salpingopharyngeus muscles are responsible for raising the pharynx and larynx during swallowing and helping to open the eustachian tube during swallowing. These muscles do not have a significant role in achieving velopharyngeal closure given their size and location. These muscles arise from the inferior border of the torus tubarius, which is at the upper level of the pharynx. They then course vertically along the lateral pharyngeal wall and under the salpingopharyngeal fold.

Musculus Uvulae Muscles

The musculus uvulae muscles contract during phonation to create a bulge, called the velar eminence, on the posterior border of the nasal surface of the velum. This bulge provides additional stiffness and helps to assure a firm velopharyngeal seal (Huang, Lee, & Rajendran, 1997; Kuehn, Folkins & Linville, 1988; Moon & Kuehn, 1996; Moon & Kuehn, 1997). The paired musculus uvulae muscles originate from the area of the palatine aponeurosis and are positioned side by side in the midline of the velum, just above the levator veli palatini muscles. They are the only intrinsic muscles of the velum (Kuehn & Moon, 2005; Moon & Kuehn, 1996). It should be noted that the name of these muscles is somewhat misleading in that they do not exist within the uvula. In fact, the uvula contains very few muscle fibers and does not contribute to velopharyngeal closure (Ettema & Kuehn, 1994).

Tensor Veli Palatini Muscles

The tensor veli palatini muscles are responsible for opening the eustachian tubes in order to enhance middle ear aeration and drainage (Ghadiali, Swarts, & Doyle, 2003). Although these muscles are the main contributors to the palatine aponeurosis, the tensor is not positioned in a way to either raise or lower the velum. Therefore, these muscles probably contribute little, if anything, to velopharyngeal closure. The tensor veli palatini muscle on each side originates from the membranous portion of the eustachian tube cartilage and the scaphoid fossa spine of the sphenoid bone (Barsoumian, Kuehn, Moon, & Canady, 1998; Schonmeyr & Sadhu, 2014). Additional slips arise from the lateral aspect of the medial pterygoid plate and the spine of the sphenoid. The tensor veli palatini muscle then courses vertically down from the skull base to pass around the pterygoid hamulus. This redirects the muscle tendon 90° medially, where it contributes to the palatine aponeurosis in the superior and anterior regions of the velum.

See **TABLE 1-1** for a summary of the primary function of each of the paired muscles.

Velopharyngeal Motor and Sensory Innervation

The motor and sensory innervation of the velopharyngeal mechanism arises from the cranial nerves in the medulla. The following section describes the specific innervation for motor movement and sensation.

Motor innervation for the muscles that contribute to velopharyngeal closure comes from the pharyngeal plexus (**FIGURE 1-22**). The pharyngeal plexus is a network of nerves that lies along the posterior wall of the pharynx and consists of the pharyngeal branches of the glossopharyngeal nerve (ninth cranial nerve [CN IX]) and the vagus nerve (tenth cranial nerve [CN X]). Innervation of the velar muscles with these nerves occurs through the brainstem nucleus ambiguus and retrofacialis (Cassell &

TABLE 1-1 **Muscles of the Velopharynx and Their Primary Functions**

Muscle	Primary Function
Levator veli palatini	Elevating the velum during velopharyngeal (VP) closure
Superior constrictor	Constricting the pharyngeal walls around the velum during VP closure
Palatopharyngeus	Medial movement of the lateral pharyngeal walls during VP closure
Palatoglossus	Depressing the velum causing VP opening for nasal sounds
Salpingopharyngeus	Elevating the pharynx and larynx and opening the eustachian tube during swallowing
Musculus uvulae	Providing bulk on the nasal surface of the velum during VP closure
Tensor veli palatini	Opening the eustachian tube during swallowing

Elkadi, 1995; Kennedy & Kuehn, 1989; Moon & Kuehn, 1996). The palatoglossus muscle has also been found to receive innervation from the hypoglossal nerve (CN XII) (Cassell & Elkadi, 1995). The tensor veli palatini, which does not contribute to velopharyngeal closure, receives motor innervation from the mandibular division of the trigeminal nerve (CN V).

Sensory innervation of both the hard and soft palate is believed to derive from the greater and lesser palatine nerves, which arise from the maxillary division of the trigeminal nerve (CN V). The faucial and pharyngeal regions of the oral cavity are innervated by the glossopharyngeal nerve (CN IX). The facial nerve (CN VII) and vagus nerve (CN X) might also contribute to sensory innervation (Perry, 2011). Although the peripheral distribution of sensory fibers may travel along different cranial nerve routes, they all appear to terminate in the spinal nucleus of the trigeminal nerve (Cassell & Elkadi, 1995). It has been reported that the cutaneous sensory nerve endings are more prolific in the anterior portion of the oral cavity but diminish in quantity as they course toward the posterior regions of the mouth (Cassell & Elkadi, 1995).

Variations in Velopharyngeal Closure
Patterns of Velopharyngeal Closure

The relative contribution to closure of each of the velopharyngeal structures varies among speakers. This is because of minor differences in muscular orientation of the soft palate and pharyngeal walls (Finkelstein, Talmi, Nachmani, Hauben, & Zohar, 1992; Finkelstein et al., 1993). As a result of these differences, three distinct patterns of velopharyngeal closure can be identified within a population of normal speakers and speakers with velopharyngeal dysfunction (Finkelstein et al., 1992; Igawa, Nishizawa, Sugihara, & Inuyama, 1998; Jordan, Schenck, Ellis, Rangarathnam, Fang, & Perry, 2017; Perry, 2011; Shprintzen, Rakoff, Skolnick, & Lavorato, 1977; Siegel-Sadewitz & Shprintzen, 1982; Skolnick & Cohn, 1989; Skolnick et al., 1973; Witzel & Posnick, 1989). This can be seen on **FIGURE 1-23**.

The most common pattern of closure is the coronal pattern. This pattern is characterized by contact of the velum against a broad area of the posterior pharyngeal wall. There may be slight anterior movement of the posterior pharyngeal wall but minimal contribution of the lateral pharyngeal walls. It is estimated that about 70%

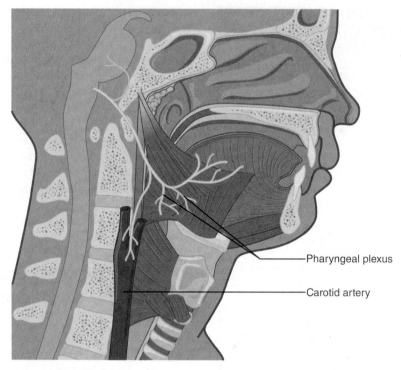

FIGURE 1-22 Position of the pharyngeal plexus.

of speakers have the coronal pattern of closure (Witzel & Posnick, 1989).

The second most common pattern of closure is the circular pattern. This pattern occurs when all the velopharyngeal structures contribute almost equally to closure, and therefore, the valve resembles a true sphincter when it closes. A Passavant's ridge is often seen in individuals with a circular pattern of closure (Skolnick & Cohn, 1989). It is estimated that about 25% of all speakers have the circular pattern of closure (Witzel & Posnick, 1989).

The least common pattern of closure is the sagittal pattern. With this pattern, the lateral pharyngeal walls move medially to meet in midline behind the velum (rather than against the velum), and there is minimal posterior displacement of the soft palate to achieve closure. This pattern seems to occur in 5% or less of speakers (Witzel & Posnick, 1989).

The variations in the basic patterns of closure among individuals are important to recognize, particularly in the evaluation process (Siegel-Sadewitz & Shprintzen, 1982; Skolnick et al., 1973). For example, on a lateral videofluoroscopy (a radiographic procedure), it may appear as if there is inadequate velopharyngeal closure with the sagittal pattern of closure, even when closure is complete, because the velum does not close against the posterior pharyngeal wall. Therefore, evaluating all of the velopharyngeal structures and their contribution to closure is important so that the basic closure pattern can be identified and considered when making treatment recommendations.

Pneumatic versus Nonpneumatic Activities

Velopharyngeal closure occurs during speech production, but it also occurs for other functions. If these functions are categorized into pneumatic versus nonpneumatic activities, a characteristic

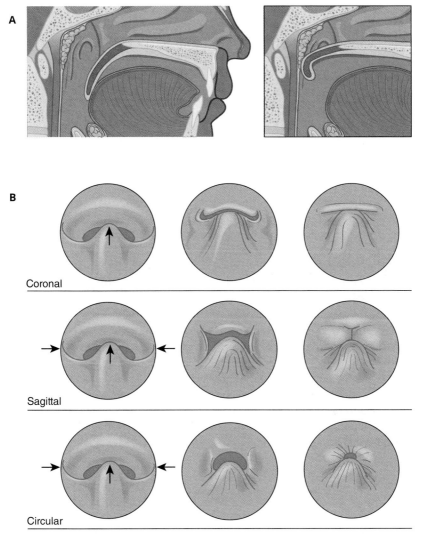

FIGURE 1-23 (A) Lateral view of VP closure as viewed through nasopharyngoscopy. **(B)** Patterns of velopharyngeal closure as viewed from above.

and distinct closure pattern can be identified for each category (Flowers & Morris, 1973; Shprintzen, Lencione, McCall, & Skolnick, 1974). In fact, there seems to be a separate neurological mechanism for closure during nonspeech activities, especially nonpneumatic activities, versus closure for speech.

Nonpneumatic activities are those that are done without airflow. They include gagging,

vomiting, and swallowing. With gagging and vomiting, the velum is raised very high in the pharynx and the lateral pharyngeal walls close firmly along their entire length. This is the only type of velopharyngeal closure that can be felt. This high and firm closure is necessary to allow substances to pass through the oral cavity without nasal regurgitation. With swallowing, the back of the tongue pushes the velum upward, and therefore, velar elevation occurs passively rather than by the contraction of the levator muscles (Flowers & Morris, 1973). It is important to note that velopharyngeal closure may be complete for nonpneumatic activities but insufficient for speech or other pneumatic activities (Shprintzen et al., 1975).

Pneumatic activities are those that utilize airflow and air pressure (both positive and negative) as a result of velopharyngeal closure. Positive pressure is necessary for blowing, whistling, singing, and speech. Negative pressure is needed for sucking and kissing. With these activities, closure occurs lower in the nasopharynx than with nonpneumatic activities.

Although closure for pneumatic activities is very different than closure for nonpneumatic activities, closure for different pneumatic activities is also physiologically different from each other (Nohara et al., 2007). Blowing, for example, requires generalized movements of the velopharyngeal structures—and levator activity for blowing is higher than for speech (Kuehn & Moon, 1994). On the other hand, speech requires precise, rapid movements of these structures. The point of contact even varies slightly for different speech sounds, as is discussed in the next section. When comparing velopharyngeal closure during singing and speech, the velopharyngeal port is closed longer and tighter in singing than in speech, particularly on the higher pitches (Austin, 1997).

Timing of Closure

Voice onset and velopharyngeal closure must be closely coordinated during speech. Velar movement for oral sounds must begin before the onset of phonation so that the velopharyngeal valve is completely closed when phonation begins. If complete closure is not achieved before activation of the sound source, then the speech will become hypernasal as a result of the escape of sound into the nasal cavity during oral speech production (Ha, Sim, Zhi, & Kuehn, 2004).

The timing of closure for an oral sound has been found to be somewhat dependent on the type of phoneme. Kent and Moll (1969) found evidence to suggest that the velar elevating gesture for a stop begins earlier and is executed more rapidly when the stop is voiceless rather than voiced. The production of nasal consonants during an utterance has an additional effect on velopharyngeal function and timing. The velum remains elevated, and closure is maintained throughout the utterance as long as oral consonants or vowels are being produced. As a nasal consonant (/m/, /n/, /ŋ/) is produced, the velum lowers quickly, and the pharyngeal walls move away from midline, thus opening the velopharyngeal valve to allow for nasal resonance. Speech segments with many oral–nasal combinations make the temporal requirements for velar movement more challenging. This can be a problem if there is tenuous velopharyngeal closure (Jones, 2006). In addition, vowels that precede or follow the nasal consonant will be slightly affected by the anticipatory lowering of the velum just before the nasal consonant and by the slight delay in raising the velum just after the nasal consonant (Bunnell, 2005). Therefore, the timing of closure requires constant fine adjustments throughout an utterance, depending on the phonemic needs. Missed timing may have implications for the perception of resonance or nasality.

Height of Closure

Even as velopharyngeal closure is maintained throughout oral speech, there are slight variations in contact because of the type of phoneme being produced and its phonemic environment (Flowers & Morris, 1973; Moll, 1962; Moon & Kuehn, 1997; Shprintzen et al., 1975; Simpson & Chin, 1981).

In general, velar heights are slightly greater for the following: consonants versus vowels, high-pressure consonants (plosives, fricatives, and affricates) versus low-pressure consonants, voiceless consonants versus voiced consonants, and high vowels versus low vowels (Moll, 1962; Moon & Kuehn, 1997). As such, velar position is constantly modified slightly with each sound production (Karnell, Linville, & Edwards, 1988).

Firmness of Closure

The exact same factors that increase the height of velar contact during speech also increase the firmness of closure. Therefore, velopharyngeal firmness is greatest when the contact is relatively high (Kuehn & Moon, 1998; Moon, Kuehn, & Huisman, 1994). Vowels adjacent to a nasal consonant, particularly when preceding the consonant, have less closure force than those adjacent to oral consonants (Moll, 1962).

Effect of Rate and Fatigue

Rapid speech can affect the efficiency of velopharyngeal movement and, thus, reduce the height and firmness of closure. This can cause an increase in the perception of hypernasality.

Muscular fatigue can also affect the height and firmness of closure, even in individuals with normal speech (Kuehn & Moon, 2000). In fact, young children are often described as "whiny" when they are tired, which is just another word for "nasal." Even blowing for an extended period of time, as when playing a wind instrument, can result in velar fatigue (Tachimura, Nohara, Satoh, & Wada, 2004).

Changes with Growth and Age

The maturational changes in the craniofacial skeleton result in changes in the relationships of the pharyngeal structures and the size of the cavities of the vocal tract (pharyngeal, oral, and nasal). The differences in the vocal tract anatomy among an infant, a child, and an adult are significant and account for the differences in the quality of the "voice" at different stages of development.

Although the cranium approaches adult size relatively early in childhood, the facial bones continue to grow into adolescence or early adulthood. The growth of the mandible and maxillary bones is somewhat affected by the development of dentition. As these structures grow and mature, they move down and forward relative to the cranium. Both the maxilla and mandible are similar in size in males and females until around 14 years of age. After that age, these facial bones continue to grow in males until around age 18, whereas there is very little additional growth in females (Tineshev, 2010; Ursi, Trotman, McNamara, & Behrents, 1993). Despite the changes in the size of the mandible and maxilla over time, there are relatively minor changes in shape, even during the various occlusal stages (Kent & Vorperian, 1995).

The velopharyngeal structures undergo significant change during the first 2 years of life. With the birth cry and early vocalizations, the velopharyngeal valve remains open. As the larynx descends and the pharynx lengthens, the velum and epiglottis begin to separate, allowing for velar movement. As such, the velopharyngeal valve begins to function during some spontaneous vocalizations between 3 and 6 months of age and is fully functional around 19 months of age (Bunton & Hoit, 2018).

In addition, the size of the pharynx changes greatly during maturation. The newborn pharynx is estimated to be approximately 4 cm long. In fact, the velum and epiglottis are in close proximity, resulting in a very short pharynx (which partly accounts for the infant's high-pitched voice). In contrast, the adult pharynx is approximately 20 cm long. It has been shown that with age and height, there is a linear increase in the length of the pharynx for both boys and girls (Rommel et al., 2003; Stellzig-Eisenhauer, 2001).

In addition to the increase in length, there is an increase of approximately 80% in the volume of the nasopharynx from infancy to adulthood. Because there is more vertical than horizontal growth, there is very little change in the anterior–posterior dimension of the nasopharynx (Kent & Vorperian, 1995; Tourne, 1991). However, there is significant change in the angle of the posterior pharyngeal wall and its relationship to the velum.

In a newborn, the oropharynx curves slightly to form the nasopharynx. At around age 5, the posterior pharyngeal wall of the nasopharynx and oropharynx meet at an oblique angle. Because of the position of the pharyngeal wall, velopharyngeal closure in children typically occurs with the back of the velum (just below the velar eminence) against the pharyngeal wall, and most likely against the adenoid tissue. By puberty, however, the inclination of the nasopharynx changes so that the posterior pharyngeal wall meets the velum at almost a right angle (Kent, 1976; Kent & Vorperian, 1995). As a result, velopharyngeal closure in adults tends to be with the top of the velum against the pharyngeal wall that is slightly above it. Also, the vertical distance between the palatal plane and cervical vertical 1 (C1) becomes greater with age, resulting in the level of velopharyngeal closure being located higher above C1 (Mason, Perry, Riski, & Fang, 2016). Fortunately, the angle of the pharyngeal wall changes at the same time as the downward and slightly forward growth of the maxilla and thus the velum. In addition, the velum increases in both length and thickness at this stage. Therefore, despite these changes in structure and velopharyngeal relationships, the competency of velopharyngeal closure is maintained.

Another factor that changes the relative dimensions of the pharyngeal space and can introduce some instability in velopharyngeal function is the presence and size of the adenoid tissue. The adenoid pad is positioned on the posterior pharyngeal wall in the area of velopharyngeal closure. In young children, the adenoid pad can be prominent in size, and in many cases, it actually assists with closure. As a result, young children actually have veloadenoidal (rather than velopharyngeal) closure (Kent & Vorperian, 1995; Maryn, Van Lierde, De Bodt, & Van Cauwenberge, 2004; Skolnick et al., 1975) (**FIGURE 1-24**).

A gradual process of involution of the adenoid tissue begins around the age of 6 but accelerates with puberty. Fortunately, the velopharyngeal mechanism is usually able to adapt

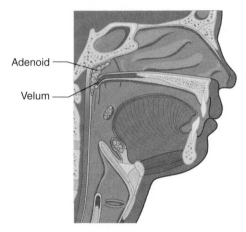

FIGURE 1-24 The adenoid pad assists in velopharyngeal closure in children.

to the anatomic changes that occur with adenoid atrophy so that velopharyngeal function is maintained. In addition, there may be an increase in velopharyngeal movement following adenoid involution—so that a more mature pattern of velopharyngeal closure is adopted (Kent & Vorperian, 1995). Finally, aging on velopharyngeal function has been studied, and the results suggest that there is virtually no deterioration in velopharyngeal function with advanced age (Hoit, Watson, Hixon, McMahon, & Johnson, 1994; Siegel-Sadewitz & Shprintzen, 1986).

Subsystems of Speech: Putting It All Together

During speech, all movements must be done quickly and with extreme accuracy. In fact, the action of every muscle for speech is influenced by the actions of other muscles in the system, and the movements of each structure are influenced by movements of other structures. In addition, every phoneme is influenced by other phonemes around it (Kollia, Gracco, & Harris, 1995). Because of this, there must be good coordination of all aspects of the physiological subsystems, which include respiration, phonation, velopharyngeal function, and articulation. To understand the importance of these subsystems and how they relate to the velopharyngeal valve, it may be helpful to review how sound is produced.

Respiration

Respiration is essential for life support, but it is also essential for speech. The air from the lungs is what provides the initiating force for phonation for consonant production. During quiet breathing, the inspiratory and expiratory phases are relatively long and usually about equal in duration. During speech, however, inspiration occurs very quickly. Subglottic air pressure is then maintained under the vocal folds during the entire phrase or sentence. The expiratory phase is much longer than the inspiratory phase and varies, depending on the length of the utterance being produced. Both the inspiratory and expiratory phases for speech are based on the phrasing of the speaker.

Phonation

Phonation (also called voicing) is the production of sound by vibration of the vocal folds. The sound created by vocal fold vibration is called the voice. The voice travels upward through the vocal tract and is then emitted through the mouth or nose during speech and singing. Voicing (or phonation) is necessary for the production of all vowels and more than half of the consonant sounds.

Phonation is initiated when air is expelled from the lungs and through the glottis. The vocal folds then close, which creates subglottic air pressure. This air pressure forces the bottom of the vocal folds open and then continues to move upward to open the top of the vocal folds. The low pressure created behind the fast-moving air column causes the bottom of the folds to close, followed by the top folds. The closure of the vocal folds cuts off the air column and releases a pulse of air. This completes one vibratory cycle. The cycles repeat for vocal fold vibration, resulting in

a type of buzzing sound (which is later modified by resonance).

During connected speech, the vocal folds must vibrate for voiced sounds, stop vibrating abruptly for voiceless sounds, and then vibrate again for the next vowel or voiced consonant (Bailly, Henrich, & Pelorson, 2010; Kent & Moll, 1969; Takemoto, Mokhtari, & Kitamura, 2010; Tsai, Chen, Shau, & Hsiao, 2009). In the simple two-syllable phrase "a cup," the vocal folds vibrate on the vowel, stop on the /k/, vibrate on the vowel, and stop again on the /p/. This requires a great deal of neuromotor coordination and control. Also, airflow must be maintained throughout the utterance so that it can continue to provide the force for phonation.

Prosody

Prosody refers to the stress, rhythm, and intonation of speech as produced by the vocal folds during phonation. Stress is related to increased laryngeal and subglottic pressure during the production of a syllable. Stressed syllables are higher in pitch and intensity, longer in duration, and produced with greater articulatory precision as compared to unstressed syllables. Rhythm refers to the alteration of stressed and unstressed syllables and the relative timing of each. Intonation refers to the frequent changes in pitch throughout an utterance, as controlled by subtle changes in vocal fold length and mass. These changes influence the rate of vibration of the vocal folds and the tension of the muscles of the larynx. Although there are changes in pitch throughout connected speech, the pitch of the voice tends to drop to a lower frequency at the end of each statement and rise to a higher frequency at the end of a question. Both stress and intonation are used for emphasis and also to help to convey meaning. For example, the words "desert" and "dessert" have different meanings that are conveyed through differences in the place of stress. When the sentence "Well, that's just fine" is uttered as if it has an exclamation point, it has a different meaning than when it is spoken as if it has a period at the end. The differences in meaning are conveyed by differences in the stress and intonation.

Resonance and Velopharyngeal Function

Once phonation has begun, the sound energy from the vocal folds travels in a superior direction through the cavities of the vocal tract, beginning with the pharyngeal cavity and ending with the oral cavity and/or nasal cavity. Resonance, as it relates to speech, is the modification of the sound from the vocal folds through selective enhancement of certain frequencies as it travels through these cavities. The frequencies that are enhanced are determined by the size and shape of the cavities.

The effect of the size and shape of the cavities of the vocal tract can be simulated by blowing across the lip of a bottle filled by water. When the bottle is mostly full, the resonating airspace is small, and the resulting sound is high in pitch. When the bottle is almost empty so that there is a larger resonating cavity, the sound is deeper in pitch and richer in perception. Although the sound source was the same, the pitch of the sound is dictated by the size of the resonating cavity.

The generation of sound and the shaping of that sound has been called the source-filter model and was first described by Gunnar Fant (Fant, 1960). This model is based on the premise that every instrument that is capable of producing sound needs at least three components: (1) a vibrating mechanism to produce sound (the source), (2) a stimulating force that can set the vibration in motion, and (3) a resonating mechanism (the filter) to selectively damp or amplify various frequencies of the sound. In human speech, the vocal folds are the vibrating mechanism (the source), subglottic air pressure is the stimulating force, and the cavities of the vocal tract are the resonators (the filters) (Baken, 1987; Sataloff, Heman-Ackah, & Hawkshaw, 2007).

Variation in the size and shape of the resonating cavities among individuals is often determined by age and gender. For example, infants have very small resonating cavities; thus, the vocal quality is very high in pitch. Women and children usually have a shorter pharynx than men; therefore, they have higher formant frequencies in their vocal product than men. An additional consideration is the wall thickness of the cavities. A thick pharyngeal wall can absorb sound, whereas a thinner wall can reflect sound. The changes in vibration that result from all these factors produce the resonance and give the perception of timbre or vocal quality (Sataloff, 1992). This is what provides the unique quality to an individual's voice.

The velopharyngeal valve influences resonance by directing the transmission of sound energy (and airflow) into the appropriate cavities during speech. During the production of oral speech sounds (all sounds with the exception of /m/, /n/, and /ŋ/), the velopharyngeal valve closes, thus blocking off the nasal cavity from the oral cavity. This allows the sound energy and airflow to be directed anteriorly into the oral cavity. During the production of nasal sounds (m/, /n/, and /ŋ/), the velopharyngeal valve opens, which allows the sound to enter the nasal cavity.

Articulation

The sound that results from phonation and resonance is further altered for individual speech sounds by the oral articulators. The oral articulators include the lips, the jaws (including the teeth), and the tongue. (The velum is also an articulator for speech.) The oral articulators alter the acoustic product for different speech sounds in two ways. First, they can vary the size and shape of the oral cavity through movement and articulatory placement. Second, the articulators can modify the manner in which the sound, and particularly the airstream, is released.

Both vowels and voiced oral consonants require oral resonance for production, and many consonants also require oral air pressure. For the production of vowels, the tongue and jaws modify the size and shape of the oral cavity, but there is little constriction of the sound energy or airflow. The differentiation of vowel sounds is determined by tongue height (high, mid, or low), tongue position (front, central, back), and lip rounding (present or absent).

On the other hand, consonants are produced by partial or complete obstruction of the oral cavity, which results in a buildup of air pressure in the oral cavity. Intraoral air pressure provides the force for the production of all pressure-sensitive consonants (plosives, fricatives, and affricates). Plosive phonemes (/p/, /b/, /t/, /d/, /k/, /g/) are produced with a buildup of intraoral pressure and then a sudden release. Fricative phonemes (/f/, /v/, /s/, /z/, /ʃ/, /ʒ/, /h/) require a gradual release of air pressure through a small or restricted opening. Affricate phonemes (/ʧ/, /ʤ/) are a combination of plosive and fricative phonemes (/ʧ/ = /t/ + /ʃ/ and /ʤ/ = /d/ + /ʒ/). As such, affricate sounds require a buildup of intraoral air pressure and then gradual release through a narrow opening. Consonants are differentiated not only by the manner of production (plosives, fricatives, affricates, liquids, and glides) but also by the place of production (bilabial, labiodental, lingual-alveolar, palatal, velar, and glottal) and voicing (voiced or voiceless).

Subsystems as "Team Players"

During speech production, each subsystem is like a member of a team. For the "team" to reach its goal of normal speech production, each subsystem must be able to execute its individual role and also learn how to work with the other "players." If it is a good player, the other team players will be more effective. If it is a poor player, this will make the job of the other team players much more difficult, and they will function less effectively. For example, velopharyngeal dysfunction can affect respiration, phonation, and articulation. It can cause an alteration of respiration during speech because the loss of airflow through the nose causes the individual to take more frequent breaths to replenish the air. Phonation may be altered if the individual compensates for inadequate oral airflow for voiceless sounds by substituting phonated sounds (i.e., n/s). On the other hand, the individual may use a breathy voice to mask the sound of hypernasality. The loss of oral airflow because of velopharyngeal dysfunction can affect articulation of pressure-sensitive consonants, causing the individual to produce sounds in the pharynx rather than the oral cavity.

SUMMARY

The anatomy of the craniofacial, intraoral, and velopharyngeal structures is well documented. On the other hand, the physiology of the velopharyngeal mechanism, particularly as it relates to speech, is very complex and not well understood. There is still much to be learned regarding the roles of the various muscles, the interaction of velopharyngeal function with articulation, and the neuromotor controls required for coordination of velopharyngeal function with the other subsystems of speech. A thorough understanding of the anatomy and physiology of the head, face, and vocal tract is particularly important in the management of speech and resonance disorders.

FOR REVIEW AND DISCUSSION

1. Why is it important to understand normal structure when working with individuals with a history of cleft lip and palate?

2. What are the facial landmarks and structures that may be relevant to the study of cleft lip?

3. Describe the internal nasal structures and the various functions of the nasal turbinates.

4. List the oral structures that can be seen when looking in the mouth.

5. List the suture lines of the hard and soft palate. Why are they called "suture" lines?

6. Describe the movement of the velopharyngeal structures and the role of the velopharyngeal muscles in closing and opening the velopharyngeal valve.

7. What are the types of velopharyngeal closure patterns among normal and abnormal speakers? Why do you think it is important to understand the basic patterns of speech when evaluating abnormal speakers?

8. Discuss the effects of type of activity, type of phoneme, rate of speech, and fatigue on velopharyngeal closure. Given the known effect of these factors on velopharyngeal closure, how would this affect the way you evaluate velopharyngeal function for speech?

9. How does velopharyngeal closure change with growth and adenoid involution? How could these changes potentially affect speech?

10. What are the physiological subsystems of speech, and how do they interact with each other for normal speech? Describe how a problem with one subsystem may affect other subsystems.

REFERENCES

Austin, S. F. (1997). Movement of the velum during speech and singing in classically trained singers. *Journal of Voice, 11*(2), 212–221.

Bailly, L., Henrich, N., & Pelorson, X. (2010). Vocal fold and ventricular fold vibration in period-doubling phonation: Physiological description and aerodynamic modeling. *Journal of the Acoustic Society of America, 127*(5), 3212–3222.

Baken, R. J. (1987). *Clinical measurement of speech and voice.* Boston, MA: College-Hill Press.

Barsoumian, R., Kuehn, D. P., Moon, J. B., & Canady, J. W. (1998). An anatomic study of the tensor veli palatini and dilatator tubae muscles in relation to the eustachian tube and velar function. *The Cleft Palate–Craniofacial Journal, 35*(2), 101–110.

Boorman, J. C., & Sommerlad, B. C. (1985). Levator palati and palatal dimples: Their anatomy, relationship, and clinical significance. *British Journal of Plastic Surgery, 38*(3), 326–332.

Brodsky, L., Moore, L., Stanievich, J., & Ogra, P. (1988). The immunology of tonsils in children: The effect of bacterial load on the presence of B- and T-cell subsets. *Laryngoscope, 98*(1), 93–98.

Bunnell, H. T. (2005). The acoustic phonetics of nasality: A practical guide to acoustic analysis. *Perspectives on Speech Science and Orofacial Disorders, 15*(2), 3–10.

Bunton, K., & Hoit, J. D. (2018). Development of velopharyngeal closure for vocalization during the first 2 years of life. *Journal of Speech, Language, and Hearing Research, 61,* 549–560.

Bzoch, K. F. (1968). Variations in velopharyngeal valving: The factor of vowel changes. *Cleft Palate Journal, 5,* 211–218.

Casey, D. M., & Emrich, L. J. (1988). Passavant's ridge in patients with soft palatectomy. *Cleft Palate Journal, 25*(1), 72–77.

Cassell, M. D., & Elkadi, H. (1995). Anatomy and physiology of the palate and velopharyngeal structures. In R. J. Shprintzen & J. Bardach (Eds.), *Cleft palate speech management: A multidisciplinary approach* (pp. 45–62). St. Louis, MO: Mosby.

Cassell, M. D., Moon, J. B., & Elkadi, H. (1990). Anatomy and physiology of the velopharynx. In J. Bardach & H. L. Morris (Eds.), *Multidisciplinary management of cleft lip and palate.* Philadelphia: Saunders.

Cheng, N. X., & Zhang, K. Q. (2004). The applied anatomic study of palatopharyngeus muscle. *Chinese Journal of Plastic Surgery, 20*(5), 384–387.

Cheng, N., Zhao, M., & Qi, K. (2006). Lateral radiographic comparison for velar movement between palatoplasty with velopharyngeal muscular reconstruction and modified Von Langenbeck's procedure. *Zhongguo Xiu Fu Chong Jian Wai Ke Za Zhi, 20*(5), 515–518.

Cunsolo, E., Marchioni, D., Leo, G., Incorvaia, C., & Presutti, L. (2010). Functional anatomy of the eustachian tube. *International Journal of Immunopathology and Pharmacology, 23*(Suppl. 1), 4–7.

Dickson, D. R. (1972). Normal and cleft palate anatomy. *Cleft Palate Journal, 9,* 280–293.

Dickson, D. R. (1975). Anatomy of the normal velopharyngeal mechanism. *Clinics in Plastic Surgery, 2*(2), 235–248.

Dickson, D. R., & Dickson, W. M. (1972). Velopharyngeal anatomy. *Journal of Speech and Hearing Research, 15*(2), 372–381.

Dickson, D. R., Grant, J. C, Sicher, H., Dubrul, E. L., & Paltan, J. (1974). Status of research in cleft palate anatomy and physiology, Part 1. *Cleft Palate Journal, 11,* 471–492.

Dickson, D. R., Grant, J. C., Sicher, H., Dubrul, E. L., & Paltan, J. (1975). Status of research in cleft lip and palate: Anatomy and physiology, Part 2. *Cleft Palate Journal, 12*(1), 131–156.

Ettema, S. L., & Kuehn, D. P. (1994). A quantitative histologic study of the normal human adult soft palate. *Journal of Speech and Hearing Research, 37,* 303–313.

Fant, G. (1960). *Acoustic theory of speech production.* The Hague, Paris: Mouton & Co.

Finkelstein, Y., Lerner, M. A., Ophir, D., Nachmani, A., Hauben, D. J., & Zohar, Y. (1993). Nasopharyngeal profile and velopharyngeal valve mechanism. *Plastic and Reconstructive Surgery, 92*(4), 603–614.

Finkelstein, Y., Talmi, Y. P., Kravitz, K., Bar-Ziv, J., Nachmani, A., Hauben, D. J., & Zohar, Y. (1991). Study of the normal and insufficient velopharyngeal valve by the "Forced Sucking Test." *Laryngoscope, 101*(11), 1203–1212.

Finkelstein, Y., Talmi, Y. P., Nachmani, A., Hauben, D. J., & Zohar, Y. (1992). On the variability of velopharyngeal valve anatomy and function: A combined peroral and nasendoscopic study. *Plastic & Reconstructive Surgery, 89*(4), 631–639.

Flowers, C. R., & Morris, H. L. (1973). Oral pharyngeal movements during swallowing and speech. *Cleft Palate Journal, 10,* 181–191.

Garcia-Garcia, A. S., Martinez-Gonzalez, J. M., Gomez-Font, R., Soto-Rivadeneira, A., & Oviedo-Roldan, L. (2010). Current status of the torus palatinus and torus mandibularis. *Medicina Oral Patología Oral y Cirugía Bucal, 15*(2), e353–e360.

Ghadiali, S. N., Swarts, J. D., & Doyle, W. J. (2003). Effect of tensor veli palatini muscle paralysis on eustachian tube mechanics. *The Annals of Otology, Rhinology, and Laryngology, 112*(8), 704–711.

Glaser, E. R., Skolnick, M. L., McWilliams, B. J., & Shprintzen, R. J. (1979). The dynamics of Passavant's ridge in subjects with and without velopharyngeal insufficiency: A multi-view videofluoroscopic study. *Cleft Palate Journal, 16*(1), 24–33.

Ha, S., Sim, H., Zhi, M., & Kuehn, D. P. (2004). An acoustic study of the temporal characteristics of nasalization in children with and without cleft palate. *The Cleft Palate-Craniofacial Journal, 41*(5), 535–543.

Hoit, J. D., Watson, P. J., Hixon, K. E., McMahon, P., & Johnson, C. L. (1994). Age and velopharyngeal function during speech production. *Journal of Speech and Hearing Research, 37*(2), 295–302.

Huang, M. H., Lee, S. T., & Rajendran, K. (1997). Structure of the musculus uvulae: Functional and surgical implications of an anatomic study. *The Cleft Palate-Craniofacial Journal, 34*(6), 466–474.

Huang, M. H., Lee, S. T., & Rajendran, K. (1998). Anatomic basis of cleft palate and velopharyngeal surgery: Implications from a fresh cadaveric study. *Plastic & Reconstructive Surgery, 101*(3), 613–627; discussion 628–629.

Hwang, K., Kim, D. J., Huan, F., Han, S. H., & Hwang, S. W. (2011). Width of the levator aponeurosis is broader than the tarsal plate. *Journal of Craniofacial Surgery, 22*(3), 1061–1063.

Igawa, H. H., Nishizawa, N., Sugihara, T., & Inuyama, Y. (1998). A fiberscopic analysis of velopharyngeal movement before and after primary palatoplasty in cleft palate infants. *Plastic & Reconstructive Surgery, 102*(3), 668–674.

Iglesias, A., Kuehn, D. P., & Morris, H. L. (1980). Simultaneous assessment of pharyngeal wall and velar displacement of selected speech sounds. *Journal of Speech and Hearing Research, 23,* 429–446.

Jones, D. L. (2006). Patterns of oral-nasal balance in normal speakers with and without cleft palate. *Folia Phoniatrica et Logopaedica, 58*(6), 383–391.

Jordan, H. N., Schenck, G. C., Ellis, C., Rangarathnam, B., Fang, X., & Perry, J. L. (2017). Examining velopharyngeal closure patterns based on anatomic variables. *Journal of Craniofacial Surgery, 28*(1), 270–274.

Kao, D. S., Soltysik, D. A., Hyde, J. S., & Gosain, A. K. (2008). Magnetic resonance imaging as an aid in the dynamic assessment of the velopharyngeal mechanism in children. *Plastic and Reconstructive Surgery, 122*(2), 572–577.

Karnell, M. P., Linville, R. N., & Edwards, B. A. (1988). Variations in velar position over time: A nasal videoendoscopic study. *Journal of Speech and Hearing Research, 31*(3), 417–424.

Kennedy, J. G., & Kuehn, D. P. (1989). Neuroanatomy of speech. In D. P. Kuehn, M. L. Lemme, & J. M. Baumgartner (Eds.), *Neural bases of speech, hearing, and language* (pp. 111–145). Boston, MA: College Hill Press.

Kent, R. D. (1976). Anatomical and neuro-muscular maturation of the speech mechanism: Evidence from acoustic studies. *Journal of Speech and Hearing Research, 19*(3), 421–447.

Kent, R. D., & Moll, K. L. (1969). Vocal-tract characteristics of the stop cognates. *Journal of the Acoustical Society of America, 46*(6), 1549–1555.

Kent, R. D., & Vorperian, H. K. (1995). Development of the craniofacial-oral-laryngeal anatomy: A review. *Journal of Medical Speech-Language Pathology, 3*(3), 145–190.

Kollia, H. B., Gracco, V. L., & Harris, K. S. (1995). Articulatory organization of mandibular, labial, and velar movements during speech. *The Journal of the Acoustical Society of America, 98*(3), 1313–1324.

Kuehn, D. P. (1979). Velopharyngeal anatomy and physiology. *Ear, Nose & Throat Journal, 58*(7), 316–321.

Kuehn, D. P., & Azzam, N. A. (1978). Anatomical characteristics of palatoglossus and the anterior faucial pillar. *Cleft Palate Journal, 15,* 349–359.

Kuehn, D. P., Folkins, J. W., & Linville, R. N. (1988). An electromyographic study of the musculus uvulae. *Cleft Palate Journal, 25*(4), 348–355.

Kuehn, D. P., & Kahane, J. C. (1990). Histologic study of the normal human adult soft palate. *Cleft Palate Journal, 27,* 26–34.

Kuehn, D. P., & Moon, J. B. (1994). Levator veli palatini muscle activity in relation to intraoral air pressure

variation. *Journal of Speech & Hearing Research, 37*(6), 1260–1270.

Kuehn, D. P., & Moon, J. B. (1998). Velopharyngeal closure force and levator veli palatini activation levels in varying phonetic contexts. *Journal of Speech, Language & Hearing Research, 41*(1), 51–62.

Kuehn, D. P., & Moon, J. B. (2000). Induced fatigue effects on velopharyngeal closure force. *Journal of Speech, Language & Hearing Research, 43*(2), 486–500.

Kuehn, D. P., & Moon, J. B. (2005). Histologic study of intravelar structures in normal human adult specimens. *The Cleft Palate–Craniofacial Journal, 42*(5), 481–489.

Lam, E., Hundert, S., & Wilkes, G. H. (2007). Lateral pharyngeal wall and velar movement and tailoring velopharyngeal surgery: Determinants of velopharyngeal incompetence resolution in patients with cleft palate. *Plastic and Reconstructive Surgery, 120*(2), 495–505; discussion 497–506.

Licameli, G. R. (2002). The eustachian tube. Update on anatomy, development, and function. *Otolaryngologic Clinics of North America, 35*(4), 803–809.

Lukens, A., Dimartino, E., Gunther, R. W., & Krombach, G. A. (2012). Functional MR imaging of the eustachian tube in patients with clinically proven dysfunction: Correlation with lesions detected on MR images. *European Radiology, 22*(3), 533–538.

Magen, H. S., Kang, A. M., Tiede, M. K., & Whalen, D. H. (2003). Posterior pharyngeal wall position in the production of speech. *Journal of Speech, Language & Hearing Research, 46*(1), 241–251.

Maryn, Y., Van Lierde, K., De Bodt, M., & Van Cauwenberge, P. (2004). The effects of adenoidectomy and tonsillectomy on speech and nasal resonance. *Folia Phoniatric Logopedia, 56*(3), 182–191.

Mason, K., Perry, J. L., Riski, J. E., & Fang, X. (2016). Age related changes between the level of velopharyngeal closure and the cervical spine. *Journal of Craniofacial Surgery, 27*(2), 498–503.

Maue-Dickson, W. (1977). Cleft lip and palate research: An updated state of the art. Section II. Anatomy and physiology. *Cleft Palate Journal, 14*(4), 270–287.

Maue-Dickson, W. (1979). The craniofacial complex in cleft lip and palate: An update review of anatomy and function. *Cleft Palate Journal, 16*(3), 291–317.

Maue-Dickson, W., & Dickson, D. R. (1980). Anatomy and physiology related to cleft palate: Current research and clinical implications. *Plastic & Reconstructive Surgery, 65*(1), 83–90.

Maue-Dickson, W., Dickson, D. R., & Rood, S. R. (1976). Anatomy of the eustachian tube and related structures in age-matched human fetuses with and without cleft palate. *Transactions of the American Academy of Ophthalmology and Otolaryngology, 82*(2), 159–164.

Mehendale, F. V. (2004). Surgical anatomy of the levator veli palatini: A previously undescribed tendonous insertion of the anterolateral fibers. *Plastic and Reconstructive Surgery, 114*(2), 307–315.

Moll, K. (1962). Velopharyngeal closure on vowels. *Journal of Speech and Hearing Research, 5,* 30–37.

Moon, J. B., & Kuehn, D. P. (1996). Anatomy and physiology of normal and disordered velopharyngeal function for speech. *National Center for Voice and Speech, 9*(April), 143–158.

Moon, J. B., & Kuehn, D. P. (1997). Anatomy and physiology of normal and disordered velopharyngeal function for speech. In K. R. Bzoch (Ed.), *Communicative disorders related to cleft lip and palate* (4th ed., pp. 45–47). Austin, TX: Pro-Ed.

Moon, J. B., & Kuehn, D. P. (2004). Anatomy and physiology of normal and disordered velopharyngeal function for speech. In K. R. Bzoch (Ed.), *Communicative disorders related to cleft lip and palate* (5th ed.). Austin, TX: Pro-Ed.

Moon, J., Kuehn, D. P., & Huisman, J. (1994). Measurement of velopharyngeal closure force during vowel production. *The Cleft Palate–Craniofacial Journal, 31,* 356–363.

Moon, J., Smith, A., Folkins, J., Lemke, J., & Gartlan, M. (1994). Coordination of velopharyngeal muscle activity during positioning of the soft palate. *The Cleft Palate–Craniofacial Journal, 31,* 45–55.

Mourino, A. P., & Weinberg, B. (1975). A cephalometric study of velar stretch in 8- and 10-year-old children. *Cleft Palate Journal, 12,* 417–435.

Nohara, K., Kotani, Y., Ojima, M., Sasao, Y., Tachimura, T., & Sakai, T. (2007). Power spectra analysis of levator veli palatini muscle electromyogram during velopharyngeal closure for swallowing, speech, and blowing. *Dysphagia, 2,* 135–139.

Nohara, K., Tachimura, T., & Wada, T. (2006). Levator veli palatini muscle fatigue during phonation in speakers with cleft palate with borderline velopharyngeal incompetence. *The Cleft Palate–Craniofacial Journal, 43,* 103–107.

Perry, J. L. (2011). Anatomy and physiology of the velopharyngeal mechanism. *Seminars in Speech and Language, 32*(2), 83–92.

Perry, J. L., & Kuehn, D. P. (2009). Magnetic resonance imaging and computer reconstruction of the velopharyngeal mechanism. *Journal of Craniofacial Surgery, 20*(Suppl. 2), 1739–1746.

Perry, J. L., Kuehn, D. P., & Sutton, B. P. (2011). Morphology of the levator veli palatini muscle using magnetic resonance imaging. *The Cleft Palate–Craniofacial Journal,* October 24, 2011. Epub ahead of print.

Pruzansky, S., & Mason, R. (1969). The "stretch factor" in soft palate function. *Journal of Dental Research, 48,* 972.

Rommel, N., Bellon, E., Hermans, R., Smet, M., De Meyer, A.-M., Feenstra, L., . . . Veereman-Wauters, G. (2003). Development of the orohypopharyngeal cavity in normal infants and young children. *The Cleft Palate–Craniofacial Journal, 40*(6), 606–611.

Sataloff, R. T. (1992, December). The human voice. *Scientific American,* 108–115.

Sataloff, R. T., Heman-Ackah, Y. D., Hawkshaw, M. J. (2007). Clinical anatomy and physiology of the voice. *Otolaryngologic Clinics of North America, 40*(5), 909–929.

Satoh, K., Wada, T., Tachimura, T., & Fukuda, J. (2005). Velar ascent and morphological factors affecting velopharyngeal function in patients with cleft palate and noncleft controls: A cephalometric study. *International Journal of Oral and Maxillofacial Surgery, 34*(2), 122–126.

Schonmeyr, B., & Sadhu, P. (2014). A review of the tensor veli palatine function and its relevance to palatoplasty. *Journal of Plastic Surgery and Hand Surgery, 48*(1), 5–9.

Seikel, J. A., King, D. W., & Drumright, D. G. (2005). *Anatomy and physiology for speech, language, and hearing* (3rd ed.). Clifton Park, NY: Thomson Delmar Learning.

Serrurier, A., & Badin, P. (2008). A three-dimensional articulatory model of the velum and nasopharyngeal wall based on MRI and CT data. *Journal of the Acoustic Society of America, 123*(4), 2335–2355.

Shimokawa, T., Yi, S. Q., Izumi, A., Ru, F., Akita, K., Sato, T., & Tanaka, S. (2004). An anatomical study of the levator veli palatini and superior constrictor with special reference to their nerve supply. *Surgical and Radiological Anatomy, 26*(2), 100–105.

Shprintzen, R. J., Lencione, R. M., McCall, G. N., & Skolnick, M. L. (1974). A three-dimensional cinefluoroscopic analysis of velopharyngeal closure during speech and nonspeech activities in normals. *Cleft Palate Journal, 11,* 412–428.

Shprintzen, R. J., McCall, G. N., Skolnick, M. L., & Lencione, R. M. (1975). Selective movement of the lateral aspects of the pharyngeal walls during velopharyngeal closure for speech, blowing, and whistling in normals. *Cleft Palate Journal, 12*(1), 51–58.

Shprintzen, R. J., Rakoff, S. J., Skolnick, M. L., & Lavorato, A. S. (1977). Incongruous movements of the velum and lateral pharyngeal walls. *Cleft Palate Journal, 14*(2), 148–157.

Siegel-Sadewitz, V. L., & Shprintzen, R. J. (1982). Nasopharyngoscopy of the normal velopharyngeal sphincter: An experiment of biofeedback. *Cleft Palate Journal, 19*(3), 194–200.

Siegel-Sadewitz, V. L., & Shprintzen, R. J. (1986). Changes in velopharyngeal valving with age. *International Journal of Pediatric Otorhinolaryngology, 11*(2), 171–182.

Simpson, R. K., & Chin, L. (1981). Velar stretch as a function of task. *Cleft Palate Journal, 18*(1), 1–9.

Skolnick, M. L., & Cohn, E. R. (1989). *Videofluoroscopic studies of speech in patients with cleft palate.* New York, NY: Springer-Verlag.

Skolnick, M. L., McCall, G., & Barnes, M. (1973). The sphincteric mechanism of velopharyngeal closure. *Cleft Palate Journal, 10,* 286–305.

Skolnick, M. L., Shprintzen, R. J., McCall, G. N., & Rakoff, S. (1975). Patterns of velopharyngeal closure in subjects with repaired cleft palate and normal speech: A multi-view videofluoroscopic analysis. *Cleft Palate Journal, 12,* 369–376.

Smith, B. E., & Kuehn, D. P. (2007). Speech evaluation of velopharyngeal dysfunction. *The Journal of Craniofacial Surgery, 18*(2), 251–261.

Smith, M. E., Scoffings, D. J., & Tysome, J. R. (2016). Imaging of the eustachian tube and its function: A systematic review. *Neuroradiology, 58*(6), 543–556.

Stellzig-Eisenhauer, A. (2001). The influence of cephalometric parameters on resonance of speech in cleft lip and palate patients. An interdisciplinary study. *Journal of Orofacial Orthopedics, 62*(3), 202–223.

Sumida, K., Yamashita, K., & Kitamura, S. (2012). Gross anatomical study of the human palatopharyngeus muscle throughout its entire course from origin to insertion. *Clinical Anatomy, 25*(3), 314–323.

Tachimura, T., Nohara, K., Satoh, K., & Wada, T. (2004). Evaluation of fatigability of the levator veli palatini muscle during continuous blowing using power spectra analysis. *The Cleft Palate–Craniofacial Journal, 41*(3), 320–326.

Takemoto, H., Mokhtari, P., & Kitamura, T. (2010). Acoustic analysis of the vocal tract during vowel production by finite-difference time-domain method. *Journal of the Acoustic Society of America, 128*(6), 3724–3738.

Tineshev, S. A. (2010). Age dynamics and secular changes of indices characterizing the neurocranium and facial cranium in ethnic Bulgarian 7-17-year-old children from the region of the Eastern Rhodopes. *Folia Med (Plovdiv), 52*(4), 32–38.

Tourne, L. P. (1991). Growth of the pharynx and its physiologic implications. *American Journal of Orthodontics and Dentofacial Orthopediatrics, 99*(2), 129–139.

Tsai, C. G., Chen, J. H., Shau, Y. W., & Hsiao, T. Y. (2009). Dynamic B-mode ultrasound imaging of vocal fold vibration during phonation. *Ultrasound in Medicine & Biology, 35*(11), 1812–1818.

Ursi, W. J., Trotman, C. A., McNamara, J. A., Jr., & Behrents, R. G. (1993). Sexual dimorphism in normal craniofacial growth. *Angle Orthodontist, 63*(1), 47–56.

Witzel, M. A., & Posnick, J. C. (1989). Patterns and location of velopharyngeal valving problems: Atypical findings on video nasopharyngoscopy. *Cleft Palate Journal, 26*(1), 63–67.

Yamawaki, Y. (2003). Forward movement of posterior pharyngeal wall on phonation. *American Journal of Otolaryngology, 24*(6), 400–404.

Yanagisawa, E., & Weaver, E. M. (1996). Passavant's ridge: Is it a functional structure? *Ear, Nose & Throat Journal, 75*(12), 766–767.

Yoshida, H., Takahashi, H., Morikawa, M., & Kobayashi, T. (2007). Anatomy of the bony portion of the eustachian tube in tubal stenosis: Multiplanar reconstruction approach. *Annals of Otology, Rhinology and Laryngology, 116*(9), 681–686.

CREDITS

Part/Chapter opener photo: © PeopleImages/Getty Images

All photos courtesy of the Cleft and Craniofacial Center at Cincinnati Children's Hospital Medical Center.

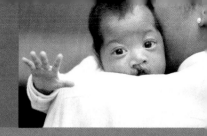

CHAPTER 2

Genetics and Patterns of Inheritance

With acknowledgment to Robert J. Hopkin for his contributions to this chapter.

CHAPTER OUTLINE

INTRODUCTION

Craniofacial anomalies, like many other conditions, tend to recur in families. The risk for recurrence, however, is variable, depending on interactions of multiple environmental and genetic factors.

The purpose of this chapter is to briefly review the modes of inheritance that may influence the occurrence of craniofacial anomalies. The first part of the chapter reviews DNA, genes, chromosomes, and the cell cycle. The second part of the chapter discusses the principles of Mendelian inheritance, including autosomal recessive, autosomal dominant, and X-linked patterns of inheritance. The last portion of the chapter focuses on complex, or non-Mendelian inheritance. Particular attention is placed on multifactorial inheritance, the pattern associated with most cases of cleft palate—or cleft lip with or without cleft palate.

Cell Anatomy

All living things contain cells, which are a fundamental building block of life. Although each tissue contains cells that are differentiated to perform specific specialized functions, all cells have certain traits in common (**FIGURE 2-1**).

A cell is a ball of protoplasm coated in a membrane. Each cell contains organelles, which perform specific functions (e.g., metabolizing energy, building complex molecules such as proteins, and breaking down waste products). The genetic material (instructions for cell and tissue functions) is contained in the nucleus, which is separated from the rest of the cell by a lipid membrane with specialized proteins. These proteins regulate transport of chemicals into and out of the nucleus.

Within the nucleus of each cell, there is another structure, called the nucleolus, in which genes are actively transcribed. The nucleus communicates directly with the endoplasmic reticulum, which is a complex system of membranes that control transport of proteins and lipids throughout the cell. The rough endoplasmic reticulum is associated with smaller organelles, called ribosomes, that put proteins together. Other important organelles include mitochondria, where energy metabolism takes place; golgi apparatus, where specialized complex molecules are formed; lysosomes, where complex molecules are broken down; and cytoskeleton, which provides structural support for the cell.

Deoxyribonucleic Acid and Genes

For centuries, scientists wondered how the information needed to organize and direct the development of an organism was transmitted from a single cell to a mature individual with complex organs and tissues. This process became more apparent with the discovery of deoxyribonucleic acid (DNA) within genes.

Deoxyribonucleic Acid

In 1869, Friedrich Miescher discovered a substance in cell nuclei that he called "nuclein." The name was eventually changed to deoxyribonucleic acid, or DNA. In 1944, Avery, Macleod, and McCarthy demonstrated that deoxyribonucleic acid, or DNA, is the substance that carries hereditary information in bacteria and that all genes carry discrete segments of DNA (Jorde, Carey, & Bamshad, 2016; McKusick, 1997).

DNA is a nucleic acid made up of building blocks called nucleotides. Nucleotides consist of a 5-carbon sugar (deoxyribose) chemically bonded to a phosphate group and a nitrogenous base. The nitrogenous base can be divided into two groups: purines (adenine and guanine) and pyrimidines (thymine and cytosine). A purine is always paired with a pyrimidine. In fact, adenine (A) is always paired with thymine (T), and guanine (G) is always paired with cytosine (C). Therefore, if one strand contains the sequence 5'GGATTCG3', the

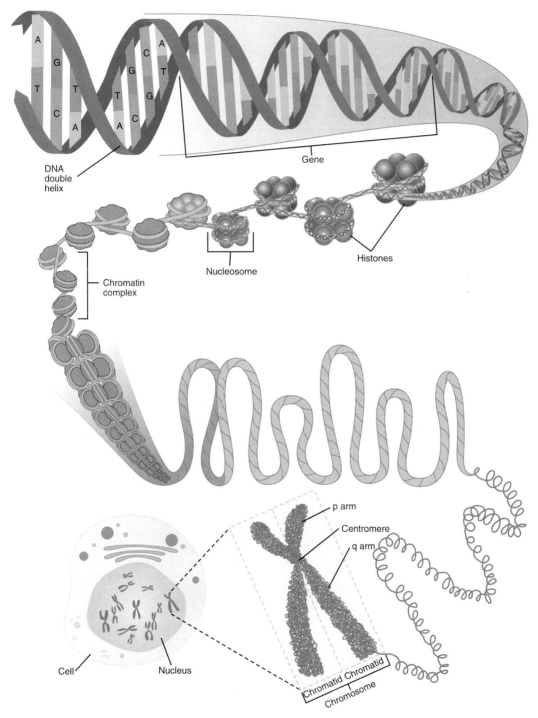

FIGURE 2-1 Diagram of a cell demonstrating that genetic material in the form of DNA is organized into chromosomes. Each chromosome contains thousands of genes.

complementary sequence would be 3'CCTAAGC5'. The numbers 5' and 3' indicate the direction of the strand. The strands are held together by hydrogen bonds between A-T pairs and C-G pairs (Strachan & Read, 1996). These nucleotides form long, unbranching polymers, which are large molecules (macromolecules) composed of repeating structural units. They are arranged in an antiparallel (going in opposite directions) double helix (coiled ladder) so that the nitrogenous bases are paired according to these specific rules.

Replication

Replication is the process of making two identical DNA molecules from one. When DNA is replicated, the double helix is unwound, and the complementary strands are separated. Nucleotides are then added sequentially to each single strand, forming new complementary strands. This results in two identical double helix molecules of DNA (Strachan & Read, 1996). This process is complex, but it must take place quickly to allow for rapid cell division and growth.

The process of replicating DNA is very carefully controlled to prevent errors. In addition, there are proofreading and repair mechanisms to preserve the exact sequence of nucleotides (Strachan & Read, 1996). Although errors are rare, they do occur. When a change in the sequence of a molecule of DNA occurs, it is referred to as a mutation. The mutation can be as small as a substitution of a single base pair or as large as the deletion of an entire chromosome. Mutations can have important consequences for the cell and the individual.

Genes

A gene is a submicroscopic functional unit of heredity consisting of a discrete segment of a DNA strand within a chromosome. Thousands of genes are found in each chromosome. The order of the nucleotides in the DNA of an individual gene determines the information coded by that gene.

In spite of the highly regulated process of DNA replication and repair, no two individuals share the exact same DNA sequence, with the exception of identical twins. In fact, much of the DNA in humans is variable. This normal variability among individuals is called polymorphism. Polymorphisms are seen in virtually all genes and contribute to the uniqueness of each individual.

Mutations of genes can lead to new variations in the DNA. Some mutations can improve function and therefore may become more common (Cummings, 1997; Jorde et al., 2016). Mutations that lead to disease tend to remain rare or are eliminated over time. In fact, mutations, deletions, and insertions of one or more nucleotides can disrupt gene function, resulting in various diseases or malformations. For example, mutations in the MSX2 gene can result in craniosynostosis. On the other hand, loss of function for the same gene leads to delayed closure of cranial sutures and persistence of fontanels into adulthood (Wilkie et al., 2000).

Chromosomes

A chromosome is a single, linear double strand of DNA with associated proteins. Human cells have 23 pairs of chromosomes for a total of 46. Each pair contains one chromosome from the mother and one from the father. *Twenty-two* of these pairs, called autosomes, are the same for both males and females. The chromosomes in the 23rd pair are referred to as sex chromosomes (X and Y) because of their role in gender determination. If a person inherits two X chromosomes (one from each parent), that person will be female. If a person inherits an X chromosome (from the mother) and a Y chromosome (from the father), the person will be male. The normal chromosomal makeup is written as 46,XX for a female and 46,XY for a male (Keagle & Brown, 1999). A karyotype is a picture of a person's chromosomes that is derived from a blood sample. A karyotype of normal human chromosomes can be seen in **FIGURE 2-2**. Together, these chromosomes contain a complete set of genetic instructions, called the genome, for cell replication and differentiation (Cummings, 1997). For more information about the human genome, see The Animated

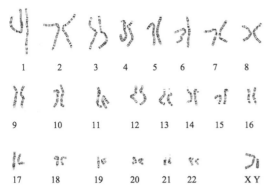

FIGURE 2-2 Karotype of normal human chromosomes. It is traditional to align chromosomes so that the "p" arm is on top.

Genome videos (Smithsonian National Museum of Natural History, n.d.).

Each chromosome has a narrowed region called a centromere, although the location of the centromere is variable. Chromosomes with a centrally located centromere are referred to as metacentric. Some centromeres are off center, leading to a short (p) arm and a long (q) arm. Chromosomes with this structure are referred to as submetacentric. Finally, the centromere may be close to one end of the chromosome. Chromosomes with this structure are referred to as acrocentric. The length of the chromosome and the location of its centromere result in a characteristic shape, which allows each chromosome to be distinguished from the others. Traditionally, chromosomes are labeled according to length, with the longest being number 1.

Chromosomal Abnormalities

Chromosomal mutations may include changes in the number of copies of an individual chromosome. The term aneuploidy refers to the presence of an abnormal number of chromosomes in a cell (e.g., a human cell with 45 or 47 chromosomes instead of the usual 46).

The loss of one copy of a chromosome results in monosomy, which is the presence of a single copy of a chromosome. The gain of an extra copy of a chromosome for a total of three chromosomes results in trisomy. Trisomies and monosomies result from a failure of one or more chromosomes to separate in cell division. This can occur in both sperm and egg development. Although the cause is not known, the risk for chromosomal abnormalities increases with advancing maternal age (Randolph, 1999). Most monosomies and trisomies end in early miscarriage.

The only monosomy that typically results in a live birth is monosomy X, or Turner syndrome. Turner syndrome (which necessarily occurs in females) is characterized by short stature, webbed neck, and lack of sexual maturation. Monosomy with just the Y chromosome results in early miscarriage.

Survival is possible for several trisomies, including trisomy for 13, 18, 21, or X. Individuals born with an extra copy of X (47,XXX) or Y (47,XXY) may be relatively healthy and difficult to distinguish from the general population. However, individuals with more than one extra copy of a sex chromosome will generally have medical and developmental problems. Those with trisomy 21 have Down syndrome. **FIGURE 2-3** shows a karyotype of a person with trisomy 13. Trisomy 13 and 18 may result in live-born infants, but they typically have multiple severe birth defects and rarely survive more than a few weeks.

In addition to abnormalities in the number of chromosomes, there can be duplications, deletions, and translocations of parts of the chromosome. These chromosomal conditions are usually associated with multiple malformations,

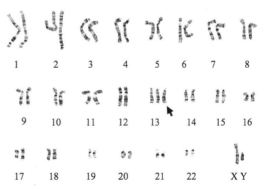

FIGURE 2-3 Karotype of human chromosomes demonstrating trisomy 13.

TABLE 2-1 Examples of Microdeletion Contiguous Gene Syndromes	
1p36 deletion syndrome	del 1p36
Wolf–Hirschhorn syndrome	del 4p16.3
Cri du chat syndrome	del 5p15
Prader–Willi syndrome	del 15q11-13
Miller–Dieker syndrome	del 17p13.3
Langer–Giedion syndrome	del 8q24
Smith–Magenis syndrome	del 17p11.2
Kallmann syndrome	del Xp22.3
X-linked ichthyosis	del Xp22.3
Jacobsen syndrome	del 11q24.1
Williams syndrome	del 7q11.23
Velocardiofacial/22q11.2 deletion syndrome	del 22q11.2

including facial clefts or other craniofacial malformations, and developmental handicaps. Combinations of deletion and duplication frequently result from an unbalanced translocation, where there is transfer of genetic material between two or more chromosomes (Gardner, Sutherland, & Shaffer, 2012; Kaiser-Rogers & Rao, 1999).

Some syndromes, referred to as contiguous gene syndromes, are caused by large deletions that contain several genes. There are many problems associated with these syndromes because of the loss of function of several important contiguous genes (Gardner et al., 2012; Jorde et al., 2016; Kaiser-Rogers & Rao, 1999). TABLE 2-1 provides a list of some microdeletion contiguous gene syndromes.

Chromosome Analysis

Chromosome analysis is performed in a cytogenetics (cell genetics) laboratory to identify abnormalities that can cause diseases or disorders. A karyotype is created by drawing blood, growing white blood cells in a culture, photographing the chromosomes, and then arranging the chromosomes in pairs by size for display and assessment.

Some chromosomal abnormalities (i.e., deletion of chromosome 22q11.2 with velocardiofacial/22q11.2 deletion syndrome) involve only very short segments that are too small to be seen using routine chromosomal analysis. With special techniques, such as fluorescence in situ hybridization (FISH), submicroscopic segments of DNA can be identified using a fluorescent dye.

Chromosomes can be specially stained to form an ideogram, which reveals a pattern of light and dark bands. The ideogram allows specific segments of the chromosome to be identified. Locations are labeled by chromosome number, the arm ("p" or "q"), and the band number. For example, a gene may be mapped to 1p36, which means that the gene is found on chromosome 1, on the short arm, and in band 36. The bands can be further subdivided in some cases, allowing for more specific localization to be described. **FIGURE 2-4** shows an ideogram of a normal chromosome 1.

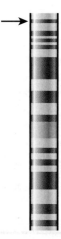

FIGURE 2-4 Ideogram (schematic drawing of the banding pattern) of chromosome 1. Note the light and dark bands. Each chromosome has a unique but consistent banding pattern that allows it to be distinguished from other chromosomes. The arrow indicates band 1p36.

When a deletion occurs, the location of the deletion can be seen on the ideogram. For example, a deletion of the short arm of chromosome 4 with a break point in band 16 in a female could be written 46,XXdel(4)(p16). **FIGURE 2-5** shows ideograms of a normal chromosome 4 and a deletion, which results in Wolf–Hirschhorn syndrome (see the chapter *Dysmorphology and Craniofacial Syndromes*).

Even with the best current staining techniques, however, the smallest bands that can be distinguished still contain multiple genes. It is not yet possible to identify individual genes on a chromosome.

In the past, it was possible to look for submicroscopic deletions only by ordering site-specific testing based on the suspected etiology. However, new technology using SNPs (single nucleotide polymorphisms) and CGH (comparative genomic hybridization) microarray analyses now allows assessment of thousands of loci simultaneously (Le Caignec et al., 2005; Schoumans et al., 2005; Ting, Ye, Thomas, Ruczinski, & Pevsner, 2006). Microarray technology makes it possible to identify small cytogenetic rearrangements that are too small to be detected with standard chromosomal analysis. These techniques can, in some cases, obtain resolution at the single gene level.

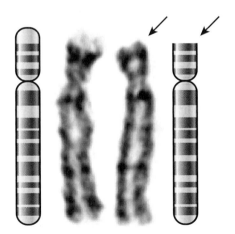

FIGURE 2-5 Ideograms of normal and deleted human chromosome 4. The arrows indicate the deleted segment at 4p16, which is associated with Wolf–Hirschhorn syndrome.

Mendelian Inheritance

In 1866, Gregor Johann Mendel outlined the common patterns of inheritance and the rules that govern them as a result of his studies on peas (McKusick, 1997). Mendelian patterns of inheritance include autosomal recessive, autosomal dominant, and X-linked inheritance. These patterns are dependent on the allele (form or copy of a gene for a trait) from each parent and whether the individual is homozygous (has two of the same alleles) or heterozygous (has two different alleles) of the gene.

Mendel described the following four rules of inheritance:

1. Genes come in pairs with one from each parent.
2. A pair of genes can have different alleles, which are variations of a gene. Some of them are dominant and will exert their effects over the other allele. Other alleles are recessive and will be manifest only when the alleles are similar or the same.
3. At meiosis (cell division), alleles segregate from each other; each gamete (male or female germ cell) carries only one allele of the pair.
4. The segregation of alleles for one gene is independent of the segregation of alleles of other genes for other traits.

These principles have remained valid (with only a few modifications) since they were first described.

To predict the effect of autosomal recessive, autosomal dominant, and X-linked inheritance on recurrence risks, a Punnett square is often used. A Punnett square is a tabular summary of possible combinations of maternal and paternal alleles to predict the probability of an offspring having a particular genotype. As such, it serves as a visual representation of Mendelian inheritance.

Pedigrees

To determine the pattern of inheritance for a condition, a pedigree can be created (Fitzsimmons, 2013).

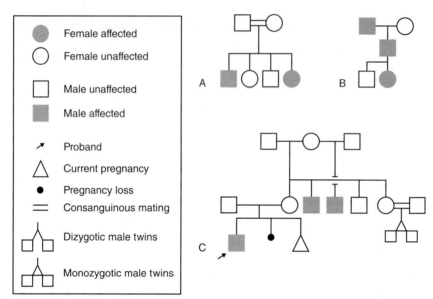

FIGURE 2-6 Three sample pedigrees. In drawing a pedigree, horizontal lines connecting two individuals indicate mating between them. Children are indicated by vertical lines with squares to indicate males and circles to indicate females. If more than one child is born to a couple, a horizontal line intersects the vertical line to allow each child to be appropriately recorded. If a parent has children with more than one partner, additional lines can be drawn as seen in the first generation of family C. Divorce or separation can be indicated by a hash mark and space in the line connecting two individuals (not shown). If more than one trait is being recorded in a family, the affected individuals can be indicated by shading only one quadrant, for example, the upper left for trait 1, the lower left for trait 2, and so on. If still more traits are recorded, different colors or patterns of shading can be added. **(A)** This pedigree demonstrates probable autosomal recessive inheritance. Note recurrence in siblings with unaffected parents and consanguinity. Multifactorial inheritance cannot be ruled out based on the information given. **(B)** This pedigree demonstrates autosomal dominant inheritance. Note father-to-son transmission and recurrence in several generations. **(C)** This pedigree demonstrates X-linked recessive inheritance. Note occurrence of multiple males born to unaffected female relatives over multiple generations.

A pedigree is a pictorial representation of the inheritance of traits or anomalies affecting family members over several generations. It allows the important findings to be recorded in a short period of time. Patterns of inheritance can be determined for most families in three to four generations. In addition, pedigrees can be simply and quickly drawn by hand during the course of a brief interview. Three sample pedigrees are illustrated in **FIGURE 2-6**.

Autosomal Recessive Inheritance

All people carry genes with mutations that are capable of causing disease. Fortunately, we

inherit two copies of each gene, one from each parent. Individuals who have one normal and one abnormal copy of the gene are heterozygous, having two different alleles. With a normal copy, they may have no detectable abnormalities. However, they will be **carriers** of the mutation and therefore could pass the abnormal allele of the gene down to their offspring. If both alleles are exactly the same (whether normal or abnormal) the individual is homozygous.

In **autosomal recessive** conditions, traits of the typical **phenotype** (group of typical characteristics associated with a genetic condition) manifest only when mutations are present in both copies of a gene. Therefore, they occur only with individuals who are either homozygous (the same mutation) or compound heterozygous (different mutations), leading to abnormalities in both alleles.

When two heterozygous carriers of an autosomal recessive condition mate, each parent has an equal probability of passing on either the normal or abnormal allele to their offspring. Therefore, the risk that the child would receive an abnormal copy of the gene from each parent and be affected with the condition is 25% for each pregnancy. In addition, there is a 50% risk that the child will receive a single copy of the mutation and become a carrier and a 25% risk that the child will receive a normal copy of the sequence of genes from both parents and be a noncarrier. If two individuals with the same autosomal recessive condition have children together, all their children will be affected because both parents have only abnormal alleles to pass on (Mueller & Cook, 1997). In all autosomal recessive conditions, males and females are affected in equal numbers. See **FIGURE 2-7** for a Punnett square of autosomal recessive inheritance. Also, see **TABLE 2-2** for a list of some autosomal recessive conditions that are associated with cleft lip or cleft palate.

There are approximately 17,000 to 23,000 different genes in each cell, and on average, each person carries six to seven potentially disease-causing mutations. Therefore, the chance that both members of a couple will carry mutations in the same

TABLE 2-2 **Examples of Autosomal Recessive Craniofacial Syndromes**
Smith–Lemli-Opitz syndrome
Meckel–Gruber syndrome
Baller–Gerold syndrome
Oral–facial–digital syndrome type II
Insley–Astley syndrome
Dubowitz syndrome
Roberts syndrome
Toriello–Carey syndrome
Varadi–Papp syndrome

gene is very small. The probability of two people carrying abnormalities in the same genes is greatly increased if they are related because relatives share genetic material. Thus, **consanguinity**, which is mating between related individuals, leads to increased risk that both members of the couple carry the same disease-causing mutations of the same genes. The closer the relationship, the more genetic material the two individuals have in common and therefore the greater the risk. This is one explanation for the high incidence of genetic disorders in isolated or inbred populations. Although the parents of individuals affected by an autosomal recessive condition are often not affected because they are merely carriers, recurrence of the condition with additional offspring is common.

In some populations, a relatively small number of original ancestors has led to a high frequency of carriers for certain disorders. This is known as a **founder effect**. When this occurs, it is often possible to trace family lines to a single common ancestor who brought a trait into a population. More frequently, a founder effect is implied by a high frequency of a few mutations in a large population. For example, three mutations account

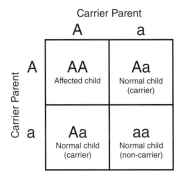

Capital letters designate a mutation.

FIGURE 2-7 Punnett square showing autosomal recessive inheritance.

for 98% of Tay-Sachs disease in the Ashkenazi Jewish population (Rutledge & Percy, 1997).

Genetic testing for carrier status can help couples in making reproductive decisions if they are from a high-risk population or there is a family history of the disorder that indicates a high probability that one or both partners may be carriers for that condition (Stevenson & Clare Davison, 2017; Uhlmann, Schuette, & Yashar, 2011). Testing is currently available for some of the more common autosomal recessive diseases, such as cystic fibrosis, sickle cell anemia, and Tay-Sachs disease. Prenatal testing for some autosomal recessive conditions is also available to distinguish affected individuals from carriers.

Autosomal Dominant Inheritance

In autosomal dominant conditions, traits of the typical phenotype manifest when mutations are present in either of the two copies of a gene. Therefore, both homozygous and heterozygous individuals will have features of the condition. As a result, pedigrees from families with autosomal dominant conditions demonstrate different findings than are seen with autosomal recessive inheritance.

When two individuals with a dominant condition mate, there is a 75% chance that they will pass the condition to their offspring because each parent is probably heterozygous (25% of offspring will inherit disease-causing mutations from each parent, 50% will inherit a single mutation, and 25% will not inherit a mutation). When an individual with a dominant condition mates with an unaffected individual, there is a 50% risk with each pregnancy of passing the condition to their offspring (who will be heterozygotes). As with autosomal recessive conditions, the number of affected males and females with autosomal dominant conditions is approximately equal. Homozygotes (persons with two abnormal alleles) for autosomal dominant disorders often have a more severe phenotype than heterozygotes. See **FIGURE 2-8** for a Punnett square

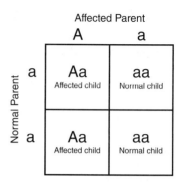

Capital letters designate a mutation.

FIGURE 2-8 Punnett square showing autosomal dominant inheritance.

TABLE 2-3 Examples of Autosomal Dominant Craniofacial Syndromes
Apert syndrome
Branchio-oto-renal syndrome
Crouzon syndrome
Distichiasis-lymphedema syndrome
Ectrodactyly–ectodermal dysplasia–cleft syndrome
Opitz Frias syndrome
Stickler syndrome
Treacher Collins syndrome
Van der Woude syndrome
Waardenburg syndrome

of autosomal dominant inheritance. Also, see **TABLE 2-3** for a list of some autosomal dominant conditions that are associated with cleft lip or cleft palate.

Autosomal dominant pedigrees often show that at least one parent is affected. If neither parent has the condition, the affected individual is presumed to carry a new mutation that is causing the condition. For some autosomal dominant conditions, the new mutation rate is high and may account for a large percentage of affected individuals, as in Pfeiffer syndrome (Winter & Baraitser, 1996).

Many autosomal dominant conditions have **variable expressivity** (variation in the phenotype associated with a single condition). This may cause affected individuals to be missed if the phenotype is not appropriately defined. For example, in Van der Woude syndrome, affected members of the same family may have lip pits, cleft lip, cleft palate, or a combination of these. Obviously, an individual with isolated lip pits could be missed if only individuals with cleft lip are identified when a family history is obtained. Most, if not all, autosomal dominant conditions demonstrate some degree of variable expressivity (Mueller & Cook, 1997).

Incomplete penetrance is the lack of a recognizable phenotype in an individual who carries a mutation that may cause an autosomal dominant trait or condition. At times, it may be difficult to distinguish between minimal expression caused by variable expressivity and true incomplete penetrance. Some families have members who have no abnormal findings (nonpenetrance) but have transmitted the trait to their children. Other individuals may have only one feature of a condition (variable expressivity) but may transmit the complete condition to their children. The factors that determine the penetrance and expressivity for a given trait are not well understood, but they include different mutations in the same gene, modification of genes that interact with the gene that causes the disorder, environmental influences, and random variation (Mueller & Cook, 1997; Murray, 1995).

Many genes have more than one function and may therefore be associated with multiple seemingly unrelated abnormalities. For example, neurofibromatosis type 1 is associated with growth of large nerve sheath tumors, called **neurofibromas**; pigmentary abnormalities of the skin; bony dysplasias; and learning disabilities. This **pleiotropy** (the phenomenon where a single mutant gene can affect multiple, unrelated systems) can contribute to the variability in genetic syndromes because each function of a gene can have either variable expression or nonpenetrance (Fitzsimmons, 2013; Mueller & Cook, 1997).

X-Linked and Y-Linked Inheritance

X-linked inheritance refers to conditions caused by mutations in genes on the X chromosome. X-linked inheritance is unique because males inherit only one allele of the X chromosome, whereas females inherit two copies.

There are many X-linked recessive conditions that affect males almost exclusively. A female is likely to have no more than mild effects, if there are any effects at all. Carrier females transmit the defective genes to 50% of their sons, who will be affected, and 50% of their daughters, who will be carriers. Affected males pass the mutation to 100% of their daughters. There is no father-to-son transmission because fathers do not give an X chromosome to their sons. See **FIGURE 2-9** for a Punnett square of X-linked inheritance with the mother as carrier and **FIGURE 2-10** for a Punnett square of X-linked inheritance with an affected father. Also,

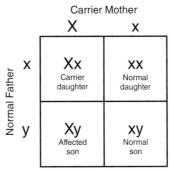

Capital letters designate a mutation.

FIGURE 2-9 Punnett square showing X-linked recessive inheritance with a carrier mother.

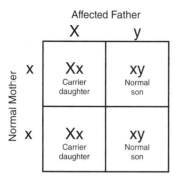

Capital letters designate a mutation.

FIGURE 2-10 Punnett square showing X-linked recessive inheritance with an affected father.

TABLE 2-4 **Examples of X-Linked Recessive Craniofacial Syndromes**
Chitayat syndrome
X-linked cleft palate
Oral–facial–digital syndrome type VIII
VATER with hydrocephaly
Lenz microphthalmia
Lowe syndrome
Oto–palato–digital syndrome type II
Simpson–Golabi–Behmel syndrome
SCARF syndrome
Say–Meyer syndrome

TABLE 2-5 **Examples of X-Linked Dominant Syndromes**
Goltz syndrome
Conradi chondrodysplasia punctate
Oral–facial–digital syndrome type I
Melnick-Needles osteodysplasty
Aicardi syndrome
Incontinentia pigmenti
X-linked hypophosphataemic rickets
Rett syndrome

see **TABLE 2-4** for a list of some X-linked conditions that are associated with cleft lip or cleft palate.

X-linked dominant inheritance is rare, with only a few known disorders. With X-linked dominant disorders (**TABLE 2-5**), all daughters of affected males inherit the disorder. Sons of affected males never inherit the disorder because they receive the Y chromosome from the father. Affected females can transmit the disorder to offspring of both sexes. There is an excess of affected females in pedigrees for X-linked dominant disorders. Many X-linked dominant disorders are lethal to affected males. See Table 2-2 for a list of some autosomal recessive conditions that are associated with cleft lip or cleft palate and craniofacial syndromes.

There are a number of X-linked conditions that cannot be clearly categorized as either recessive or dominant. They affect females who are heterozygous, but they may affect males more severely. This group of disorders is often lumped with X-linked recessive disorders in the medical literature but should more appropriately be referred to simply as X-linked. Some examples of this pattern include Aarskog syndrome, Opitz BBBG syndrome, Alport syndrome, Coffin–Lowry syndrome, fragile X syndrome, and Fabry disease. This group of disorders is characterized by variable expressivity and high levels of nonpenetrance in females but with complete penetrance and more uniform expression in males.

Of course, Y-linked disorders affect only males. Because there are relatively few genes on the Y chromosome and the only major Y-linked traits are for male gender and sperm production, the transmission of other types of traits from a father to his son is considered diagnostic of autosomal dominant inheritance.

Non-Mendelian Inheritance

Many disorders that recur in families do not follow the basic rules of Mendelian inheritance. The remainder of this chapter reviews some of the mechanisms involved in the inheritance of these disorders.

Multifactorial Inheritance

Some human disorders result from an interaction of multiple genes with environmental influences. This is called multifactorial inheritance. Environmental factors known to increase risks for birth defects are called teratogens. Common examples of teratogens include alcohol, cigarette smoke, anti-epileptic medications, maternal diabetes, and congenital infections. Most, if not all, teratogens exert their effects by interfering with the regulation of gene expression.

Inherited traits and abnormalities associated with multifactorial inheritance can be divided into two categories: continuous variation and threshold. Continuous variation traits include height, weight, intelligence, and blood pressure. These traits are not easily distinguished from normal variation because the boundary between normal and abnormal is arbitrary. In contrast, threshold abnormalities involve a trait that is either present or absent. As the number of risk factors for the trait increases, the additive risk ultimately crosses a threshold, resulting in expression of the trait. Threshold abnormalities include various birth defects. In the case of cleft lip, with or without cleft palate, many possible risk factors have been identified that can have an additive effect. These include variations in 4 to 12 candidate genes, which include TGFA, RARA, BCL3, and END1 (Lidral & Moreno, 2005) and many environmental teratogens. See TABLE 2-6 for a list of multifactorial abnormalities/disorders.

Some inherited disorders show a tendency to have more severe manifestations or an earlier age of onset with succeeding generations. This phenomenon, known as anticipation, is typically

TABLE 2-6 Examples of Multifactorial Abnormalities/Disorders
Cleft lip with or without cleft palate
Cleft palate
Velopharyngeal insufficiency
Diabetes mellitus
Alzheimer disease
Alcoholism
Atherosclerotic heart disease
Cognitive disability
Colon cancer
Bipolar disease

caused by large expansions of nucleotide repeats, most commonly the nucleotides of CAG. As the number of repeats expands, it becomes unstable so that in the next generation there is a tendency for the number of repeats to be greater. This, in turn, leads to an earlier age of onset and a more severe phenotype. Disorders of anticipation include fragile X syndrome, Huntington's disease, spinocerebellar ataxias, and other adult-onset neurodegenerative disorders.

Some disorders can also be affected by whether the abnormal gene was inherited maternally or paternally. This phenomenon is called imprinting (Butler, 2002; Tilghman, 1999). If a gene is maternally imprinted, the allele inherited from the mother is not expressed. The opposite is true if the gene is paternally imprinted. This has been demonstrated to occur in Beckwith–Wiedemann syndrome, Prader–Willi syndrome, Angelman syndrome, and Russell–Silver syndrome.

The risk for recurrence of a multifactorial trait in family members can be estimated by doing population studies. The estimated recurrence risk for a family with one individual with cleft palate is 3% to 5%. If there are two affected first-degree relatives, the risk goes up to approximately 9% to 15%, depending on which family members have cleft lip (Curtis, Fraser, & Warburton, 1961; Wyszynski, Zeiger, Tilli, Bailey-Wilson, & Beaty, 1998). The reason for the range depends on the gender of the persons affected, how closely related the affected individuals are to the pregnancy, and the severity of the cleft (Grosen et al., 2010).

Multifactorial inheritance is very difficult to study because it is complicated by heterogeneity, small effects of each risk factor, incomplete penetrance, and complex interactions. On the other hand, some of the most common human diseases are a result of multifactorial inheritance. Fortunately, recent advances in informatics and genetics have greatly increased the ability to study the additive effects of multiple genetic factors and interacting factors related to specific birth defects. The study of the structure, function, evolution, and mapping of genomes, referred to as genomics, began with the Human Genome Project. Genomics is also allowing analysis of very large amounts of data in a short period of time so that it is now possible to sequence the entire genome of an individual for diagnostic purposes.

SUMMARY

The basics of genetics and the principles of inheritance that are covered in this chapter are fundamental to the understanding of the etiology of craniofacial malformations and the risk for recurrence. In addition, an understanding of the basis of malformation syndromes is important for appropriate management of the patient and counseling for the family regarding prognosis for the affected child and recurrence risk. As new insights are discovered into the causes of genetic diseases and birth defects, it will become increasingly important to understand these principles and apply them for improved management of each affected patient and family.

FOR REVIEW AND DISCUSSION

1. Describe the "anatomy" of a chromosome and all its contents.

2. How many chromosomes are in human cells? Describe how the 23rd pair of chromosomes determines gender.

3. What is meant by monosomy and trisomy? What common syndrome is due to trisomy 21?

4. What is a karyotype? How is it done? What information can it give the clinician?

5. Which is likely to cause more abnormalities—a chromosomal defect or single gene defect? Why do you think that is the case?

6. Define heterozygous and homozygous? Explain how they relate to autosomal recessive and autosomal dominant inheritance?

7. Cleft palate is often described as the result of multifactorial inheritance. Explain what that means and what factors might cause cleft lip/palate.

8. What is X-linked inheritance? Is it more serious in boys or girls? Why?

9. What is a pedigree? What can it tell you, and why should it be done for individuals with a craniofacial anomaly?

10. What is a phenotype? How does it relate to variable expressivity? Why is it important to know about variable expressivity when evaluating a genetic syndrome in a family?

REFERENCES

Butler, M. G. (2002). Imprinting disorders: Non-Mendelian mechanisms affecting growth. *Journal of Pediatric Endocrinology,* 5(Suppl. 5), 1279–1288.

Cummings, M. (1997). *Human heredity* (4th ed.). Eagan, MD: West/Wadsworth.

Curtis, E., Fraser, F., & Warburton, D. (1961). Congenital cleft lip and palate. *American Journal of Diseases in Childhood, 102,* 853–857.

Fitzsimmons, J. S. (2013). *A handbook of clinical genetics.* Waltham, MA: Butterworth-Heinemann.

Gardner, R. J. M., Sutherland, G. R., & Shaffer, L. G. (2012). *Chromosome abnormalities and genetic counseling* (4th ed). New York, NY: Oxford University Press.

Grosen, D., Chevrier, C., Skytthe, A., Bille, C., Mølsted, K., Sivertsen, A., . . . Christensen, K. (2010). A cohort study of recurrence patterns among more than 54,000 relatives or oral cleft cases in Denmark: Support for the multifactorial threshold model of inheritance. *Journal of Medical Genetics, 47*(3), 162–168.

Jorde, L. B., Carey, J. C., & Bamshad, M. J. (2016). *Medical genetics* (5th ed.). Philadelphia, PA: Elsevier, Inc.

Kaiser-Rogers, K., & Rao, K. (1999). Structural chromosomal rearrangements. In S. Gersen & M. Keagle (Eds.), *The principles of clinical cytogenetics* (pp. 191–228). Totowa, NJ: Humana Press.

Keagle, M., & Brown, J. (1999). DNA, chromosomes, and cell division. In S. Gersen & M. Keagle (Eds.), *The principles of clinical cytogenetics* (pp. 11–30). Totowa, NJ: Humana Press.

Le Caignec, C., Boceno, M., Saugier-Veber, P., Jacquemont, S., Joubert, M., David, A., . . . Rival, J. (2005). Detection of genomic imbalances by array-based comparative genomic hybridization in fetuses with multiple malformations. *Journal of Medical Genetics, 42,* 121–128.

Lidral, A. C., & Moreno L. M. (2005). Progress toward discerning the genetics of cleft lip. *Current Opinion in Pediatrics, 17,* 731–739.

McKusick, V. (1997). History of medical genetics. In D. Rimoin, J. Connor, & R. Pyeritz (Eds.), *Emery and Rimoin's principles and practice of medical genetics* (3rd ed., vol. 1, pp. 1–30). New York, NY: Churchill Livingstone.

Mueller, R., & Cook, J. (1997). Mendelian inheritance. In D. Rimoin, J. Connor, & R. Pyeritz (Eds.), *Emery and Rimoin's principles and practice of medical genetics* (3rd ed., vol. 1, pp. 87–102). New York, NY: Churchill Livingstone.

Murray, J. C. (1995). Face facts: Genes, environment, and clefts. *American Journal of Human Genetics, 57*(2), 227–232.

Randolph, L. (1999). Prenatal cytogenetics. In S. Gersen & M. Keagle (Eds.), *The principles of clinical cytogenetics* (pp. 259–316). Totowa, NJ: Humana Press.

Rutledge, S., & Percy, A. (1997). Gangliosidoses and related lipid storage diseases. In D. Rimoin, J. Connor, & R. Pyeritz (Eds.), *Emery and Rimoin's principles and practice of medical genetics* (3rd ed., vol. 2, pp. 2105–2130). New York, NY: Churchill Livingstone.

Schoumans, J., Ruivenkamp, C., Holmberg, E., Kyllerman, M., Anderlid, B. M., & Nordenskjöld, M. (2005). Detection of chromosomal imbalances in children with idiopathic mental retardation by array-based comparative genomic hybridization (array-CGH). *Journal of Medical Genetics, 42,* 699–705.

Smithsonian National Museum of Natural History in partnership with the NIH National Human Genome Research Institute. (n.d.). *The animated genome.* Retrieved from https://unlockinglifescode.org/media/animations/659#660

Stevenson, A. C., & Clare Davison, B. C. (2017). *Genetic counselling* (2nd ed.). Philadelphia, PA: Elsevier, Inc.

Strachan, T., & Read, A. (1996). *Human molecular genetics.* New York, NY: Wiley-Liss.

Tilghman, S. M. (1999). The sins of the fathers and mothers: Genomic imprinting in mammalian development. *Cell, 96*(2), 185–193.

Ting, J. C., Ye, Y., Thomas, G. H., Ruczinski, L., & Pevsner, J. (2006). Analysis and visualization of chromosomal abnormalities in SNP data with SNPscan. *Bioinformatics, 7*(1), 25.

Uhlmann, W. R., Schuette, J. L., & Yashar, B. (2011). *A guide to genetic counseling* (2nd ed.). Indianapolis, IN: John Wiley & Sons.

Wilkie, A. O., Tang, Z., Elanko, N., Walsh, S., Twigg, S. R., Hurst, J. A., . . . Maxson, R. E. (2000). Functional haploinsufficiency of the human homeobox gene MSX2 causes defects in skull ossification. *Nature Genetics, 24*(4), 387–390.

Winter, R., & Baraitser, M. (1996). *London dysmorphology database* (1) [Compact Disc]. London, UK: Oxford Medical Databases.

Wyszynski, D. F., Zeiger, J., Tilli, M. T., Bailey-Wilson, J. E., & Beaty, T. H. (1998). Survey of genetic counselors and clinical geneticists regarding recurrence risks for families with nonsyndromic cleft lip with or without cleft palate. *American Journal of Medical Genetics, 79*(3), 184–190.

CREDITS

Chapter opener photo: © PeopleImages/Getty Images
Figure 2-2 and Figure 2-3: Courtesy of Ruthann Blough Pfau, PhD, Dayton Children's Hospital.

All other photos courtesy of the Cleft and Craniofacial Center at Cincinnati Children's Hospital Medical Center.

CHAPTER 3

Clefts of the Lip and Palate

CHAPTER OUTLINE

INTRODUCTION

A cleft is an abnormal opening or fissure in an anatomical structure that is normally closed. Cleft lip and/or palate (CL/P) is a congenital condition in that it is noted at birth.

Cleft lip and/or cleft palate is the second most common birth defect in the United States and the most common congenital defect of the face. A cleft of the lip affects facial aesthetics, whereas a cleft of the palate can affect feeding, middle ear function, speech, and resonance. An isolated cleft palate or submucous cleft is often associated with craniofacial syndromes that include other anomalies. Clefts vary in type and severity but almost always follow the path of the normal embryological suture lines.

This chapter begins with a description of the embryological development of the lip and palate. This information is helpful in understanding the various causes and classification of clefts, which are further described. Particular emphasis is placed on submucous cleft palate because this anomaly is not always easy to identify, yet it can cause problems with speech and resonance. Finally, the potential functional disorders that can occur secondary to each type of cleft are discussed.

Embryological Development

A basic knowledge of embryological development and the sequence of lip and palate formation helps the clinician to understand why clefts occur as they do. This knowledge also relates to how clefts are described and classified.

Embryological development of the face and palate is dependent on the formation of neural crest cells in the embryo. These cells migrate at different rates and times to form the structures of the face and oral cavity. A delay or disruption in this migration can result in a cleft.

Embryological closure of the lip (and alveolar ridge) begins around 7 weeks' gestation, whereas closure of the hard palate and velum starts around 9 weeks' gestation. In both cases, the fusion begins at the incisive foramen and then moves outward (**FIGURE 3-1**).

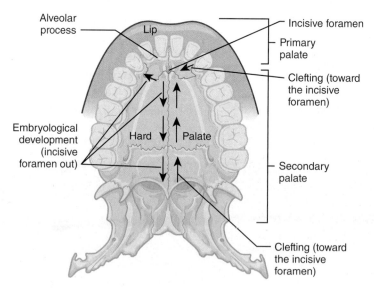

FIGURE 3-1 Embryological development and patterns of clefting. Embryological development proceeds from the incisive foramen out to the periphery. Clefting patterns begin at the periphery and follow the lines of normal embryological fusion toward the incisive foramen to the point of the disruption. The classification of clefts is based on embryological development, with the incisive foramen as the dividing point between the primary palate and secondary palate.

The alveolar ridge is actually the first structure to fuse. Beginning at the area of the incisive foramen, fusion proceeds in an anterior direction to form the alveolar ridge through the fusion of the premaxilla with the maxillary bones at the bilateral incisive suture lines. Closure then proceeds to form the base of the external nose and then downward to form the upper lip. The prolabium and two lateral lip segments of the upper lip are then fused, forming the philtrum and philtral ridges. The last part of the upper lip to be completed is the vermilion.

Prior to palatal fusion, the tongue is in a superior and posterior position in the nasopharynx. In addition, the palatal bones are vertical and positioned on each side of the tongue. Around the 7 or 8 weeks' gestation, the mandible begins to drop down and forward, bringing the tongue down and forward with it. Once the tongue is out of the way, the palatal bones move from a vertical to a horizontal position. The palatal bones then begin to fuse with the premaxilla at the area of the incisive foramen. The process of fusion in this case moves in a posterior direction to fuse the palatal bones in midline along the median palatine suture line to complete the formation of the hard palate. The vomer bone, which forms a portion of the nasal septum, moves downward to fuse with the superior surface of the hard palate, thus completing the separation of the nasal cavity into two halves. Once the hard palate is formed, the velum is fused in midline, forming the median raphe. Lastly, the uvula is formed. Fusion of the hard palate and velum is usually complete by 12 weeks' gestation.

Causes of Clefts

Clefts of the lip and palate occur as a result of a disruption or delay in cell migration or palatal shelf movement during embryological development. As a result, there is failure of fusion at the embryological suture lines. Clefts can be caused by either an inherited (genetic or chromosomal) condition and/or environmental factors during pregnancy. Inherited conditions are considered endogenous (internal) factors, and environmental causes are considered exogenous (external) factors.

The etiology of a cleft in a single individual is complex. This is because there are several genes that, when defective, can cause a genetic predisposition for a cleft. However, the defective gene(s) may not actually cause a cleft unless there are also specific environmental factors that trigger the gene's expression. A combination of both endogenous and exogenous factors in the etiology of the cleft is called multifactorial inheritance.

Inherited (Endogenous) Factors

A considerable amount of research has been done to find the genes that cause or predispose a fetus to have nonsyndromic CL/P. Specific genes that are active during early craniofacial development have been implicated in the etiology of CL/P, including transforming growth factor-alpha retinoic acid receptor; transforming growth factor beta; MSX1 (Lidral et al., 1998); and IRF6, the gene (Adeyemo & Butali, 2017; Rahimov, Jugessur, & Murray, 2012; Zucchero et al., 2004). To date, 17 genes have been found to be associated with nonsyndromic orofacial clefts.

Once a couple has a child with a cleft, their risk of having another child with a cleft is 3% to 5%, or a 30- to 45-fold increase over a typical risk. The recurrence risk for CL/P is also elevated for affected individuals and their siblings when they have children. The recurrence risk increases with each additional child born with a cleft. (See the chapter *Genetics and Patterns of Inheritance* for more information on inheritance of clefts related to craniofacial syndromes.)

Environmental (Exogenous) Factors

Environmental (exogenous) factors that can cause clefts include teratogens or physical interference of fetal development. Teratogens are substances that can cause congenital malformations. Teratogens that have been associated with CL/P include cigarette smoke (Honein, Paulozzi, & Watkins,

2001; Reiter et al., 2012); alcohol; certain drugs (e.g., Dilantin, valium, anticonvulsants, and corticosteroids) (Edwards et al., 2003); lead pollution (Vinceti et al., 2001); viruses, including rubella and even influenza (Metneki, Puho, & Czeizel, 2005); maternal nutritional deficiencies, including a lack of vitamin B-6 (Munger et al., 2004); and maternal obesity (Moore, Singer, Bradlee, Rothman, & Milunsky, 2000). In the past, folic acid deficiency was thought to be a cause of orofacial clefts because it is important for embryonic and fetal development of the neural tube. However, recent studies have found that folic acid fortification during pregnancy does not reduce the incidence of clefting in large populations (Bille, Knudsen, & Christensen, 2005; Castilla, Orioli, Lopez-Camelo, Dutra Mda, & Nazer-Herrera, 2003; Hashmi, Waller, Langlois, Canfield, & Hecht, 2005; Munger et al., 2004; Ray, Meier, Vermeulen, Wyatt, & Cole, 2003).

As previously mentioned, physical interference is another exogenous factor that can affect embryonic development. This can include fetal positioning or crowding and placental factors. In addition, micrognathia (small mandible) can result in physical interference with palatal fusion. For example, with Pierre Robin sequence, the mandible is abnormally small and does not move down and forward at the appropriate time. Therefore, the back of the tongue remains high in the nasopharynx. If the back of the tongue is in this position when the hard palate and velum begin to fuse, the tongue will interfere with fusion. This causes a wide, bell-shaped cleft palate as the velum forms around the base of the tongue. (See the chapter *Dysmorphology and Craniofacial Syndromes* for more information about Pierre Robin sequence.)

Another cause of physical disruption of embryonic development is amniotic bands. Amniotic bands are strands of tissue that occur when the amnion (the membrane surrounding the embryo and fetus) ruptures. These strands can attach to various body parts and act as tourniquets, cutting off blood supply to the developing structures. This can result in amputations of developing limbs or digits, clefts of the lip or palate, and other oral and facial deformities.

Types and Classification of Clefts

Orofacial clefts can be of the lip only, the palate only, or both. A cleft lip occurs when there is failure of parts of the lip and often the alveolar ridge to come together early in the life of a fetus. A cleft palate occurs when the midline of the roof of the mouth does not fuse normally during fetal development, leaving an opening between the oral cavity and the nasal cavity. Clefts of the lip and palate vary in length and width, depending on the degree of fusion of the individual parts. In addition, the structures surrounding the cleft are often hypoplastic in that the tissues (i.e., bone, muscles, and nerves) are underdeveloped in their formation.

Both types of clefts follow their respective embryological suture lines (see the chapter *Anatomy and Physiology*). Because embryological fusion goes from the incisive foramen out (forward for the alveolar ridge and lip and backward for the hard palate and velum), anything that disrupts that process will cause a cleft along the embryological suture line from that point all the way to the periphery (lip or uvula). Therefore, as can be seen in Figure 3-1, clefts begin at the periphery and follow the lines of normal embryological fusion toward the incisive foramen to the point of the disruption in fusion. A complete cleft (of the lip or palate) is one that follows the embryological fusion line(s) and extends all the way to the incisive foramen. An incomplete cleft (of the lip or palate) is one that does not extend all the way to the incisive foramen.

Because there are different types of clefts with different combinations and levels of severity, the naming and classification of clefts can be a challenge. Although several classification systems have been proposed over the years, the system that has gained the most universal acceptance is the one proposed by Kernahan and Stark (1958), who recommended that clefts be classified based on embryological development. As such, there are two basic categories of clefts: clefts of the primary palate and clefts of the secondary palate, with the incisive foramen as the dividing point between the two. This division can be viewed schematically on the right side of Figure 3-1.

The primary palate consists of the structures that are anterior to the incisive foramen and fuse around 7 weeks' gestation. These structures include the alveolar ridge and the lip (even though the terminology is primary "palate"). The secondary palate consists of the structures that are posterior to the incisive foramen and fuse around 9 weeks' gestation. These structures include the hard palate (excluding the alveolar ridge), the velum, and the uvula. Clefts can be of the primary palate, secondary palate, or both.

Although this basic classification system is used most commonly by professionals, a modification of the Kernahan and Stark classification system was later proposed by Kernahan (1971). This model uses a "striped-Y" figure as a means of identifying both the type and the extent of the cleft, as noted in **FIGURE 3-2**. The upper "arms" of the Y represent the incisive suture lines of the primary palate, and the base of the Y represents the median palatine suture line of the secondary palate. The center point where the arms and the base connect represents the area of the incisive foramen.

The arms of the Y are divided into segments, with the right side numbered as 1, 2, and 3 and the left side numbered as 4, 5, and 6. The most top segment of each arm represents the lip, the middle segment represents the alveolar ridge, and the bottom segment represents the area between the alveolar ridge and the incisive foramen. The base of the Y is also divided into numbered segments, where 7 and 8 represent the hard palate and 9 represents the velum.

By darkening the affected segments on this diagram, a visual representation can be made of not just the type of cleft (primary and/or secondary palate) but also the extent of the cleft (complete or incomplete). If there is a submucous cleft, the affected segments are marked with crosshatches.

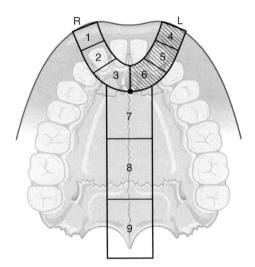

FIGURE 3-2 The Kernahan striped Y for cleft classification. The upper arms of the Y represent the primary palate, and the base represents the secondary palate. The most anterior segment represents the lip, the middle segment represents the alveolus, and the posterior segment represents the area between the alveolus and the incisive foramen. The secondary palate (hard and soft palate) is also divided into sections to represent the areas of the velum and hard palate. The segments affected by the cleft are darkened on the diagram so that a visual representation can be made of the type and extent of the cleft. If there is a submucous cleft, the affected segments are marked with crosshatches.

Clefts of the Primary Palate

As previously mentioned, clefts of the primary palate affect structures anterior to the incisive foramen. Therefore, clefts of the primary palate affect the lip (and often the nose) and can extend into the alveolar ridge.

Types and Severity

A cleft of the primary palate follows the embryological suture lines, which include the philtral ridges above the upper lip and below the nose, and the incisive suture lines of the alveolar ridge. The cleft can be narrow or very wide.

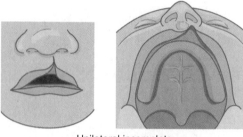

Unilateral incomplete

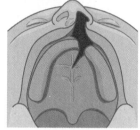

Unilateral complete

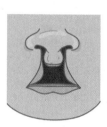
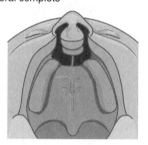

Bilateral complete

FIGURE 3-3 Types of clefts of the primary palate. Note the short columella and the distortion of the ala on the affected side.

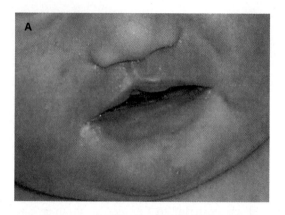

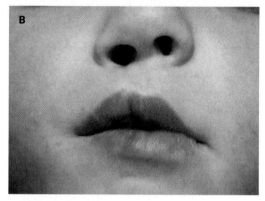

FIGURE 3-4 Forme fruste (also known as a microform cleft), which is a very mild form of incomplete cleft of the primary palate and is somewhat analogous to a bifid uvula of the secondary palate.

Clefts of the primary palate can be incomplete or complete (**FIGURE 3-3**). An incomplete cleft of the primary palate is one that does not extend all the way to the incisive foramen. It can be as minor as a forme fruste (also called microform cleft), which can cause only a small notch in the upper lip (**FIGURE 3-4**). A forme fruste is often analogous to a submucous cleft palate in that the overlying tissue of the lip may be intact while the underlying tissues are incompletely developed. Another type of incomplete cleft lip is a Simonart's band (**FIGURE 3-5**), which is a band of tissue that bridges

a cleft lip. It may be the result of partial fusion that has separated. This finding is of no clinical significance, and therefore the treatment is the same as with a more common type of cleft lip.

A complete cleft of the primary palate is one that extends through the entire lip, nostril sill, and alveolar ridge to the incisive foramen. (When the term "complete cleft lip" is used, it usually refers to a complete cleft of the primary palate, which also includes the alveolar ridge.) Because this type of cleft is more extensive, it has a bigger effect on the structures.

Because the incisive suture lines and the philtral ridges are bilateral, a cleft of the primary palate

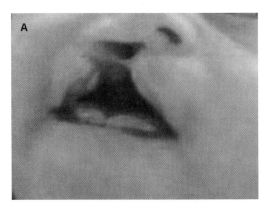 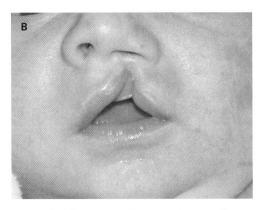

FIGURE 3-5 Simonart's band, which is a strand of soft tissue partially filling the gap between the medial and lateral portions of a cleft lip.

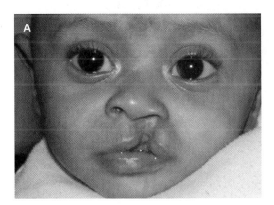 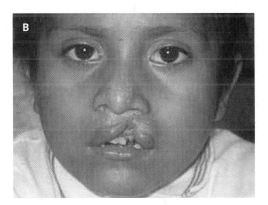

FIGURE 3-6 Unilateral incomplete cleft of the primary palate.

can be unilateral (on either the right or left side) or bilateral (on both sides). If the cleft is unilateral, it most often occurs on the left side (Jensen, Kreiborg, Dahl, & Fogh-Andersen, 1988; Kim & Baek, 2006). **FIGURE 3-6** illustrates examples of a unilateral incomplete cleft of the lip and alveolar ridge. **FIGURE 3-7** shows examples of a bilateral incomplete cleft. **FIGURE 3-8** shows examples of a unilateral complete cleft of the primary palate.

When there is a bilateral complete cleft of the primary palate (that extends to the incisive foramen on both sides), the cleft isolates both the philtrum (now called the prolabium) and the triangular-shaped premaxilla bone. In many cases, these structures are positioned in an extremely anterior position at birth so that they appear to extend from the tip of the nose. **FIGURE 3-9** shows children with a bilateral complete cleft of the primary palate. In most cases, the prolabium appears as tissue that is attached to the tip of the nose, and the premaxilla is isolated and in an anterior position.

Clefts of the primary palate cause more than just a separation of the tissues. These clefts also cause hypoplasia (underdevelopment) of the nearby tissues and a misalignment of the related structures. By examining an unrepaired cleft lip closely, it is apparent that all the structures are present, including the philtral dimple and both of the philtral ridges, but the cleft courses just to the

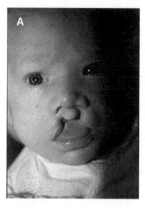
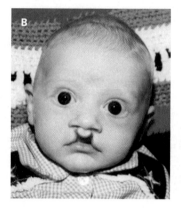
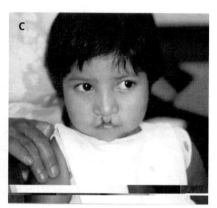

FIGURE 3-7 Bilateral incomplete cleft of the primary palate (lip and alveolus). Note the distortion of the nose.

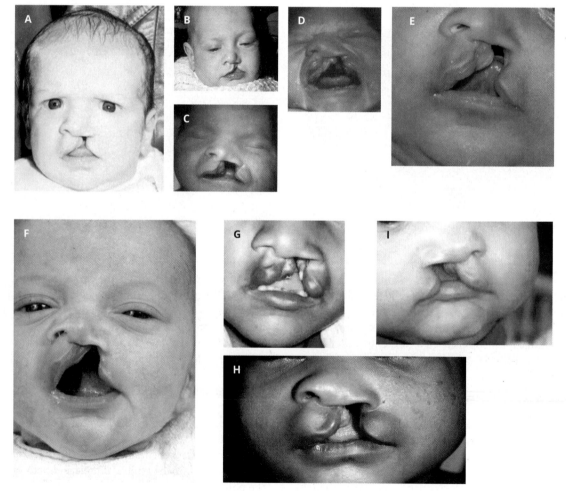

FIGURE 3-8 Unilateral complete cleft of the primary palate (lip and alveolus).

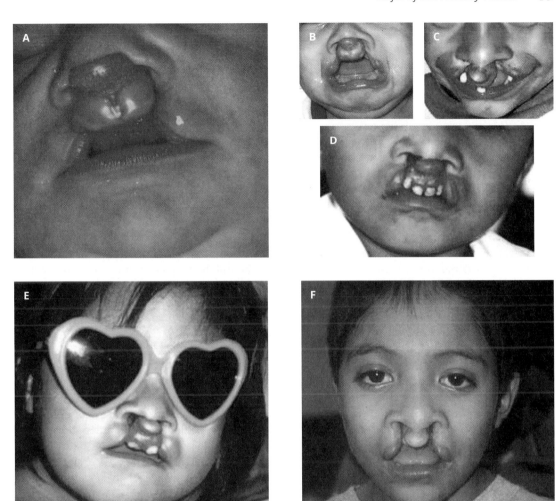

FIGURE 3-9 Bilateral complete cleft lip.

lateral side of the philtral ridge. On the cleft side(s), the lip is short, and the Cupid's bow is twisted up into the cleft. If the cleft goes through the entire lip, the upper portion of the orbicularis oris muscle is discontinuous and also misaligned in that it curves upward along the edges of the vermilion.

Finally, a cleft of the primary palate often affects the formation of the nose, even if it is an incomplete cleft and does not reach the nasal sill. The nasal ala on the affected side(s) is often spread laterally because of the separation of the lip. This causes the nose to appear very wide and flattened. In addition, the formation of the columella is often affected. If the cleft is unilateral, the columella on the cleft side will be short and positioned obliquely, with its base deviated toward the noncleft side. When the cleft is bilateral and complete, the columella is often so short that it is virtually nonexistent, giving the appearance that the prolabium and premaxilla are attached to the tip of the nose. Although even a short, incomplete cleft can affect the nose somewhat, the formation of the nose is most affected when the cleft is more extensive and/or wide.

Children who have had a repair of a cleft of the primary palate usually have a residual nasolabial fistula (also known as an intentional fistula) located in the alveolar ridge just under the labial sulcus (furrow between the lip and gum) of the upper lip. This fistula is left open deliberately by the surgeon during the initial repair to allow for unrestricted maxillary growth for a period of time. It is later closed by an alveolar bone graft just before the permanent teeth begin to erupt. (See the chapter *Dental Anomalies*.)

Effects on Function

The effects of a cleft of the primary palate on function vary, depending on the severity. An incomplete cleft of the primary palate causes aesthetic concerns but rarely causes any functional problems. In contrast, a complete cleft of the primary palate can cause dental and occlusal abnormalities, a small oral cavity size, and dental interference with speech sound production. The nasal cavity is smaller in individuals with unilateral cleft lip and palate than in those with bilateral clefts because of the skewing of the nasal septum toward the unaffected side. Although the nasal cavity continues to grow with age, it remains about 30% smaller than normal because of the inherent hypoplasia of the structures and the restrictive effects of surgical correction (Drake, Davis, & Warren, 1993; Reiser, Andlin-Sobocki, Mani, & Holmstrom, 2011). Reduced nasal cavity

size can affect nasal breathing and resonance during speech.

Clefts of the Secondary Palate

As previously mentioned, clefts of the secondary palate affect structures posterior to the incisive foramen. Therefore, clefts of the secondary palate affect the uvula and can affect the velum and hard palate.

Types and Severity

A cleft of the secondary palate follows the median raphe and the midline palatine suture of the hard palate. As such, clefts of the secondary palate are always in the midline and therefore cannot be unilateral or bilateral. Clefts of the secondary palate vary in width. They can be very narrow or very wide.

As with clefts of the primary palate, clefts of the secondary palate can also be incomplete or complete (**FIGURE 3-10**). An incomplete cleft of the secondary palate is one that does not extend all the way to the incisive foramen. It can be as slight as a line in the midline of the uvula or a bifid uvula. **FIGURE 3-11** shows examples of an incomplete cleft of the secondary palate. A more extensive incomplete cleft palate may extend into the velum or even partially into the hard palate.

A complete cleft of the secondary palate is one that extends through the uvula, velum, and

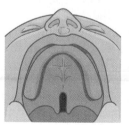 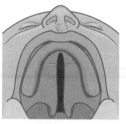 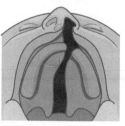 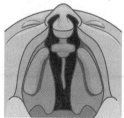

Incomplete cleft palate   Complete cleft palate   Unilateral complete cleft lip and palate   Bilateral complete cleft lip and palate

FIGURE 3-10 Various types of cleft palate.

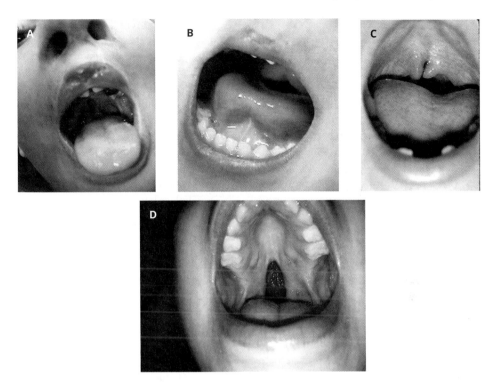

FIGURE 3-11 Incomplete cleft palate.

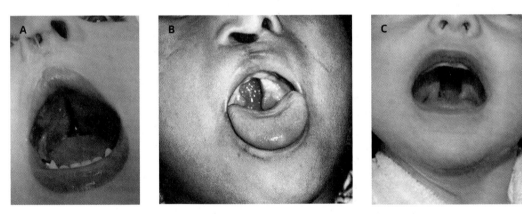

FIGURE 3-12 Complete cleft palate.

hard palate and then follows the median palatine suture line through the hard palate all the way to the incisive foramen. **FIGURE 3-12** shows examples of a complete cleft of the palate. When there is a complete cleft of the palate, the velar aponeurosis is absent, and the orientation of the levator veli palatini, palatopharyngeus, and musculus uvulae muscles is altered (Dickson, 1972; Koch, Grzonka, & Koch, 1998; Rittler et al., 2011). Although the origins of the levator veli palatini muscles are normal, the muscle insertions are necessarily abnormal as a result of the open cleft. Instead of a midline insertion, there is a diastasis (separation) of the paired levator veli palatini muscles. Therefore, the muscles insert onto the posterior border of the cleft hard palate, instead of in midline, thus rendering these muscles essentially nonfunctional (Dickson, 1972; Dickson, Grant, Sicher, Dubrul, & Paltan, 1974; Dickson, Grant, Sicher, Dubrul, & Paltan, 1975; Maue-Dickson, 1979; Maue-Dickson & Dickson, 1980; Mehendale, 2004). Even fibers of the palatopharyngeus muscle insert abnormally into the hard palate. In addition, the musculus uvulae muscles are typically hypoplastic. This abnormal configuration of muscles because of cleft palate has been referred to as the cleft muscle of Veau. In **FIGURE 3-13**, Figure 3-13A shows the orientation of the velar muscles in a normal palate and velum. Figure 3-13B shows the abnormal orientation of the muscles when there is a cleft.

A cleft palate often occurs with a cleft lip. **FIGURE 3-14** shows examples of a bilateral complete cleft lip and cleft palate. Because of the bilateral complete cleft of the primary palate, the prolabium and premaxilla are isolated and in an anterior position. The vomer portion of the nasal septum can be viewed through the cleft of the palate. The vomer bone, which forms the bottom part of the nasal septum, is usually attached to the larger of the two palatal segments when combined with a unilateral cleft of the primary palate and is not attached to either segment when combined with a bilateral cleft of the primary palate.

Cleft palate can also be isolated (cleft palate only). An isolated cleft palate is more often associated with a craniofacial syndrome and thus with other structural anomalies and functional issues. **FIGURE 3-15** shows a cleft palate with no involvement of the primary palate. A wide, bell-shaped cleft palate with no cleft lip is characteristic of Pierre Robin sequence. As previously mentioned, Pierre Robin sequence can be caused by physical interference of mandibular growth in utero. However, it can also be the result of genetic causes of micrognathia (a small mandible), as is

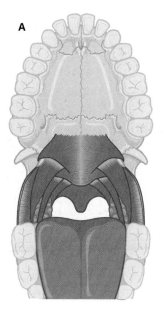 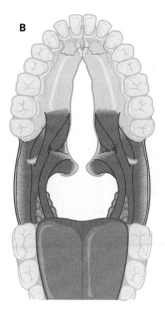

FIGURE 3-13 (A) Illustration of normal velar musculature. Note that the muscles insert in midline. **(B)** Abnormal velar musculature as a result of a cleft palate. Note that the fibers of the levator veli palatini muscles, and even the palatopharyngeus muscles, insert into the posterior border of the hard palate. This abnormal orientation is called the cleft muscle of Veau.

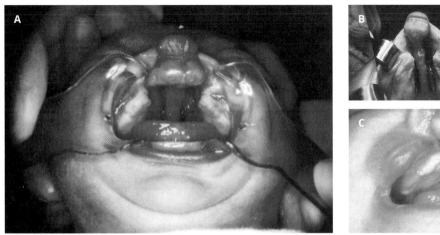
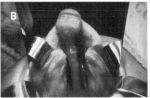
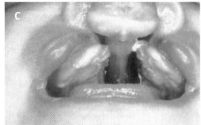

FIGURE 3-14 Bilateral complete cleft of the primary palate and secondary palate. Note the prolabium, premaxilla, and the nasal septum.

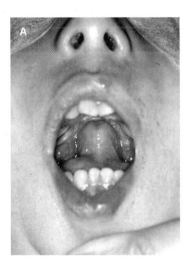
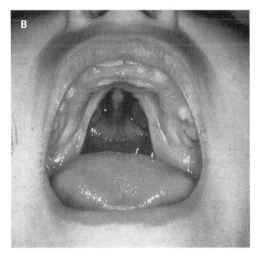

FIGURE 3-15 Wide, bell-shaped cleft palate with no cleft lip. This is characteristic of Pierre Robin sequence.

characteristic of several syndromes (e.g., velo-cardiofacial/22q11.2 deletion syndrome Stickler syndrome, and Treacher Collins syndrome).

Effects on Function

A cleft of the secondary palate can cause several functional problems, including significant difficulty with sucking and nasal regurgitation when feeding, disorders of speech and/or resonance, issues related to oronasal (palatal) fistulas, conductive hearing loss from chronic middle ear effusion, and airway obstruction from a reduction in the nasal and/or pharyngeal cavity space. When the cleft palate is associated with a craniofacial syndrome, there may also be neurological involvement, which can affect language development and cognitive function.

Newborns with cleft palate usually experience initial problems with feeding because of the inability to achieve suction. They also experience nasal regurgitation during feeding. Both are because of the abnormal coupling of the nasal and oral cavities as a result of the open cleft. (See the chapter *Early Feeding Problems*.)

Children with cleft palate are at risk for disorders of speech production and resonance as a result of velopharyngeal insufficiency (a form of velopharyngeal dysfunction due to abnormal structure; see the chapter *Speech/Resonance Disorders and Velopharyngeal Dysfunction*). Although the goal of cleft palate surgery is to correct the orientation of the muscles and lengthen the velum for normal velopharyngeal function, about 20% to 30% of individuals with a history of cleft palate are likely to have velopharyngeal insufficiency, despite the surgical repair (Bardach, 1995). This can be caused from either a short velum or poor velar movement as a result of abnormal insertion of the levator muscles.

Some patients will develop a palatal fistula (also known as an oronasal fistula) in the palate after the palate is repaired (Bykowski, Naran, Winger, & Losee, 2015). This should not be confused with an unrepaired incomplete cleft. This type of fistula is actually a result of a partial dehiscence (or breakdown) of the cleft repair. The fistula can be located anywhere in the hard palate or velum but will always be located along the embryological or surgical suture lines (**FIGURE 3-16**). The effect of the fistula on function depends on its size and location. Anterior fistulas can cause nasal regurgitation of liquids and, if large, soft foods. Anterior fistulas can also cause nasal emission during speech and, if large, hypernasality.

Children with clefts of the secondary palate frequently have dysfunction of the tensor veli palatini muscles, which are designed to open the eustachian tubes. This malfunction causes chronic middle ear effusion. Therefore, affected children have more frequent bouts of otitis media and secondary conductive hearing loss than their unaffected peers (Sheer, Swarts, & Ghadiali, 2010) (see the chapter *Facial, Oral, and Pharyngeal Anomalies*).

Upper airway obstruction with mouth breathing is very common in patients with a

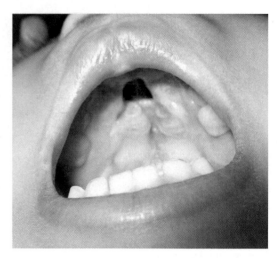

FIGURE 3-16 Oronasal (palatal) fistula. An oronasal fistula is a hole in the palate that occurs because of a partial dehiscence (or breakdown) of the cleft repair. The fistula can be located anywhere in the hard palate or velum along the suture lines. Fistulas are particularly common in the area of the incisive foramen, as seen in this case.

history of cleft palate (Liu, Warren, Drake, & Davis, 1992; Rosé, Thissen, Otten, & Jonas, 2003; Warren & Drake, 1993; Warren, Hairfield, & Dalston, 1990; Warren, Hairfield, & Dalston, 1991). This can be because of a nasal septal deviation that can alter nasal cavity size (Sandham & Murray, 1993). It can also be from a decrease in depth of the nasopharynx because of the posterior displacement of the maxilla (Fukushiro & Trindade, 2005; Satoh, Wada, Tachimura, & Fukuda, 2005; Smahel, Kasalova, & Skvarilova, 1991; Smahel & Mullerova, 1992). Airway obstruction is a particular concern in patients with Pierre Robin sequence because the micrognathia causes glossoptosis (the posterior displacement of the tongue so that it is in the pharynx).

When a cleft palate is associated with a craniofacial syndrome, there are usually other craniofacial anomalies that affect generalized function. For example, underlying brain abnormalities may affect speech, feeding, language, and cognition. In addition, anomalies of the ears may affect hearing.

Submucous Cleft Palate

A submucous cleft palate is a congenital defect in which the oral surface of the secondary palate is intact, but the underlying structure of the palate is incompletely developed because of delayed fusion of the nasal surface of the palate as compared to the oral surface. As a result, a submucous cleft is usually more apparent on the nasal surface of the velum, as observed through nasopharyngoscopy, than on the oral surface. It can be theorized that fusion of the oral surface of the velum slightly precedes fusion of the nasal surface, which is why a submucous cleft sometimes occurs.

Types and Severity

As with other types of clefts, a submucous cleft can be incomplete or complete. If the submucous cleft is incomplete, it may be as minor as a hypoplastic or malformed uvula with no involvement of the velum. If complete, the submucous cleft courses under the mucosa of the entire velum and hard palate to the area of the incisive foramen. **FIGURE 3-17** shows various degrees of severity of a submucous cleft and the effect of the defect on the musculature.

Despite an intact oral surface, a submucous cleft can cause the levator veli palatini muscles to attach to the posterior border of the hard palate, rather than interdigitating with each other in the midline of the velum. In addition, the musculus uvulae muscles may be hypoplastic, as noted through nasopharyngoscopy. Therefore, during phonation, the nasal surface of the velum appears flat, or even concave, instead of the normal convex shape. Just like an isolated (open) cleft palate, a submucous cleft often occurs as part of a generalized syndrome with multiple other craniofacial malformations and resultant functional issues (Reiter, Haase, & Brosch, 2010; Sekhon, Ethunandan, Markus, Krishnan, & Rao, 2011).

Overt Submucous Cleft

An overt submucous cleft palate is one that can be seen on the oral surface of the palate during an intraoral examination. The diagnosis is made by observation of one or more of the following classic characteristics: a bifid or hypoplastic uvula, a zona pellucida in the velum, "tenting" of the velum during phonation, and a notch that can be palpated in the posterior border of the hard palate. **FIGURE 3-18** shows many examples of a submucous cleft.

Abnormalities of the uvula vary in appearance. In some cases, the uvula is clearly bifid, with two distinct pendulous structures instead of a single pedicle (Figures 3-18A, 3-18F, and 3-18G). In other cases, a bifurcation is not easily appreciated, although there may be a faint line in the middle (Figure 3-18B) or the uvula may appear to be hypoplastic. A bifid or hypoplastic uvula can be an isolated anomaly (as an incomplete cleft) with no further involvement of the velum and hard palate. However, the observation of a bifid or hypoplastic uvula suggests that embryological development was disrupted at some point during secondary palate formation. Therefore, when it is noted, it is important to rule out an associated submucous cleft that extends into the velum.

A zona pellucida is a bluish area that can sometimes be seen in the midline of the velum when there is a submucous cleft (Figures 3-18A, 3-18B, and 3-18G). This area is the result of thin mucosa with a lack of the normal underlying muscle mass.

A common sign of a submucous cleft is "tenting" of the velum during phonation and a lack of a velar dimple (Figures 3-18C and 3-18D). Both of these observations are a result of the diastasis of the paired levator veli palatini muscles and the insertion of these muscles into the posterior border of the hard palate. With phonation, this abnormal muscle insertion makes the velum appear to "tent up" toward the hard palate. In some cases, this V-shaped abnormality can be viewed underneath the surface of the mucoperiosteum, all the way to the area of the incisive foramen. Sometimes, the defect is not as obvious and may just look like a minor defect in the velum (Figure 3-18E).

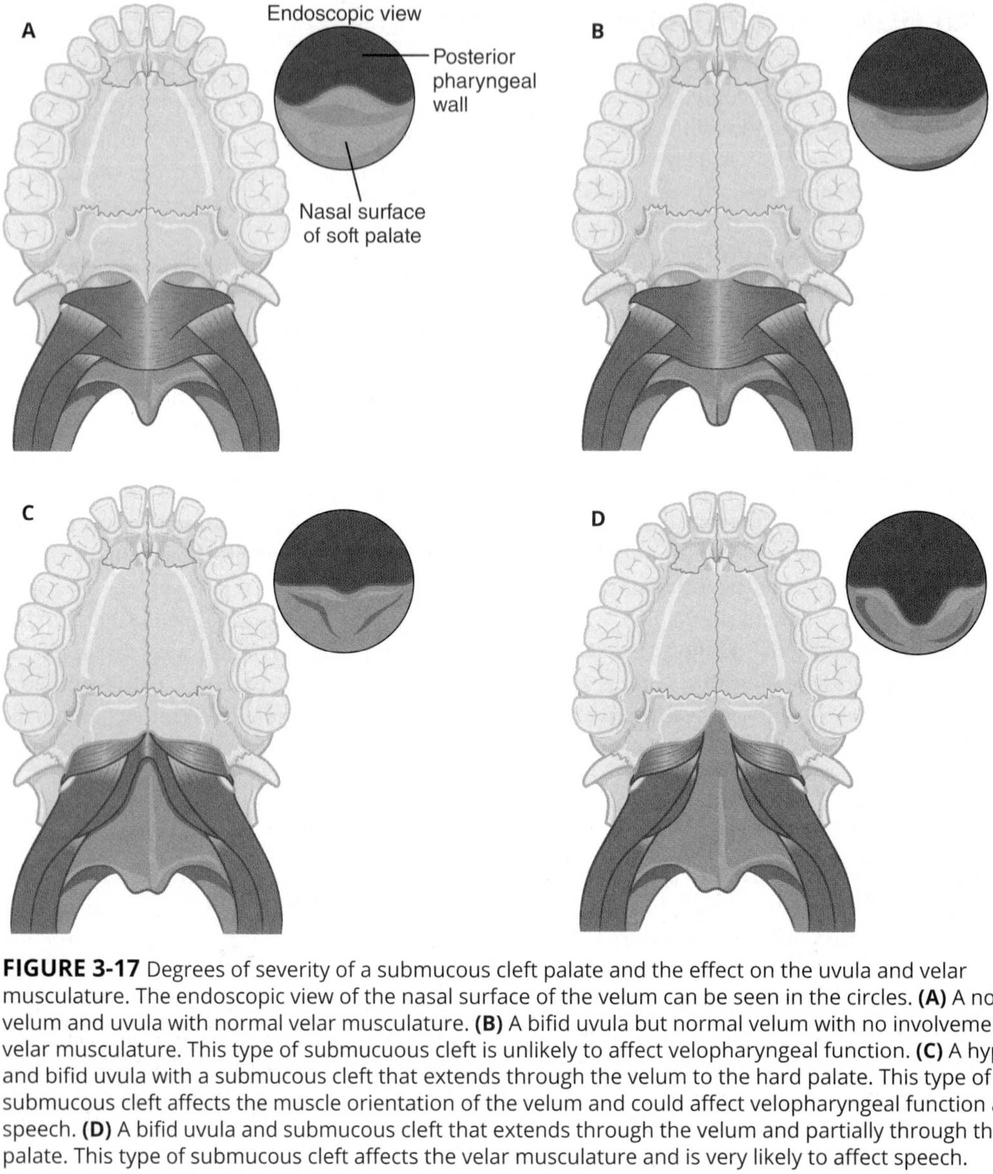

FIGURE 3-17 Degrees of severity of a submucous cleft palate and the effect on the uvula and velar musculature. The endoscopic view of the nasal surface of the velum can be seen in the circles. **(A)** A normal velum and uvula with normal velar musculature. **(B)** A bifid uvula but normal velum with no involvement of the velar musculature. This type of submucuous cleft is unlikely to affect velopharyngeal function. **(C)** A hypoplastic and bifid uvula with a submucous cleft that extends through the velum to the hard palate. This type of submucous cleft affects the muscle orientation of the velum and could affect velopharyngeal function and thus speech. **(D)** A bifid uvula and submucous cleft that extends through the velum and partially through the hard palate. This type of submucous cleft affects the velar musculature and is very likely to affect speech.

If the submucous cleft extends through at least part of the hard palate, a notch in the midline of the posterior border of the hard palate can usually be felt through palpation. A notch in the hard palate may be present, even when an intraoral examination shows an apparently intact uvula and velum (Malata, Cooter, & Batchelor, 1993; Shprintzen, Schwartz, Daniller, & Hoch, 1985).

Occult Submucous Cleft

An occult submucous cleft is a "hidden" defect in the velum because it is not apparent on the

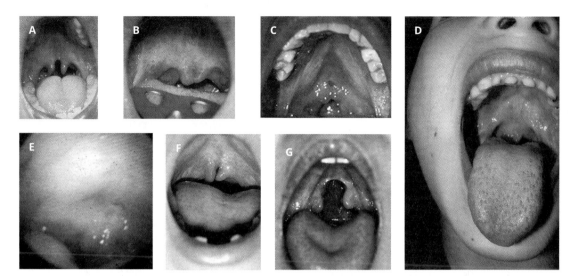

FIGURE 3-18 Submucous cleft. **(A)** Note the bifid uvula and zona pellucida. **(B)** Note the hypoplastic uvula with a faint line in the middle and the zona pellucida. **(C)** Note the diastasis of the velar musculature and how the muscles insert into the hard palate, resulting in an inverted V shape. **(D)** Note the subtle inverted V during velar elevation, indicating an abnormality in the insertion of the levator veli palatini muscle. **(E)** Note the hypoplastic uvula with a thin line in the middle. **(F)** Note the bifid uvula and subtle abnormality in the velum. **(G)** Note the overt cleft of the uvula and velum and submucous cleft of the hard palate.

oral surface of the velum (Abdel-Aziz, Dewidar, El-Hoshy, & Aziz, 2009). In fact, it can be appreciated only by viewing the nasal surface of the velum through nasopharyngoscopy. A nasopharyngoscopy view of an occult submucous cleft often shows a V-shaped midline defect with a flattening or depression in the area of the velar eminence. **FIGURE 3-19** is an endoscopic view of a velum showing the nasal surface. On the posterior edge of the velum, there is a small indentation, and on the nasal surface, there is a depression rather than a rounded bulky mass of the musculus uvulae muscles. These characteristics, and the absence of an abnormality on the oral surface, are typical of an occult submucous cleft.

The occult submucous cleft is not embryologically or genetically different from other variations of the submucous cleft. Instead, the occult submucous cleft represents a point on the continuum of severity of submucous cleft and cleft palate. Therefore, individuals with an occult submucous cleft have some of the same abnormalities as those with an overt submucous cleft

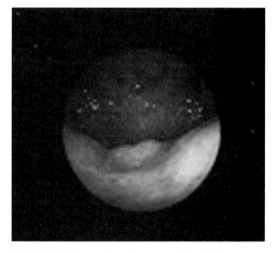

FIGURE 3-19 Occult submucous cleft. This is an endoscopic view of the velum showing the nasal surface. It can be seen that the edge of the velum has a depression rather than the rounded muscle mass of the musculus uvulae muscles. This depression is an indication of a submucous cleft. This is an occult (hidden) submucous cleft because there was no abnormality noted on the oral surface of the velum.

and even open cleft palate. The musculus uvulae muscles are often either absent or deficient (Croft, Shprintzen, Daniller, & Lewin, 1978; Finkelstein, Hauben, Talmi, Nachmani, & Zohar, 1992; Rourke, Weinberg, Marazita, & Jabbour, 2017), and there is often abnormal insertion of the levator muscles into the hard palate.

Effects on Function

The effect of a submucous cleft on function depends on the extent of the defect. If the submucous cleft extends very far into the velum, it can result in velopharyngeal insufficiency with hypernasal speech (Reiter, Brosch, Wefel, Schlomer, & Haase, 2011; Shprintzen et al., 1985). Studies have shown that overall, one-fourth to one-half of individuals with submucous cleft will have associated velopharyngeal dysfunction (Bagatin, 1985; Garcia Velasco, Ysunza, Hernandez, & Marquez, 1988; Kono, Young, & Holtmann, 1981; Sullivan, Vasudavan, Marrinan, & Mulliken, 2011). In addition, there may be nasal regurgitation with swallowing, especially during the first year of life and an increased risk for middle ear disease with conductive hearing loss from abnormalities of the tensor veli palatini muscle (Garcia Velasco et al., 1988; Sheahan, Miller, Earley, Sheahan, & Blayney, 2004).

Although individuals with a submucous cleft are at risk for dysfunction of the velopharyngeal valve, many people with this abnormality have normal speech, normal middle ear function, and no history of nasal regurgitation with swallowing (Park et al., 2000). McWilliams (1991) studied a group of 130 patients with submucous cleft and found that 44% remained asymptomatic into adulthood. Therefore, the mere presence of a submucous cleft should not be a concern if there is normal speech. It is important, however, that the individual and the family are counseled regarding this abnormality, for several reasons. The family should be informed that a full adenoidectomy with a submucous cleft is usually contraindicated because of the risk that this will cause velopharyngeal

insufficiency (Saunders, Hartley, Sell, & Sommerlad, 2004). In addition, the family should be counseled regarding the genetic risk for additional offspring with submucous cleft, cleft palate, or associated syndromes.

Treatment of Submucous Cleft

Surgical correction of a submucous cleft palate is not routinely done as with an open cleft palate because many children with a submucous cleft will develop normal speech. Surgical correction is considered only after speech has developed and velopharyngeal insufficiency has been diagnosed (Abdel-Aziz et al., 2009; Chen, Wu, & Noordhoff, 1994; Garcia Velasco et al., 1988; Gosain, Conley, Marks, Larson, 1996). For optimal speech results, surgical correction should be done as soon as possible after the diagnosis, however (Reiter et al., 2011).

Facial Clefts

Facial cleft is a collective term that includes not only clefts of the lip and palate but other less common types of clefts of the face as well. Facial clefts can affect any of the facial structures, including the forehead, eyes, ears, nose, cheeks, mouth, and jaws. As with clefts of the lip and palate, facial clefts vary considerably in terms of the extent of the cleft and the effect on the soft tissue and bone. However, most facial clefts are severe and are accompanied by many other anomalies.

Types and Severity

Facial clefts are typically described using the Tessier classification system (Tessier, 1976). This system was developed by Paul Tessier, who was a French plastic surgeon and is considered the father of modern craniofacial surgery. Using numbers from 0–14, with the midline designated as 0, the location and extent of the cleft can be described. These 15 types of clefts are often put into 4 groups, based on their general position: midline clefts, paramedian clefts, orbital clefts, and oblique (lateral) clefts (**FIGURE 3-20**).

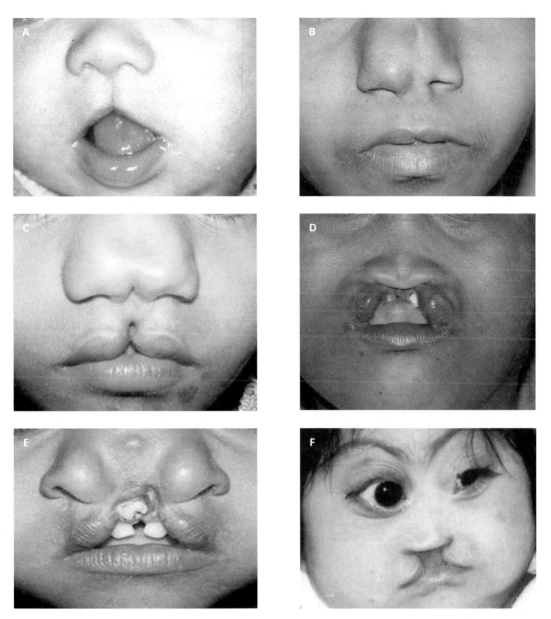

FIGURE 3-20 Midline facial clefts of various degrees of severity. **(A)** Mild midline cleft of the lip only. **(B)–(E)** Midline facial clefts that affect the nose. **(F)** Midline facial cleft with holoprosencephaly, which is a condition in which there is failure of the forebrain to divide into the two hemispheres.

A midline (median) facial cleft can be very mild so that there is only a notch in the midline of the vermilion or a slight cleft of the upper lip (Figure 3-20A). However, midline clefts are often associated with a spectrum of other midline anomalies, such as bifid nose (Miller, Grinberg, & Wang, 1999; Patel & Tantri, 2010), frontonasal dysplasia (abnormal tissue development)

(Hodgkins et al., 1998), and hypertelorism (wide spacing between the eyes) (Figure 3-20 B–E). Midline clefts can also affect brain development, causing cranial base anomalies, an encephalocele (a congenital gap in the skull, with herniation of brain tissue into the nose or palate), or an absent corpus callosum (the nerve fibers that allow communication between the cerebral hemispheres). In severe cases, a midline cleft may be associated with holoprosencephaly (failure of the forebrain to divide into two hemispheres) (Figure 3-20F).

An oblique cleft begins at the mouth and then courses laterally, horizontally, and upward so that it may affect the facial bones, nasal structures, orbits, and even the ears. As shown in **FIGURE 3-21**, a oblique cleft can be unilateral (Figure 3-21A) or bilateral (Figure 3-21B) (Kuriyama, Udagawa, Yoshimoto, Ichinose, & Suzuki, 2008). More extensive conditions of clefts may also be described anatomically, such as "oro-occular cleft" and "fronto-nasal dysplasia."

As with cleft lip and palate, facial clefts are caused by a variety of factors that disrupt neural crest cell migration, resulting in the lack of fusion of the facial bones. In addition, amniotic bands are often responsible for certain types of facial clefts (Hukki et al., 2004).

Effects on Function

Facial clefts can actually affect any part of the face or head. Therefore, the effect on function is variable. However, these clefts often affect a variety of functional areas, including cognition, language, speech, resonance, hearing, feeding, and swallowing.

Incidence of Clefts

Incidence of Cleft Lip and Palate

In epidemiology, the term prevalence refers to the number of cases of a disease or disorder that are present in a particular population at a given

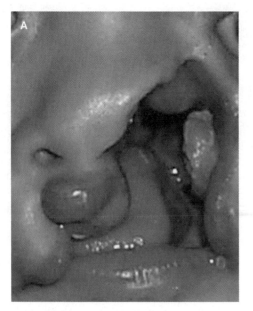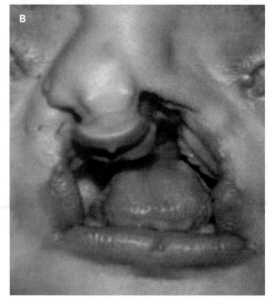

FIGURE 3-21 Oblique facial clefts. **(A)** Unilateral. **(B)** Bilateral.

time. In contrast, the term incidence refers to the number of new cases of a disease or disorder in a given population, such as the number of persons becoming ill with a certain disease. Although some studies report numbers using the word "prevalence," the word "incidence," meaning the number of new births, is used in this text.

Epidemiological estimates of the incidence of nonsyndromic clefts of the lip and/or palate around the world vary greatly because of a variety of factors. These include differences in the sample populations, genetic differences by racial background, the surveillance methodology, the inclusion criteria of the studies (e.g., live births only or including fetal deaths), and the clinical classification of clefts (International Perinatal Database of Typical Oral Clefts [IPDTOC] Working Group, 2011; Mitchell, 2009).

As a result of these differences, the reported incidence estimates of orofacial clefts range from 7.75 to 10.63 per 10,000 live births (Parker et al., 2010; Tanaka, Mahabir, Jupiter, & Menezes, 2012). Cleft lip, with or without cleft palate, is more prevalent than cleft palate alone (Gorlin, Cohen, & Hennekam, 2001; Mossey & Little, 2002; Rahimov et al., 2012). Overall, oral clefts in any form (i.e., cleft lip, cleft lip and palate, or isolated cleft palate) have been estimated to occur in about 1 in every 700 live births (Kadir et al., 2017; World Health Organization [WHO], 2001). In the United States, cleft lip and palate is the second most common birth defect (Parker et al., 2010).

There is evidence to show that there are differences between males and females in the incidence and types of clefts typically presented. Overall, boys are affected more frequently than girls by a ratio of 3:2 (Sekhon et al., 2011; Wyszynski, Beaty, & Maestri, 1996). Cleft lip, with or without cleft palate, occurs about twice as often in males than in females and is usually more severe in males. On the other hand, cleft palate occurs about twice as often in females as in males (Jensen et al., 1988; Maresova, Veleminska, & Mullerova, 2004; Mossey, Little, Munger, Dixon, & Shaw, 2009). Although the reason for these differences between

genders is not clearly understood, it has been speculated that it could be related to differences in the timing of the development of the lip and palate in the embryo. Burdi and Silvey (1969) found that, in the male human embryo, the horizontal positioning and subsequent closure of the secondary palate occur earlier than in the female embryo. Because the palatal shelves are open longer in the female, there is a greater period of time during which there is susceptibility to environmental teratogens.

The incidence of clefts also varies significantly depending on racial background. The incidence is highest in Native Americans (1 in 300), then Asians (1 in 500), and then Caucasians (1 in 800). The incidence of clefts is lowest in those of African descent (1 in 2000) (Gorlin et al., 2001).

About 10% to 15% of individuals with cleft lip (with or without cleft palate) have a related syndrome. In contrast, 40% to 50% of individuals with cleft palate have only a related syndrome. In fact, there are about 400 recognized syndromes that include cleft palate as one of their features. When cleft palate occurs as part of a syndrome, there are usually other associated craniofacial malformations as well as other malformations and medical conditions (Beriaghi et al., 2009; Jones, 1988; Shprintzen et al., 1985).

Incidence of Submucous Cleft

Several studies have reported the incidence of bifid uvula in a primarily Caucasian population to be between 0.2% and 2.0% (Bagatin, 1985; Gorlin, Cervenka, & Pruzansky, 1971; Wharton & Mowrer, 1992). One study compared the occurrence of bifid uvula in four races and found the relative frequency by race is similar to the relative frequency of cleft lip and palate (Shapiro, Meskin, Cervenka, & Pruzansky, 1971).

Several studies have attempted to determine the incidence of submucous cleft in the general population (Bagatin, 1985; Gosain, Conley, Santoro, & Denny, 1999). Gosain and colleagues (1996) summarized the results of several studies in the literature and stated that incidence of the classic characteristics of submucous cleft palate among the general population is between 0.02% and 0.08%.

Although a submucous cleft may be noticed at birth or soon after, especially if there are early feeding problems, an occult submucous cleft is usually not discovered unless the child has evidence of hypernasality. In some cases, the defect is not noted for years or is never discovered, especially if it is asymptomatic and not causing any problems with speech. Therefore, the incidence of occult submucous cleft is not known.

The incidence of submucous cleft palate in individuals with clefts of the primary palate has been found to be significantly greater than the incidence of submucous cleft palate found in the general population (Gosain et al., 1999; Kono et al., 1981). Because of this increased risk, it is important for individuals with cleft lip to be thoroughly examined for submucous cleft. Early detection of submucous cleft associated with cleft lip is important for the prevention of middle ear problems and for the proper management of velopharyngeal insufficiency, if it occurs.

Incidence of Facial Clefts

Fortunately, facial clefts are very rare. The exact incidence of facial clefts is unknown, and estimates vary greatly because of the rarity of their occurrence and the lack of standard methods of data collection (Cooper, Ratay, & Marazita, 2006; Darzi & Chowdri, 1993).

SUMMARY

Cleft lip and palate is a common birth defect that presents in a variety of ways. When a cleft occurs, it is the result of a disruption in embryological development. There are different types of clefts, such as clefts of the primary palate and clefts of the secondary palate. There are also different degrees of severity, from a notch in the lip to a bilateral complete cleft of the lip and alveolar ridge or from a bifid uvula to complete cleft palate. A submucous cleft is a type of cleft that is not readily apparent because it affects the underlying structures of the velum while leaving the oral surface intact. Many craniofacial syndromes include cleft palate as part of the phenotype.

As will be noted in subsequent chapters, cleft lip and cleft palate can affect the development of communication skills in a variety of ways. Therefore, healthcare providers, particularly members of a cleft palate or craniofacial team, need to be aware of this so that appropriate intervention can be initiated.

FOR REVIEW AND DISCUSSION

1. Beginning with the incisive foramen, describe the process and direction of embryological development of the lip and palate.

2. What are possible causes of clefts? Given these causes, what do you think could be done to reduce the risk of clefting in a population?

3. What is meant by the terms "primary palate" and "secondary palate"? What structures are included? How does this classification system relate to embryological development?

4. List different types of clefts of the primary palate. What are the potential functional problems with regard to these clefts? What professional disciplines may be involved in treatment?

5. List different types of clefts of the secondary palate. What are the potential functional

problems with regard to these clefts? What professional disciplines may be involved in treatment?

6. Describe the possible characteristics of a submucous cleft palate. Why is this type of cleft often undetected at birth? Discuss the occurrence of submucous cleft as it relates to embryological development.

7. What structures may be involved in a facial cleft? In addition to the obvious aesthetic concerns, what are some reasons that these types of clefts are of particular concern?

REFERENCES

Abdel-Aziz, M., Dewidar, H., El-Hoshy, H., & Aziz, A. A. (2009). Treatment of persistent post-adenoidectomy velopharyngeal insufficiency by sphincter pharyngoplasty. *International Journal of Pediatric Otorhinolaryngology, 73*(10), 1329–1333.

Adeyemo, W. L., & Butali, A. (2017). Genetics and genomics etiology of nonsyndromic orofacial clefts. *Molecular Genetics & Genomic Medicine, 5*(1), 3–7.

Bagatin, M. (1985). Submucous cleft palate. *Journal of Maxillofacial Surgery, 13*(1), 37–38.

Bardach, J. (1995). Secondary surgery for velopharyngeal insufficiency. In R. J. Shprintzen & J. Bardach (Eds.), *Cleft palate speech management: A multidisciplinary approach* (pp. 277–294). St. Louis, MO: Mosby.

Beriaghi, S., Meyers, S. L., Jensen, S. A., Kaimal, S., Chan, C. M., & Schaefer, G. B. (2009). Cleft lip and palate: Association with other congenital malformations. *The Journal of Clinical Pediatric Dentistry, 33*(3), 207–210.

Bille, C., Knudsen, L. B., & Christensen, K. (2005). Changing lifestyles and oral clefts occurrence in Denmark. *The Cleft Palate–Craniofacial Journal, 42*(3), 255–259.

Burdi, A. R., & Silvey, R. G. (1969). Sexual differences in closure of the human palatal shelves. *Cleft Palate Journal, 6*, 1–7.

Bykowski, M. R., Naran, S., Winger, D. G., & Losee, J. E. (2015). The rate of oronasal fistula following primary cleft palate surgery: A meta-analysis. *Cleft Palate–Craniofacial Journal, 52*(4), e81–e87.

Castilla, E. E., Orioli, I. M., Lopez-Camelo, J. S., Dutra Mda, G., & Nazer-Herrera, J. (2003). Preliminary data on changes in neural tube defect prevalence rates after folic acid fortification in South America. *American Journal of Medical Genetics Part A, 123*(2), 123–128.

Chen, K. T., Wu, J., & Noordhoff, S. M. (1994). Submucous cleft palate. *Chang Keng I Hsueh: Chang Gung Medical Journal, 17*(2), 131–137.

Cooper, M. E., Ratay, J. S., & Marazita, M. L. (2006). Asian oral-facial cleft birth prevalence. *The Cleft Palate–Craniofacial Journal, 43*(5), 580–589.

Croft, C. B., Shprintzen, R. J., Daniller, A. L., & Lewin, M. L. (1978). The occult submucous cleft palate and the musculus uvulae. *Cleft Palate Journal, 15*, 150–154.

Darzi, M. A., & Chowdri, N. A. (1993). Oblique facial clefts: A report of Tessier numbers 3, 4, 5, and 9 clefts. *The Cleft Palate–Craniofacial Journal, 30*(4), 414–415.

Dickson, D. R. (1972). Normal and cleft palate anatomy. *Cleft Palate Journal, 9*, 280–293.

Dickson, D. R., Grant, J. C., Sicher, H., Dubrul, E. L., & Paltan, J. (1974). Status of research in cleft palate anatomy and physiology, Part 1. *Cleft Palate Journal, 11*, 471–492.

Dickson, D. R., Grant, J. C., Sicher, H., Dubrul, E. L., & Paltan, J. (1975). Status of research in cleft lip and palate: Anatomy and physiology, Part 2. *Cleft Palate Journal, 12*, 131–156.

Drake, A. F., Davis, J. U., & Warren, D. W. (1993). Nasal airway size in cleft and noncleft children. *Laryngoscope, 103*(8), 915–917.

Edwards, M. J., Agho, K., Attia, J., Diaz, P., Hayes, T., Illingworth, A., Roddick L. G. (2003). Case-control study of cleft lip or palate after maternal use of topical corticosteroids during pregnancy. *American Journal of Medical Genetics Part A, 120*(4), 459–463.

Finkelstein, Y., Hauben, D. J., Talmi, Y. P., Nachmani, A., & Zohar, Y. (1992). Occult and overt submucous cleft palate: From peroral examination to nasendoscopy and back again. *International Journal of Pediatric Otorhinolaryngology, 23*(1), 25–34.

Fukushiro, A. P., & Trindade, I. E. (2005). Nasal airway dimensions of adults with cleft lip and palate: Differences among cleft types. *Cleft Palate Journal, 42*(4), 396–402.

Garcia Velasco, M., Ysunza, A., Hernandez, X., & Marquez, C. (1988). Diagnosis and treatment of submucous cleft palate: A review of 108 cases. *Cleft Palate Journal, 25*(2), 171–173.

Gorlin, R. J., Cervenka, J., & Pruzansky, S. (1971). Facial clefting and its syndromes. *Birth Defects Original Article Series, 7*(7), 3–49.

Gorlin, R., Cohen, M. J., & Hennekam, R. C. M. (2001). *Syndromes of the head and neck* (4th ed.). New York, NY: Oxford University Press.

Gosain, A. K., Conley, S. F., Marks, S., & Larson, D. L. (1996). Submucous cleft palate: Diagnostic methods and outcomes of surgical treatment. *Plastic & Reconstructive Surgery, 97*(7), 1497–1509.

Gosain, A. K., Conley, S. F., Santoro, T. D., & Denny, A. D. (1999). A prospective evaluation of the prevalence of submucous cleft palate in patients with isolated cleft lip versus controls. *Plastic & Reconstructive Surgery, 103*(7), 1857–1863.

Hashmi, S. S., Waller, D. K., Langlois, P., Canfield, M., & Hecht, J. T. (2005). Prevalence of nonsyndromic oral clefts in Texas: 1995–1999. *American Journal of Medical Genetics, Part A, 134*(4), 368–372.

Hodgkins, P., Lees, M., Lawson, J., Reardon, W., Leitch, J., Thorogood, P., . . . Taylor, D. (1998). Optic disc anomalies and frontonasal dysplasia. *British Journal of Ophthalmology, 82*(3), 290–293.

Honein, M. A., Paulozzi, L. J., & Watkins, M. L. (2001). Maternal smoking and birth defects: Validity of birth certificate data for effect estimation. *Public Health Reports, 116*(4), 327–335.

Hukki, J., Balan, P., Ceponiene, R., Kantola-Sorsa, E., Saarinen, P., & Wikstrom, H. (2004). A case study of amnion rupture sequence with acalvaria, blindness, and clefting: Clinical and psychological profiles. *Journal of Craniofacial Surgery, 15*(2), 185–191.

International Perinatal Database of Typical Oral Clefts (IPDTOC) Working Group. (2011). Prevalence at birth of cleft lip with or without cleft palate: Data from the International Perinatal Database of Typical Oral Clefts (IPDTOC). *The Cleft Palate–Craniofacial Journal, 48*, 66–81.

Jensen, B. L., Kreiborg, S., Dahl, E., & Fogh-Andersen, P. (1988). Cleft lip and palate in Denmark, 1976–1981: Epidemiology, variability, and early somatic development. *Cleft Palate Journal, 25*(3), 258–269.

Jones, M. C. (1988). Etiology of facial clefts: Prospective evaluation of 428 patients. *Cleft Palate Journal, 25*(1), 16–20.

Kadir, A., Mossey, P. A., Blencowe, H., Moorthie, S., Lawn, J. E., Mastroiacovo, P., & Modell, B. (2017). Systematic review and meta-analysis of the birth prevalence of orofacial clefts in low- and middle-income countries. *The Cleft Palate–Craniofacial Journal, 54*(5), 571–581.

Kernahan, D. A. (1971). The striped Y-A symbolic classification for cleft lip and palate. *Plastic & Reconstructive Surgery, 47*(5), 469–470.

Kernahan, D. A., & Stark, R. B. (1958). A new classification for cleft lip and cleft palate. *Plastic & Reconstructive Surgery, 22*, 435.

Kim, N. Y., & Baek, S. H. (2006). Cleft sidedness and congenitally missing or malformed permanent maxillary lateral incisors in Korean patients with unilateral cleft lip and alveolus or unilateral cleft lip and palate. *American Journal of Orthodontics and Dentofacial Orthopedics, 130*(6), 752–758.

Koch, K. H., Grzonka, M. A., & Koch, J. (1998). Pathology of the palatal aponeurosis in cleft palate. *The Cleft Palate–Craniofacial Journal, 35*(6), 530–534.

Kono, D., Young, L., & Holtmann, B. (1981). The association of submucous cleft palate and clefting of the primary palate. *Cleft Palate Journal, 18*(3), 207–209.

Kuriyama, M., Udagawa, A., Yoshimoto, S., Ichinose, M., & Suzuki, H. (2008). Tessier number 7 cleft with oblique clefts of bilateral soft palates and rare symmetric structure of zygomatic arch. *Journal of Plastic, Reconstructive & Aesthetic Surgery, 61*(4), 447–450.

Lidral, A. C., Romitti, P. A., Basart, A. M., Doetschman, T., Leysens, N. J., Daack-Hirsch, S., . . . Murray, J. C. (1998). Association of MSX1 and TGFB3 with nonsyndromic clefting in humans. *American Journal of Human Genetics, 63*(2), 557–568.

Liu, H., Warren, D. W., Drake, A. F., & Davis, J. U. (1992). Is nasal airway size a marker for susceptibility toward clefting? *The Cleft Palate–Craniofacial Journal, 29*(4), 336–339.

Malata, C. M., Cooter, R. D., & Batchelor, A. G. (1993). Submucous cleft palate with a discontinuous bony deformity. *The Cleft Palate–Craniofacial Journal, 30*(6), 590–592.

Maresova, K., Veleminska, J., & Mullerova, Z. (2004). The development of intracranial relations in patients with complete unilateral cleft lip and palate in relation to surgery method and gender aspect. *Acta Chirurgiae Plasticae, 46*(3), 89–94.

Maue-Dickson, W. (1979). The craniofacial complex in cleft lip and palate: An update review of anatomy and function. *Cleft Palate Journal, 16*(3), 291–317.

Maue-Dickson, W., & Dickson, D. R. (1980). Anatomy and physiology related to cleft palate: Current research and clinical implications. *Plastic & Reconstructive Surgery, 65*(1), 83–90.

McWilliams, B. J. (1991). Submucous clefts of the palate: How likely are they to be symptomatic? *The Cleft Palate–Craniofacial Journal, 28*(3), 247–249; discussion 250–251.

Mehendale, F. V. (2004). Surgical anatomy of the levator veli palatini: A previously undescribed tendinous insertion of the anterolateral fibers. *Plastic & Reconstructive Surgery, 114*(2), 307–315.

Metneki, J., Puho, E., & Czeizel, A. E. (2005). Maternal diseases and isolated orofacial clefts in Hungary. *Birth Defects Research, 73*(9), 617–623.

Miller, P. J., Grinberg, D., & Wang, T. D. (1999). Midline cleft. Treatment of the bifid nose. *Archives of Facial Plastic Surgery, 1*(3), 200–203.

Mitchell, L. E. (2009). Epidemiology of cleft lip and palate. In J. E. Lossee & R. E. Kirschner (Eds.), *Comprehensive Cleft Care* (pp. 35–42). New York, NY: McGraw-Hill.

Moore, L. L., Singer, M. R., Bradlee, M. L., Rothman, K. J., & Milunsky, A. (2000). A prospective study of the risk of congenital defects associated with maternal obesity and diabetes mellitus. *Epidemiology, 11*(6), 689–694.

Mossey, P. A., & Little, J. (2002). Epidemiology of oral clefts: An international perspective. In D. F. Wyszynski (Ed.), *Cleft lip and palate: From origin to treatment* (pp. 127–144). New York, NY: Oxford University Press.

Mossey, P. A., Little, J., Munger, R. G., Dixon, M. J., & Shaw, W. C. (2009). Cleft lip and palate. *Lancet, 374*(9703), 1773–1785.

Munger, R. G., Sauberlich, H. E., Corcoran, C., Nepomuceno, B., Daack-Hirsch, S., & Solon, F. S. (2004). Maternal vitamin B-6 and folate status and risk of oral cleft birth defects in the Philippines. *Birth Defects Research, 70*(7), 464–471.

Park, S., Saso, Y., Ito, O., Tokioka, K., Kato, K., Nitta, N., Kitano, I. (2000). A retrospective study of speech development in patients with submucous cleft palate treated by four operations. *Scandinavian Journal of Plastic and Reconstructive Surgery and Hand Surgery, 34*(2), 131–136.

Parker, S. E., Mai, C. T., Canfield, M. A., Rickard, R., Wang, Y., Meyer, R. E., … Correa, A. (2010). Updated national birth prevalence estimates for selected birth defects in the United States, 2004-2006. *Birth Defects Research Part A: Clinical and Molecular Teratology, 88*, 1008–1016.

Patel, N. P., & Tantri, M. D. (2010). Median cleft of the upper lip: A rare case. *The Cleft Palate–Craniofacial Journal, 47*(6), 642–644.

Rahimov, F., Jugessur, A., & Murray, J. C. (2012). Genetics of nonsyndromic orofacial clefts. *The Cleft Palate–Craniofacial Journal, 49*(1), 73–91.

Ray, J. G., Meier, C., Vermeulen, M. J., Wyatt, P. R., & Cole, D. E. (2003). Association between folic acid food fortification and congenital orofacial clefts. *Journal of Pediatrics, 143*(6), 805–807.

Reiser, E., Andlin-Sobocki, A., Mani, M., & Holmstrom, M. (2011). Initial size of cleft does not correlate with size and function of nasal airway in adults with unilateral cleft lip and palate. *Journal of Plastic Surgery and Hand Surgery, 45*(3), 129–135.

Reiter, R., Brosch, S., Ludeke, M., Fischbein, E., Haase, S., Pickhard, A., & Maier, C. (2012). Genetic and environmental risk factors for submucous cleft palate. *European Journal of Oral Sciences, 120*(2), 97–103.

Reiter, R., Brosch, S., Wefel, H., Schlomer, G., & Haase, S. (2011). The submucous cleft palate: Diagnosis and therapy. *International Journal of Pediatric Otorhinolaryngology, 75*(1), 85–88.

Reiter, R., Haase, S., & Brosch, S. (2010). Submucous cleft palate: An often late diagnosed malformation. *Laryngo-Rhino-Otologie, 89*(1), 29–33.

Rittler, M., Cosentino, V., Lopez-Camelo, J. S., Murray, J. C., Wehby, G., & Castilla, E. E. (2011). Associated anomalies among infants with oral clefts at birth and during a 1-year follow-up. *American Journal of Medical Genetics Part A, 155A*(7), 1588–1596.

Rosé, E., Thissen, U., Otten, J. E., & Jonas, I. (2003). Cephalometric assessment of the posterior airway space in patients with cleft palate after palatoplasty. *The Cleft Palate–Craniofacial Journal, 40*(5), 498–503.

Rourke, R., Weinberg, S. M., Marazita, M. L., & Jabbour, N. (2017). Diagnosing subtle palatal anomalies: Validation of video-analysis and assessment protocol for diagnosing occult submucous cleft palate. *International Journal of Pediatric Otorhinolaryngology, 100*, 242–246.

Sandham, A., & Murray, J. A. (1993). Nasal septal deformity in unilateral cleft lip and palate. *The Cleft Palate–Craniofacial Journal, 30*(2), 222–226.

Satoh, K., Wada, T., Tachimura, T., & Fukuda, J. (2005). Velar ascent and morphological factors affecting velophalyngeal function in patients with cleft palate and noncleft controls: A cephalometric study. *International Journal of Oral and Maxillofacial Surgery, 34*(2), 122–126.

Saunders, N. C., Hartley, B. E., Sell, D., & Sommerlad, B. (2004). Velopharyngeal insufficiency following adenoidectomy. *Clinical Otolaryngology and Allied Sciences, 29*(6), 686–688.

Sekhon, P., Ethunandan, M., Markus, A., Krishnan, G., & Rao, B. (2011). Congenital anomalies associated with cleft lip and palate: An analysis of 1632 consecutive patients. *The Cleft Palate–Craniofacial Journal, 48*(4), 371–378.

Shapiro, B. L., Meskin, L. H., Cervenka, J., & Pruzansky, S. (1971). Cleft uvula: A micro-form of facial clefts and its genetic basis. *Birth Defects Original Article Series, 7*(7), 80–82.

Sheahan, P., Miller, I., Earley, M. J., Sheahan, J. N., & Blayney, A. W. (2004). Middle ear disease in children with congenital velopharyngeal insufficiency. *The Cleft Palate–Craniofacial Journal, 41*(4), 364–367.

Sheer, F. J., Swarts, J. D., & Ghadiali, S. N. (2010). Finite element analysis of eustachian tube function in cleft palate infants based on histological reconstructions. *The Cleft Palate–Craniofacial Journal, 147*(6), 600–610.

Shprintzen, R. J., Schwartz, R. H., Daniller, A., & Hoch, L. (1985). Morphologic significance of bifid uvula. *Pediatrics, 75*(3), 553–561.

Smahel, Z., Kasalova, P., & Skvarilova, B. (1991). Morphometric nasopharyngeal characteristics in facial clefts. *Journal of Craniofacial Genetics and Developmental Biology, 11*(1), 24–32.

Smahel, Z., & Mullerova, I. (1992). Nasopharyngeal characteristics in children with cleft lip and palate. *The Cleft Palate–Craniofacial Journal, 29*(3), 282–286.

Sullivan, S. R., Vasudavan, S., Marrinan, E. M., & Mulliken, J. B. (2011). Submucous cleft palate and velopharyngeal insufficiency: Comparison of speech outcomes using three operative techniques by one surgeon. *The Cleft Palate–Craniofacial Journal, 48*(5), 561–570.

Tanaka, S. A., Mahabir, R. G., Jupiter, D. C., & Menezes, J. M. (2012). Updating the epidemiology of cleft lip with or without cleft palate. *Plastic and Reconstructive Surgery, 129,* 511e–517e.

Tessier, P. (1976). Anatomical classification of facial, cranio-facial and latero-facial clefts. *Journal of Maxillofacial Surgery, 4*(2), 69–92.

Vinceti, M., Rovesti, S., Bergomi, M., Calzolari, E., Candela, S., Campagna, A., . . . Vivoli, G. (2001). Risk of birth defects in a population exposed to environmental lead pollution. *Science of the Total Environment, 278*(1–3), 23–30.

Warren, D. W., & Drake, A. F. (1993). Cleft nose: Form and function. *Clinics in Plastic Surgery, 20*(4), 769–779.

Warren, D. W., Hairfield, W. M., & Dalston, E. T. (1990). The relationship between nasal airway size and nasal-oral breathing in cleft lip and palate. *Cleft Palate Journal, 27*(1), 46–51; discussion 51–52.

Warren, D. W., Hairfield, W. M., & Dalston, E. T. (1991). Nasal airway impairment: The oral response in cleft palate patients. *American Journal of Orthodontics & Dentofacial Orthopedics, 99*(4), 346–353.

Wharton, P., & Mowrer, D. E. (1992). Prevalence of cleft uvula among school children in kindergarten through grade five. *The Cleft Palate–Craniofacial Journal, 29*(1), 10–12; discussion 13–14.

World Health Organization. (2001, December). *Global registry and database on craniofacial anomalies: Report of a WHO registry meeting on craniofacial anomalies.* Bauru, Brazil: Author.

Wyszynski, D. F., Beaty, T. H., & Maestri, N. E. (1996). Genetics of nonsyndromic oral clefts revisited. *The Cleft Palate–Craniofacial Journal, 33*(5), 406–417.

Zucchero, T. M., Cooper, M. E., Maher, B. S., Daack-Hirsch, S., Nepomuceno, B., Ribeiro, L., . . . Murray, J. C. (2004). Interferon regulatory factor 6 (IRF6) gene variants and the risk of isolated cleft lip or palate. *New England Journal of Medicine, 351*(8), 769–780.

CREDITS

Chapter opener photo: © PeopleImages/Getty Images Figure 3-20 (A–E) and Figure 3-21 (A–B): Courtesy Likith V. Reddy, Texas A&M College of Dentistry, and Srinivas Gosla Reddy, Hyderabad, India.

All other photos courtesy of the Cleft and Craniofacial Center at Cincinnati Children's Hospital Medical Center.

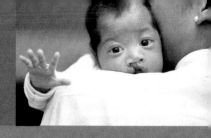

CHAPTER 4

Dysmorphology and Craniofacial Syndromes

With acknowledgment to Howard M. Saal for his contributions to this chapter.

CHAPTER OUTLINE

INTRODUCTION

Congenital anomalies occur in 3% to 5% of all live births and are among the most common causes of hospitalization in childhood. Although cleft lip and palate make up a significant percentage of congenital anomalies, other craniofacial anomalies can occur that have a significant effect on both aesthetics, function, and the child's health. In fact, there are over 400 distinct syndromes associated with facial clefts.

Craniofacial anomalies, particularly those associated with a syndrome, are often a result of a genetic condition. Therefore, it is important that each child born with these anomalies has a complete genetic evaluation and follow-up evaluations as the child grows and develops.

One purpose of this chapter is to discuss the types and causes of dysmorphology. A list of dysmorphic characteristics commonly seen with craniofacial conditions is provided. In addition, the most common craniofacial syndromes are described, and many more are listed in **APPENDIX 4A**. Finally, the components of a complete genetics evaluation are discussed, along with the information that is important to obtain in order to arrive at a genetics diagnosis.

Dysmorphology

Dysmorphology is defined as the study of abnormal shape or form. Morphogenesis is the process of embryonic tissue formation. Dysmorphogenesis describes errors in the process of morphogenesis, which result in dysmorphic (abnormally formed) features. Factors that can cause these dysmorphic features include intrinsic genetic factors or external nongenetic forces during fetal development.

The diagnosis of many genetic and craniofacial disorders depends upon the identification of specific dysmorphic features, including both major and minor anomalies. Major anomalies are those that cause significant medical and/or cosmetic issues and usually require medical intervention. On the other hand, minor anomalies are those that have diagnostic significance but have a minimal effect on the patient and therefore usually require no intervention.

Malformations and Deformations

There are a variety of potential malformations and deformations associated with cleft lip/palate and craniofacial syndromes (Seto-Salvia & Stanier, 2014). A list of some of them with their definitions can be found in TABLE 4-1.

A malformation is a morphologic anomaly that is the result of a genetic etiology (Jones, 2006). If there are genetic factors that cause

dysplasia (abnormal growth or development of a tissue or organ), this will lead to a malformation. Most craniofacial anomalies (including cleft lip and most cases of cleft palate) are malformations.

In contrast, a deformation (deformity) is a morphologic anomaly that occurs when external forces disrupt the development of an intrinsically (genetically) normal structure during fetal development (Jones, 2006). This disruption causes a breakdown or interference with the normal developmental process. Examples of deformations include clubfoot, occasionally micrognathia (a small or underdeveloped mandible), and plagiocephaly (abnormal flattening of the skull, usually on the back side).

One cause of deformations is fetal exposure to teratogens. Common teratogens that cause birth defects include alcohol, cigarette smoke, anticonvulsants (such as hydantoin, valproic acid, and carbamazepine), and vitamin A analogs (such as retinoic acid).

Another cause of deformations is physical disruption to normal development in utero. For example, amniotic bands occur when the amnion (the membrane surrounding the embryo and fetus) ruptures, leaving strands of tissue floating in the amniotic cavity. These strands can attach to limbs, the head, or other body parts and act as tourniquets, cutting off blood supply to developing structures. This results in amputations of limbs and digits, cleft lip, and other oral and facial deformities (**FIGURE 4-1**).

TABLE 4-1 Terms Related to Dsymorphology and Craniofacial Anomalies

General Terms

- Malformation: a result of genetic or chromosomal factors
- Deformation: a result of mechanical factors or teratogens
- Disruption: a factor that causes embryological development to cease
- Micro: small
- Macro: large
- Somia: body
- Fistula: abnormal opening into a cavity
- Stenosis: narrowing of any canal
- Atresia: congenital closure of an opening, passage, or cavity
- Hypertrophy: overgrowth of a structure
- Atrophy: shrinkage or degeneration of a structure
- Dysplasia: abnormal tissue development
- Hyperplasia (hyperplastic): overdevelopment of a structure
- Hypoplasia (hypoplastic): defective formation or incomplete development of a structure
- Sequence: the occurrence of a pattern of anomalies that occur because of a single cause
- Syndrome: a pattern of multiple malformations that regularly appear together and are pathogenically related
- Association: two or more anomalies that appear together frequently in a population but have no known similar genetic cause

Anomalies of the Eyes

- Ocular or ophtha: eye
- Canthus: corner of the eye
- Palpebra: eyelids
- Palpebral fissures: eye slits
- Myopia: nearsightedness
- Coloboma: congenital notch in the lower eyelid, iris, or retina
- Hypertelorism: wide-spaced eyes
- Hypotelorism: narrow-spaced eyes
- Exophthalmus: eyes are extruded ("bug eyes")
- Mongoloid slant: upward slant of the eyes
- Antimongoloid slant: downward slant of the eyes (as in Treacher Collins syndrome)
- Epicanthal folds: folds of skin extending from the root of the nose to the eyebrow and covering the inner corner of the eye. This is normal in the Asian population.

Anomalies of the Ears

- Otic: relating to the ear (otitis, otolaryngologist, otorrhea, microtia, etc.)
- Preauricular tags: projection of scalp and skin tags in cheek
- Microtia: small or absent external ear or middle ear anomalies
- Auditory atresia: congenital closure of the auditory canal

Anomalies of the Nose

- Choanal atresia: closure of the choana or back of the nose
- Stenotic naris: narrowing of the nostril
- Deviated septum: septum is not straight in the midline

Anomalies of the Mouth

- Stomia: related to the mouth
- Microstomia: small mouth
- Macrostomia: large mouth

(continues)

TABLE 4-1 Terms Related to Dsymorphology and Craniofacial Anomalies *(continued)*

Anomalies of the Tongue

- Lingual: related to the tongue
- Lingual frenulum: small fold that attaches the tongue to the floor of the mouth to stabilize it during movement
- Ankyloglossia (aka tongue-tie): short or anterior attachment of the lingual frenulum
- Glossoptosis: posterior position of the tongue
- Macroglossia: very large tongue
- Microglossia: very small tongue

Anomalies of the Dentition and Occlusion (see the chapter **Dental Anomalies** *for additional terms)*

- Malocclusion: improper dental or skeletal relationship of the arches
- Crossbite: the maxillary tooth or teeth are inside the arch of the mandibular teeth
- Overbite: the teeth overlap too much, and the bite is deep
- Overjet: maxillary incisors are labioverted, or stick out toward the lips
- Underjet: maxillary incisors are linguoverted, or face inward toward tongue
- Open bite: the maxillary teeth do not come together to overlap or occlude with the mandibular teeth
- Diastema: space or opening between the teeth, usually the middle teeth

Anomalies of the Mandible

- Micrognathia: small mandible
- Retrognathia: retrusive mandible
- Prognathia: protrusive mandible

Anomalies of the Facial Bones

- Malar hypoplasia: lack of cheekbone development
- Midface/maxillary retrusion or deficiency: causes concavity of the midface

Anomalies of the Larynx

- Laryngomalacia: abnormally soft laryngeal structures, usually improve with development
- Tracheoesophageal fistula: congenital opening between the trachea and the esophagus, resulting in aspiration with feeding
- Laryngeal web: web between the vocal folds, usually in the anterior portion of the larynx

Anomalies of the Cranium

- Frontal bossing: a prominent forehead
- Craniosynostosis: premature closure of the cranial sutures, causing the cranium to be abnormally shaped (e.g., Crouzon, Apert)
- Brachycephaly: short, flattened skull with broad forehead and wide face from coronal synostosis
- Dolichocephaly: long, narrow skull seen with prematurity
- Holoprosencephaly: failure of the prosencephalon (forebrain) to divide into double lobes; often occurs with midline clefts
- Microcephaly: small head circumference in comparison to age-matched peers
- Plagiocephaly: asymmetric skull
- Scaphocephaly: long, narrow skull and frontal bossing from sagittal synostosis
- Trigonocephaly: top of skull is triangular shaped with pointed forehead

Anomalies of the Fingers and Toes

- Digits: fingers (including the thumbs) and toes
- Brachiodactyly: short digits
- Clinodactyly: curved digits
- Syndactyly: fusion of digits

Cardiac Anomalies
- VSD: ventricular septal defect
- ASD: atrial septal defect
- Tetralogy of Fallot: most common form of heart disease
  - VSD
  - Dextroposition (right-sided) of aorta
  - Right ventricular hypertrophy
  - Pulmonary stenosis

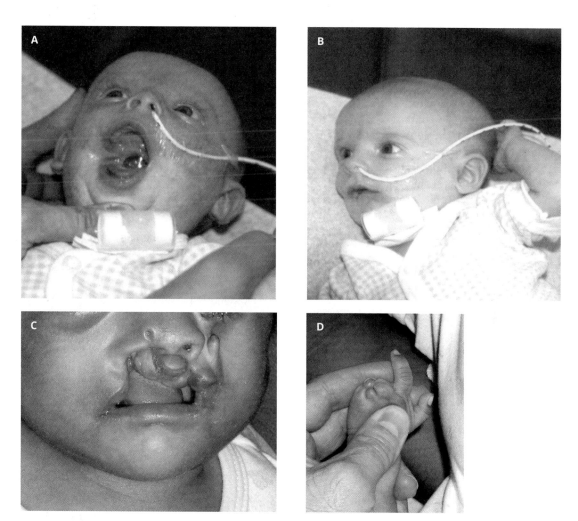

FIGURE 4-1 Amniotic band deformities. **(A)** Oral deformity from amniotic bands. **(B)** Micrognathia from amniotic bands. **(C)** Facial cleft and deformity from amniotic bands. **(D)** Finger amputations from amniotic bands.

Syndromes, Associations, and Sequences

A syndrome is a pattern of multiple anomalies that are pathogenically related and therefore have a common known or suspected cause. Many children with craniofacial conditions have underlying syndromes as the cause of the specific craniofacial anomaly. Because craniofacial syndromes affect the facial features, they can cause affected individuals to look alike, even when there is no familial relationship. Recognizing a specific syndrome is important for medical management and is a focus of genetic counseling.

An association is a nonrandom occurrence of a pattern of multiple anomalies in two or more individuals. In contrast to a syndrome, the etiology of an association has not yet been identified, and therefore the recurrence risks are not known. One example is VATER (vertebral, anal, tracheo-esophageal, and renal) association, which includes vertebral anomalies; anorectal anomalies (imperforate anus); tracheoesophageal fistula; and renal, radial, and other limb anomalies.

In contrast to a syndrome or an association, a sequence in medicine is defined as a series of ordered consequences from a single cause. The initiating cause may be an inherited anomaly (resulting in a malformation) or an outside force (often resulting in a deformation). Regardless, the causal factor causes a "sequence" of consequences. An example of this is Pierre Robin sequence, which is further described later in this chapter.

Craniofacial Syndromes and Conditions

Although most clefts are isolated birth defects, some are caused by underlying genetic syndromes or conditions. In fact, it has been estimated that there are over 400 distinct syndromes associated with facial clefts (Gorlin, Cohen, & Hennekam, 2001). These craniofacial syndromes are diagnosed based on the pattern of major and minor malformations (Jones & Jones, 2009). In addition to known syndromes, approximately 40% to 50% of patients seen by a geneticist have a cluster of malformations that are either rare or possibly unique. These patients are diagnosed as having a provisionally unique syndrome until other patients with the same pattern of anomalies are identified and reported.

Genetic syndromes should be suspected when multiple family members are affected with clefts or when there are additional anomalies associated with the patient's cleft. A craniofacial syndrome should also be suspected in all patients with cleft palate only (CPO) or submucous cleft. This is because underlying syndromes with other anomalies occur much more often in patients with CPO than in those with clefts involving the lip. In fact, the London Dysmorphology Database lists 485 syndromes, excluding chromosome disorders, in which CPO may be a feature (Baraitser & Winter, 1991; Baraitser & Winter, 2002). In addition, a prospective analysis done by the Craniofacial Center at Cincinnati Children's showed that approximately 55% of all cases of CPO were syndromic or had additional anomalies (Stanier & Moore, 2004).

Appendix 4A shows many of the cleft and craniofacial conditions that are seen in a craniofacial center, along with their typical features and concerns. In addition, TABLE 4-2 shows syndromes primarily associated with cleft lip with or without cleft palate and those associated primarily with cleft palate only.

The following is a more in-depth discussion of a few of these craniofacial conditions.

Beckwith–Wiedemann Syndrome

Beckwith–Wiedemann syndrome (**FIGURE 4-2**) is a genetic disorder that results in prenatal and postnatal overgrowth of structures. Children with Beckwith–Wiedemann syndrome are usually large for gestational age (often more than 10 pounds at birth). Some are born with an umbilical hernia or

TABLE 4-2 Syndromes Commonly Associated with Cleft Lip (with or without Cleft Palate) and Cleft Palate Only

Cleft Lip (with or without Cleft Palate)	Cleft Palate Only
Amniotic bands	CHARGE syndrome
CHARGE syndrome	Fetal hydantoin syndrome
Fetal alcohol syndrome	Hemifacial microsomia
Hemifacial microsomia	Kabuki syndrome
Opitz syndrome	Stickler syndrome
Oral–facial–digital syndrome type I (OFD I)	Van der Woude syndrome
Popliteal pterygium syndrome	Velocardiofacial/22q11.2 deletion syndrome
Trisomy 13	
Van der Woude syndrome	
Wolf–Hirschhorn syndrome	

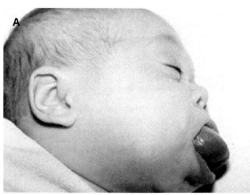

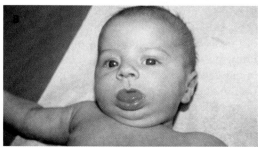

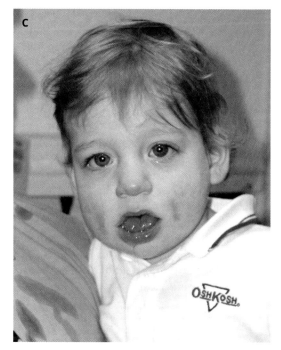

FIGURE 4-2 Beckwith–Wiedemann syndrome with macroglossia. Macroglossia causes breathing and feeding difficulties for newborns. If not adequately treated, it is likely to cause speech problems.

even an omphalocele, where part of the intestine is outside of the abdomen in the region of the umbilical cord. There is a risk for severe neonatal hypoglycemia (low blood sugar), which can result in seizures and even be life threatening.

Patients with Beckwith–Wiedemann syndrome often have accelerated growth during early childhood, which can result in hemihypertrophy, where one side of the body grows faster and larger than the other side. A major feature of this syndrome is macroglossia (very large tongue). The large tongue can cause Pierre Robin sequence with cleft palate (Dios, Posse, Sanroman, & Garcia, 2000; Laroche, Testelin, & Devauchelle, 2005).

Children with Beckwith–Wiedemann syndrome have a significant risk of developing a Wilms tumor (a malignant tumor of the kidney), a hepatoblastoma (a malignant tumor of the liver), or other malignant tumors in the abdomen. The risk for developing such tumors is between 5% and 8%, with most cases occurring before 8 years. For this reason, a child with Beckwith–Wiedemann syndrome should receive renal and abdominal ultrasound examinations at least every 4 months.

Development in Beckwith–Wiedemann syndrome is usually normal, although there is a risk for developmental delay if neonatal hypoglycemia is prolonged. The large tongue may contribute to abnormal cranial and dental growth, including prognathism (a large mandible). The large tongue often causes obstructive breathing, feeding problems, and speech problems. Resonance can be affected by a cleft palate but also by the size of the tongue, which can block the transmission of acoustic energy in the oral cavity. For these reasons, some children with Beckwith–Wiedemann syndrome require a partial glossectomy (surgical reduction of the tongue) (Shuman, Beckwith, Smith, & Weksberg, 2016).

CHARGE Syndrome

CHARGE syndrome (**FIGURE 4-3**) is an acronym for coloboma, heart defect, choanal atresia,

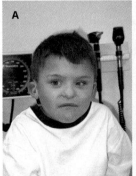
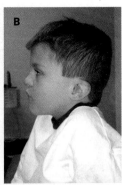
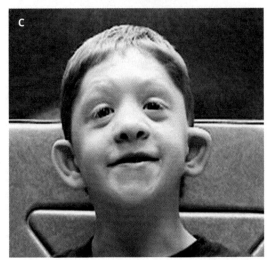

FIGURE 4-3 CHARGE syndrome. **(A)** There is a defect in the left eye and a hearing aid on the child's right ear. **(B)** Note the mild ear anomaly. **(C)** Note the ear anomalies.

retarded growth and/or development, genitourinary anomalies, and ear anomalies and/or deafness (Hsueh, Yang, Lu, & Hsu, 2004). A diagnosis of CHARGE syndrome requires at least four of the six clinical features, and one of the features must be the presence of choanal atresia (a blockage at the back of the nasal passage) or colobomas (congenital defects of the eye, such as a notch in the lower eyelid or defects of the iris or retina).

The colobomas of CHARGE syndrome usually affect the retina, causing significant visual impairment (McMain et al., 2008; Plomp et al.,

1998). The heart defects are often very serious and life threatening. There may be abnormalities or absence of the pituitary gland, which affects growth and genitourinary development. Genitourinary anomalies are usually related to micropenis (small penis) or cryptorchidism (undescended testicles). There may also be delayed or absent puberty. External ear anomalies, hearing loss, and deafness are very common as well. Although some individuals with CHARGE syndrome have normal intelligence, brain anomalies and severe intellectual disability are seen in most patients. Cleft lip and/or cleft palate occurs in many patients with CHARGE syndrome (Jongmans et al., 2006; Saal, 2016). Speech and language disorders commonly occur because of cleft palate, intellectual disability, and hearing loss/deafness.

Down Syndrome (Trisomy 21)

Down syndrome (also called trisomy 21) is the most common of all chromosome disorders, with an incidence of 1 in 700 live births. It occurs when the baby is born with an extra copy of chromosome 21.

Down syndrome is associated with mild to moderate intellectual disability. In addition, Down syndrome has characteristic facial features, which include upward slanting palpebral fissures (eye slits), epicanthal folds (folds of skin over the medial portion of the palpebral fissures) at the inner canthus (corner of the eye), micrognathia, macroglossia, broad face, short neck, and low-set ears. There may also be hypotonia; short stature; and an increased risk for hypothyroidism, leukemia, middle ear disease, and celiac disease. Approximately 50% of individuals with Down syndrome are born with a congenital heart defect. Cleft lip and/or cleft palate occur infrequently in Down syndrome. However, affected individuals have speech and language disorders because of poor oral-motor function, conductive hearing loss, and intellectual impairment (Bull, 2011).

Fetal Alcohol Syndrome

Fetal alcohol syndrome (FAS) is caused by exposure to significant amounts of alcohol during gestation, particularly during the first trimester (**FIGURE 4-4**). Although the precise amount of alcohol intake necessary to cause fetal alcohol syndrome remains unknown, it is generally accepted that women who consume two alcoholic drinks daily during pregnancy are at risk for delivering babies with small birth size. The intake of more drinks per day can cause other serious clinical complications (Jones, 2006).

The classic signs of fetal alcohol syndrome include low birth weight, microcephaly (small head size), dysmorphic facial features with narrow palpebral fissures, thin upper lip, short nose, flat philtrum, and occasionally cleft lip and/or cleft palate. Congenital heart defects are common, particularly ventricular septal defect (VSD) (a hole in the wall that separates the lower chambers of the heart). Developmental delays and intellectual disabilities are almost universal. The average intelligence quotient in this population has been estimated to be 63 (Jones, 2006). In addition, older children with fetal alcohol

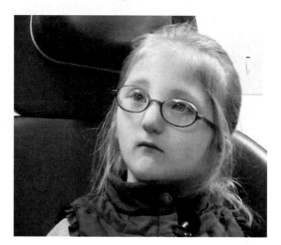

FIGURE 4-4 Fetal alcohol syndrome. Features typically include microcephaly, dysmorphic facial features with narrow palpebral fissures, thin upper lip, short nose, and flat philtrum.

syndrome often have severe behavior problems, including hyperactivity, distractibility, poor judgment, and difficulty interpreting social cues (Jones, 2006; Nash, Sheard, Rovet, & Koren, 2008; Saal, 2016; Streissguth et al., 1991).

Hemifacial Microsomia

Hemifacial microsomia (**FIGURE 4-5**) is a condition with numerous names, including oculo–auriculo–vertebral (OAV), facio–auriculo–vertebral (FAV) spectrum, and Goldenhar syndrome if there are epibulbar lipodermoids (fatty cysts) on the sclera (white portion) of the eyeball. This is a relatively common multiple anomaly disorder with a birth incidence of 1 in 3000 to 5000 live births (Jones, 2006). Most cases are sporadic, although some familial cases have been reported.

The primary feature of hemifacial microsomia is hypoplasia (underdevelopment or defective formation) of the maxilla, mandible, and ear on the affected side(s). Hemifacial microsomia is usually unilateral (hence the name), although about 30% of the cases have bilateral involvement (Gorlin et al., 2001). The right side tends to be affected more often than the left, and boys are affected more frequently than girls (Jones, 2006).

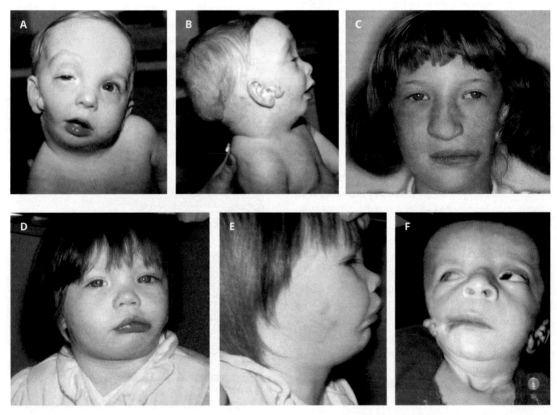

FIGURE 4-5 Hemifacial microsomia. **(A)** Note the severe facial asymmetry. **(B)** The lateral view shows severe dysplasia of the right ear and an ear tag. **(C)** and **(D)** Note the facial asymmetry and the slight cleft of the corner of the mouth on the affected side. **(E)** Note the atretic ear. **(F)** Note the skin tags and the cleft in the corner of the mouth.

The hypoplasia of hemifacial microsomia may affect the temporomandibular joint, limiting the extent of mouth opening. An intraoral evaluation may reveal an occlusal cant (a sloping transverse occlusal plane caused by inadequate vertical maxillary growth on one side) and unilateral velar paresis. Cleft lip and/or cleft palate are seen in about 15% of affected patients. There can also be weakness of the facial nerve (cranial nerve VII) on the affected side. Ear involvement ranges from mild dysplasia to anotia (absence of the external auditory canal). Anomalies of the eyes can occur, including colobomas of the upper eyelid or retina and microphthalmia (small eyes).

Brain anomalies can be seen in this population, including hydrocephalus (fluid accumulation in the brain), encephalocele (protrusion of the brain through an opening in the skull), and absence of the corpus callosum (band of nerve fibers joining the hemispheres of the brain). Vertebral anomalies are found in about 15% of cases and usually involve the cervical vertebrae. Serious heart defects and kidney abnormalities can occur, leading to significant morbidity (Strömland et al., 2007).

Although most patients with hemifacial microsomia have normal intelligence, learning disabilities and intellectual disability may occur if there are anomalies of the brain. Speech disorders are common because of dental malocclusion, limited mouth opening, cleft palate, and velar paralysis or paresis.

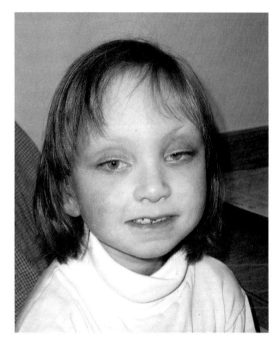

FIGURE 4-6 Kabuki syndrome. Note the wide palpebral fissures (eye openings) with eversion (turning out) of the lateral portion of the lower lid, external ear anomalies, arched eyebrows, and a broad nasal tip.

Kabuki Syndrome

Kabuki syndrome (**FIGURE 4-6**), also called Kabuki makeup syndrome after the dramatic appearance of the Kabuki actors, is a distinctive genetic condition. Facial features include wide palpebral fissures with eversion (turning out) of the lateral portion of the lower lid, external ear anomalies, arched eyebrows, and a broad nasal tip. Other anomalies can include cleft palate and submucous cleft palate, vertebral anomalies, congenital heart defects, and low muscle tone

(Hannibal et al., 2011). Speech and language are usually affected by mild to moderate intellectual impairment and cleft palate, if present.

Moebius Syndrome

Moebius syndrome (**FIGURE 4-7**) is a nonprogressive neurological disorder that includes paralysis of the facial nerve (seventh cranial nerve [CN VII]) and sometimes other cranial nerves. Individuals with Moebius syndrome cannot smile, frown, or move their eyes laterally. As a result, they have no facial expression (Figure 4-7A). Many individuals with Moebius syndrome also have micrognathia, microstomia, a short or unusually shaped tongue, cleft palate, limb abnormalities, and digit and dental abnormalities, such as missing or misaligned teeth (Figure 4-7B).

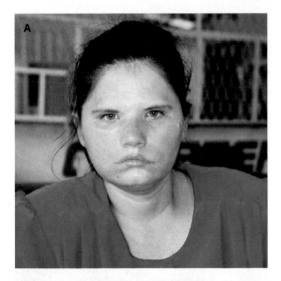

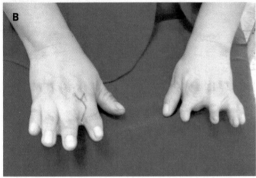

FIGURE 4-7 Moebius syndrome. **(A)** Note the lack of expression in the face. **(B)** There is syndactyly (webbing) of the fingers.

The lack of facial movement affects the child's bilabial competence and therefore ability to produce bilabial and labiodental sounds. Other sounds many also be affected by the small tongue.

Neurofibromatosis Type 1

Neurofibromatosis type 1 (NF1) (**FIGURE 4-8**) is one of the most common autosomal dominant genetic disorders, with a prevalence of approximately 1 in 3000 individuals (Friedman, Birch, & Greene, 1993). The diagnosis of neurofibromatosis type 1 is usually made by clinical evaluation and

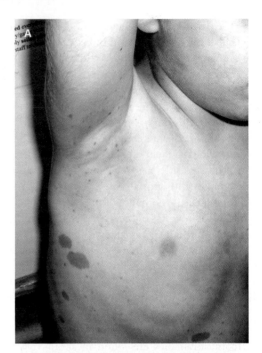

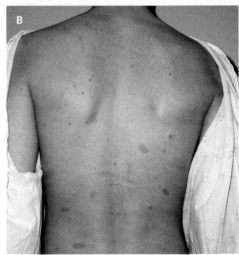

FIGURE 4-8 Neurofibromatosis. Note the café au lait spots on the skin.

the presence of two or more clinical features out of seven. The seven features are (1) six or more café au lait macules (pigmented spots the color of coffee with milk); (2) two or more neurofibromas (benign tumors that grow on nerves) or a single plexiform (spongy) neurofibroma; (3) freckling in the axillae or the inguinal region; (4) an optic pathway tumor (diagnosed with magnetic resonance imaging [MRI]); (5) two or more Lisch nodules (small hamartomas or benign tumors) of the iris; (6) osseous lesions of the sphenoid wing of the cranium or long bone bowing (usually of the tibia); (7) a first-degree relative with neurofibromatosis type 1 diagnosed with the preceding criteria (Viskochil, 2002).

Although patients with NF1 rarely have craniofacial anomalies, a significant number have velopharyngeal incompetence from brainstem tumors (Zhang et al., 2012). In fact, NF1 is the second most common syndrome seen in the VPI Clinic at Cincinnati Children's. In addition to velopharyngeal incompetence (which is a neurological form of VPI) these children often have delays in speech sound and language development (Thompson, Viskochil, Stevenson, & Chapman, 2010).

Opitz G Syndrome

Opitz G syndrome (**FIGURE 4-9**) is a condition that has many names, including hypertelorism-hypospadias syndrome, Opitz BBB syndrome, and Opitz-Frias syndrome. The typical manifestations of Opitz G syndrome are hypertelorism and hypospadias in affected males (where the orifice of the penis is proximal to its normal location). Other features may include imperforate anus, cryptorchidism, congenital heart defects, inguinal hernias, intellectual disability, and learning disabilities.

One characteristic that can be very serious is a laryngeal cleft. This abnormality in the development of the larynx can lead to swallowing disorders, aspiration pneumonia, and speech problems. Many patients require long-term tracheostomy management as a result. Clefts are frequently seen in this population. In fact, Opitz G syndrome is the second most common

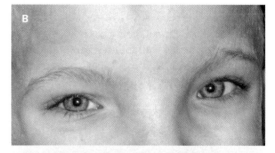
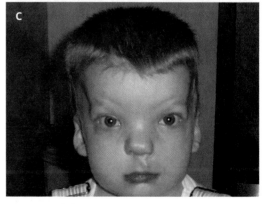

FIGURE 4-9 Opitz syndrome. In all cases, note the hypertelorism (wide-spaced eyes) and evidence of cleft lip.

identifiable cause of syndromic clefts at the Craniofacial Center at Cincinnati Children's.

Oral–Facial–Digital Syndrome Type I

Oral–facial–digital syndrome type I (OFD I) (**FIGURE 4-10**) is an X-linked dominant condition. Therefore, affected females can have affected daughters, but it is usually lethal in males (Goodship, Platt, Smith, & Burn, 1991; Prattichizzo et al., 2008). Infants born with this condition often have a midline cleft lip with multiple oral frenula (oral tissue webs), cleft palate, and tongue abnormalities that include lobulations and notching (Figure 4-10B). There is often hypertelorism, with a broad nose and hair that is coarse and sparse. There may be abnormal or missing teeth with decreased enamel. Digital anomalies include brachydactyly (short fingers), variable degrees of syndactyly (fusion or webbing of the digits), or clinodactyly (curved or bent digits). Renal anomalies may be seen, including the presence of renal cysts. Brain anomalies have been reported, including hydrocephalus and absence of the corpus callosum.

Developmental disabilities are common in this population, especially in the presence of brain anomalies (Jones, 2006). Speech and language difficulties are generally related to the cleft palate and developmental disabilities.

Pierre Robin Sequence

Pierre Robin (pronounced ro bæn') sequence is caused by micrognathia (**FIGURE 4-11**). Micrognathia is a common genetic malformation that occurs as part of several craniofacial syndromes (e.g., Stickler syndrome, Treacher Collins syndrome, velocardiofacial/22q11.2 deletion syndrome (VCFS/22q deletion syndrome), and fetal alcohol syndrome). Micrognathia can also be a deformation as a result of physical forces that inhibit mandibular growth in utero. The risk of recurrence of micrognathia, and associated Pierre Robin sequence, is elevated only if the cause was from a genetic condition.

With normal embryological development, the mandible begins to drop down and forward around the 7th or 8th week of gestation. This brings the tongue down and forward with it. Once the tongue is out of the way, the hard palate and then velum are able to fuse. If the mandible (which contains the tongue) remains very small and does not grow down and forward at the appropriate time, this will result in glossoptosis posterior displacement of the tongue in the nasopharynx. Because of its high

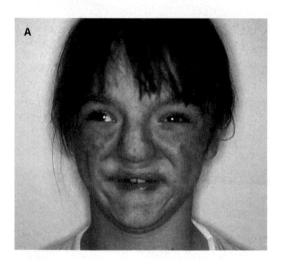
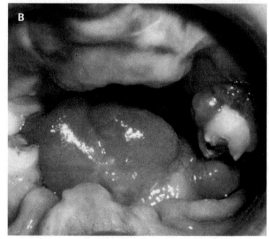

FIGURE 4-10 Oral–facial–digital syndrome type 1. Note the lobulations and fissures of the tongue.

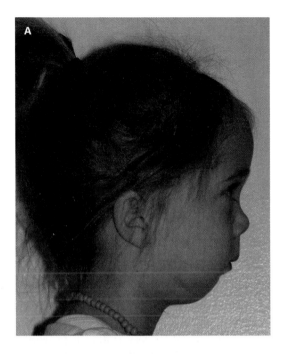

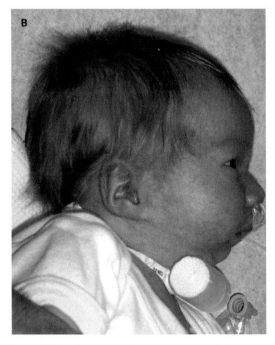

FIGURE 4-11 Pierre Robin sequence with the characteristic micrognathia (small mandible).

position in the pharynx, the tongue will interfere with fusion of the hard palate and velum, causing a wide, bell-shaped cleft palate. Therefore, the triad of anomalies that are typical with Pierre Robin sequence include micrognathia, which causes glossoptosis, which causes cleft palate (Figure 4-11A).

Because of the glossoptosis, newborns with Pierre Robin sequence often have severe upper airway obstruction that can be life threatening. There are many approaches to airway management for affected infants, and the treatment must be individualized for each child. The first approach is to keep the infant in a prone position because gravity causes the tongue to fall forward, relieving the glossoptosis for some infants. Sometimes, it is necessary to use a nasopharyngeal airway tube, which goes through the nose and the pharynx below the region of tongue obstruction. This tube may be needed until 3 or 4 months of age. Some infants do not respond adequately to such conservative treatments. These infants require a tracheostomy, which is the surgical placement of a tube directly in the trachea to bypass the area of obstruction (Figure 4-11B). Usually the tracheostomy tube remains in place until after the palate is repaired, or until about 14 months. Unfortunately, the presence of the tracheostomy tube interferes with vocalizations, often leading to further speech issues in addition to those related to the cleft palate.

A newer procedure to manage patients with glossoptosis is mandibular distraction (Fritz & Sidman, 2004; Hong, McNeil, Kearns, & Magit, 2012; Sidman, Sampson, & Templeton, 2001). With this procedure, an osteotomy (fracture or cut) is created on both sides of the mandible, and the two segments of the mandible are separated. They are pulled apart gradually (over several days or weeks) until there is adequate lengthening of the mandible to open the pharynx and relieve the obstruction. This procedure can be done in early infancy and usually results in normal respiration and feeding.

Most infants with Pierre Robin sequence also have early feeding problems. Some of these infants respond to short periods of feeding with a nasogastric tube (NG tube), which is placed through the nose into the stomach. In more severe cases, a gastrostomy tube (G-tube), which is placed directly into the stomach, is needed.

Stickler Syndrome

Stickler syndrome (**FIGURE 4-12**) is the most common cause of micrognathia, which results in Pierre Robin sequence with cleft palate. It is an autosomal dominant disorder with variable expressivity, so individuals with this condition may have just a few clinical features of this syndrome, or they may be severely affected.

In addition to micrognathia, Stickler syndrome includes other characteristic facial features. These include a flat facial profile, epicanthal folds, a small nose, flat nasal bridge, and midface hypoplasia. Individuals with Stickler syndrome often have high myopia (severe nearsightedness), which is usually progressive. There is also a high risk for retinal detachments, so these patients must

be followed closely by an ophthalmologist. Most individuals with Stickler syndrome have a high-frequency hearing loss, which may be complicated by the conductive hearing loss secondary to middle ear effusion because of the cleft palate (Antunes, Alonso, & Paula, 2012; Nowak, 1998). Therefore, they should be followed with serial audiograms. Finally, there is a risk for early-onset osteoarthritis.

Development is usually normal with Stickler syndrome, and affected individuals are not at risk for learning disabilities. Speech and language problems are usually related to the cleft palate; hearing loss; and in some instances, problems secondary to tracheostomy.

Treacher Collins Syndrome

Treacher Collins syndrome (**FIGURE 4-13**) is also called mandibulofacial dysostosis. It is an autosomal dominant condition with variable expressivity, which makes it difficult to predict the outcome of offspring of affected individuals.

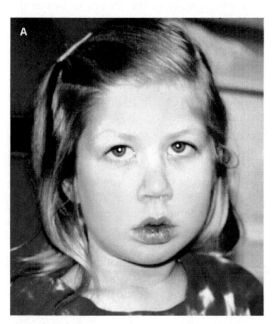
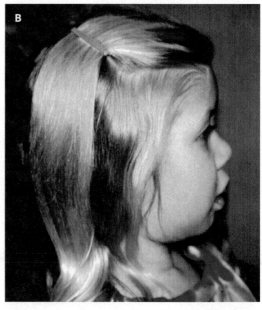

FIGURE 4-12 Stickler syndrome. **(A)** This girl has the characteristic features of a flat facial profile, small nose, and flat nasal bridge. **(B)** Note the micrognathia. She was also born with Pierre Robin sequence from the micrognathia, which is typical of this syndrome.

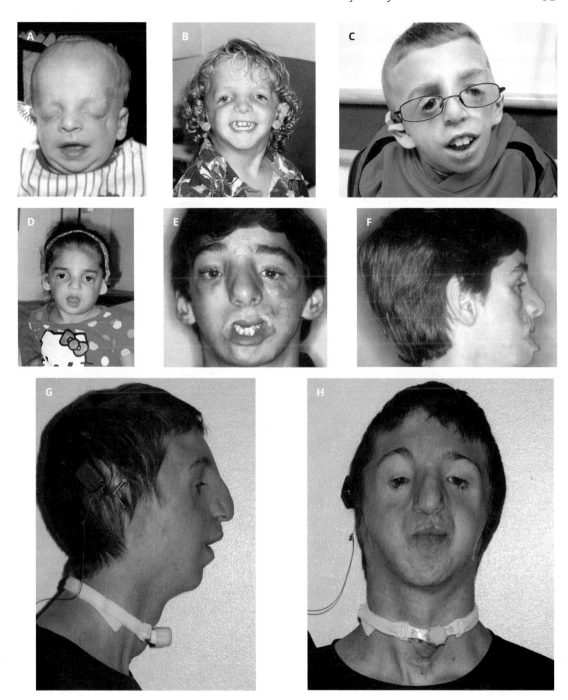

FIGURE 4-13 Treacher Collins syndrome. These children show typical characteristics, including micrognathia, severe hypoplasia of the zygomatic arches, down-slanting palpebral fissures, and secondary low-set ears. Hearing loss is common, as noted by the hearing aids.

The classic features of Treacher Collins syndrome include downward-slanting palpebral fissures, colobomas of the lower eyelids, micrognathia, hypoplasia of the maxilla and zygomatic arches, macrostomia (a large mouth), microtia (small or dysplastic ear), and atresia of the external auditory canal (Martelli-Junior et al., 2009; Posnick & Ruiz, 2000). Conductive hearing loss is common from middle ear anomalies. Treacher Collins syndrome usually includes Pierre Robin sequence, although most individuals with this condition do not have clefts, despite pronounced micrognathia.

Intelligence is usually normal in this population. Speech disorders are common from the hearing loss and micrognathia. The speech disorders are exacerbated when cleft palate or airway obstruction is also present.

Trisomy 13

Trisomy 13 (**FIGURE 4-14**) is a disorder where the baby is born with an extra copy of chromosome 13. The incidence of this disorder is about 1 in 5000 live births (Jones, 2006).

Trisomy 13 is associated with multiple serious life-endangering birth defects, including severe brain anomalies, congenital heart defects, polydactyly (extra fingers and/or toes), spina bifida, and severe eye defects. Unilateral or bilateral cleft lip/palate is seen in 60% to 80% of cases (Jones, 2006). Many infants with trisomy 13 have a midline cleft lip and midline facial deformities. This usually denotes holoprosencephaly, which is the failure of the brain to divide into the two hemispheres. Over 90% of affected children die before their first birthday, usually from a central nervous system or cardiac event. Therefore, patients with trisomy 13 are rarely seen in a craniofacial center.

Children who do survive for several years are usually severely to profoundly intellectually disabled and require a great deal of care. They tend to have severe feeding difficulties that require nasogastric feeding. Because most children with trisomy 13 do not survive beyond

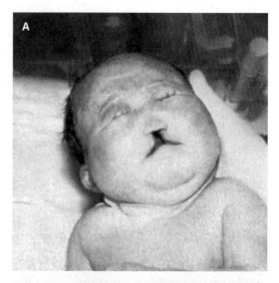

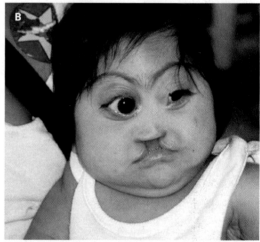

FIGURE 4-14 (A) A newborn female with trisomy 13 and holoprosencephaly. Note the midline cleft. **(B)** A child with a midline cleft and holoprosencephaly.

1 year of age, a gastrostomy is rarely performed to assist with feeding.

Van der Woude Syndrome

Van der Woude syndrome (**FIGURE 4-15**) is characterized by cleft lip and/or cleft palate and missing teeth. What is particularly unique to this syndrome, however, it that there are bilateral lip pits on the lower lip (Jones, 2006)

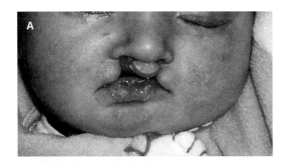

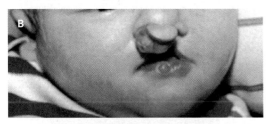

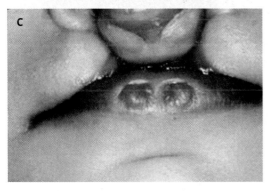

FIGURE 4-15 Van der Woude syndrome. Each child was born with a bilateral cleft lip and palate. The bilateral lip pits on the lower lip are a diagnostic feature of this syndrome. This is an autosomal dominate syndrome and therefore has a 50% recurrence risk.

(Figure 4-15B and C). This is important to recognize because Van der Woude syndrome is an autosomal dominant syndrome. Therefore, the recurrence risk with this syndrome is 50%, rather than the typical 3% to 5% when there is a nonsyndromic cleft.

Individuals with Van der Woude syndrome typically have normal development and intellect. However, they often have speech problems related to the cleft.

Velocardiofacial/22q11.2 Deletion Syndrome

Velocardiofacial syndrome (VCFS), also known as 22q11.2 deletion syndrome (22q), and even DiGeorge syndrome, is the most common syndrome associated with cleft palate and/or velopharyngeal dysfunction (**FIGURE 4-16**). The incidence of VCFS/22q deletion syndrome is estimated to be approximately 1 in 2000 to 4000 live births (Kobrynski & Sullivan, 2007; Shprintzen, 2000). In the VPI Clinic at Cincinnati Children's, VCFS/22q deletion syndrome is diagnosed in about 20% of patients with velopharyngeal dysfunction in the absence of overt cleft palate. Because these children are at high risk for feeding, language, speech, resonance, and voice disorders, speech-language pathologists should be particularly knowledgeable about this syndrome.

VCFS/22q deletion syndrome is caused by a gene deletion on the long arm (q arm) of chromosome 22, in the area of band 11 (thus 22q11.2 deletion syndrome). This can be diagnosed with a fluorescence in situ hybridization (FISH) test or a microarray analysis. Although most individuals with VCFS/22q deletion syndrome demonstrate this deletion, approximately 10% of patients with the syndrome do not have a demonstrable deletion. It is assumed that these individuals have a mutation or genetic rearrangement of the critical region on chromosome 22 that cannot yet be detected by current diagnostic tests. Most identified cases represent new deletions with no prior family history, but 10% to 20% of cases have a parent with features of the syndrome.

More than 180 different features have been reported with VCFS/22q deletion syndrome. The most common characteristics are velopharyngeal dysfunction (velo), congenital heart defects (cardio), and dysmorphic (facial) features (Goldmuntz, 2005; Shprintzen, 1994; Shprintzen, 2000; Vantrappen et al., 1999).

Velopharyngeal dysfunction in individuals with VCFS/22q deletion syndrome may be because of an overt cleft palate (often associated with Pierre Robin sequence), a submucous cleft, or hypotonia

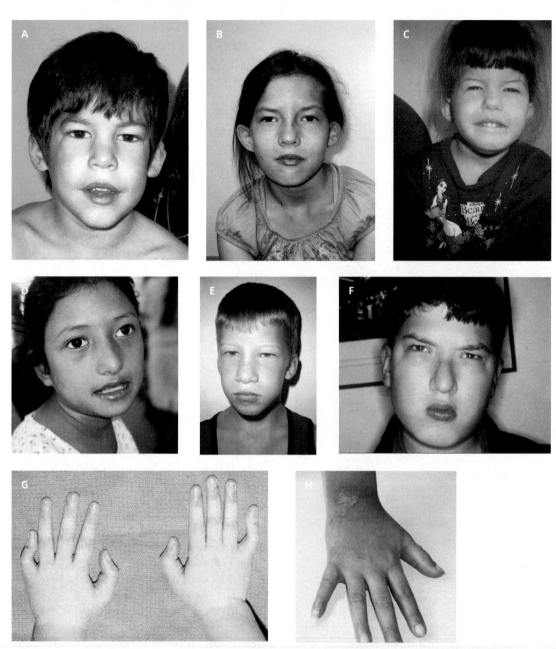

FIGURE 4-16 Velocardiofacial/22q11.2 deletion syndrome. **(A)–(F)** Note the long, narrow face; broad nasal tip; narrow palpebral fissures (eye openings); and ear anomalies. **(G)** and **(H)** Long, tapered fingers are characteristic of this syndrome.

of the velopharyngeal structures. Velopharyngeal dysfunction is the most common feature of VCFS/22q deletion syndrome in that almost all affected children have it to some degree. If a pharyngoplasty is needed for velopharyngeal dysfunction, the prognosis for total correction is somewhat guarded because of the pharyngeal hypotonia.

Congenital cardiac anomalies associated with VCFS/22q deletion syndrome often include ventricular septal defects (VSD), atrial septal defects (ASD), and pulmonary artery stenosis. Vascular anomalies are also common, including right-sided aortic arch, tortuosity of the retinal blood vessels, and medial displacement of the carotid arteries (Even-Or, Wohlgelernter, & Gross, 2005; Johnson, Gentry, Rice, & Mount, 2010; Ross, Witzel, Armstrong, & Thomson, 1996; Witt, Miller, Marsh, Muntz, & Grames, 1998). In fact, pulsation of the carotid arteries can often be viewed on the pharyngeal wall through nasopharyngoscopy. Because medial displacement of the carotid arteries is common in this population, surgeons must be sure to examine the posterior pharyngeal wall closely prior to placement of a pharyngeal flap. Abnormalities of the heart and related blood vessels are called conotruncal defects because of their location and development. In the population of children born with conotruncal heart defects, 10% to 15% have VCFS/22q deletion syndrome. Therefore, any child with a cleft palate or VPI and a congenital heart defect should be evaluated for VCFS/22q deletion syndrome (Goldmuntz, 2005; Marino, Digilio, Toscano, Giannotti, & Dallapiccola, 1999; Ryan et al., 1997).

There are many physical characteristics associated with VCFS/22q deletion syndrome. These include the following facial features: a long, narrow face often from vertical maxillary excess; narrow palpebral fissures; flattened malar eminence (cheekbone); a broad nasal root; a bulbous nasal tip; a thin upper lip; micrognathia, often causing Class II malocclusion; minor auricular anomalies; and microcephaly (Dyce et al., 2002) (Figure 4-16A–F). Additional physical features include short stature, usually below the 10th

percentile; long, tapered fingers (Figure 4-16G and H); and hyperextensibility of the joints.

Individuals with VCFS/22q deletion syndrome can have a myriad of medical problems, including kidney or urinary tract anomalies; laryngotracheal anomalies, such as a laryngeal web; umbilical or inguinal hernias; chronic middle ear effusion, presumably from tensor veli palatini dysfunction; upper airway obstruction caused by a narrow airway; endocrine problems, which are related to retarded growth; and poor immunity from abnormal T-lymphocyte function (Dyce et al., 2002). A subgroup of patients have hypoplasia or absence of the thymus (the organ in the chest that is the source of T-lymphocytes) or parathyroid glands (which make a hormone to regulate calcium levels in the blood) (Fomin et al., 2010; Stevens, Carey, & Shigeoka, 1990). The hypocalcemia can be the cause of seizures in these patients (Chao, Chao, Hwang, & Chung, 2009; Ryan et al., 1997; Tsai, Lian, & Chen, 2009).

VCFS/22q deletion syndrome is associated with brain anomalies that affect neurodevelopment. As such, affected infants often have hypotonia and poor oral-motor skills. As they grow, they often demonstrate gross and fine motor dysfunction, oral apraxia, and childhood apraxia of speech (CAS) (Kummer, Lee, Stutz, Maroney, & Brandt, 2007). Cognitive problems are common with VCFS/22q deletion syndrome. There can be mild to moderate mental disability, specific learning disabilities, reading difficulty, and problems with comprehension of abstract concepts (Antshel, Conchelos, Lanzetta, Fremont, & Kates, 2005; Jacobson et al., 2010; Kok & Solman, 1995). Educational goals must therefore focus on the development of language and communication skills.

Individuals with VCFS/22q deletion syndrome often have social, behavioral, and psychiatric issues (Swillen et al., 1997). They can have a seemingly outgoing personality but social disinhibition. Pragmatic disorders are common in this population. Particularly concerning is the risk for psychiatric disorders, such as depression, bipolar disorder, and even schizophrenia and schizo-affective disorder (Heineman-de Boer, Van Haelst, Cordia-de Haan, & Beemer, 1999; Karayiorgou et al., 1995). Psychiatric issues typically begin to occur during adolescence.

Wolf–Hirschhorn Syndrome (4p Syndrome)

Wolf–Hirschhorn syndrome is a chromosome disorder that is caused by a deletion or missing portion of the short arm of chromosome 4 (hence, 4p syndrome). Affected patients have a distinctive facial appearance, likened to a Greek helmet because of the presence of hypertelorism, and a prominent nasal bridge. A cleft lip and/or palate is a common feature. Most patients are very small, grow poorly, and have microcephaly. They may have heart defects, and seizures are very common. Developmental disabilities are universal in this disorder. Most patients have severe to profound intellectual disability and significant communication disorders (Jones, 2006).

Craniosynostosis Syndromes

Craniosynostosis is the premature fusion of one or more cranial sutures, which causes the skull to grow abnormally. This results in a misshaped head. Although not as common as cleft lip and/or cleft palate, craniosynostosis occurs in about 1 in 2000 to 2500 live births (Hunter & Rudd, 1976; Hunter & Rudd, 1977; Kimonis, Gold, Hoffman, Panchal, & Boyadjiev, 2007).

The distortion of the skull from craniosynostosis depends on the sutures that are involved. Premature closure of the coronal suture causes brachycephaly, where there is no anterior–posterior growth of the skull, while the lateral growth continues. This results in a short and flattened skull, a broad forehead, and wide face. On the other hand, premature closure of the sagittal suture causes scaphocephaly, where there is no lateral growth of the skull, while the AP growth

continues. This results in a long, narrow skull and frontal bossing (a prominent, protruding forehead). (The long, narrow skull that is often seen with prematurity is called dolichocephaly. This typically resolves on its own.) When multiple sutures are involved, asymmetry of the skull, called plagiocephaly, results.

Most cases of craniosynostosis are limited to the fusion of a single cranial suture, with no additional anomalies. Children with isolated craniosynostosis have an excellent prognosis for normal health, growth, and neurodevelopment. When craniosynostosis involves more than one suture, however, or when there are other congenital anomalies, it is likely to be a result of a syndrome.

Craniosynostosis syndromes have a genetic etiology and are typically inherited in an autosomal dominant manner, with a 50% recurrence risk (Robin, 1999; Wilkie, 1997). The prognosis for children who have a craniosynostosis syndrome is more guarded than with isolated craniosynostosis. If brain development is impaired by the restricted growth of the cranium or there is an increase in intracranial pressure (ICP), intellectual disability can result. Craniotomy and skull reshaping procedures are often required, both for normal brain development and function and to improve the aesthetics.

There are over 100 syndromes that include craniosynostosis as a feature (Cohen, 1991; Gorlin et al., 2001; Rice, 2008). Appendix 4A shows several of the craniosynostosis syndromes that are seen in a craniofacial center, along with their typical features and concerns. The following is a more in-depth discussion of a few of these syndromes.

Apert Syndrome

Apert syndrome (**FIGURE 4-17**) is caused by coronal synostosis. Its features include midface hypoplasia and shallow orbits, resulting in exophthalmos (protrusion of the eyeballs). There is also hypertelorism, strabismus, and a beaked-shape nose (Cohen & Kreiborg, 1992; Jones, 2006). There can be a cleft palate or a very

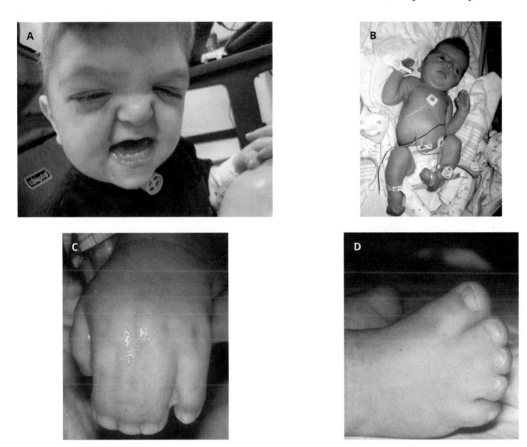

FIGURE 4-17 Apert syndrome. This syndrome includes craniosynostosis and syndactyly (webbing) of the fingers and toes of all four extremities.

narrow palate, causing dental crowding (Hohoff, Joos, Meyer, Ehmer, & Stamm, 2007). Narrowing of the upper nasal and pharyngeal airway or choanal stenosis is common and results in significant upper airway obstruction and hyponasality. Finally, individuals with Apert syndrome have syndactyly of the fingers and toes. The webbing may be of soft tissue, but it can also include the bone (Figure 4-17C and D).

Although normal intelligence is found in some patients, most patients with Apert syndrome have some degree of developmental disability, including mild to moderate intellectual disability. Communication disorders are common, including speech sound disorders from the small oral cavity and narrow palate and hyponasality secondary to upper airway obstruction.

Crouzon Syndrome

Crouzon syndrome (**FIGURE 4-18**) is the most common craniosynostosis syndrome. It is also caused by premature closure of the coronal sutures. This creates facial features that are similar to those in Apert syndrome, including midface hypoplasia, shallow orbits, exophthalmos, hypertelorism, and strabismus. Cleft palate and submucous cleft palate can occur, but not frequently (Jones, 2006; Robin, 1999).

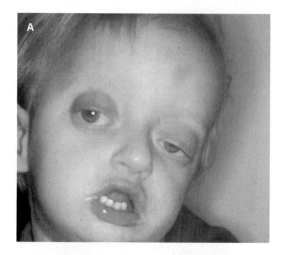

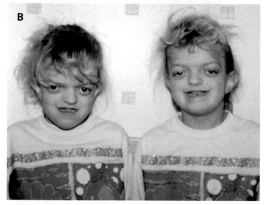

FIGURE 4-18 Crouzon syndrome. Typical characteristics of this condition include a wide forehead; a wide and flattened face; and shallow orbits, which cause proptosis of the eyes.

In contrast to Apert syndrome, there are no digital anomalies with Crouzon syndrome. Developmental disabilities can occur if there is hydrocephalus or agenesis of the corpus callosum. However, children with Crouzon syndrome usually exhibit normal development and intelligence.

Pfeiffer Syndrome

Pfeiffer syndrome is genetically heterogeneous (caused by different genes). In most patients with classic Pfeiffer syndrome, the craniofacial features are similar to those seen in Crouzon syndrome,

including coronal craniosynostosis, midface hypoplasia, shallow orbits with exophthalmos, and hypertelorism (Plomp et al., 1998). However, Pfeiffer syndrome type 1 also includes broad thumbs and great toes with variable degrees of syndactyly. Hearing loss and cleft palate are occasionally seen. Intelligence is usually normal.

Pfeiffer syndrome type 2 and type 3 are more serious, with limb contractures, airway obstruction, and occasional gastrointestinal disorders. Pfeiffer syndrome type 2 involves multiple sutures, resulting in a "cloverleaf skull" and severe midface hypoplasia and exophthalmos. Pfeiffer syndrome type 3 is usually associated with tracheal anomalies and upper airway stenosis (Stone, Trevenen, Mitchell, & Rudd, 1990). Intellectual disability, often severe, is seen in almost all children with Pfeiffer syndrome type 2 and type 3. Death in early childhood is common, especially in Pfeiffer syndrome type 2, which is more likely to be associated with cloverleaf skull and more serious upper airway obstruction.

Saethre-Chotzen Syndrome

Saethre-Chotzen syndrome is known to cause variable degrees of craniosynostosis, especially coronal synostosis. Facial features can be variable but often include ptosis (drooping of the eyelids), midface hypoplasia, a crumpled appearance to the top of the external ear, and mild digit anomalies (e.g., syndactyly or brachydactyly). Some individuals have broad thumbs and/or great toes with medial deviation of the great toes. A small number of individuals will have cleft palate or submucous cleft palate (Stoler, Rogers, & Mulliken, 2009).

Intelligence in Saethre-Chotzen syndrome is often normal, although there is an increased risk for developmental disabilities, including intellectual disability. Most patients do not have significant speech or language difficulties unless they have cleft palate or intellectual disability.

The Genetics Evaluation

The purpose of the genetics evaluation is to (1) to make a diagnosis; (2) determine the natural history of the condition, which will assist with anticipatory management for medical and developmental issues; (3) determine recurrence risks and prenatal counseling for the parents and other close family members; and (4) provide genetic psychosocial counseling and family support, which is often the most important function of the genetics evaluation. It is clear that the genetics evaluation is an important component of the early management of a child born with a craniofacial disorder, and the findings can significantly influence long-term medical and educational management and ultimate outcomes.

The genetics evaluation is somewhat different from the standard medical evaluation because greater emphasis is placed on the pregnancy and family history (Abuelo, 2002; Jones & Jones, 2009; McDonald-McGinn, Driscoll, & Matthews, 2009; Saal, 2016; Yoon, Pham, & Dipple, 2016). Additionally, most cases of craniofacial disorders are treated as chronic conditions with a need for long-term, integrated management.

Prenatal History

The prenatal history is particularly important to determine whether the fetus had any exposure to teratogens, which are chemical or physical agents that can interfere with the normal embryological processes. Teratogens can include drugs, radiation, viruses, or any other outside agent that can result in abnormal fetal development. Therefore, information regarding maternal exposure (e.g., medications or radiation) and maternal illnesses (e.g., infections or diabetes) during pregnancy can be helpful in determining a diagnosis.

Several common medications can act as teratogens and cause orofacial and other disorders if taken during pregnancy. These include anticonvulsants, corticosteroids, and benzodiazepines (for anxiety or insomnia) (Mitchell, 2009). Some medications that are teratogens, such as anticonvulsants, are still prescribed to pregnant women because their benefit in controlling seizures outweighs the risks for fetal anomalies. Alcohol and smoking are other significant teratogens that cause developmental disabilities and growth delays and are associated with cleft lip, cleft palate, and Pierre Robin sequence.

Medical History

The medical history of the newborn with a craniofacial anomaly should include perinatal complications, such as respiratory problems, feeding difficulties, or seizures. Information about birth weight, length, and head circumference is important because, although many syndromes are associated with low birth weight or small head size, others, such as Beckwith–Wiedemann syndrome, are associated with large body size for gestational age. All congenital anomalies should be documented in the medical history because certain birth defects (e.g., eye anomalies, genital anomalies, and heart defects) can give clues as to the possibility of an underlying genetic syndrome.

For the older child, it is important to determine whether he or she has been previously diagnosed with a syndrome, disorder, or medical condition. The examination results from other medical disciplines (e.g., ophthalmology, audiology, neurology, and speech pathology) are important to obtain. Finally, the medical history should include a list of major illnesses, hospitalizations, and surgeries along with a list of current and past medications.

Developmental History

The developmental history should include information about early milestones, especially those regarding gross motor, fine motor, and language development. A history of early intervention and therapy (e.g., speech therapy, occupational therapy, physical therapy) should be obtained. It is important to ask about school performance and whether the child has needed special education services. If developmental or intelligence testing has been done, it is helpful to have the results. Finally, if a grade was repeated, it is important to know the reasons (e.g., school absences from illness or medical interventions, learning problems, or issues with behavior).

Feeding History

Early feeding problems are common in infants with cleft palate and other craniofacial conditions. Infants with nonsyndromic cleft palate have feeding difficulty because of the inability to achieve suction with an open palate. These feeding problems are usually resolved quickly with simple feeding modifications. Other anatomic disorders related to feeding difficulty include tongue-based airway obstruction, which occurs with Pierre Robin sequence, choanal atresia or stenosis, and submucous cleft palate. If the infant has persistent feeding problems beyond the first week of life for unknown reasons, there may be an underlying neurological condition. In this case, further evaluation with a feeding specialist or a feeding team is beneficial.

The evaluation of the older child should include a history of feeding difficulties and feeding modifications. It is also important to determine whether any current feeding challenges exist and how they are being managed.

Family History

The need for a comprehensive family history is what really distinguishes the genetics evaluation from a standard medical evaluation. A pedigree, which is a pictorial representation of family members and their line of descent, is developed (see the chapter *Genetics and Patterns of Inheritance*, Figure 2-6). This can be used by the geneticist to analyze the patterns of inheritance, particularly for certain traits or anomalies. If possible, it is important to extend the pedigree to four generations. It can be valuable to identify whether any of the parents are related in any way (called consanguinity) because this can give insight into rare autosomal recessive disorders. The presence of multifactorial disorders, such as cleft lip or cleft palate, may be seen in other first- and second-degree relatives and may alter the genetic counseling regarding recurrence risks.

Any and all medical problems in relatives are noted, with special attention to infertility or miscarriages, birth defects (e.g., cleft lip, cleft palate, and congenital heart defects), major medical disorders or illnesses, and early deaths. Developmental disabilities in the family are also important to note.

Physical Examination

The physical examination of the child with a cleft or craniofacial condition is fairly straightforward and standard. However, special attention is given to growth parameters (weight, height or length, and head circumference). Microcephaly, which is a small head size, is important to note because it can indicate poor brain growth or development. Children with microcephaly often have underlying genetic conditions and are at greater risk for developmental disabilities. Poor weight gain may indicate poor feeding or possibly a genetic condition associated with small stature, such as a chromosome disorder.

In addition to a focus on growth, the geneticist performs an examination to identify dysmorphic features, which can be indicative of a specific disorder or syndrome. This may include measurements of the eyes, ears, mouth, nose, and numerous other structures. It is important to identify specific dermatoglyphics (creases on the hands or abnormalities in the fingerprints), which can give clues to early developmental problems. A specific neurologic examination is also done because it can give insight regarding the child's muscle tone, level of function, and degree of social interaction.

Photographs are taken of the patient at each visit. It is often helpful to look at earlier photographs that the parents bring to the visit as well as photographs of other family members. It is also beneficial to examine the parents and siblings for features similar to those of the patient.

Laboratory and Imaging Studies

After the history is reviewed and the examination is completed, it is necessary to determine whether laboratory studies are needed. Laboratory studies can help to confirm or rule out a syndrome that is suspected based on the patient's clinical features.

If a specific chromosome anomaly is suspected (e.g., trisomy 13; Down syndrome, which is also known as trisomy 21; or Turner syndrome), then specific testing with chromosome analysis is done. If VCFS/22q deletion syndrome is suspected, then a fluorescence in situ hybridization (FISH) study is performed to confirm the deletion on chromosome 22q11.2 (Bartsch et al., 2003; Oh, Workman, & Wong, 2007).

Many children with chromosome disorders have rare deletions and duplications. When a chromosome disorder is suspected because of multiple congenital anomalies and/or the presence of developmental delays or intellectual disabilities, the most useful diagnostic test is a microarray analysis. This is a DNA-based study that can identify most chromosome anomalies, including submicroscopic duplications and deletions (Manning & Hudgins, 2010).

In addition to the laboratory studies, it is often helpful to obtain X-rays to determine bone maturation or to identify specific skeletal syndromes. An MRI scan of the brain can help identify structural anomalies in children with serious developmental disorders, microcephaly, or neurological symptoms.

Finally, referrals to other physicians may be necessary as part of a complete genetics assessment. An ophthalmology examination should be done for all children with cleft palate only because myopia (nearsightedness) is a clue to the diagnosis of Stickler syndrome and may be severe enough to cause retinal detachment. Children with suspected heart defects, such as those with VCFS/22q deletion syndrome, should have an echocardiogram. If a heart anomaly is found, the child should be evaluated by a cardiologist.

Genetic Counseling

After all the above are completed, the family is seen for genetic counseling regarding the issues of heredity and development. Part of the process involves discussion of the natural history of the condition, which helps them to understand what to expect in the future and plan for medical interventions. In addition, families often have questions regarding the cause of the condition and the recurrence risks for themselves, their child, and other family members. For many genetic disorders, recurrence risks are known and can be shared with the family. There is ongoing research to determine the relative recurrence risk of cleft lip and palate on the basis of not only genetic background but also based on various environmental influences (e.g., smoking, alcohol use, and dietary factors). This will be useful in genetic counseling in the future and possibly for the development of future preventive measures (Kohli & Kohli, 2012).

In addition to discussing recurrence risks, it is also important to identify prenatal testing and reproductive options for the condition. Amniocentesis can be performed for prenatal identification of chromosome anomalies and specific known genetic disorders, using molecular analysis. For some birth defects, such as cleft lip with or without cleft palate, fetal ultrasound studies can be done. Unfortunately, prenatal therapy for most birth defects is not available.

Because many genetic disorders have associated developmental disabilities, referrals for developmental testing, including a speech and language evaluation, are often indicated. It is also important to plan for school interventions, with referrals for special services in the appropriate school system or community agency as necessary.

Psychosocial Counseling

Last, the genetics evaluator should recognize the difficulty of having a child with a birth defect and offer psychosocial supports for the family. It is essential to identify community and national resources for the family, such as local, state, and national support groups and meetings. Specific websites can be shared with the family members to help them find educational and support resources.

SUMMARY

To ensure that patients receive the services they need, it is important that all healthcare providers recognize dysmorphic craniofacial features and have knowledge about how these anomalies can affect the patient's function and health. This is important so that appropriate diagnostic testing is done, which can lead to more effective treatment planning.

All patients who present with craniofacial anomalies should be seen for a complete genetics evaluation to determine the underlying etiology.

Syndrome diagnosis is important for several reasons. Knowing the genetic diagnosis helps the family anticipate potential medical, developmental, and communication problems that are typically associated with the syndrome. Knowing the recurrence risk also helps with family planning. Finally, syndrome identification helps professionals from the craniofacial team and the family plan appropriate medical, surgical, therapeutic, and educational interventions to achieve the best possible outcome for the child.

FOR REVIEW AND DISCUSSION

1. Why should healthcare providers be observant of craniofacial anomalies?

2. What is the difference between a deformation and malformation? Which one has an increased recurrence risk?

3. Define syndrome, association, and sequence.

4. What does the presence of bilateral lip pits indicate, and why is it important to identify the lip pits?

5. Describe some syndromes that are associated with cleft palate.

6. List some craniofacial anomalies that will particularly affect the development of communication skills.

7. What anomaly causes Pierre Robin sequence? Describe how this anomaly causes a series of other malformations.

8. What is the difference between Pierre Robin sequence and Stickler syndrome? Which is more serious and why?

9. What are the characteristics of VCFS/22q deletion syndrome? Why do you think identification of this syndrome often occurs in the school years rather than in infancy?

10. What is craniosynostosis? What are some syndromes that involve craniosynostosis? What are potential functional problems with craniosynostosis syndromes?

11. Why is a genetics evaluation recommended for children born with cleft lip and palate? Why is it particularly important for children born with cleft palate only (without cleft lip)?

12. Describe the components of a genetics evaluation and why each component is important.

REFERENCES

Abuelo, D. (2002). Genetic evaluation and counseling for craniofacial anomalies. *Medicine & Health Rhode Island, 85*(12), 373–378.

Antshel, K. M., Conchelos, J., Lanzetta, G., Fremont, W., & Kates, W. R. (2005). Behavior and corpus callosum morphology relationships in velocardiofacial syndrome (22q11.2 deletion syndrome). *Psychiatry Research, 138*(3), 235–245.

Antunes, R. B., Alonso, N., & Paula, R. G. (2012). Importance of early diagnosis of Stickler syndrome in newborns. *Journal of Plastic Reconstructive and Aesthetic Surgery, 65*(8), 1029–1034.

Baraitser, M., & Winter, R. (1991). Update on the London Dysmorphology Database. *The Cleft Palate-Craniofacial Journal, 28*(3), 318.

Baraitser, M., & Winter, R. M. (2002). London Dysmorphology Database, London Neurogenetics Database and Dysmorphology Photo Library on CD-ROM [Version 3]. Oxford: Oxford University Press.

Bartsch, O., Nemeckova, M., Kocarek, E., Wagner, A., Puchmajerova, A., Poppe, M., . . . Goetz, P. (2003). DiGeorge/velocardiofacial syndrome: FISH studies of chromosomes 22q11 and 10p14, and clinical reports on the proximal 22q11 deletion. *American Journal of Medical Genetics A, 117A*(1), 1–5.

Bull, M. J., & Committee on Genetics. (2011). Health supervision for children with Down syndrome. *Pediatrics, 128*(2), 393–496.

Chao, P. H., Chao, M. C., Hwang, K. P., & Chung, M. Y. (2009). Hypocalcemia impacts heart failure control in DiGeorge 2 syndrome. *Acta Paediatrica, 98*(1), 195–198.

Cohen, M. M., Jr. (1991). Etiopathogenesis of craniosynostosis. *Neurosurgery Clinics of North America, 2*(3), 507–513.

Cohen, M. M., Jr., & Kreiborg, S. (1992). Upper and lower airway compromise in the Apert syndrome. *American Journal of Medical Genetics, 44*(1), 90–93.

Dios, P. D., Posse, J. L., Sanroman, J. F., & Garcia, E. V. (2000). Treatment of macroglossia in a child with Beckwith-Wiedemann syndrome. *Journal of Oral and Maxillofacial Surgery, 58*(9), 1058–1061.

Dyce, O., McDonald-McGinn, D., Kirschner, R. E., Zackai, E., Young, K., & Jacobs, I. N. (2002). Otolaryngologic manifestations of the 22q11.l deletion syndrome. *Archives of Otolaryngology-Head & Neck Surgery, 128*(12), 1408–1412.

Even-Or, E., Wohlgelernter, J., & Gross, M. (2005). Medial displacement of the internal carotid arteries in velocardiofacial syndrome. *Israel Medical Association Journal, 7*(11), 749–750.

Fomin, A. B., Pastorino, A. C., Kim, C. A., Pereira, C. A., Carneiro-Sampaio, M., & Abe-Jacob, C. M. (2010). DiGeorge Syndrome: A not so rare disease. *Clinics, 65*(9), 865–869.

Friedman, J. M., Birch, P., & Greene, C. (1993). National Neurofibromatosis Foundation International Database. *American Journal of Medical Genetics, 45*(1), 88–91.

Fritz, M. A., & Sidman, J. D. (2004). Distraction osteogenesis of the mandible. *Current Opinion in Otolaryngology & Head & Neck Surgery, 12*(6), 513–518.

Goldmuntz, E. (2005). DiGeorge syndrome: New insights. *Clinics in Perinatology, 32*(4), 963–978.

Goodship, J., Platt, J., Smith, R., & Burn, J. (1991). A male with type I orofaciodigital syndrome. *Journal of Medical Genetics, 28*(10), 691–694.

Gorlin, R., Cohen, M. J., & Hennekam, R. C. M. (2001). *Syndromes of the head and neck* (4th ed.). New York, NY: Oxford University Press.

Hannibal, M. C., Buckingham, K. J., Ng, S. B., Ming, J. E., Beck, A. E., McMillin, M. J., . . . Bamshad, M. J. (2011). Spectrum of MLL2 (ALR) mutations in 110 cases of Kabuki syndrome. *American Journal of Medical Genetics A, 155A*(7), 1511–1516.

Heineman-de Boer, J. A., Van Haelst, M. J., Cordia-de Haan, M., & Beemer, F. A. (1999). Behavior problems and personality aspects of 40 children with velocardiofacial syndrome. *Genetic Counseling, 10*(1), 89–93.

Hohoff, A., Joos, U., Meyer, U., Ehmer, U., & Stamm, T. (2007). The spectrum of Apert syndrome: Phenotype, particularities in orthodontic treatment, and characteristics of orthognathic surgery. *Head & Face Medicine, 3*, 10.

Hong, P., McNeil, M., Kearns, D. B., & Magit, A. E. (2012). Mandibular distraction osteogenesis in children with Pierre Robin sequence: Impact on health-related quality of life. *International Journal of Pediatric Otorhinolaryngology, 76*(8), 1159–1163.

Hsueh, K. F., Yang, C. S., Lu, J. H., & Hsu, W. M. (2004). Clinical characteristics of CHARGE syndrome. *Journal of Chinese Medical Association, 67*(10), 542–546.

Hunter, A. G., & Rudd, N. L. (1976). Craniosynostosis. I. Sagittal synostosis: Its genetics and associated clinical findings in 214 patients who lacked involvement of the coronal suture(s). *Teratology, 14*(2), 185–193.

Hunter, A. G., & Rudd, N. L. (1977). Craniosynostosis. II. Coronal synostosis: Its familial characteristics and associated clinical findings in 109 patients lacking bilateral polysyndactyly or syndactyly. *Teratology, 15*(3), 301–309.

Jacobson, C., Shearer, J., Habel, A., Kane, F., Tsakanikos, E., & Kravariti, E. (2010). Core neuropsychological characteristics of children and adolescents with 22q11.2 deletion. *Journal of Intellectual Disability Research, 54*(8), 701–713.

Johnson, M. D., Gentry, L. R., Rice, G. M., & Mount, D. L. (2010). A case of congenitally absent left internal carotid artery: Vascular malformations in 22q11.2 deletion syndrome. *The Cleft Palate–Craniofacial Journal, 47*(3), 314–317.

Jones, K. L. (2006). *Smith's recognizable patterns of human malformation* (6th ed.). Philadelphia, PA: Elsevier.

Jones, M. C., & Jones, K. L. (2009). Syndromes of orofacial clefting. In J. E. Lossee & R. E. Kirschner (Eds.), *Comprehensive cleft care* (pp. 107–127). New York, NY: McGraw-Hill.

Jongmans, M. C., Admiraal, R. J., van der Donk, K. P., Vissers, L. E., Baas, A. F., Kapusta, L., . . . van Raven-swaaij, C. M. (2006). CHARGE syndrome: The phenotypic spectrum of mutations in the CHD7 gene. *Journal of Medical Genetics, 43*(4), 306–314.

Karayiorgou, M., Morris, M. A., Morrow, B., Shprint-zen, R. J., Goldberg, R., Borrow, J., . . . Lasseter, V. K. (1995). Schizophrenia susceptibility associated with interstitial deletions of chromosome 22q11. *Proceedings of the National Academy of Sciences of the United States of America, 92*(17), 7612–7616.

Kimonis, V., Gold, J. A., Hoffman, T. L., Panchal, J., & Boyadjiev, S. A. (2007). Genetics of craniosynostosis. *Seminars in Pediatric Neurology, 14*(3), 150–161.

Kobrynski, L. J., & Sullivan, K. E. (2007). Velocardiofacial syndrome, DiGeorge syndrome: The chromosome 22q11.2 deletion syndromes. *Lancet, 370*(9596), 1443–1452.

Kohli, S. S., & Kohli, V. S. (2012). A comprehensive review of the genetic basis of cleft lip and palate. *Journal of Oral and Maxillofacial Pathology, 16*(1), 64–72.

Kok, L. L., & Solman, R. T. (1995). Velocardiofacial syndrome: Learning difficulties and intervention. *Journal of Medical Genetics, 32*(8), 612–618.

Kummer, A. W., Lee, L., Stutz, L., Maroney, A., & Brandt, J. W. (2007). The prevalence of apraxic characteristics in patients with velocardiofacial syndrome as compared to other populations. *The Cleft Palate–Craniofacial Journal, 44*(2), 175–181.

Laroche, C., Testelin, S., & Devauchelle, B. (2005). Cleft palate and Beckwith-Wiedemann syndrome. *The Cleft Palate–Craniofacial Journal, 42*(2), 212–217.

Manning, M., & Hudgins, L. (2010). Array-based technology and recommendations for utilization in medical genetics practice for detection of chromosomal abnormalities. *Genetics in Medicine, 12*(11), 742–745.

Marino, B., Digilio, M. C., Toscano, A., Giannotti, A., & Dallapiccola, B. (1999). Congenital heart defects in patients with DiGeorge/velocardiofacial syndrome and del22q11. *Genetic Counseling, 10*(1), 25–33.

Martelli-Junior, H., Coletta, R. D., Miranda, R. T., Barros, L. M., Swerts, M. S., & Bonan, P. R. (2009). Orofacial features of Treacher Collins syndrome. *Medicina Oral Patologia Oral y Cirugia Bucal, 14*(7), E344–E348.

McDonald-McGinn, D. M., Driscoll, D. A., & Matthews, M. (2009). Prenatal and genetic counseling. In J. E. Lossee & R. E. Kirschner (Eds.), *Comprehensive cleft care* (pp. 71–82). New York, NY: McGraw-Hill.

McMain, K., Blake, K., Smith, I., Johnson, J., Wood, E., Tremblay, F., & Robitaille, J. (2008). Ocular features of CHARGE syndrome. *Journal of the American Association for Pediatric Ophthalmology and Strabismus, 12*(5), 460–465.

Mitchell, L. E. (2009). Epidemiology of cleft lip and palate. In J. E. Lossee & R. E. Kirschner (Eds.), *Comprehensive Cleft Care* (pp. 35–42). New York, NY: McGraw-Hill.

Nash, K., Sheard, E., Rovet, J., & Koren, G. (2008). Understanding fetal alcohol spectrum disorders (FASDs): Toward identification of a behavioral phenotype. *The Scientific World Journal, 8*, 873–882.

Nowak, C. B. (1998). Genetics and hearing loss: A review of Stickler syndrome. *Journal of Communication Disorders, 31*(5), 437–454.

Oh, A. K., Workman, L. A., & Wong, G. B. (2007). Clinical correlation of chromosome 22q11.2 fluorescent in situ hybridization analysis and velocardiofacial syndrome. *The Cleft Palate–Craniofacial Journal, 44*(1), 62–66.

Plomp, A. S., Hamel, B. C., Cobben, J. M., Verloes, A., Offermans, J. P., Lajeunie, E., & de Die-Smulders, C. E. (1998). Pfeiffer syndrome type 2: Further delineation and review of the literature. *American Journal of Medical Genetics, 75*(3), 245–251.

Posnick, J. C., & Ruiz, R. L. (2000). Treacher Collins syndrome: Current evaluation, treatment, and future directions. *The Cleft Palate–Craniofacial Journal, 37*(5), 434.

Prattichizzo, C., Macca, M., Novelli, V., Giorgio, G., Barra, A., & Franco, B. (2008). Mutational spectrum of the oral-facial-digital type 1 syndrome: A study on a large collection of patients. *Human Mutation, 29*(10), 1237–1246.

Rice, D. P. (2008). Clinical features of syndromic craniosynostosis. *Frontiers of Oral Biology, 12*, 91–106.

Robin, N. H. (1999). Molecular genetic advances in understanding craniosynostosis. *Plastic and Reconstructive Surgery, 103*(3), 1060–1070.

Ross, D. A., Witzel, M. A., Armstrong, D. C, & Thomson, H. G. (1996). Is pharyngoplasty a risk in velocardiofacial syndrome? An assessment of medially displaced carotid arteries. *Plastic and Reconstructive Surgery, 98*(7), 1182–1190.

Ryan, A. K., Goodship, J. A., Wilson, D. L., Philip, N., Levy, A., Seidel, H., . . . Scrambler, P. J. (1997). Spectrum of clinical features associated with interstitial chromosome 22q11 deletions: A European collaborative study. *Journal of Medical Genetics, 34*(10), 798–804.

Saal, H. M. (2016). Genetic evaluation for craniofacial conditions. *Facial Plastic Surgery Clinics of North America, 24*(4), 405–425.

Seto-Salvia, N., & Stanier, P. (2014). Genetics of cleft lip and/or cleft palate: Association with other common anomalies. *European Journal of Medical Genetics, 57*(8), 381–393.

Shprintzen, R. J. (1994). Velocardiofacial syndrome and DiGeorge sequence. *Journal of Medical Genetics, 31*(5), 423–424.

Shprintzen, R. J. (2000). Velocardiofacial syndrome. *Otolaryngologic Clinics of North America, 33*(6), 1217–1240.

Shuman, C., Beckwith, J. B., Smith, A. C., & Weksberg, R. (2016). Beckwith–Wiedemann syndrome. In M. P. Adam, H. H. Ardinger, R. A. Pagon, S. E. Wallace, L. J. H. Bean, K. Stephens, & A. Amemiya (Eds.), *GeneReviews Seattle*. Seattle, WA: University of Washington, Seattle. https://www.ncbi.nlm.nih.gov/books/NBK1394/

Sidman, J. D., Sampson, D., & Templeton, B. (2001). Distraction osteogenesis of the mandible for airway obstruction in children. *Laryngoscope, 111*(7), 1137–1146.

Stanier, P., & Moore, G. E. (2004). Genetics of cleft lip and palate: Syndromic genes contribute to the incidence of non-syndromic clefts. *Human Molecular Genetics, 13*(Spec. No. 1), R73–R81.

Stevens, C. A., Carey, J. C., & Shigeoka, A. O. (1990). DiGeorge anomaly and velocardiofacial syndrome. *Pediatrics, 85*(4), 526–530.

Stoler, J. M., Rogers, G. F., & Mulliken, J. B. (2009). The frequency of palatal anomalies in Saethre-Chotzen syndrome. *The Cleft Palate–Craniofacial Journal, 46*(3), 280–284.

Stone, P., Trevenen, C. L., Mitchell, L., & Rudd, N. (1990). Congenital tracheal stenosis in Pfeiffer syndrome. *Clinical Genetics, 38*(2), 145–148.

Streissguth, A. P., Aase, J. M., Clarren, S. K., Randels, S. P., LaDue, R. A., & Smith, D. F. (1991). Fetal alcohol syndrome in adolescents and adults. *Journal of the American Medical Association, 265*(15), 1961–1967.

Strömland, K., Miller, M., Sjögreen, L., Johansson, M., Joelsson, B. M., Billstedt, E., . . . Granström, G. (2007). Oculo-auriculo-vertebral spectrum: Associated anomalies, functional deficits and possible developmental risk factors. *American Journal of Medical Genetics A, 143A*(12), 1317–1325.

Swillen, A., Devriendt, K., Legius, E., Eyskens, B., Dumoulin, M., Gewillig, M., Fryns, J. P. (1997). Intelligence and psychosocial adjustment in velocardiofacial syndrome: A study of 37 children and adolescents with VCFS. *Journal of Medical Genetics, 34*(6), 453–458.

Thompson, H. L., Viskochil, D. H., Stevenson, D. A., & Chapman, K. L. (2010). Speech-language characteristics of children with neurofibromatosis type 1. *American Journal of Medical Genetics A, 152A*(2), 284–290.

Tsai, P. L., Lian, L. M., & Chen, W. H. (2009). Hypocalcemic seizure mistaken for idiopathic epilepsy in two cases of DiGeorge syndrome (chromosome 22q11 deletion syndrome). *Acta Neurology Taiwan, 18*(4), 272–275.

Vantrappen, G., Devriendt, K., Swillen, A., Rommel, N., Vogels, A., Eyskens, B., . . . Fryns, J. P. (1999). Presenting symptoms and clinical features in 130 patients with the velocardiofacial syndrome. *Genetic Counseling, 10*(1), 3–9.

Viskochil, D. (2002). Genetics of neurofibromatosis 1 and the NF1 gene. *Journal of Child Neurology, 17*(8), 562–570; discussion 571–562, 646–551.

Wilkie, A. O. (1997). Craniosynostosis: Genes and mechanisms. *Human Molecular Genetics, 6*(10), 1647–1656.

Witt, P. D., Miller, D. C., Marsh, J. L., Muntz, H. R., & Grames, L. M. (1998). Limited value of preoperative cervical vascular imaging in patients with velocardiofacial syndrome. *Plastic and Reconstructive Surgery, 101*(5), 1184–1195; discussion 1196–1199.

Yoon, A. J., Pham, B. N., & Dipple, K. M. (2016). Genetic screening in patients with craniofacial malformations. *Journal of Pediatric Genetics, 5*(4), 220–224.

Zhang, I., Husein, M., Dworschak-Stokan, A., Jung, J., Matic, D. B., Siu, V., . . . Doyle, P. C. (2012). Neurofibromatosis and velopharyngeal insufficiency: Is there an association? *Journal of Otolaryngology-Head & Neck Surgery, 41*(1), 58–64.

CREDITS

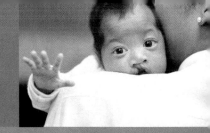

APPENDIX 4A

Craniofacial Syndromes and Conditions

Amniotic Bands	
Etiology	Caused by restricted development of parts of the fetus from constriction of amniotic bands
Inheritance	Sporadic; from fetal environment so no risk of inheritance
Phenotypic features	Clefts: Bands can affect development of the lip or palate if they are in the mouth Craniofacial features: facial deformities if the bands restrict the face Other features: clubfoot deformity; limb, hand, and finger anomalies or amputations
Communication concerns	Communication disorders related to cleft palate

Apert Syndrome (also known as Acrocephalosyndactly Type I)	
Etiology	Mutation of a gene on the long arm of chromosome 10 (10q25.3-q26). Causes premature closure of the coronal sutures so that the skull grows laterally but not anteriorly.
Inheritance	Autosomal dominant: 50% recurrence risk
Phenotypic features	Clefts: Cleft palate occurs infrequently Craniofacial features: similar to Crouzon syndrome, including a prominent forehead with a flat occiput, exophthalmos, hypertelorism, antimongoloid slant, strabismus and midface hypoplasia/retrusion, Class III malocclusion, low-set ears, upper airway obstruction Other features: syndactyly of fingers and toes, developmental disabilities
Communication concerns	Communication disorders related to upper airway obstruction, intellectual impairment, cleft palate, and class III malocclusion

Beckwith–Wiedemann Syndrome

Etiology	Some are from mutations in the short arm of chromosome 11 (11p15).
Inheritance	Sporadic
Phenotypic features	Craniofacial features: hypertrophic facial features, macroglossia Other features: large at birth, neonatal hypoglycemia; organ macromegaly; hemihypertrophy; umbilical hernia; omphalocele; abnormalities of kidneys, pancreas, and adrenal cortex; at risk for Wilms tumor, hepatablastoma, and malignant tumors of the abdomen. Macroglossia can cause feeding issues; upper airway obstruction and sleep apnea; dental malocclusion; and ultimately, prognathia.
Communication concerns	Communication disorders related to macroglossia and dental malocclusion

CHARGE Syndrome

Etiology	Sporadic. Caused by mutations on the CHD7 gene (located on chromosome 8) or mutations on chromosomes 7 and 8
Inheritance	Autosomal dominant: 50% recurrence risk
Phenotypic features	Clefts: Pierre Robin sequence, cleft lip and palate Primary features: coloboma; heart disease; atresia of the choanae; retarded growth and development; genital anomalies, cryptorchidism, micropenis, hypogonadism, delayed puberty; ear anomalies, hearing loss and deafness Other features: micrognathia, brain and cranial nerve anomalies, abnormal or absent pituitary gland, and developmental disability
Communication concerns	Communication disorders related to hearing loss, cleft palate, and the presence of neurological dysfunction

Crouzon Syndrome

Etiology	Mutation along the long arm of chromosome 10 (10q25.3-q26). Causes premature closure of the coronal sutures so that the skull grows laterally but not anteriorly.
Inheritance	Autosomal dominant: 50% recurrence risk
Phenotypic features	Clefts: Cleft palate and submucous cleft palate are occasionally seen in these patients Craniofacial features: features similar to Apert syndrome, including broad forehead, flat occiput, exophthalmos, hypertelorism, antimongoloid slant, strabismus and midface hypoplasia/retrusion, class III malocclusion, low-set ears Other features: can have hydrocephalus or agenesis of the corpus callosum; occasional developmental disabilities
Communication concerns	Communication disorders related to developmental disabilities or brain anomalies (if present), cleft palate, class III malocclusion, and upper airway obstruction

Down Syndrome (also known as Trisomy 21)

Etiology	Extra copy of chromosome 21
Inheritance	Sporadic
Phenotypic features	Clefts: Clefts are not part of this syndrome. Craniofacial features: upward slanting of the palpebral fissures with epicanthal folds on the inner corner of the eyes, micrognathia, macroglossia and/or protruding tongue, broad face, short neck, low-set ears Other features: short limbs resulting in short stature, a crease across one or both palms, hypotonia, congenital heart defects, gastroesophageal reflux, breathing issues and obstructive sleep apnea, mild to moderate mental retardation
Communication concerns	Communication disorders related to developmental disability and large or hypotonic tongue

Ectrodactyly–Ectodermal Dysplasia–Cleft Syndrome (EEC Syndrome)

Etiology	Genetic defect on the long arm of chromosome 7 (7q11.2-q21.3)
Inheritance	Autosomal dominant: 50% recurrence risk
Phenotypic features	Clefts: Cleft lip and cleft palate are common Craniofacial features: partial anodontia or microdontia, maxillary and malar hypoplasia, photophobia, defects of the lacrimal duct system, ossicular anomalies Other features: ectrodactyly (deficiency or absence of one or more central digits of the hand or foot), sometimes referred to as a "lobster-claw" deformity; ectodermal dysplasia (dry skin and mucosa; dry, sparse hair); absent sweat glands
Communication concerns	Voice issues, particularly breathiness, from lack of vocal fold hydration. Communication disorders related to the cleft and conductive hearing loss.

Fetal Alcohol Syndrome (FAS)

Etiology	Teratogenic (usually 4–6 alcoholic drinks per day)
Inheritance	Teratogenic, so no risk of inheritance
Phenotypic features	Clefts: Pierre Robin sequence, cleft palate, and cleft lip Craniofacial features: short palpebral fissures; short nose, flat philtrum, and thin upper lip; microcephaly Other features: small size at birth; heart defects, including ventricular septal defect (VSD) and atrial septal defect (ASD); cognitive impairment (average intelligence is about 65); severe behavior problems, hyperactivity, poor judgment, difficulty interpreting social cues, behavioral problems
Communication concerns	Communication disorders related to cognitive impairment and neurological dysfunction

Fetal Hydantoin Syndrome (also known as Fetal Dilantin Syndrome)

Etiology	Teratogenic from use of Dilantin for seizures during pregnancy
Inheritance	Teratogenic, so no risk of inheritance
Phenotypic features	Clefts: Clefts are not part of this syndrome Craniofacial features: microcephaly and minor dysmorphic craniofacial features Other features: intrauterine growth restriction, limb defects, hypoplastic nails, developmental delay or cognitive impairment
Communication concerns	Communication disorders related to developmental delay or cognitive impairment

Hemifacial Microsomia (HFM) (also known as Oculo-Auriculo-Vertebral [OAV] Dysplasia, Facio-Auriculo-Vertebral Spectrum [FAV], or Goldenhar Syndrome)

Etiology	Sporadic
Inheritance	Autosomal dominant: 50% recurrence risk
Phenotypic features	Clefts: cleft lip and/or palate in about 15% of cases Craniofacial features: facial asymmetry from unilateral hypoplasia of the face or malar, maxillary, and/or mandibular processes; cleft-like extension of corner of mouth; ear anomalies, including microtia or anotia and preauricular tags or pits; eye anomalies, including colobomas of upper eyelid, epibulbar lipodermoids, microphthalmia; dysplasia or aplasia of temporomandibular joint, affecting the opening of the mouth and excursion of mandible Other features: cervical vertebral anomalies Note: Hemifacial microsomia is usually unilateral but can be bilateral, although more severe on one side.
Communication concerns	Communication disorders related to velopharyngeal insufficiency or incompetence, hearing loss, or asymmetric oral structures

Kabuki Syndrome (also known as Kubuki Makeup Syndrome)

Etiology	Caused by mutations in the KMT2D gene
Inheritance	Autosomal dominant: 50% recurrence risk
Phenotypic features	Clefts: cleft palate or submucous cleft Craniofacial features: characteristic facial features, microcephaly, dental anomalies Other features: vertebral anomalies, short stature, congenital heart defects, hypotonia
Communication concerns	Communication disorders related to mild to moderate intellectual impairment and cleft palate, if present

Moebius Syndrome	
Etiology	Absence or underdevelopment of abducent nerve (sixth cranial nerve [CN VI]) and facial nerve (seventh cranial nerve [CN VII])
Inheritance	Rarely inherited; incidence is 2 to 20 cases per million births
Phenotypic features	Clefts: Clefts are not part of this syndrome Craniofacial features: lack of movement of the face, resulting in a flat, "mask-type" facies; strabismus; occasional hearing loss if cranial nerve VIII is affected; occasional breathing and/or swallowing problems Other features: micrognathia; microstomia; a short or unusually shaped tongue; cleft palate; limb abnormalities; dental abnormalities, such as missing or misaligned teeth
Communication concerns	Communication disorders related to the inability to produce bilabial and sometimes labiodental sounds for speech; inability to smile, move the eyes or mouth, or show facial expression; possible hearing problems

Neurofibromatosis Type 1 (NF1) (also known as von Recklinghausen Disease)	
Etiology	A genetic mutation in a gene called NF1
Inheritance	Autosomal dominant: 50% recurrence risk
Phenotypic features	Clefts: Clefts are not part of this syndrome Craniofacial features: no abnormalities Other features: café au lait macules, neurofibromas
Communication concerns	There is often velopharyngeal incompetence from brainstem tumors.

Opitz G Syndrome (also known as BBB Syndrome, Opitz-Frias Syndrome, Hypertelorism-Hypospadias Syndrome)	
Etiology	One form is caused by a mutation in the MID1 gene on the X chromosome. Another form is caused by a mutation in an unidentified gene on chromosome 22.
Inheritance	If X-linked: recessive inheritance If related to chromosome 22: autosomal dominant: 50% recurrence risk
Phenotypic features	Clefts: laryngeal cleft, cleft lip, cleft palate Craniofacial features: hypertelorism, flat nasal bridge, thin upper lip, low-set ears Other features: hypospadias, cryptorchidism, imperforate anus, heart defects, inguinal hernias, absent corpus callosum, learning disabilities and mental retardation
Communication concerns	Communication disorders related to long-term tracheostomy management, cleft palate, learning disabilities and mental retardation

Oral–Facial–Digital Syndrome Type I (OFD I)	
Etiology	X-linked
Inheritance	Autosomal dominant in females: 50% recurrence risk; usually lethal in males
Phenotypic features	Clefts: cleft lip, cleft palate, midline cleft lip Craniofacial features: hypertelorism, lobulated tongue, multiple hyperplastic oral frenula, notching in alveolar ridge, broad nose, hydrocephalus, absence of corpus callosum Other features: syndactyly or clinodactyly; dry skin and dry, sparse hair; missing teeth; renal cysts; cognitive impairment or developmental disabilities
Communication concerns	Communication disorders related to the cleft, cognitive impairment, or developmental disabilities. The lobulated tongue does not usually affect speech.

Pfeiffer Syndrome	
Etiology	Mutation in the fibroblast growth factor receptor (FGFR genes) on the short arm of chromosome 8 (8p11.2-p12). Causes premature closure of the coronal sutures.
Inheritance	Autosomal dominant: 50% recurrence risk
Phenotypic features	Clefts: cleft palate is rare Craniofacial features: coronal craniosynostosis, midface hypoplasia, shallow orbits with exophthalmos, hypertelorism, tracheal anomalies and upper airway stenosis, hearing loss Other features: broad thumbs and great toes Note: Type 1 is most common; type 2 and type 3 have the same clinical features but are more severe. The craniosynostosis involves multiple sutures, giving the skull a cloverleaf appearance. Death in early childhood is common.
Communication concerns	Communication disorders related to cognitive impairment or hearing loss

Pierre Robin Sequence	
Etiology	Micrognathia that may be from crowding in utero or may be genetic as part of a syndrome (e.g., Stickler syndrome or velocardiofacial/22q11.2 deletion syndrome). Micrognathia interferes with the downward progression of the tongue and the closure of the velum.
Inheritance	Depends on whether it is from genetic factors secondary to a syndrome or mechanical factors in utero
Phenotypic features	Clefts: usually a wide, bell-shaped cleft palate Craniofacial features: micrognathia; glossoptosis; airway and feeding issues, particularly at birth Other features: none
Communication concerns	Communication disorders related to the cleft and airway obstruction

Popliteal Pterygium Syndrome

Etiology	Mutations of the interferon regulatory factor 6 (IRF6) gene on the long arm of chromosome 1 (1q32.3-q41)
Inheritance	Autosomal dominant: 50% recurrence risk
Phenotypic features	Clefts: usually includes cleft lip and cleft palate Craniofacial features: lip pits near the center of the lower lip, tissue connecting the eyelids or jaws, missing teeth Other features: webs of skin behind the knee; abnormal genitals, including cryptorchidism; learning disabilities or mild cognitive problems
Communication concerns	Communication disorders related to jaw restriction, learning disabilities, or cognitive problems

Saethre-Chotzen Syndrome (also known as Acrocephalosyndactyly Type 3 or Chotzen Syndrome)

Etiology	Complete or partial deletion of the TWIST gene. Causes premature closure of the coronal sutures so that the skull grows laterally but not anteriorly.
Inheritance	Autosomal dominant: 50% recurrence risk
Phenotypic features	Clefts: cleft palate or submucous cleft palate Craniofacial features: coronal synostosis, ptosis of the eyelids, midface hypoplasia, external ear anomalies Other features: Cognitive impairment occurs infrequently.
Communication concerns	Communication disorders related to cleft palate or cognitive impairment, if present

Stickler Syndrome

Etiology	Mutations on the short arm of chromosome 6 (6p21)
Inheritance	Autosomal dominant: 50% recurrence risk
Phenotypic features	Clefts: usually includes cleft palate only Craniofacial features: Pierre Robin sequence with the characteristics of micrognathia, glossoptosis, and wide, bell-shaped cleft palate; a wide, flat face with midface hypoplasia; epicanthal folds; sensorineural hearing loss, high myopia, and risk for retinal detachments Other features: early onset of osteoarthritis and other joint disorders
Communication concerns	Communication disorders related to cleft palate and hearing loss

Treacher Collins Syndrome

Etiology	Mutations on the long arm of chromosome 5 (5q32-q33.3)
Inheritance	Autosomal dominant: 50% recurrence risk
Phenotypic features	Clefts: Clefts occur infrequently, despite Pierre Robin sequence with pronounced micrognathia Craniofacial features: downward slanting of the palpebral fissures, colobomas of the lower eyelids, microtia or middle ear anomalies, hypoplastic zygomatic arches and malar hypoplasia, macrostomia or microstomia, micrognathia, glossoptosis
Communication concerns	Communication disorders related to conductive hearing loss and micrognathia

Trisomy 13

Etiology	Duplication of chromosome 13
Inheritance	Chromosomal, usually sporadic
Phenotypic features	Clefts: cleft lip and palate. May have a midline cleft. Craniofacial features: severe eye defects, midline facial deformities Other features: severe brain anomalies, including holoprosencephaly; congenital heart defects; polydactyly; spina bifida; severe to profound cognitive impairment
Communication concerns	Most infants die before their first birthday.

Van der Woude Syndrome

Etiology	Mutation of interferon regulatory growth factor 6 (IRF6) gene on the long arm of chromosome 1 (1q.32-41)
Inheritance	Autosomal dominant: 50% recurrence risk
Phenotypic features	Clefts: cleft lip and palate Craniofacial features: bilateral lip pits on the lower lip, missing teeth
Communication concerns	Communication disorders related to the cleft

Velocardiofacial/22q11.2 Deletion Syndrome or (VCFS/22q Deletion Syndrome; also known as DiGeorge Syndrome)

Etiology	Second most common genetic syndrome, following Down syndrome
Inheritance	Chromosomal, autosomal dominant: 50% recurrence risk
Phenotypic features	Primary features:

Primary features:

- Velo: velopharyngeal dysfunction causing hypernasality, usually secondary to an occult submucous cleft or pharyngeal hypotonia
- Cardio: Minor cardiac and vascular anomalies, including ventricular septal defect (VSD), atrial septal defect (ASD), patent ductus arteriosis (PDA), pulmonary stenosis, tetralogy of Fallot, right-sided aortic arch, medially displaced internal carotid arteries, and tortuosity of the retinal arteries. Parents often report a history of heart murmur at birth.
- Facial: microcephaly; long face with vertical maxillary excess; micrognathia (small jaw) or retruded mandible, often with a class II malocclusion; nasal anomalies, including wide nasal bridge, narrow alar base, and bulbous nasal tip; narrow palpebral fissures (slit-like eyes); malar flatness; thin upper lip; minor auricular anomalies; abundant scalp hair

Other features: long, slender digits; hyperextensibility of the joints; short stature, usually below the 10th percentile in weight and height; Pierre Robin sequence (cleft palate, micrognathia, glossoptosis with airway obstruction); umbilical and inguinal hernias; laryngeal web; gross and fine motor delays; various brain anomalies; social disinhibition; risk of onset of psychosis in adolescence; learning disabilities and concrete thinking; mild to moderate cognitive impairment

Communication concerns	Communication disorders related to velopharyngeal insufficiency, pharyngeal hypotonia, verbal apraxia, conductive and/or sensorineural hearing loss, laryngeal anomalies and developmental disabilities

Wolf–Hirschhorn Syndrome

Etiology	Deletion or missing portion of short arm of chromosome 4
Inheritance	Usually sporadic, autosomal dominant: 50% recurrence risk
Phenotypic features	Clefts: cleft palate is common Craniofacial features: distinctive facial appearance, which is likened to a Greek helmet; hypertelorism; coloboma of the iris; prominent nasal bridge; microcephaly; micrognathia; short philtrum; dysplastic ears and periauricular tag; occasional hearing loss Other features: congenital heart defects; small stature and poor growth; renal anomalies; hypotonia; developmental disabilities or severe to profound cognitive impairment
Communication concerns	Communication disorders related to developmental disabilities and cognitive impairment and hearing loss, if present

CREDITS

Appendix opener photo: PeopleImages/Getty Images

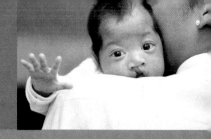

CHAPTER 5

Facial, Oral, and Pharyngeal Anomalies

With acknowledgment to J. Paul Willging for his contributions to this chapter.

CHAPTER OUTLINE

INTRODUCTION

Children who are born with clefts and other congenital craniofacial anomalies have issues with both aesthetics and function. In addition, they can be affected by acquired diseases and conditions of the face, ear, nose, and throat that further interfere with function. In fact, children with congenital craniofacial anomalies are at greater risk for some of these conditions (e.g., chronic middle ear effusion and upper airway obstruction) than children in the general population.

The purpose of this chapter is to review congenital anomalies and acquired conditions of the face, oral cavity, and pharyngeal cavity and discuss how each of these affect function. Because the ear, nose, and throat are important for speech production and general communication, abnormalities of these structures are a particular concern.

The Ear

Children born with craniofacial anomalies may have associated malformations of the external or middle ear. Abnormalities of the inner ear are less common but can occur. Malformations of the external ear only affect aesthetics, whereas malformations of the middle and inner ear can cause hearing loss that ultimately affects the ability to communicate.

External Ear

Patients with craniofacial anomalies, especially those with syndromes, often have microtia, which is a malformation of the pinna (Alasti & Van Camp, 2009; Brent, 1999; Luquetti, Heike, Hing, Cunningham, & Cox, 2011) (**FIGURE 5-1**). When there is microtia of the external ear, it is not uncommon to also find aural atresia (also called auditory atresia), which is a closure or absence of the external auditory canal. In fact, the more severely malformed the pinna is, the greater the chances are for significant problems within the external auditory canal and even involving the tympanic membrane (eardrum) and ossicles (Kountakis, Helidonis, & Jahrsdoerfer, 1995).

Aural atresia is commonly found in Treacher Collins syndrome, hemifacial microsomia, and Nager syndrome. It results in a conductive hearing loss because the sound energy cannot travel directly through the external auditory canal to the tympanic membrane (also called the eardrum) and therefore cannot reach the inner ear.

Children with bilateral aural atresia require bone conduction hearing aids. These may be conventional aids that make contact with the skull by means of a headband, or they may be bone-anchored hearing aids (BAHAs), which are implanted into the bone of the skull (osseointegrated) for a rigid attachment. Bone conduction hearing aids directly vibrate the end organ within the cochlea. Children with unilateral aural atresia generally do not require a hearing aid if their hearing is normal in the unaffected ear. It is of interest that children with aural atresia rarely experience ear infections. The explanation for this is not known.

Reconstruction of the external auditory canal (in addition to the middle ear structures, including the tympanic membrane and ossicular chain) can be done in the early school years. Patients with bilateral aural atresia benefit from reconstruction with an improvement in hearing. Patients with unilateral atresia are often reconstructed, but the benefits are less easily quantifiable. The risk of this surgical procedure lies in the potential damage to CN VII, or the seventh cranial nerve (facial nerve) (Chang, Lee, Choi, & Song, 2007), which is the facial nerve that provides motor innervation for the facial muscles. Damage to the nerve can cause partial or complete paralysis that may be temporary or permanent, depending on the degree of injury. Computed tomography (CT) scans of the temporal bone can be used to predict the course of the facial nerve in atretic ears, but these scans are not always of value. A rating scale has been developed to predict the hearing outcome of the surgical

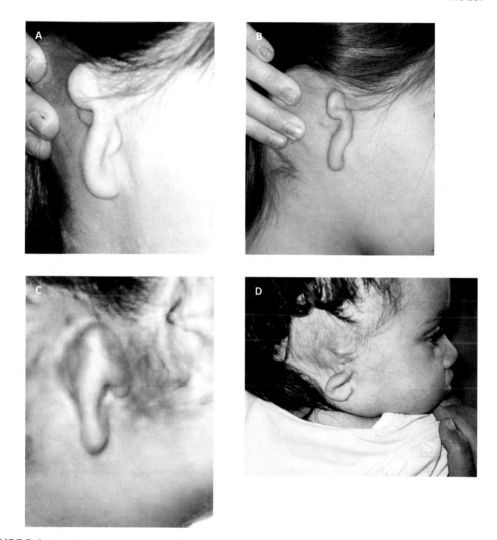

FIGURE 5-1 Microtia. The more severe the external deformity, the more likely it is that the middle ear cannot be reconstructed, despite the fact that the external ear and middle ear develop from different sites of origin.

correction of the external auditory canal and tympanic membrane based on the overall development of the middle ear space, the size and position of the ossicles, the presence of the stapes, and the position of the facial nerve. If surgical correction of the aural atresia is being considered, it should be done after surgical reconstruction of the pinna to repair the microtia. On the other hand, a BAHA can provide normal hearing, without risk to the facial nerve (**FIGURE 5-2**). Because of this advantage, a BAHA is more commonly recommended than surgical repair of the ear canal.

Middle Ear

When malformations are found in the external ear, there are often malformations or anomalies of the middle ear structures as well (Kosling, Omenzetter, & Bartel-Friedrich, 2009; Sheahan, Miller, Earley, Sheahan, & Blayney, 2004). For example,

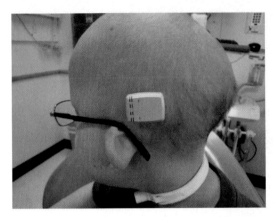

FIGURE 5-2 A bone-anchored hearing aid (BAHA). These aids can provide normal hearing for patients with atresia, without risk to the facial nerve, as is the case with surgery.

abnormal formation of the ossicles in addition to external ear malformations is common in Crouzon, Apert, and Goldenhar syndromes. In some cases, there is fusion of the ossicles to the surrounding bone. When the ossicles are abnormally formed or fused, it affects the transmission of sound to the inner ear, causing a conductive hearing loss.

As previously mentioned, surgical correction of abnormalities of the middle ear, including the tympanic membrane and ossicles, can be done in the early school years. In addition, bone conduction hearing aids allow correction of most kinds of conductive hearing loss.

Eustachian Tube

The eustachian tube connects the middle ear with the nasopharynx. This tube is closed at rest and opens when the tensor veli palatini muscle, which is attached directly to the cartilage of the eustachian tube, contracts in the act of swallowing or yawning. As the eustachian tube opens, it provides ventilation to the middle ear and mastoid cavities, equalizes middle ear pressure with that of the environment, and allows fluids to drain out of the middle ear space.

When the eustachian tube fails to open normally, the lack of drainage and buildup of negative pressure can cause middle ear effusion (a collection of fluid within the middle ear space). If the eustachian tube begins to function, the fluids will be absorbed by the lymphatics in the middle ear mucosa, and the normal condition will be restored. If the eustachian tube continues to malfunction, however, the middle ear effusion will persist. Bacteria can ascend the eustachian tube and grow in this effusion, leading to an ear infection called acute otitis media (**FIGURE 5-3**).

Acute otitis media is a common disease process in children. In fact, all young children, even those without ear anomalies, are at risk for middle ear disease, and half of children under the age of 3 will have had at least one episode of acute otitis media. This is because in children under the age of 6, the eustachian tubes lie in a horizontal plane between the nasopharynx and the middle ear. This horizontal orientation impairs middle ear drainage and allows for reflux of secretions from the pharynx into the tube. In addition, the eustachian tubes are oriented in such a way that the tensor veli palatini muscles are directed at an unfavorable angle to open the tubes. Both of

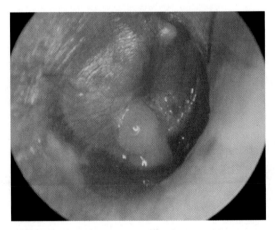

FIGURE 5-3 Acute otitis media. The infected middle ear fluid can be seen exuding from the hole created in the eardrum. This can be treated with a myringotomy.

these anatomic relationships predispose children to a tendency for ear infections. As growth and development occur, the skull base flexes upon itself, moving the origin of the eustachian tube musculature into a more favorable orientation for the opening of the tube. The palate also drops in relation to the ear, resulting in a 45° angulation of the eustachian tube. This angulation prevents some of the reflux of nasopharyngeal secretions into the eustachian tube, thereby minimizing the occurrence of infections (**FIGURE 5-4**).

In addition to the normal risk for middle ear disease, children with cleft palate or other craniofacial anomalies are at increased risk for persistent middle ear effusion or recurrent otitis media (Alper et al., 2011; Alper et al., 2012; da Silva, Collares, & da Costa, 2010; Sapci, Mercangoz, Evcimik, Karavus, & Gozke, 2008; Sheahan et al., 2004). This is because with a cleft palate or submucous cleft, there is often associated dysplasia of the tensor veli palatini muscles, thus affecting their function. In addition, patients with a cleft palate or other craniofacial conditions may have abnormally shaped eustachian tube cartilages with abnormal attachment to the tensor veli palatini muscles. Both of these abnormalities add to the risk for chronic middle ear disease (da Silva

et al., 2010; Durr & Shapiro, 1989; Heller, Gens, Croft, & Moe, 1978; Paradise, 1976; Paradise et al., 1974; Paradise & Bluestone, 1974; Trujillo, 1994).

Acute otitis media usually causes a high fever and severe ear pain. As a result, the affected child is often inconsolable. Occasionally, the tympanic membrane ruptures from both the increased pressure produced by the inflammatory process in the middle ear and the toxic effect of the bacterial infection.

In addition to causing discomfort and pain, acute otitis media causes a conductive hearing loss because of the diminished mobility of the tympanic membrane vibrating the ossicles in the middle ear. The extent of the conductive hearing loss is variable, ranging from 5 to 55 decibels, according to the physical nature of the effusion.

One serious potential complication of acute or chronic otitis media is mastoiditis, which is an infection of the mastoid process of the temporal bone. This infection is essentially a closed-space abscess that can cause erosion of the bone, leading to potentially life-threatening complications. The infection often extends laterally behind the ear, causing the ear to protrude from the side of the head. It can also erode medially, causing meningitis, brain abscess, or facial nerve paralysis.

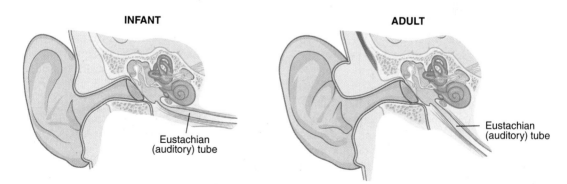

INFANT

ADULT

Eustachian (auditory) tube

Eustachian (auditory) tube

FIGURE 5-4 Angulation of the eustachian tube in an infant and an adult. The angulation of the eustachian tube changes with growth and development. In a young child, the eustachian tube ascends up to the middle ear at a 10° angle. In the adult, this angle changes to 45°. The orientation of the musculature around the eustachian tube also changes over time, improving the ability to ventilate the middle ear with age.

SPEECH NOTES

Conductive Hearing Loss

It is unlikely that mild conductive hearing loss will cause a speech and/or language disorder, but diminished hearing can delay speech and language acquisition (Baudonck, Van Lierde, Dhooge, & Corthals, 2011; Coez et al., 2010; Ertmer, 2011; Fitzpatrick, Crawford, Ni, & Durieux-Smith, 2011; Moeller et al., 2010; Rosenfeld et al., 2016). Auditory stimulation is particularly important during the first year of life. During this time, the neurons in the auditory brainstem are maturing, and the neural connections are being formed (Sininger, Doyle, & Moore, 1999). If sensory input to the auditory nervous system is interrupted during early development, it can have a detrimental effect on speech and language learning (Rvachew, Slawinski, Williams, & Green, 1999). Hearing must always be evaluated in the presence of speech and language difficulties to ensure that there is normal auditory function before initiation of therapeutic intervention for speech and language disorders.

Sensorineural hearing loss is another potential serious complication of repeated ear infections. The toxins produced by the bacteria may enter the cochlea through the delicate membranes in the inner ear. With repeated exposure to these toxins, the hair cells of the cochlea may be damaged, leading to a permanent hearing loss.

Acute otitis media is treated with oral antibiotics that sterilize the middle ear effusion and result in rapid resolution of the child's ear symptoms. Antibiotics treat the infection but do not make the fluid dissipate. The middle ear fluid persists in children after the infection has been resolved for about 1 month in 40% of patients, up to 2 months in 20% of patients, and about 3 months in 5% of patients (Liu, Sun, & Zhao, 2001; Teele, Klein, & Rosner, 1980). While the fluid remains in the middle ear space, there will be a mild conductive

hearing loss. Once the eustachian tube begins to function normally, allowing a return to normal middle ear pressure and normal aeration function, the fluid in the middle ear is absorbed. In the meantime, antibiotics may help prevent additional infections from developing, but again, they have no effect in the resolution of the effusion.

The treatment for recurrent acute otitis media often includes multiple courses of antibiotics. However, the potential for the development of antibiotic-resistant bacteria increases with the number of antibiotics prescribed and the total duration of antibiotic treatment. Chronic antibiotic use in the treatment of noninfected middle ear effusion has been one of the major factors in the development of antibiotic-resistant bacteria.

Surgical intervention is recommended if the child has had six or more episodes of acute otitis media or a middle ear effusion that persists for 3 months or longer and is associated with a conductive hearing loss. The surgical treatment includes a myringotomy and insertion of pressure-equalizing tubes (American Academy of Family Physicians, American Academy of Otolaryngology Head and Neck Surgery, & American Academy of Pediatrics Subcommittee on Otitis Media with Effusion, 2004; Rosenfeld et al., 2004). A myringotomy is a small, surgical incision that is made in the tympanic membrane to allow for drainage of middle ear fluid. Ventilation tubes, also called pressure-equalizing (PE) tubes (**FIGURE 5-5**), are surgically inserted in

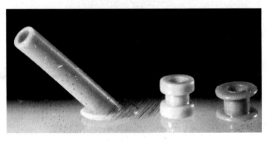

FIGURE 5-5 Examples of types of ventilation tubes, also called pressure-equalizing (PE) tubes.

the tympanic membrane to provide an alternate route for air to enter the middle ear space when the eustachian tube is nonfunctional. Ventilation tubes do not correct the underlying problems related to recurrent otitis media. Instead, they bypass the eustachian tube function until growth and development have progressed to the point where normal eustachian tube function can be achieved. If normal pressures can be established in the middle ear, the effusion will resolve and not recur. In addition, the irritation effect of the effusion on the mucosa resolves, leading to a normal middle ear system. The conductive hearing loss from the effusion also disappears, returning hearing to normal.

Ventilation tubes typically remain in the tympanic membrane for a length of time determined by their size. The longer the flanges of the tube, the longer their retention will be. The tubes generally extrude within 1 to 2 years. As the tube is expelled, the tympanic membrane heals. Ventilation tubes are generally required only once in the majority (80%) of patients requiring their placement. If recurring ear infections are again encountered after the ventilation tubes have extruded, another set of tubes can be inserted.

An adenoidectomy is often considered in conjunction with the second set of tubes. Because the eustachian tubes open just to the side of the adenoid in the nasopharynx, an enlarged adenoid may obstruct the eustachian tube openings, contributing to continued middle ear pathology (Nguyen, Manoukian, Yoskovitch, & Al-Sebeih, 2004). When this is the case, an adenoidectomy can be beneficial in establishing improved eustachian tube function (Gates, Avery, Prihoda, & Cooper, 1987; Grimmer & Poe, 2005).

For patients with cleft palate and other craniofacial anomalies, a particularly aggressive approach to the management of recurrent otitis media is required, given their increased risk. This includes early insertion of ventilation tubes. In fact, this can be done prophylactically with a lip repair. However, ventilation tube insertion is generally done at the time of the palate repair because earlier insertion increases the rate of chronic drainage through the tubes. Following palatoplasty, eustachian tube function usually improves, and the incidence of ear infections decreases, although not to the level of children without cleft palate. Also, as with children without cleft palate, there is gradual resolution of chronic otitis media with age (Alper et al., 2016).

Inner Ear

Structural malformations of the inner ear occur independent of other structural problems involving the pinna, external auditory canal, tympanic membrane, or middle ear. Abnormal development of the otic capsule within the temporal bone leads to abnormal development of the cochlea and semicircular canals. Abnormalities of the inner ear are uncommon but may be associated with craniofacial anomalies, especially with certain syndromes (e.g., Stickler syndrome, Treacher Collins syndrome, and hemifacial microsomia). Inner ear abnormalities typically cause a disruption of nerve impulses within the inner ear or through the brainstem to the auditory cortex, resulting in a sensorineural hearing loss. A hearing aid for one or both ears is often effective. Cochlear implants are offered as a means to treat sensorineural hearing loss in patients who derive no benefit from conventional hearing aids (Moores, 2005).

Audiologic Care

Because children born with clefts or other craniofacial anomalies often have congenital abnormalities of the auditory structures, they are at increased risk for ear disease and hearing loss. Hearing loss may occur intermittently or become permanent. It can range from mild to severe. Hearing loss can significantly affect speech and language development, education, social interactions, and even vocational opportunities. Therefore, children with craniofacial anomalies should be followed by an audiologist and otolaryngologist for periodic evaluations and treatment as necessary.

The American Cleft Palate–Craniofacial Association has specific recommendations for audiologic management of children born with a cleft lip/palate or other craniofacial differences (ACPA, 2018). They are as follows[a]:

- A record of the newborn's hearing screen should be obtained after discharge from the birth facility. If the newborn did not pass the screen, a complete audiological diagnostic evaluation should be performed by three months of age.
- The timing of audiological follow-up examinations should be determined on the basis of the child's history of ear disease and/or hearing loss. Audiological followup examinations should continue through adulthood as necessary.
- Audiological evaluations should begin at approximately nine months of age, and include a behavioral audiologic evaluation. Behavioral tests should be repeated at least every six to twelve months until the child is five years of age. After age five, if the hearing test is consistently within normal limit, then audiologic evaluations should be conducted annually until adolescence.
- If an individual with a craniofacial difference presents with a hearing loss of any type or degree (conductive, sensorineural, mixed, mild, moderate or severe) the schedule of audiological testing will change based on the audiologist's discretion.
- At each audiological visit, behavioral and physiologic audiological testing should be conducted. Behavioral evaluations include pure tone and, when possible, speech audiometry. Physiologic tests should include acoustic emittance testing (tympanometry and middle ear reflexes) and otoacoustic emissions (OAEs).
- All children undergoing myringotomies and placement of ventilation (pressure-equalizing) tubes should be seen for audiologic assessment regularly.
- When a persistent hearing loss is identified, amplification (hearing aid, bone-anchored hearing aids [BAHA], cochlear implants, and auditory training or frequency modulation [FM] systems) should be considered.
- When a hearing loss occurs in the presence of microtia or atresia of the outer or middle ear, either unilaterally or bilaterally, conventional bone conduction amplification should be considered. Depending upon the degree of loss, candidacy, and patient preference, a bone-anchored hearing system (auditory osseointegrated implant) may be considered as a treatment option.
- Once amplification has been provided, routine audiologic follow-up is necessary to monitor hearing status and the function of the amplification system.
- For any child with a documented hearing loss, an immediate referral should be made to the child's school district for appropriate educational services.

Facial Structures

Every year, thousands of children are born with cleft lip (and/or cleft palate) or other anomalies of the facial structures. Facial anomalies affect overall aesthetics and can result in a certain amount of stigma for the individual. In addition, many facial anomalies can impair vital functions of daily life (e.g., speech, hearing, vision, and feeding). The following section describes some of the more common facial anomalies and their potential effect on function.

Nose

Anomalies of the nose are common in patients with cleft lip/palate and craniofacial syndromes.

---

[a]   Reprinted with permission from American Cleft Palate–Craniofacial Association. (2018). Parameters for evaluation and treatment of patients with cleft lip/palate or other craniofacial differences. Chapel Hill, NC: American Cleft Palate–Craniofacial Association. doi: 10.1177/1055665617739564.

These anomalies can affect both aesthetics and function. For example, clefts of the primary palate often cause asymmetry of the nose and reduced projection of the nasal tip, which affect aesthetics. Anomalies of the inside of the nose often affect function, in particular, breathing and resonance.

There are several anomalies that can affect the anterior or posterior openings of the nasal cavity. For example, one naris or both nares (the anterior openings) may be partially or completely stenosed secondary to a cleft lip repair. Other nasal anomalies include unilateral or bilateral pyriform aperture stenosis, which is a narrowing of the pyriform aperture (the opening to the bony portion of the nasal cavity). This can be caused by overgrowth of the maxilla (Brown, Myer, & Manning, 1989; Visvanathan & Wynne, 2012). At the back of the nose, the choanae (posterior openings) can be blocked by enlarged adenoids. Even more concerning is that the choanae may be narrowed in a condition known as choanal stenosis, or completely closed, as in choanal atresia. These abnormalities can be either unilateral or bilateral.

Because neonates are obligatory nasal breathers, bilateral choanal atresia is particularly problematic. When the infants are unsuccessful with nasal respiration, they become fussy and eventually begin to cry. They are able to breathe well while crying. As they settle down, however, they are again unsuccessful with nasal respiration, and the cycle repeats. Without early surgical intervention, this cyclical cyanosis (bluish skin color from a lack of oxygen) can lead to death from exhaustion. Choanal atresia occurs more commonly in females and has an incidence of 1 in about 8000 births (Kubba, Bennett, & Bailey, 2004). About half of patients with choanal atresia have other congenital abnormalities.

A deviated nasal septum is commonly associated with clefts, particularly with unilateral clefts of the lip and palate. With a cleft palate, there is not the normal midline groove on the nasal aspect of the maxilla in which the vomer can insert for

stabilization. Although the nasal septum is not stabilized in a bilateral cleft, it typically remains in midline. With a unilateral cleft, however, the septum generally deviates into the nasal cavity of the cleft side. A deviated septum may also occur during birth if the nose of the neonate is forced against the pelvis during delivery, causing the septum to slip off the maxillary groove.

Finally, some children experience chronic sinus problems. When this occurs, evaluation of the sinuses is typically done through a CT scan, as can be seen in **FIGURE 5-6**. Unlike acute sinusitis, which may resolve with

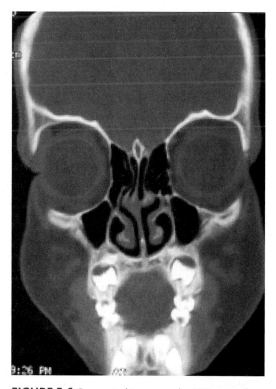

FIGURE 5-6 Computed tomography (CT) scan of the nose and paranasal sinuses. The sinuses are air-filled spaces that are found in the cheeks and between the eyes. This scan shows the nasal cavities separated by the nasal septum. The turbinates are the small bones arising from the lateral aspect of the nasal cavity.

SPEECH NOTES

Obstruction of the Nasal Cavity

Both anterior and posterior obstruction of the nasal cavity can affect the flow of air for normal nasal breathing and can also affect resonance. Anterior obstruction from a deviated septum, pyriform aperture stenosis, or stenosis of the nares can cause nasal cul-de-sac resonance. This is typically noted on nasal sounds but is also noted on oral sounds if there is a moderate to severe degree of velopharyngeal insufficiency. Obstruction of the posterior choanae by scarring or an enlarged adenoid pad can cause hyponasality. This is most noticeable on nasal sounds but can affect vowels to a mild degree.

medication, chronic sinusitis often requires surgical intervention.

Maxilla

Maxillary retrusion (also known as **midface deficiency**) is a common anomaly in individuals with a repaired cleft lip and palate. It is characterized by a small upper jaw (maxilla) relative to a normal lower jaw (mandible). It is almost always associated with an **anterior crossbite** (the maxillary teeth are inside the mandibular teeth) and **Class III malocclusion** (the maxilla is behind the mandible) (see the chapter *Dental Anomalies* for more information). Maxillary retrusion is felt to be caused by an inherent dysplasia of the maxilla from the cleft, which makes it short, and possible restriction in maxillary growth with the surgical repair, which makes it retrusive (Kawakami, Yagi, & Takada, 2002) (**FIGURE 5-7**).

Because the maxilla forms the floor of the nose, a short maxilla causes the nasal cavity to be relatively small. A retrusive maxilla causes the pharynx to be very shallow. Both of these conditions can have a negative effect on the patency of the upper airway.

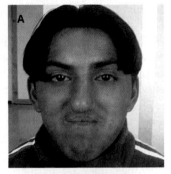

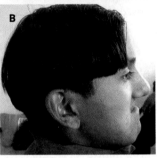

FIGURE 5-7 Maxillary retrusion. This is a common issue with cleft lip and palate.

SPEECH NOTES

Maxillary Retrusion

With normal occlusion, the maxillary teeth overlap the mandibular teeth, the tongue remains within the mandibular arch just under the alveolar ridge, and the tongue tip has sufficient room for elevation. When there is maxillary retrusion, however, the tongue tip may be anterior to the maxillary alveolar ridge and the maxillary incisors. When this is the case, the production of anterior sounds, such as sibilants (/s/, /z/, /ʃ/, /ʒ/, /tʃ/, /dʒ/), lingual-alveolars (/t/, /d/, /n/, /l/), labiodentals (/f/ and /v/), and even bilabials (/p/, /b/, /m/) can be affected. See the chapter *Dental Anomalies* for more information regarding the effects of occlusion on speech.

The retrusion of the maxilla affects the size of the nasal cavity and the depth of the pharynx. In addition to its effect on breathing, it can affect the quality of resonance.

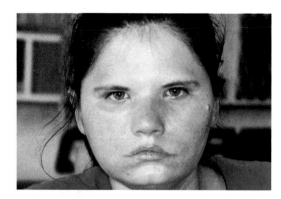

FIGURE 5-8 Moebius. Note the mask-like facies.

Facial Nerve

Facial paralysis may occur as a result of an injury (surgical or traumatic), infection (viral or bacterial), or **Bell's palsy** (a temporary unilateral facial paralysis thought to be caused by trauma) (Chen & Wong, 2005; Peitersen, 1992; Terzis & Anesti, 2011; Yetter, Ogren, Moore, & Yonkers, 1990). It may also be from congenital abnormalities of the nerve or associated muscles, as in hemifacial microsomia, which is usually unilateral, or Moebius syndrome, which is bilateral and results in a mask-like facies (**FIGURE 5-8**).

Oral Cavity

The oral cavity extends from the lips anteriorly to the faucial pillars posteriorly. Anomalies of the oral cavity are common and can have a significant effect on speech. Dental anomalies are discussed in the chapter *Dental Anomalies* and therefore are not covered in this chapter.

Lips

The lips function in eating, drinking, speech, and prevention of sialorrhea (drooling). For aesthetic reasons and normal function, the individual should be able to achieve and maintain bilabial closure during normal nasal breathing.

A common problem following a cleft lip repair is a short upper lip. The lip may be deficient in tissue because of the basic dysmorphology from the cleft lip, and it may also be shortened secondary to the contractile effects of the scar from the cleft lip repair. If the premaxilla is protrusive, the relative shortening of the lip appears more pronounced. **FIGURE 5-9** shows a child with a short upper lip caused by scarring. She is able to achieve bilabial closure only with effort.

SPEECH NOTES

Facial Paralysis

Facial paralysis causes a lack of facial expression and lip movement, which affects feeding and speech (Goldberg, DeLorie, Zuker, & Manktelow, 2003; Meyerson & Foushee, 1978). Facial paralysis also affects the ability to produce bilabial and possibly labiodental phonemes. Tongue movement is usually unaffected. The individual may learn to compensate by producing bilabial sounds with the tongue tip. Some individuals become very adept at producing the sound in a way that is acoustically similar to the labial sound.

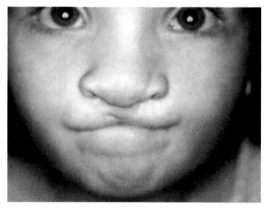

FIGURE 5-9 Short upper lip. This causes difficulty with bilabial competence at rest and with bilabial sound production.

SPEECH NOTES

Lips

When the upper lip is short and/or the premaxilla is protrusive, there may be **bilabial incompetence**, which is the inability to close the lips naturally at rest. If lip closure is difficult to accomplish at rest, there will also be difficulties with the production of bilabial sounds (/p/, /b/, /m/) with speech. Even if bilabial closure can be achieved with effort, this will not occur consistently during connected speech.

Many individuals compensate for the inability to produce bilabial sounds by producing these sounds with labiodental placement. This usually results in little auditory distortion, but this placement can be visually distracting to the listener.

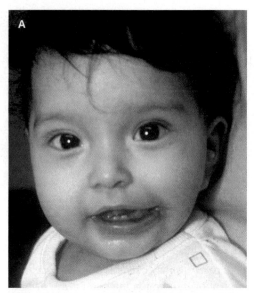

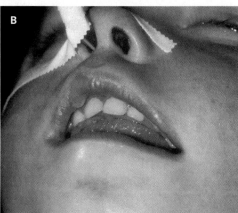

FIGURE 5-10 Macrostomia.

There are several additional anomalies of the upper lip that can occur following a cleft lip repair, including vermilion tissue above the white roll, asymmetry of the lip, and a flattening of Cupid's bow. If the orbicularis oris muscle around the lips is not approximated during the lip repair, the discontinuity of these muscle bundles will become apparent over time. Bulges just lateral to the area of the philtrum will be seen as a result.

Mouth

Congenital abnormalities of the size and shape of the mouth can occur, especially with some syndromes. Note that the suffix "stomia" is used for the word "mouth." This is not to be confused with the suffix "somia," which refers to body.

Macrostomia refers to an excessively large mouth opening. This is particularly common with hemifacial microsomia, where one corner of the mouth can extend into the cheek, making the mouth opening on that particular side large and distorted in appearance (**FIGURE 5-10**). On the other hand, **microstomia** refers to a small mouth opening (**FIGURE 5-11**). Microstomia can be congenital but can also be acquired because of injuries or burns. This is because scarring can cause severe contractures of the mouth.

Tongue

Lingual (tongue) anomalies are associated with certain syndromes. **Macroglossia** is a condition in which the tongue is abnormally large, and it

Macrostomia and Microstomia

Macrostomia does not cause speech problems. On the other hand, if the microstomia is severe enough to affect mouth opening, it can affect articulation and cause oral cul-de-sac resonance (or "mumbling") (see the chapter *Speech/ Resonance Disorders and Velopharyngeal Dysfunction* for more information).

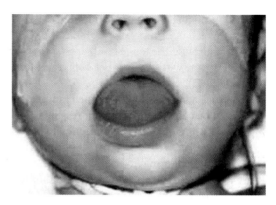

FIGURE 5-12 Macroglossia secondary to Beckwith–Wiedemann syndrome. This photo demonstrates macroglossia with severe discrepancy between the size of the oral cavity and the size of the tongue.

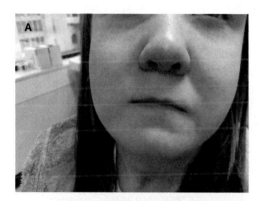

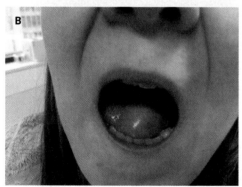

FIGURE 5-11 Microstomia.

Macroglossia and Microglossia

Macroglossia can interfere with the production of bilabial and labiodental sounds. It can also affect production of lingual-alveolar sounds if it causes the tongue tip to extend past the maxillary incisors. This position can result in either a frontal or lateral distortion of sibilants (Topouzelis, Iliopoulos, & Kolokitha, 2011; Van Borsel, Van Snick, & Leroy, 1999). It can also contribute to the use of palatal–dorsal articulation, especially if the tongue tip rests anterior to the alveolar ridge. Macroglossia also affects resonance. Because the tongue fills most of the oral cavity, there is little space for normal oral resonance of the sound. This results in an oral or pharyngeal cul-de-sac resonance.

In contrast to macroglossia, microglossia is a relatively small tongue for the oral cavity space. It usually has no detrimental effect on speech, unless the tongue is not able to reach the alveolar ridge for articulation.

is one of the main characteristics of Beckwith–Wiedemann syndrome (**FIGURE 5-12**).

Because the tongue is too large to fit in the oral cavity, it protrudes past the alveolar ridge, causing an open-mouth posture. The chronic open-mouth posture can also contribute to excessive drooling. As the dentition develops, an anterior open bite may occur because the tongue is in the area where the teeth are erupting. The biggest concern, at least initially, is the effect it can have on the airway.

Other lingual anomalies include a lobulated tongue, which is common in oral–facial–digital (OFD) syndrome. The tongue may appear to have multiple lobes, with fissures between each lobe (**FIGURE 5-13**).

Finally, a discussion of lingual anomalies would not be complete without addressing ankyloglossia. Ankyloglossia, commonly referred to as tongue-tie (**FIGURE 5-14**), is a condition where there is abnormal restriction of tongue-tip movement from either a short lingual frenulum (Figure 5-14A) or a frenulum that is attached near the tip of the tongue (Figure 5-14B and C). Ankyloglossia is usually congenital, but it can also occur after radical oral surgery.

The diagnostic criteria for ankyloglossia include (1) the person cannot elevate the tongue tip to the alveolar ridge with the mouth

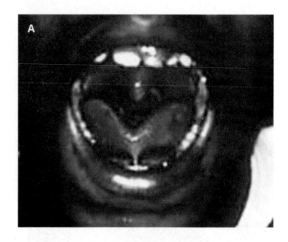

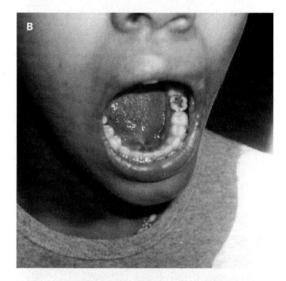

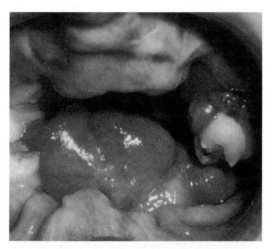

FIGURE 5-13 Lobulations of the tongue. This is a characteristic of oral–facial–digital (OFD) syndrome.

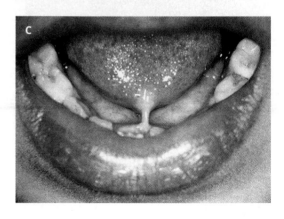

SPEECH NOTES

Lobulated Tongue

A lobulated tongue usually does not affect lingual mobility and therefore rarely affects speech.

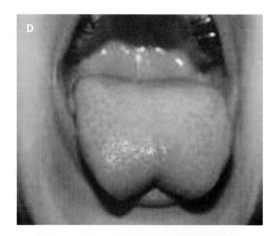

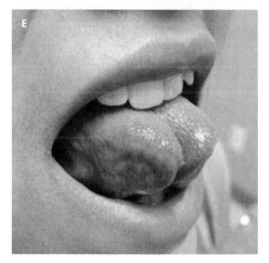

FIGURE 5-14 Ankyloglossia. Ankyloglossia is a condition describing the attachment of the lingual frenulum to the anterior tongue tip. It may impede normal tongue mobility but rarely requires intervention for speech purposes.

open (Figure 5-14A); (2) the person cannot protrude the tongue tip past the mandibular incisors (or mandibular gingiva) (Figure 5-14D); and (3) with protrusion, the tip of the tongue is heart shaped, with a midline indentation (Figure 5-14D and E).

Ankyloglossia can cause a variety of issues. A short lingual frenulum can affect the infant's ability to latch on to the nipple for feeding.

Although ankyloglossia is common in neonates, it tends to correct itself as the child grows (Garcia Pola, Gonzalez Garcia, Garcia Martin, Gallas, & Seoane Leston, 2002). Ankyloglossia later in life can affect the person's ability to move a bolus in the mouth, particularly if the bolus is in the buccal sulcus (area between the teeth and cheeks) (Kern, 1991). Infrequently, a short lingual frenulum can pull the gingiva away from bottom teeth between the mandibular incisors, causing dental issues. Ankyloglossia can affect aesthetics, making some affected individuals self-conscious. It can even affect "French kissing." Although it is commonly assumed that ankyloglossia can affect speech, there is no clear evidence to support that assumption.

SPEECH NOTES

Ankyloglossia

Ankyloglossia has less effect on speech than most laypeople (and even some professionals) assume. This is because very little tongue tip excursion is needed for normal speech production (AHRQ, 2015; Kummer, 2005; Moller, 1994). In English, the most the tongue tip needs to elevate to the alveolar ridge (without the mouth widely open) is for the /l/ sound. If that is not possible, the /l/ can be produced with the tongue tip down and dorsum up. The farthest that the tongue needs to protrude is against the back of the maxillary incisors for /θ/ and /ð/ sounds. It does not need to protrude beyond the mandibular incisors.

It has been suggested the lingual trill sound in other languages (as in Spanish) may be affected by ankyloglossia. This remains to be proven.

Because ankyloglossia rarely causes problems with speech, frenulectomy is usually not indicated for speech purposes, except perhaps if there is oral-motor dysfunction. However, it may be indicated for the reasons previously mentioned, particularly for feeding problems.

Palate

Palatal arch anomalies are common in individuals with cleft palate or other craniofacial syndromes. There may be abnormalities in the height, width, and configuration of the palatal arch. The palatal vault may be low and flat because of collapsed lateral palatal segments, or it may be very high and narrow, causing crowding of the teeth and tongue. A narrow, high-arched palate is often seen in children who have had an endotracheal tube at birth.

A fistula (pl. fistulae or fistulas) is an abnormal opening or passageway between two epithelialized organs that do not normally connect. A palatal fistula (also called an oronasal fistula) is an opening between the oral surface of the palate or velum and the nasal cavity (**FIGURE 5-15**). Palatal fistulas occur as an unintentional postoperative breakdown of the cleft repair because of inadequate healing. In addition, maxillary advancement, and sometimes growth, can cause a small, asymptomatic fistula to open further and become symptomatic.

Although fistulas can occur anywhere along the palatal suture lines, a common site for a fistula is at the junction of the hard and soft palate. If there was a bilateral complete cleft of the lip and palate, fistulas are also commonly seen at the junction of the premaxilla and lateral segments of the maxilla.

A nasolabial fistula is an opening in the alveolus (high in the gum ridge just under the upper lip). It is sometimes called an intentional fistula. This is because it is often left deliberately by the surgeon during the initial lip and alveolar ridge repair to allow for unrestricted maxillary

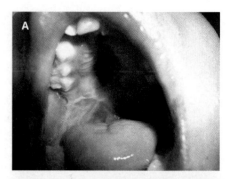

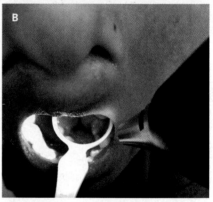

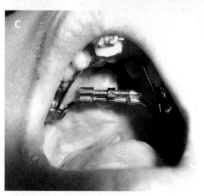

FIGURE 5-15 Oronasal (palatal) fistula.

growth for a period of time (Folk, D'Antonio, & Hardesty, 1997). The nasolabial fistula is later closed by an alveolar bone graft when permanent teeth begin to erupt.

Depending on its location and size, a fistula may be asymptomatic for speech yet may cause regurgitation of fluids (and sometimes food) into the nasal cavity. In particular, it is common for a

SPEECH NOTES

Fistulas

A nasolabial fistula does not affect speech because it is located under the lip and out of the way of the airflow and speech sound articulation.

The effect of an oronasal fistula on speech depends on both its size and location. Anterior fistulas will affect speech more than posterior fistulas because the upward movement of the tongue can push air into the opening. A small palatal fistula is usually not symptomatic because during production of most speech phonemes, the course of the airflow is horizontal to the fistula opening. If the fistula is in the area of the incisive foramen however, nasal emission on lingual-alveolar sounds may be noted because as the tongue tip elevates for the sound production, it may push the airstream into the fistula. A medium-sized fistula can cause consistent nasal air emission on all sounds, particularly anterior sounds. There may also be compensatory productions to either close the fistula with the tongue or to articulate sounds behind the fistula, before the air leak. A very large fistula causes hypernasality, in addition to nasal emission.

Research has shown that an anterior leak of air through an open fistula can affect the function of the velopharyngeal valve as well (Isberg & Henningsson, 1987; Tachimura, Hara, Koh, & Wada, 1997). Therefore, evaluation of velopharyngeal function must be done with this in mind.

Palatal fistulas are typically surgically closed with the bone graft, which is timed with the eruption of teeth. If the fistula is causing both nasal emission and hypernasality, an obturator can be used until the fistula can be surgically repaired.

nasolabial fistula to cause slight regurgitation of food (particularly chocolate and red sauce) in the corresponding nostril. A large palatal fistula can cause food to become stuck in the opening and even in the nasal cavity.

Tonsils and Adenoids

There are actually three types of "tonsils": the palatine tonsils (usually known as just the "tonsils"), which are located between the anterior and posterior faucial pillars in the oral cavity; the pharyngeal tonsil, also known as the "adenoids," which resides in the nasopharynx; and the lingual tonsil, which is located at the base of the tongue. Tonsils are composed of lymphatic tissue and serve as part of the body's immune system in children.

Tonsils and adenoids start to grow after birth and are at their largest when a child is around 6 years old. By age 7 to 8, this tissue starts to shrink, and by the late teens, they are usually barely visible. Most adults have minimal, if any, tonsil or adenoid tissue.

In addition to their role in the immune system, adenoids can actually assist with velopharyngeal closure because of their location in the nasopharynx. In fact, young children with a prominent adenoid pad usually have veloadenoidal closure rather than velopharyngeal closure (Maryn, Van Lierde, De Bodt, & Van Cauwenberge, 2004).

Tonsil and adenoid tissue is particularly prone to hypertrophy (abnormal enlargement of a part of the body caused by enlargement of its constituent cells) in young children. The etiology for the overgrowth of this tissue is unknown, but it is thought to be secondary to chronic stimulation from infection or allergic sources. Adenoid and/or tonsillar hypertrophy often causes upper airway obstruction and abnormal resonance, which is further described as follows.

Tonsillar Hypertrophy

Hypertrophy of the faucial tonsils is typically graded on a 4-point scale. Tonsils that are 1+ in size are contained within the faucial pillars; tonsils that are 2+ extend minimally beyond the faucial pillars; tonsils that are 3+ obstruct the oropharyngeal inlet to a moderate degree; and tonsils that are 4+ in size touch in the midline (**FIGURE 5-16**).

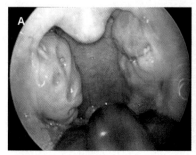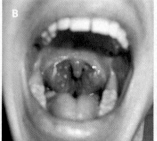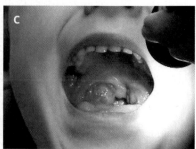

FIGURE 5-16 Hypertrophic tonsils. **(A)** and **(B)** Grade 3+ tonsils. **(C)** Grade 4+ tonsils.

SPEECH NOTES

Tonsillar Hypertrophy

Enlarged tonsils can affect speech and resonance in several ways:

- If one tonsil (or both of the tonsils) pushes posteriorly against the posterior faucial pillar, it can limit the function of the palatopharyngeus muscle and therefore affect lateral pharyngeal wall movement. This typically causes a small velopharyngeal opening, resulting in nasal emission.
- If the tonsils expand posteriorly so they are in the pharynx, they can affect the transmission of sound into the nasal cavity, resulting in hyponasality.
- Occasionally, a tonsil extends into the pharynx and then upward so that it is between the velum and posterior pharyngeal wall during velopharyngeal closure. This usually results in an incomplete velopharyngeal seal with small gaps on either side of the interfering tonsil. These small gaps typically cause audible nasal emission/rustle (see Figure 10-18B and Figure 10-18C in the chapter *Speech/ Resonance Disorders and Velopharyngeal Dysfunction*) (Finkelstein, Bar-Ziv, Nachmani, Berger, & Ophir, 1993; Kummer, Billmire, & Myer, 1993; MacKenzie-Stepner, Witzel, Stringer, & Laskin, 1987; Shprintzen, Sher, & Croft, 1987).
- If the tonsils expand toward midline, resulting in "kissing tonsils," they will block sound and airflow from entering the oral cavity, thus causing pharyngeal cul-de-sac resonance (see the chapter *Speech/ Resonance Disorders and Velopharyngeal Dysfunction* for more information about resonance).
- If the tonsils expand anteriorly, articulation of posterior sounds (e.g., /k/ and /g/) can be affected. As a result, the individual may compensate by fronting (i.e., t/k, d/g).
- If there is airway obstruction with tonsillar hypertrophy, regardless of the direction of expansion, the tongue is often displaced down and forward in order to open the airway. This can cause fronting of sibilants and even fronting of lingual-alveolar sounds.

Overall, hypertrophic tonsils can cause a mixture of hyponasality, pharyngeal cul-de-sac resonance, nasal emission, and abnormal articulation—sometimes in the same patient (Al-Shamaa, Jefferson, & Ball, 2003; Feilberg, Sorensen, & Eriksen, 1993; Oulis, Vadiakas, Ekonomides, & Dratsa, 1994; Singh, Gathwala, Pathania, Singh, & Yadav, 1994) (see the chapter *Speech/Resonance Disorders and Velopharyngeal Dysfunction* for more information). In addition, they can cause difficulty passing food from the oral cavity to the pharynx during swallowing because of the blockage at the back of the oral cavity. The treatment for these speech, resonance, and swallowing problems is tonsillectomy.

Occasionally, one tonsil will be significantly larger than the other (**FIGURE 5-17**). This abnormal growth pattern can be a cause of concern and should be further investigated.

Tonsils that are excessively large (grade 3+ or larger) may expand anteriorly, medially, or posteriorly. If they expand posteriorly, they may intrude into the oropharynx. In severe cases,

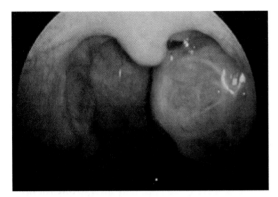

FIGURE 5-17 A large tonsil on the patient's left side. Asymmetric tonsils are a cause for concern because a tumor may be causing the abnormal growth pattern. In this example, the left tonsil is a grade 4+, whereas the right tonsil is a grade 1+.

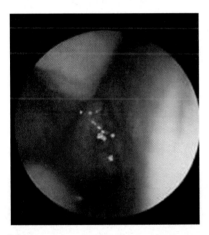

FIGURE 5-18 Adenoid tissue blocking the choana. This can have a significant effect on nasal respiration and also affect nasal resonance.

they may even expand upward into the nasopharynx, thus interfering with velopharyngeal function.

Adenoid Hypertrophy

Adenoid hypertrophy can cause obstruction of the nasopharyngeal airway and can even block the choanal openings at the back of the nasal cavity (**FIGURE 5-18**). This can cause upper airway obstruction, characterized by mouth breathing, snoring, and even sleep apnea.

Lingual Tonsil Hypertrophy

Lingual tonsil hypertrophy occurs infrequently and rarely becomes large enough to require removal. However, lingual tonsil hypertrophy can be a particular problem for children with Down syndrome (Al-Shamaa et al., 2003; Donnelly, Shott, LaRose, Chini, & Amin, 2004) (**FIGURE 5-19**).

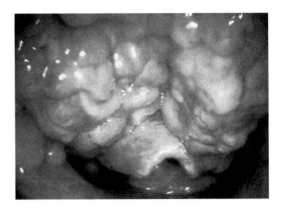

FIGURE 5-19 Lingual tonsils. Lingual tonsils are located in the base of the tongue. When enlarged, they can cause significant obstruction of airway. In this case, the larynx cannot be seen because of the enlargement of the lingual tonsils, which completely fill the vallecula.

Adenotonsillar hypertrophy is the enlargement of both the tonsil and adenoid tissue. Adenotonsillar hypertrophy may be relative in that it can occur with normal-sized tonsils and adenoid tissue but with relatively small adjacent structures. For example, patients with midface hypoplasia, as in Crouzon, Apert, and Down syndromes, may have an adenoid pad situated in a relatively small nasopharynx, creating obstructive symptoms. A similar problem may occur in patients with micrognathia (as is common in Pierre Robin sequence) where normal tonsil and adenoid tissue combined with a narrow oropharyngeal inlet and glossoptosis can create upper airway obstruction.

Adenoid Atrophy

Almost all children are able to maintain velopharyngeal closure as the adenoid tissue begins to gradually atrophy. However, children with a history of cleft palate, submucous cleft, or tenuous velopharyngeal closure may begin to show evidence of mild velopharyngeal insufficiency, particularly around puberty. If this occurs, surgical intervention is needed for correction (Mason & Warren, 1980; Siegel-Sadewitz & Shprintzen, 1986).

Laryngeal Anomalies

Congenital laryngeal anomalies (i.e., laryngomalacia, laryngeal web, laryngoesophageal cleft, and vocal fold paralysis) are common in children born with craniofacial syndromes. Laryngomalacia is a congenital softening of the tissues of the larynx above the vocal folds. It is the most common cause of noisy breathing in infancy. For most infants, this resolves without treatment by 18 to 20 months of age. A laryngeal web is characterized by tissue between the vocal folds near the anterior commissure (**FIGURE 5-20**). It can cause shortness of breath, a weak cry, stridor (a high-pitched, wheezing sound), poor feeding, hoarseness, and aphonia. Surgical treatment is needed to break the web to eliminate airway obstruction. A laryngeal web is a common phenotypic feature of velocardiofacial/22q11.2 deletion syndrome. A laryngoesophageal cleft is characterized by an opening between the larynx and the esophagus. This can cause aspiration of food or liquids when the child swallows. Therefore, it requires immediate surgical correction. Congenital vocal fold paralysis is the absence of movement of one or both vocal folds caused by dysfunction of the motor nerve supply to the larynx. The symptoms include stridor, a weak cry or voice, feeding difficulties, and aspiration. Treatment may include surgery, depending on a patient's symptoms, particularly the extent of airway compromise

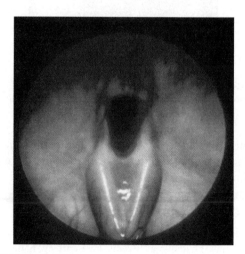

FIGURE 5-20 Laryngeal web. A laryngeal web can cause significant breathing problems. Affected patients often have very strident breathing. A laryngeal web is often seen with velocardiofacial/22q11.2 deletion syndrome.

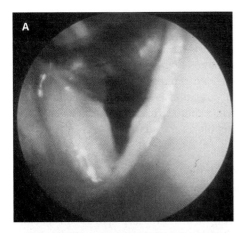

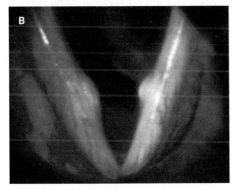

FIGURE 5-21 Vocal nodules.

and aspiration. Finally, children with congenital anomalies are not immune to acquired conditions, such as vocal nodules (**FIGURE 5-21**).

Upper Airway Obstruction

As previously mentioned, upper airway obstruction in children is commonly caused by tonsillar and/or adenoid hypertrophy. Evidence of airway obstruction is often visible on the child's face. The typical adenoid facies (which can be seen with tonsillar hypertrophy as well) is characterized by an open-mouth posture, anterior tongue position, the forward and downward position of the mandible, facial elongation, suborbital coloring ("black eyes"), puffy eyes, and the appearance of pinched nostrils. Symptoms of airway obstruction from adenoid and/or tonsillar hypertrophy

may also include stertorous (a heavy snoring sound) breathing, chronic mouth breathing, loud snoring, and even obstructive sleep apnea.

Obstructive sleep apnea (OSA) is a disorder that is characterized by long pauses in breathing during sleep from upper airway obstruction. An obstructive sleep apnea event is a period when the person is exerting muscular forces to inspire but is unsuccessful in moving air into the lungs because of a blockage in the upper airway. The obstructed airway is further compromised during deep sleep by generalized hypotonia that causes collapse of the hypopharyngeal structures. In a supine position, the tongue base retrodisplaces, causing further compromise of the airway. Common characteristics of sleep apnea include restlessness during sleep and constant tossing and turning to find a position where breathing requires less effort. When observed in children, this is significant and requires attention. Polysomnography (an overnight sleep study) is used to diagnosis sleep disturbances to determine appropriate treatment.

The diagnosis of obstructive sleep apnea is a confirmation that the individual's sleep is inadequate, causing the person to be tired during the day. This can impair concentration, memory, and daily function at school (or work). It can also cause hyperactivity, behavior issues, and learning problems in children. Sleep apnea contributes to a long-term risk for weight issues, cardiovascular disease, heart attack, stroke, hypertension, and depression. Because of the short- and long-term effects that sleep apnea can have on learning, quality of life, and even long-term health, it should be considered in all children with craniofacial anomalies and actively treated whenever it is diagnosed (Carter & Watenpaugh, 2008; Jayaraman, Sharafkhaneh, Hirshkowitz, & Sharafkhaneh, 2008). Following are treatment methods to relieve or eliminate upper airway obstruction.

Tracheostomy

A tracheostomy is a surgical procedure that is done to relieve conditions that cause life-threatening airway obstruction. It is often done for infants soon after birth.

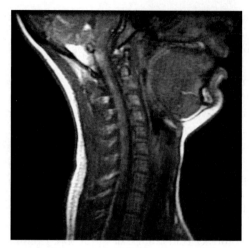

FIGURE 5-22 Glossoptosis. The radiograph shows a tongue base that is blocking the pharynx, causing significant airway obstruction.

The tracheostomy procedure is done by making a vertical incision in the midline of the neck overlying the trachea. The trachea is then incised vertically, usually through the third and fourth rings, creating an opening in the anterior wall. A tracheostomy tube is then inserted into the tracheal opening, and the edges of the opening are sutured to the skin in the neck. This creates a surgically created stoma (an opening into a hollow organ) through which the patient can breathe.

Tracheostomy is often indicated for certain congenital anomalies, such as subglottic stenosis, tracheal stenosis, or laryngeal web. Infants born with Pierre Robin sequence are often candidates for tracheostomy caused by the airway problems that occur as a result of the small mandible (micrognathia) and glossoptosis (**FIGURE 5-22**). Tracheostomy is also indicated for patients who cannot adequately raise secretions from their airway and therefore need frequent suctioning. This includes patients who are unconscious and those who are unable to cough because of paralysis or significant chest pain.

Mandibular Distraction

Mandibular distraction can be done to help relieve tongue-based upper airway obstruction in newborns. It is usually started in the first few weeks of life. Bone cuts are made through the mandible at an angle on both sides. Distraction devices are then used to pull the jaw forward. New bone rapidly forms to fill in the gap on both sides, thus creating a longer mandible. This provides more space for the tongue so that it no longer blocks the airway.

Tonsillectomy

Tonsillectomy is indicated for hypertrophic tonsils that are affecting speech and resonance or causing obstructive sleep apnea. Tonsillectomy is also indicated for recurrent tonsillitis or peritonsillar abscess.

Because the tonsils reside in the oral cavity, they do not contribute to velopharyngeal function. Therefore, tonsillectomy is *not* contraindicated for patients with cleft palate, submucous

SPEECH NOTES

Tonsillectomy

Tonsillectomy typically results in either no effect on speech or a positive effect. The positive effect may be the elimination of cul-de-sac resonance by removing the blockage at the entrance to the oral cavity. It can also eliminate nasal emission from the interference of the tonsils in velopharyngeal closure.

Despite this, hypernasality has been reported following tonsillectomy in a few rare cases (Gibb & Stewart, 1975; Haapanen, Ignatius, Rihkanen, & Ertama, 1994; Mora et al., 2009; Subramaniam & Kumar, 2009). This can be caused by either abnormal scarring of the faucial pillars, which can restrict lateral or pharyngeal wall movement, or a postoperative "protection response" secondary to the pain of the procedure. With this protection response, the patient avoids velopharyngeal movement for both swallowing and speech; this avoidance can remain as a habit long after the pain is gone. Fortunately, this is easy to correct with only a few speech therapy sessions.

cleft, or velopharyngeal insufficiency (D'Antonio, Snyder, & Samadani, 1996; Paulson, Macarthur, Beaulieu, Brockman, & Milczuk, 2012). When a tonsillectomy is done, the tonsils are removed in their entirety, including the capsule deep under the tonsil. Therefore, they do not grow back.

Adenoidectomy

The indications for adenoidectomy include hyponasality, intractable middle ear effusion, or obstructive sleep apnea (Abdel-Aziz, 2012; Darrow & Siemens, 2002). With adenoidectomy, the capsule deep to the adenoid pad is left in place because it protects the underlying bone of the skull base. Because the capsule is left in place, some regrowth of the adenoid can occur over time.

Continuous Positive Airway Pressure

Frequently, continuous positive airway pressure therapy is required for long-term treatment of obstructive sleep apnea. Continuous positive airway pressure (CPAP) is a method to keep the nasopharyngeal airway open during sleep by applying mild air pressure on a continuous basis through the nose and pharynx. The CPAP equipment consists of a face mask and an air pressure generator. The patient wears the mask over the

SPEECH NOTES

Adenoidectomy

The irregular surface that occurs with adenoid regrowth after adenoidectomy can affect the firmness of the veloadenoidal seal during speech. This usually causes a small velopharyngeal opening during speech and thus nasal emission. This small velopharyngeal opening may disappear in time as the adenoid pad begins to atrophy before puberty. In some cases, however, another partial adenoidectomy to smooth the surface may be considered.

Velopharyngeal insufficiency following adenoidectomy is a risk, although the risk is minimal for most children (Abdel-Aziz, Dewidar, El-Hoshy, & Aziz, 2009; Donnelly, 1994; Fernandes, Grobbelaar, Hudson, & Lentin, 1996; Parton & Jones, 1998; Pulkkinen, Ranta, Heliovaara, & Haapanen, 2002; Ren, Isberg, & Henningsson, 1995; Saunders, Hartley, Sell, & Sommerlad, 2004; Witzel, Rich, Margar-Bacal & Cox, 1986). The risk has been estimated to be between 1 in 500 and 1 in 3000 (Stewart, Ahmed, Razzell, & Watson, 2002).

Temporary velopharyngeal insufficiency during the first few weeks following adenoidectomy is very common. With removal of the adenoid pad, the soft palate must extend farther posteriorly, or the lateral walls must extend farther medially to achieve closure. Most children are able to accomplish this adjustment in velopharyngeal function within a few days or weeks. If hypernasality and/or nasal emission persists beyond 6 to 8 weeks, however, it is unlikely that it will resolve spontaneously. In these cases, surgical repair by a surgeon experienced with cleft palate is required. It should be noted that speech therapy will not correct hypernasality or nasal emission following adenoidectomy because the cause is abnormal structure, not abnormal function.

There are several risk factors for velopharyngeal insufficiency following adenoidectomy. The biggest risk factor is a cleft palate or a submucous cleft. In fact, patients who have hypernasality after adenoidectomy are frequently found to have an occult submucous cleft on further inspection (Parton & Jones, 1998; Saunders et al., 2004; Schmaman, Jordaan, & Jammine, 1998). Other risk factors include a family history of cleft palate or hypernasality, sucking difficulties as an infant, and oral-motor dysfunction or other neuromuscular problems.

If the patient has upper airway obstruction from enlarged adenoids yet has one or more of these risk factors, a conservative superior half adenoidectomy can be performed (Finkelstein, Wexler, Nachmani, & Ophir, 2002). With this procedure, the airway obstruction is reduced by removing the superior half of the adenoid tissue, which can obstruct the choanae, while maintaining adequate tissue inferiorly for the velum to close against for speech.

nose during sleep, and a certain level of pressure, usually in the range of 6 to 20 cm H_2O, is delivered to the pharynx through the nose. This forces the pharyngeal airway open and prevents pharyngeal collapse during respiration. Although CPAP is effective in overcoming the effects of obstructive sleep apnea, long-term nightly use of the machine leads to a high degree of noncompliance over time.

Uvulopalatopharyngoplasty

In the pediatric population, upper airway obstruction is primarily caused by adenotonsillar hypertrophy and is therefore treated by adenotonsillectomy. In teenagers and adults, however, the tonsils and adenoids are very small and therefore are not likely to cause obstruction. Obstructive sleep apnea in older patients is often secondary to redundant mucosa of the soft palate and posterior pharyngeal wall, causing the oropharyngeal inlet to be small. In these cases, the treatment of the obstruction is a surgical procedure called **uvulopalatopharyngoplasty (UPPP)** (Aneeza et al., 2011; Blythe, Henrich, & Pillsbury, 1995; Croft & Golding-Wood, 1990; Han, Xu, Hu, & Zhang, 2012; Kavey, Whyte, Blitzer, & Gidro-Frank, 1990; Yanagisawa & Weaver, 1997).

As part of the UPPP, the remaining tonsil tissue is removed, and the anterior and posterior tonsillar pillars are sewn together to open the oropharyngeal inlet. The free margin of the soft palate is resected along with the uvula, and the raw edges of the soft palate are sewn together, shortening the soft palate. Although snoring is usually markedly improved as a result of this procedure, the overall effect on the sleep apnea is often disappointing.

There are a few other surgical procedures that can be done for obstructive sleep apnea. They include moving the tongue base anteriorly; reducing the size of the tongue base; or bringing the mandible forward, along with the tongue.

SPEECH NOTES

Uvulopalatopharyngoplasty

If done properly, uvulopalatopharyngoplasty (UPPP) does not have a negative effect on velopharyngeal function and thus on resonance. This is because the velar tissue that is removed is below the area of normal velar contact with the posterior pharyngeal wall. However, if the surgeon is too aggressive and removes too much of the velum under its bend, it can affect the patient's resonance and also cause nasal regurgitation during swallowing (Rihkanen & Soini, 1992; Salas-Provance & Kuehn, 1990; Tewary & Cable, 1993).

CASE REPORT

Upper Airway Obstruction, Hypernasality, and Continuous Positive Airway Pressure

Tam was a Vietnamese male born with bilateral complete cleft lip and palate. The cleft lip was closed in Vietnam, but the palate was left unrepaired. When Tam entered the United States at the age of 21, the palate was still open, and he did not speak any English. Soon after arriving in this country, the palate was repaired, and a pharyngeal flap (to correct velopharyngeal insufficiency) was done. Although the prognosis for correcting speech is guarded when the palate is closed that late, Tam exceeded all expectations. He received several months of speech therapy following his surgery and quickly developed oral production of speech sounds while learning English.

Tam was seen for an evaluation in the VPI Clinic several years later, at the age of 27. At that time, articulation was normal for the production of all speech sounds. Resonance was found to be mildly hypernasal, and there was barely audible nasal air emission during the production of pressure-sensitive phonemes. Overall, Tam was happy with his speech. However, he reported difficulty with nasal breathing and significant snoring at night, which was the primary reason for his return. A sleep study was done, which confirmed obstructive sleep apnea (OSA).

A nasopharyngoscopy (endoscopy) assessment showed the cause of these symptoms. Although the pharyngeal flap was an appropriate width and in good position, there was a leak in the left port during speech, causing slight nasal emission. At the same time, the lateral ports on either side of the flap were too small for normal nasal breathing and the likely cause for the OSA.

With this combination of symptoms, determining the appropriate treatment is a challenge. If the left port were narrowed further to eliminate the nasal emission during speech, it would increase the airway problems. On the other hand, opening the ports to improve nasal breathing would increase the nasal emission and probably cause hypernasality.

After discussing the options with Tam, he decided to forgo further surgical intervention. Instead, he began using continuous positive airway pressure (CPAP) at night, which resulted in significant improvement in his sleep. With this option, the flap could be left intact for speech, yet the airway was forced open at night for sleep.

SUMMARY

Facial, oral, and pharyngeal anomalies can be congenital or acquired. It is important to recognize that these types of anomalies can cause airway obstruction, feeding/swallowing dysfunction, speech disorders, and abnormal resonance. Although many laypeople, and even professionals, believe that ankyloglossia is a cause of abnormal speech, there is no current evidence to support that belief.

Clinical providers should understand how the tonsils and adenoids affect speech and resonance and how surgical removal of this tissue can have a positive, or sometimes negative, effect on speech and resonance. Finally, speech-language pathologists and otolaryngologists need to work together to adequately diagnose and treat disorders that are caused by facial, oral, and pharyngeal anomalies.

FOR REVIEW AND DISCUSSION

1. Describe the potential malformations of the ears in patients who have craniofacial anomalies.

2. Describe normal eustachian tube function, including the action of the muscle. What happens if the eustachian tube does not function normally?

3. Why are young children more prone to otitis media than adults? Why are children with cleft palate particularly at risk for chronic middle ear effusion and recurrent otitis media? What can be done prophylactically for children who are at particular risk?

4. Describe potential malformations of the nose. How could these malformations affect resonance? If there is abnormal resonance, is the individual a candidate for speech therapy? Why or why not?

5. How does maxillary retrusion affect the nose and pharynx? How does that affect function?

6. What potential problems can be caused by ankyloglossia? Why is ankyloglossia unlikely to cause speech problems?

7. How does macroglossia affect speech and resonance?

8. Describe the location of the tonsils and adenoids. Why are irregular adenoids a potential problem for speech?

9. What are the potential effects of tonsillar hypertrophy on speech and resonance? What are the potential effects of adenoid hypertrophy on speech and resonance?

10. Describe the potential benefits of tonsillectomy. Describe the potential risks and benefits of adenoidectomy. What is the treatment of post-adenoidectomy velopharyngeal insufficiency?

11. Why is it important to discuss the tonsils and adenoids separately? Why do you think people confuse the risk and benefits of tonsillectomy versus adenoidectomy?

12. What are treatment options for upper airway obstruction? When is tracheostomy appropriate? When is uvulopalatopharyngoplasty (UPPP) appropriate? When is CPAP appropriate?

REFERENCES

Abdel-Aziz, M. (2012). The effectiveness of tonsillectomy and partial adenoidectomy on obstructive sleep apnea in cleft palate patients. *Laryngoscope, 122*(11), 2563–2567.

Abdel-Aziz, M., Dewidar, H., El-Hoshy, H., & Aziz, A. A. (2009). Treatment of persistent post-adenoidectomy velopharyngeal insufficiency by sphincter pharyngoplasty. *International Journal of Pediatric Otorhinolaryngology, 73*(10), 1329–1333.

Agency for Healthcare Research and Quality (AHRQ). (2015). Treatments for ankyloglossia and ankyloglossia with concomitant lip-tie. *Comparative Effectiveness Review, 149.* Retrieved from https://www.ncbi.nlm.nih.gov/books/NBK299120/

Alasti, F., & Van Camp, G. (2009). Genetics of microtia and associated syndromes. *Journal of Medical Genetics, 46*(6), 361–369.

Alper, C. M., Losee, J., Mandel, E. M., Seroky, J. T., Swarts, J. D., & Doyle, W. J. (2011). Post-palatoplasty eustachian tube function in young children with cleft palate. *The Cleft Palate–Craniofacial Journal, 49*(4), 504–507.

Alper, C. M., Losee, J. E., Mandel, E. M., Seroky, J. T., Swarts, J. D., & Doyle, W. J. (2012). Pre- and post-palatoplasty eustachian tube function in infants with cleft palate. *International Journal of Pediatric Otorhinolaryngology, 76*(3), 388–391.

Alper, C. M., Losee, J. E., Seroky, J. T., Mandel, E. M., Richert, B. C., & Doyle, W. J. (2016). Resolution of otitis media with effusion in children with cleft palate followed through five years of age. *The Cleft Palate–Craniofacial Journal, 53*(5), 607–613.

Al-Shamaa, M., Jefferson, P., & Ball, D. R. (2003). Lingual tonsil hypertrophy: Airway management. *Anaesthesia, 58*(11), 1134–1135.

American Academy of Family Physicians, American Academy of Otolaryngology Head and Neck Surgery, & American Academy of Pediatrics Subcommittee on Otitis Media with Effusion. (2004). Otitis media with effusion. *Pediatrics, 113*(5), 1412–1429.

American Cleft Palate–Craniofacial Association (ACPA). (2018). Parameters for evaluation and treatment of patients with cleft lip/palate or other craniofacial differences. Retrieved from http://acpa-cpf.org/team-care/standardscat/parameters-of-care/. Accessed February 4, 2018.

Aneeza, W. H., Marina, M. B., Razif, M. Y., Azimatun, N. A., Asma, A., & Sani, A. (2011). Effects of uvulopalatopharyngoplasty: A seven year review. *Medical Journal of Malaysia, 66*(2), 129–132.

Baudonck, N., Van Lierde, K., Dhooge, I., & Corthals, P. (2011). A comparison of vowel productions in prelingually deaf children using cochlear implants, severe hearing-impaired children using conventional hearing aids and normal-hearing children. *Folia Phoniatrica et Logopaedica, 63*(3), 154–160.

Blythe, W. R., Henrich, D. E., & Pillsbury, H. C. (1995). Outpatient uvuloplasty: An inexpensive, single-staged procedure for the relief of symptomatic snoring. *Otolaryngology–Head and Neck Surgery, 113*(1), 1–4.

Brent, B. (1999). The pediatrician's role in caring for patients with congenital microtia and atresia. *Pediatric Annals, 28*(2), 374–383.

Brown, O. E., Myer, C. M., III, & Manning, S. C. (1989). Congenital nasal pyriform aperture stenosis. *Laryngoscope, 99*(1), 86–91.

Carter, R., III, & Watenpaugh, D. E. (2008). Obesity and obstructive sleep apnea: Or is it OSA and obesity? *Pathophysiology, 15*(2), 71–77.

Chang, S. O., Lee, J. H., Choi, B. Y., & Song, J. J. (2007). Long term results of postoperative canal stenosis in congenital aural atresia surgery. *Acta Otolaryngologica* (558), 15–21.

Chen, W. X., & Wong, V. (2005). Prognosis of Bell's palsy in children: Analysis of 29 cases. *Brain and Development, 27*(7), 504–508.

Coez, A., Belin, P., Bizaguet, E., Ferrary, E., Zilbovicius, M., & Samson, Y. (2010). Hearing loss severity: Impaired processing of formant transition duration. *Neuropsychologia, 48*(10), 3057–3061.

Croft, C. B., & Golding-Wood, D. G. (1990). Uses and complications of uvulopalatopharyngoplasty. *Journal of Laryngology and Otology, 104*(11), 871–875.

D'Antonio, L. L., Snyder, L. S., & Samadani, S. (1996). Tonsillectomy in children with or at risk for velopharyngeal insufficiency: Effects on speech. *Otolaryngology–Head and Neck Surgery, 115*(4), 319–323.

Darrow, D. H., & Siemens, C. (2002). Indications for tonsillectomy and adenoidectomy. *Laryngoscope, 112*(8, Suppl. 100, Pt. 2), 6–10.

da Silva, D. P., Collares, M. V., & da Costa, S. S. (2010). Effects of velopharyngeal dysfunction on middle ear of repaired cleft palate patients. *The Cleft Palate–Craniofacial Journal, 47*(3), 225–233.

Donnelly, L. F., Shott, S. R., LaRose, C. R., Chini, B. A., & Amin, R. S. (2004). Causes of persistent obstructive sleep apnea despite previous tonsillectomy and adenoidectomy in children with Down syndrome as depicted on static and dynamic cine MRI. *American Journal of Roentgenology, 183*(1), 175–181.

Donnelly, M. J. (1994). Hypernasality following adenoid removal. *Irish Journal of Medical Science, 163*(5), 225–227.

Durr, D. G., & Shapiro, R. S. (1989). Otologic manifestations in congenital velopharyngeal insufficiency. *American Journal of Diseases of Children, 143*(1), 75–77.

Ertmer, D. J. (2011). Assessing speech intelligibility in children with hearing loss: Toward revitalizing a valuable clinical tool. *Language, Speech, and Hearing Services in Schools, 42*(1), 52–58.

Feilberg, V. L., Sorensen, J. N., & Eriksen, H. O. (1993). Hypertrophic tonsils, upper airway obstruction and cardiac complications: A combined otological, medical and anesthesiological problem. *Ugeskrift for Laeger, 155*(38), 3003–3005.

Fernandes, D. B., Grobbelaar, A. O., Hudson, D. A., & Lentin, R. (1996). Velopharyngeal incompetence after adenotonsillectomy in noncleft patients. *British Journal of Oral and Maxillofacial Surgery, 34*(5), 364–367.

Finkelstein, Y., Bar-Ziv, J., Nachmani, A., Berger, G., & Ophir, D. (1993). Peritonsillar abscess as a cause of transient velopharyngeal insufficiency. *The Cleft Palate–Craniofacial Journal, 30*(4), 421–428.

Finkelstein, Y., Wexler, D. B., Nachmani, A., & Ophir, D. (2002). Endoscopic partial adenoidectomy for children with submucous cleft palate. *The Cleft Palate–Craniofacial Journal, 39*(5), 479–486.

Fitzpatrick, E. M., Crawford, L., Ni, A., & Durieux-Smith, A. (2011). A descriptive analysis of language and speech skills in 4- to 5-yr-old children with hearing loss. *Ear and Hearing, 32*(5), 605–616.

Folk, S. N., D'Antonio, L. L., & Hardesty, R. A. (1997). Secondary cleft deformities. *Clinics in Plastic Surgery, 24*(3), 599–611.

Garcia Pola, M. J., Gonzalez Garcia, M., Garcia Martin, J. M., Gallas, M., & Seoane Leston, J. (2002). A study of pathology associated with short lingual frenum. *Journal of Dentistry for Children, 69*(1), 59–62.

Gates, G., Avery, C., Prihoda, T., & Cooper, J. J. (1987, December 3). Effectiveness of adenoidectomy and tympanostomy tubes in the treatment of chronic otitis media with effusion. *New England Journal of Medicine, 317*, 1444–1451.

Gibb, A. G., & Stewart, I. A. (1975). Hypernasality following tonsil dissection: Hysterical aetiology. *Journal of Laryngology and Otology, 89*(7), 779–781.

Goldberg, C., DeLorie, R., Zuker, R. M., & Manktelow, R. T. (2003). The effects of gracilis muscle transplantation on speech in children with Moebius syndrome. *Journal of Craniofacial Surgery, 14*(5), 687–690.

Grimmer, J. F., & Poe, D. S. (2005). Update on eustachian tube dysfunction and the patulous eustachian tube. *Current Opinion in Otolaryngology & Head and Neck Surgery, 13*(5), 277–282.

Haapanen, M. L., Ignatius, J., Rihkanen, H., & Ertama, L. (1994). Velopharyngeal insufficiency following palatine tonsillectomy. *European Archives of Oto-Rhino-Laryngology, 251*(3), 186–189.

Han, D., Xu, W., Hu, R., & Zhang, L. (2012). Voice function following Han's uvulopalatopharyngoplasty. *Journal of Laryngology and Otology, 126*(1), 47–51.

Heller, J. C., Gens, G. W., Croft, C. B., & Moe, D. G. (1978). Conductive hearing loss in patients with velopharyngeal insufficiency. *Cleft Palate Journal, 15*(3), 246–253.

Isberg, A., & Henningsson, G. (1987). Influence of palatal fistulas on velopharyngeal movements: A cineradiographic study. *Plastic and Reconstructive Surgery, 79*(4), 525–530.

Jayaraman, G., Sharafkhaneh, H., Hirshkowitz, M., & Sharafkhaneh, A. (2008). Pharmacotherapy of obstructive sleep apnea. *Therapeutic Advances in Respiratory Disease, 2*(6), 375–386.

Kavey, N. B., Whyte, J., Blitzer, A., & Gidro-Frank, S. (1990). Postsurgical evaluation of uvulopalatopharyngoplasty: Two case reports. *Sleep, 13*(1), 79–84.

Kawakami, M., Yagi, T., & Takada, K. (2002). Maxillary expansion and protraction in correction of midface retrusion in a complete unilateral cleft lip and palate patient. *Angle Orthodontics, 72*(4), 355–361.

Kern, I. (1991, July 1). Tongue tie. *Medical Journal of Australia, 155,* 33–34.

Kosling, S., Omenzetter, M., & Bartel-Friedrich, S. (2009). Congenital malformations of the external and middle ear. *European Journal of Radiology, 69*(2), 269–279.

Kountakis, S., Helidonis, E., & Jahrsdoerfer, R. (1995). Microtia grade as an indicator of middle ear development in aural atresia. *Archives of Otolaryngology–Head & Neck Surgery, 121*(8), 885–886.

Kubba, H., Bennett, A., & Bailey, C. M. (2004). An update on choanal atresia surgery at Great Ormond Street Hospital for Children: Preliminary results with Mitomycin C and the KTP laser. *International Journal of Pediatric Otorhinolaryngology, 68*(7), 939–945.

Kummer, A. W. (2005, December 27). To clip or not to clip? That's the question. *The ASHA Leader, 10*(17), 6–7, 30.

Kummer, A. W., Billmire, D. A., & Myer, C. M. D. (1993). Hypertrophic tonsils: The effect on resonance and velopharyngeal closure. *Plastic and Reconstructive Surgery, 91*(4), 608–611.

Liu, L., Sun, Y., & Zhao, W. (2001). The effects of otitis media with effusion and hearing loss on the speech outcome after cleft palate surgery. *Zhonghua Kou Qiang Yi Xue Za Zhi, 36*(6), 424–426.

Luquetti, D. V., Heike, C. L., Hing, A. V., Cunningham, M. L., & Cox, T. C. (2011). Microtia: Epidemiology and genetics. *American Journal of Medical Genetics Part A, 158A*(1), 124–139.

MacKenzie-Stepner, K., Witzel, M. A., Stringer, D. A., & Laskin, R. (1987). Velopharyngeal insufficiency due to hypertrophic tonsils: A report of two cases. *International Journal of Pediatric Otorhinolaryngology, 14*(1), 57–63.

Maryn, Y., Van Lierde, K., De Bodt, M., & Van Cauwenberge, P. (2004). The effects of adenoidectomy and tonsillectomy on speech and nasal resonance. *Folia Phoniatrica et Logopedica, 56*(3), 182–191.

Mason, R. M., & Warren, D. W. (1980). Adenoid involution and developing hypernasality in cleft palate. *Journal of Speech and Hearing Disorders, 45*(4), 469–480.

Meyerson, M. D., & Foushee, D. R. (1978). Speech, language and hearing in Moebius syndrome: A study of 22 patients. *Developmental Medicine & Child Neurology, 20*(3), 357–365.

Moeller, M.P., McCleary, E., Putman, C., Tyler-Krings, A., Hoover, B., & Stelmachowicz, P. (2010). Longitudinal development of phonology and morphology in children with late-identified mild-moderate sensorineural hearing loss. *Ear and Hearing, 31*(5), 625–635.

Moller, K. T. (1994). Dental-occlusal and other oral conditions and speech. In J. E. Bernthal & N. W. Bankson (Eds.), *Child phonology: Characteristics, assessment, and intervention with special populations* (pp. 3–28). New York, NY: Thieme Medical Publishers.

Moores, D. F. (2005). Cochlear implants: An update. *American Annals of the Deaf, 150*(4), 327–328.

Mora, R., Jankowska, B., Mora, F., Crippa, B., Dellepiane, M., & Salami, A. (2009). Effects of tonsillectomy on speech and voice. *Journal of Voice, 23*(5), 614–618.

Nguyen, L. H., Manoukian, J. J., Yoskovitch, A., & Al-Sebeih, K. H. (2004). Adenoidectomy: Selection criteria for surgical cases of otitis media. *Laryngoscope, 114*(5), 863–866.

Oulis, C. J., Vadiakas, G. P., Ekonomides, J., & Dratsa, J. (1994). The effect of hypertrophic adenoids and tonsils on the development of posterior crossbite and oral habits. *Journal of Clinical Pediatric Dentistry, 18*(3), 197–201.

Paradise, J. L. (1976). Management of middle ear effusions in infants with cleft palate. *Annals of Otology,*

Rhinology, and Laryngology, 85(2, Suppl. 25, Pt. 2), 285–288.

Paradise, J. L., Alberti, P. W., Bluestone, C. D., Cheek, D. B., Lis, E. F., & Stool, S. E. (1974). Pediatric and otologic aspects of clinical research in cleft palate. *Clinics in Pediatrics (Philadelphia), 13*(7), 587–593.

Paradise, J. L., & Bluestone, C. D. (1974). Early treatment of the universal otitis media of infants with cleft palate. *Pediatrics, 53*(1), 48–54.

Parton, M. J., & Jones, A. S. (1998). Hypernasality following adenoidectomy: A significant and avoidable complication. *Clinics in Otolaryngology, 23*(1), 18–19.

Paulson, L. M., Macarthur, C. J., Beaulieu, K. B., Brockman, J. H., & Milczuk, H. A. (2012). Speech outcomes after tonsillectomy in patients with known velopharyngeal insufficiency. *International Journal of Otolaryngology, 2012.* doi:10.1155/2012/912767

Peitersen, E. (1992). Natural history of Bell's palsy. *Acta Oto-Laryngologica, 492*(Suppl.), 122–124.

Pulkkinen, J., Ranta, R., Heliovaara, A., & Haapanen, M. L. (2002). Craniofacial characteristics and velopharyngeal function in cleft lip/palate children with and without adenoidectomy. *European Archives of Oto-Rhino-Laryngology, 259*(2), 100–104.

Ren, Y. F., Isberg, A., & Henningsson, G. (1995). Velopharyngeal incompetence and persistent hypernasality after adenoidectomy in children without palatal defect. *The Cleft Palate–Craniofacial Journal, 32*(6), 476–482.

Rihkanen, H., & Soini, I. (1992). Changes in voice characteristics after uvulopalatopharyngoplasty. *European Archives of Otorhinolaryngology, 249*(6), 322–324.

Rosenfeld, R. M., Culpepper, L., Doyle, K. J., Grundfast, K. M., Hoberman, A., Kenna, M. A., . . . Yawn, B. (2004). Clinical practice guideline: Otitis media with effusion. *Otolaryngology–Head & Neck Surgery, 130*(5, Suppl.), 95–118.

Rosenfeld, R., Shin, J., Schwartz, S., Coggins, R., Gagnon, G., Hackell, J., . . . Corrigan, M. D. (2016). Clinical practice guideline: Otitis media with effusion (Update). *Otolaryngology–Head and Neck Surgery, 154,* S1–S41.

Rvachew, S., Slawinski, E., Williams, M., & Green, C. (1999). The impact of early onset otitis media on babbling and early language development. *Journal of the Acoustical Society of America, 105*(1), 467–475.

Salas-Provance, M. B., & Kuehn, D. P. (1990). Speech status following uvulopalatopharyngoplasty. *Chest, 97*(1), 111–117.

Sapci, T., Mercangoz, E., Evcimik, M. F., Karavus, A., & Gozke, E. (2008). The evaluation of the tensor veli palatini muscle function with electromyography in chronic middle ear diseases. *European Archives of Oto-Rhino-Laryngology, 265*(3), 271–278.

Saunders, N. C., Hartley, B. E., Sell, D., & Sommerlad, B. (2004). Velopharyngeal insufficiency following adenoidectomy. *Clinical Otolaryngology & Allied Sciences, 29*(6), 686–688.

Schmaman, L., Jordaan, H., & Jammine, G. H. (1998). Risk factors for permanent hypernasality after adenoidectomy. *South African Medical Journal, 88*(3), 266–269.

Sheahan, P., Miller, L., Earley, M. J., Sheahan, J. N., & Blayney, A. W. (2004). Middle ear disease in children with congenital velopharyngeal insufficiency. *The Cleft Palate–Craniofacial Journal, 41*(4), 364–367.

Shprintzen, R. J., Sher, A. E., & Croft, C. B. (1987). Hypernasal speech caused by tonsillar hypertrophy. *International Journal of Pediatric Otorhinolaryngology, 14*(1), 45–56.

Siegel-Sadewitz, V. L., & Shprintzen, R. J. (1986). Changes in velopharyngeal valving with age. *International Journal of Pediatric Otorhinolaryngology, 11*(2), 171–182.

Singh, I., Gathwala, G., Pathania, R., Singh, J., & Yadav, S. P. (1994). Hypertrophic tonsils causing articulation defect. *Indian Journal of Pediatrics, 61*(1), 106–107.

Sininger, Y., Doyle, K., & Moore, J. (1999). The case for early identification of hearing loss in children: Auditory system development, experimental auditory deprivation, and development of speech perception and hearing. *Pediatric Clinics of North America, 46*(2), 1–14.

Stewart, K. J., Ahmed, R. E., Razzell, R. E., & Watson, A. C. H. (2002). Altered speech following adenoidectomy: A 20 year experience. *British Journal of Plastic Surgery, 55,* 469–473.

Subramaniam, V., & Kumar, P. (2009). Impact of tonsillectomy with or without adenoidectomy on the acoustic parameters of the voice: A comparative study. *Archives of Otolaryngology–Head & Neck Surgery, 135*(10), 966–969.

Tachimura, T., Hara, H., Koh, H., & Wada, T. (1997). Effect of temporary closure of oronasal fistulae on levator veli palatini muscle activity. *The Cleft Palate–Craniofacial Journal, 34*(6), 505–511.

Teele, D., Klein, J., & Rosner, B. (1980). Epidemiology of otitis media in children. *Annals of Otology, Rhinology, and Laryngology, 89*(3, Suppl.), 5–6.

Terzis, J. K., & Anesti, K. (2011). Experience with developmental facial paralysis: Part I. Diagnosis and associated stigmata. *Plastic and Reconstructive Surgery, 128*(5), 488e–497e.

Tewary, A. K., & Cable, H. R. (1993). Speech changes following uvulopalatopharyngoplasty. *Clinical Otolaryngology and Allied Sciences, 18*(5), 390–391.

Topouzelis, N., Iliopoulos, C., & Kolokitha, O. E. (2011). Macroglossia. *International Dental Journal, 61*(2), 63–69.

Trujillo, L. (1994). Prevention of conductive hearing loss in cleft palate patients. *Folia Phoniatrica et Logopedica, 46*(3), 123–126.

Van Borsel, J., Van Snick, K., & Leroy, J. (1999). Macroglossia and speech in Beckwith-Wiedemann syndrome: A sample survey study. *International Journal of Language & Communication Disorders, 34*(2), 209–221.

Visvanathan, V., & Wynne, D. M. (2012). Congenital nasal pyriform aperture stenosis: A report of 10 cases and literature review. *International Journal of Pediatric Otorhinolaryngology, 76*(1), 28–30.

Witzel, M. A., Rich, R. H., Margar-Bacal, F., & Cox, C. (1986). Velopharyngeal insufficiency after adenoidectomy: An 8-year review. *International Journal of Pediatric Otorhinolaryngology, 11*(1), 15–20.

Yanagisawa, E., & Weaver, E. M. (1997). An unusual appearance of velopharyngeal closure in a post-uvulopalatopharyngoplasty patient. *Ear, Nose & Throat Journal, 76*(1), 14–15.

Yetter, M. F., Ogren, F. P., Moore, G. F., & Yonkers, A. J. (1990). Bell's palsy: A facial nerve paralysis diagnosis of exclusion. *Nebraska Medical Journal, 75*(5), 109–116.

CREDITS

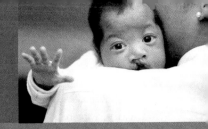

CHAPTER 6

Dental Anomalies

With acknowledgment to Richard Campbell and Murray Dock for their contributions to this chapter.

CHAPTER OUTLINE

INTRODUCTION

Children with cleft of the primary palate or other craniofacial conditions commonly have anomalies of the teeth and jaws (Akcam, Evirgen, Uslu, & Toygar Memikoğlu, 2010; Aljamal, Hazza'a, & Rawashdeh, 2010; Tannure et al., 2012). Their dental problems can include any combination of missing or extra teeth; crowded, impacted, or rotated teeth; or dental crossbite. These children may also have jaw problems, ranging from simple to complex. Jaw problems in this population include any combination of upper or lower jaw deficiency; upper or lower jaw excess; deep overbite; anterior or posterior open bite; and anterior or posterior crossbite. Both dental and occlusal anomalies have the potential to cause obligatory speech distortions or result in the use of compensatory articulation productions during speech.

Dental management of these patients requires coordination among several dental specialists, including pediatric dentists, orthodontists, oral-maxillofacial surgeons, and prosthodontists (Kirschner & LaRossa, 2000; Kuijpers-Jagtman, Borstlap-Engels, Spauwen, & Borstlap, 2000; Mouradian, Omnell, & Williams, 1999; Strong, 2002; Turvey, Vig, & Fonseca, 1996; Vasan, 1999; Wangsrimongkol & Jansawang, 2010). Together, these professionals monitor and treat problems of the developing dentition, occlusion, and facial growth of the patient with cleft lip and/or palate (Strauss, 1998; Strauss, 1999). In addition, close cooperation between the dental specialists and the speech-language pathologist leads to a more holistic management of the patient with dental abnormalities.

This chapter begins with a review of normal dentition and occlusion. Dental and occlusal abnormalities are then described, along with their effects on speech production. Finally, the stages of dental development and dental treatment are discussed.

There are a variety of terms that are used to describe normal and abnormal dentition and occlusion. A list of some of them with their definitions can be found in TABLE 6-1.

TABLE 6-1 Terms Related to Normal and Abnormal Dentition and Occlusion

Dental Adjectives

- Buccal: for the buccinator muscle of the cheeks; pertaining to, in the direction of, or adjacent to the cheek; the part of the dental arch that is posterior to the canine teeth and on the side of the teeth
- Labial: relating to the lip; the outer part of the dental arch that touches the lip
- Lingual: related to the tongue; also the inner part of the upper and lower dental arch that is in contact with the tongue
- Palatal: the inner part of the upper and lower dental arch that is in proximity to the surface of the hard palate
- Distal: away from the center of the body, midline, or point of origin
- Mesial: the direction toward the midline, following the curvature of the dental arch
- Proximal: close to the center of the body, midline, or point of origin

Dentition

- Dentition: pertains to the arrangement of the teeth in the mouth
- Deciduous teeth: baby teeth
- Succedaneous teeth: permanent adult teeth
- Incisors: two central and two lateral in each arch
- Cusps: points on the teeth
- Cuspids: teeth that have one point or cusp; also known as canines; two in each arch
- Bicuspids: teeth that typically have two cusps
- First bicuspids: first premolars
- Second bicuspids: second premolars
- Central fossa (pl. fossae): the valley between the buccal and lingual cusps of a tooth
- Deciduous teeth: primary, or "baby," teeth; 10 teeth in each arch
- Succedaneous teeth: secondary or permanent teeth; 16 teeth in each arch
- Mixed dentition: presence of both primary and secondary teeth
- 6-year molars: first molars
- 12-year molars: second molars
- Wisdom teeth: third molars

Occlusion and Malocclusion

- Condyle: jaw joint
- Dental occlusion: the manner in which the maxillary teeth and mandibular teeth fit together, or the bite; in normal occlusion, the upper arch overlaps the lower arch when they come together at rest
- Malocclusion: abnormal dental or skeletal relationship of the maxillary and mandibular teeth so that the arches do not close together normally during biting
- Skeletal relationship: the way the jaws (not just the teeth) come together
- Micrognathia: when the lower jaw is small
- Midface (maxillary) retrusion: when the maxillary jaw is dysplastic and/or retrusive
- Prognathia (prognathism): when the lower jaw is large
- Retrognathia: when the lower jaw is small relative to the upper jaw
- Angle's Classification System:
  - Class I occlusion: Normal dental arch relationship, although the teeth may be misaligned; the mesiobuccal (front outside) cusp of the first maxillary molar fits in the buccal (outside) groove of the first mandibular molar.
  - Class II malocclusion: Abnormal dental arch relationship where the mesiobuccal (front outside) cusp of the first maxillary molar is anterior to the buccal (outside) groove of the first mandibular molar; the mandibular arch is too far behind the maxillary arch, often caused by micrognathia.
  - Class III malocclusion: Abnormal dental arch relationship where the mesiobuccal (front outside) cusp of the first maxillary molar is posterior to the buccal (outside) groove of the first mandibular molar; the mandibular arch is too far in front of the maxillary arch because of either maxillary retrusion or mandibular prognathism.

Crossbites

- Single tooth crossbite: crossbite that involves only one upper and one lower tooth
- Anterior crossbite: a condition where a maxillary tooth or teeth, such as the central incisors, lateral incisors, or canines, are inside the mandibular arch; commonly seen in patients with dental or skeletal Class III malocclusion
- Lateral (also known as posterior) crossbite: involves any combination of teeth distal (posterior) to the canines and usually occurs because the maxilla is too narrow
- Complete crossbite: when the maxilla is very narrow and, as a result, the entire maxillary arch is inside the mandibular arch during occlusion

Dental Anomalies

- Diastema: a space or opening between the teeth, usually the upper central incisors
- Ectopic teeth: normal teeth that erupt in an abnormal position
- Supernumerary teeth: extra teeth; usually erupt in the line of the cleft
- Labioversion: malposition of an anterior tooth from the normal line of occlusion toward the lips
- Linguoversion: malposition of an anterior tooth from the normal line of occlusion toward the tongue
- Open bite: when one or more maxillary teeth fail to occlude with the opposing mandibular teeth; primarily affects the anterior dentition (anterior open bite) and less commonly the posterior dentition (lateral open bite)
- Overbite: the vertical overlap of the upper and lower incisors; can be measured in millimeters but is often reported as a percentage of coverage of the lower incisors by the upper incisors; normal overbite is approximately 2 mm, or about 25%; greater amounts are called either deep overbite or deep bite
- Deep bite: when the upper teeth overlap more than 25% of the lower teeth; the lower incisors may be in contact with the alveolar ridge of the palate
- Underbite: the abnormal vertical overlap of the lower incisors over the upper incisors
- Overjet: normal horizontal (or anterior–posterior) relationship between the upper and lower incisors is about 2 mm with upper incisors and lower incisors in light contact; excessive overjet is where the maxillary incisors are labioverted, or stick out toward the lips
- Underjet: a reversal of the normal incisor position, with the maxillary incisors linguoverted, or facing inward toward the tongue; also called linguoversion or anterior crossbite

(continues)

TABLE 6-1 **Terms Related to Normal and Abnormal Dentition and Occlusion** *(continued)*

Clefts
- Noncleft segment: greater segment on the noncleft side in unilateral clefts of the primary palate

Evaluation and Treatment
- Pedodontist: a pediatric dentist
- Prosthodontist: a dental professional who makes dentures, palatal obturators, palatal lifts, etc.
- Cephalometric radiograph (cephalograms): a standardized lateral skull film used to measure the jaw relationship and the soft tissue profile of the forehead, nose, lips, and chin; often used in orthodontic and orthognathic surgery planning; often referred to as cephalograms
- NAM: nasal alveolar molding
- Lip adhesion: temporary surgical closure
- Distraction osteogenesis: a method for increasing bone length that involves making a corticotomy in the middle of a bone and then slowly pulling the cut ends apart (distracting) with a mechanical device; new bone is able to regenerate between the cut ends, obviating the need for bone grafts; can be used for maxillary or mandibular advancement
- Premaxillary orthopedics: infant oral orthopedics
- Gingivoperiosteoplasty: a procedure to close the cleft of the alveolus with raised gingival flaps and the underlying periosteum on each edge of the cleft; raw surfaces are advanced and sewn together to allow the bone progenitor cells to lay down bone as the patient grows
- Corticotomy: a partial cut in the bone
- Rapid palatal expander (RPE): a palatal expansion device that consists of two or four molar bands and a jackscrew connecting them in the middle of the palate; turning the screw creates the necessary force to widen the dental arches
- Reverse pull headgear (or face mask): a nonsurgical option for correction of maxillary retrusion

Normal Dentition and Dental Occlusion

Dentition includes two arches of teeth—the upper (or maxillary) arch and the lower (or mandibular) arch. All teeth are paired, with one of each type of tooth on the right side and a matching tooth on the left side.

The first set of teeth, called **deciduous teeth**, consists of the 20 primary teeth, with 10 in each arch (**FIGURE 6-1**). In one arch, starting from the midline and moving **distally** (away from the center or point of origin), the pairs are central incisors, lateral incisors, canines (also known as cuspids), primary first molars, and primary second molars.

Deciduous teeth are eventually shed and replaced by permanent adult teeth. This second set of teeth, sometimes called **succedaneous teeth**, consists of 32 teeth, with 16 in each arch (**FIGURE 6-2**). In one arch, starting from the midline and proceeding distally, the pairs are central incisors, lateral incisors, canines (cuspids), first

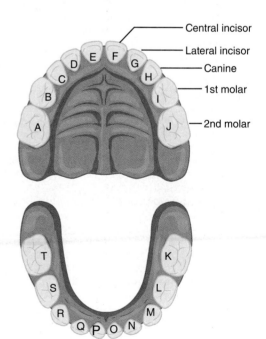

FIGURE 6-1 Occlusal view of all 20 primary teeth.

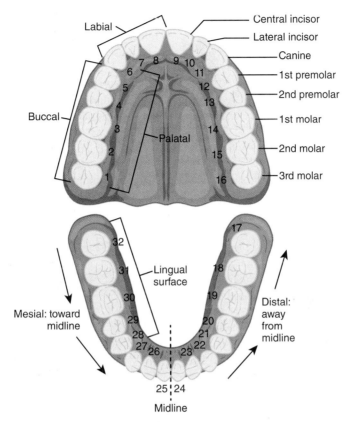

FIGURE 6-2 Occlusal view of all 32 permanent teeth.

premolars (first bicuspids), second premolars (second bicuspids), first molars (6-year molars), second molars (12-year molars), and third molars (wisdom teeth).

In addition to anatomical names for the teeth, dental professionals often use a system to label each individual tooth in both sets. With this system, the primary teeth are lettered A through T, and the permanent teeth are numbered 1 through 32.

Many terms are used to describe the position of the teeth in the arch (see Figure 6-2). The dental **midline** is at the apex of the dental arch, where the left and right halves join. The direction toward the midline is **mesial**. The direction away from the midline is **distal**. The outer part of the arch that touches the lip is **labial**. The part of the arch that is posterior to the canine teeth is frequently referred to as **buccal** (for the buccinator

muscle in the cheeks). The inner part of the upper and lower arches is often referred to as **lingual** because it is next to the tongue, although some clinicians refer to the inner part of the upper arch as **palatal** because of its proximity to the hard palate.

The shape of each tooth depends on its type. For example, incisor teeth are somewhat shovel shaped, and their biting surfaces are thin, knife-like edges. They are used for biting. The remaining teeth have rounded points, known as **cusps**, which are used for chewing.

The number of cusps depends on the type of tooth and its position in the arch. Canines have one cusp, premolars (bicuspids) have two cusps, upper molars have four cusps, and lower molars have four or five cusps. Variations in the number of cusps do occur but are usually of no consequence. Cusps are arranged in rows, one on the

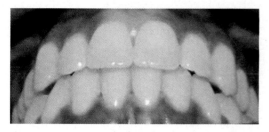

FIGURE 6-3 Normal dental occlusion with the normal overlap of the upper teeth over the lower teeth.

outside (buccal or labial) and one to the inside (palatal or lingual) of the tooth. The area between the cusps is called the central fossa.

Dental occlusion refers to the bite, or the manner in which both arches of the teeth fit together. Normal occlusion of the upper to the lower teeth, called a Class I occlusion, is important for aesthetics, biting and chewing, and speech.

When there is normal occlusion, the upper arch partially overlaps the lower arch so that the cusps of one arch fit into the fossae of the opposing arch (**FIGURE 6-3**). In addition, the

SPEECH NOTES

Normal Dentition and Dental Occlusion

When there is normal dental occlusion:

- The lips come together easily at rest for bilabial competence, which is important for production of bilabial sounds.
- The lower lip is able to approximate maxillary teeth for production of labiodental sounds.
- The jaws (maxilla and mandible) are appropriately aligned so that the tongue tip rests under the alveolar ridge and behind the maxillary incisors. As a result of this position, the tongue tip is able to move up and down and back and forth for all lingual sounds (interdental, lingual-alveolar, and palatal phonemes) without dental interference.

incisors have a specific horizontal and vertical relationship. The horizontal (anterior–posterior) relationship between the incisors, called overjet, refers to how far the upper incisor teeth are ahead of the lower incisors. A normal amount of overjet is about 2 mm, as measured from the labial surface of the lower incisor to the labial surface of the upper incisor, with the teeth in occlusion. The vertical overlap of the upper and lower incisors is called overbite. Normal overbite is approximately 2 mm, or about 25% of the length of the lower incisors.

Dental Anomalies
Abnormal Incisor Relationships

As previously noted, a certain amount of overjet and overbite of the incisors is normal. When the amount exceeds the norms, however, it can affect both aesthetics and speech.

An overjet is considered abnormal when the horizontal relationship between the incisors, with the upper and lower incisors in light contact, exceeds 2 mm (**FIGURE 6-4**). Underjet (also called anterior crossbite or linguoversion) refers to a reversal of the normal upper to lower incisor relationship so that the upper incisors are inside (or lingual to) the lower incisors (**FIGURE 6-5**). Like overjet, underjet is measured in millimeters.

An overbite is when there is excessive overlap of the upper incisors over the lower incisors. An overbite is considered abnormal when the upper incisors overlap the lower incisors by more than 2 mm, or about 25% (**FIGURE 6-6**). Greater amounts of overbite are associated with a deep overbite, or deep bite. If the upper teeth completely overlap the lower or the lower incisors are in contact with the palate, this would be a 100% overbite. Underbite (deep bite) is when the upper teeth are inside the lower teeth and there is excessive vertical overlap of the lower incisors over the upper incisors.

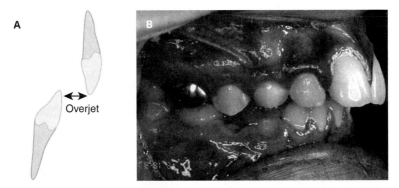

FIGURE 6-4 Overjet. **(A)** Overjet is the horizontal overlap of the incisors. **(B)** Abnormal overjet from incisor protrusion can be seen in this example.

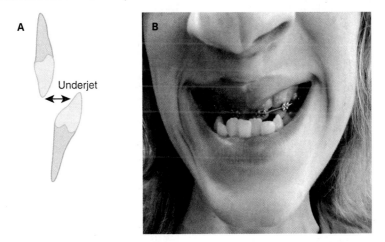

FIGURE 6-5 (A) Underjet is when the upper incisors are lingual to the lower incisors. **(B)** This patient demonstrates severe underjet.

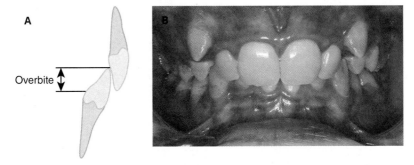

FIGURE 6-6 Overbite. **(A)** An overbite is measured as the vertical overlap of the incisors from the incisal edges and is often expressed as a percentage of overbite. **(B)** In this instance the upper incisors almost completely overlap the lower incisors, making a deep bite.

A **diastema** is a space or opening between the teeth. It usually refers to a space between the maxillary central incisors (**FIGURE 6-7**). It affects aesthetics but has no effect on function.

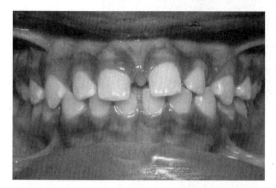

FIGURE 6-7 Diastema. A diastema is a space or opening between any of the teeth. Clinicians commonly use the term diastema to indicate the space between the maxillary central incisors, as seen in this case.

SPEECH NOTES

Abnormal Incisor Relationships

Overjet: Severe overjet of incisors may affect bilabial competence at rest and alter the production of bilabial sounds during speech. Individuals may attempt to compensate by using a labiodental placement for bilabial sounds.

Underjet: Underjet, causing an anterior crossbite, can cause the maxillary teeth to interfere with tongue tip placement for sibilants. This may result in an obligatory lateral distortion. In contrast, if the speaker compensates by opening the teeth, a frontal distortion usually occurs.

Overbite and underbite: Both an overbite and underbite can shorten the vertical dimension of the oral cavity during occlusion, causing lingual crowding and possible lateral distortion of sibilant sounds. The individual may compensate by opening the teeth slightly to increase the vertical dimension.

Diastema: A diastema is merely a cosmetic issue and has no effect on speech.

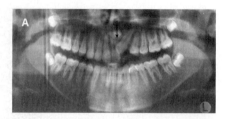

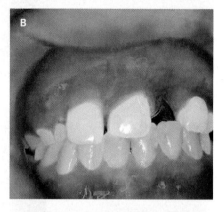

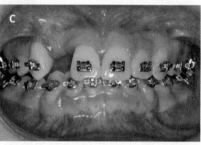

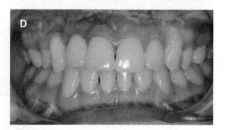

FIGURE 6-8 Missing teeth from the cleft site. **(A)** A panoramic X-ray demonstrating a permanent tooth missing from the cleft site. The upper left lateral incisor (tooth #10) is frequently missing, as it is in this case (see the arrow), and the upper left canine has moved into its place. **(B)** The lateral incisor and canine are both missing. **(C)** The lateral incisor is missing. **(D)** The missing lateral incisor in C is replaced with an implant and a crown.

Missing, Malpositioned, and Malformed Teeth

Because clefts of the primary palate follow the incisive suture lines, teeth that normally border these suture lines (the lateral incisors and canines) are often missing, abnormal, or malpositioned.

A common finding in this patient population is an absence of the lateral incisor and/or canine (**FIGURE 6-8**) (Camporesi, Baccetti, Marinelli, Defraia, & Franchi, 2010). These teeth may be either congenitally absent or lost because of a lack of bony support. Even children with a history of submucous cleft have an increased frequency of missing teeth or other dental abnormalities (Heliovaara, Ranta, & Rautio, 2004). Fortunately, missing permanent teeth can be replaced with an implant and a crown (Figure 6-8D).

Even when present, teeth in the line of the cleft may be abnormally small, malformed, or rotated (Figure 6-8A and **FIGURE 6-9**).

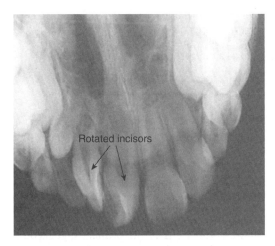

FIGURE 6-9 Rotated teeth in the cleft site. An occlusal X-ray demonstrates that teeth in the line of the cleft are frequently malpositioned or rotated about the long axis of the roots. In this view, the maxillary right central and lateral incisors (see arrows) are rotated approximately 90° each so that the lingual surfaces of their crowns are facing each other. By comparison, the maxillary left central and lateral incisors are nearly normal with almost no rotation (on the right side of this view). Note that there is also a supernumerary tooth distal to the rotated incisors.

Central incisors and lateral incisors are most often affected and are usually rotated toward the cleft. The incisors may also be fused at the roots.

Finally, there may be a **supernumerary tooth** (extra tooth) (**FIGURE 6-10A**) or **ectopic tooth** (tooth that erupts in abnormal positions) (**FIGURE 6-10B**). These teeth may remain unerupted or be displaced palatally or labially in the line of the cleft.

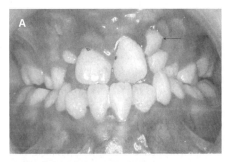

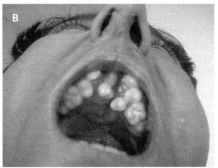

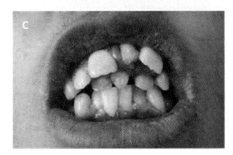

FIGURE 6-10 Supernumerary and ectopic teeth. **(A)** An extra tooth may occur in the line of the cleft, as in this case of a supernumerary primary incisor, distal and superior to the patient's maxillary left central incisor (see arrow). **(B)** Multiple ectopic teeth in the area of lingual movement for speech. **(C)** Another case of ectopic teeth.

SPEECH NOTES

Missing, Malpositioned, and Malformed Teeth

Missing teeth: Most people believe that the teeth are necessary for speech production, particularly for **sibilant phonemes** (/s/, /z/, /ʃ/, /ʒ/, /ʧ/, /ʤ/) because we close our teeth for production. Actually, sibilants are not produced by forcing airstream through the closed teeth. Instead, they are produced by forcing the airstream through the narrow opening between the tongue tip and alveolar ridge. The reason that we close the teeth for production is to elevate the mandible, which positions the tongue tip just under the alveolar ridge. Similarly, teeth are not necessary for labiodental sounds (/f/, /v/) because these sounds can be produced with the bottom lip against the top gum ridge.

Because teeth are not necessary for normal speech, even edentulous people are able to articulate clearly. In addition, when there is premature loss of the deciduous teeth from decay, it should not affect speech development (Gable, Kummer, Lee, Creaghead, & Moore, 1995).

Malpositioned teeth: Although teeth are not necessary for normal speech, they may cause speech problems by interfering with bilabial or lingual sound production because of their abnormal position (Shprintzen, Siegel-Sadewitz, Amato, & Goldberg, 1985). Many speech sounds can be affected because most consonants are produced in the front of the oral cavity by the tongue tip or the lips (Shprintzen et al., 1985). Dental abnormalities most commonly affect the following groups of phonemes: sibilant phonemes (/s/, /z/, /ʃ/, /ʒ/, /ʧ/, /ʤ/), lingual-alveolar phonemes (/t/, /d/, /n/, /l/), bilabial phonemes (/p/, /b/, /m/), and labiodental phonemes (/f/, /v/).

Abnormalities of the dentition may affect speech by causing obligatory distortions and/or compensatory errors (Trost-Cardamone, 1997). **Obligatory distortions** (also known as **passive speech characteristics**) occur when articulation placement is normal, but the structural abnormalities (in this case, the teeth) interfere with the airstream or sound, resulting in a speech distortion. **Compensatory errors** (also known as **active speech characteristics**) occur when articulation is altered to compensate for structural abnormalities. This results in a substitution error. There does not appear to be a direct relationship between the severity of the malocclusion and the severity of the misarticulations or distortions. Instead, an individual's ability to adapt to structural abnormalities plays a significant role in the amount of speech distortion (Johnson & Sandy, 1999).

Rotated, supernumerary, or ectopic teeth may interfere with tongue tip movement during speech. Even when placement of the tongue tip is normal, the teeth can divert the airstream laterally, causing an obligatory lateral distortion on sibilants and even lingual-alveolar phonemes. If the individual pulls the tongue back to compensate, it causes the dorsum of the tongue to touch the palate. This placement also diverts the airstream laterally, resulting in a lateral distortion.

Malformed teeth: Malformed teeth do not affect speech production.

Open Bite

Open bite occurs when one or more maxillary teeth fail to occlude with the opposing mandibular teeth (**FIGURE 6-11**). Open bites primarily affect the anterior dentition (anterior open bite) and less commonly the posterior dentition (lateral open bite). Causes of open bite include poor occlusion from digit or pacifier sucking habits or skeletal discrepancies. Open bites are sealed by the tongue on swallowing, which is often confused as tongue thrust (Proffit, Fields, Sarver, & Ackerman, 2013).

Crossbite

Crossbite is a common dental abnormality in children with clefts of the primary and secondary palate. In crossbite, the normal overlap of the upper teeth to the lower teeth is reversed so that the upper teeth are inside the lower teeth.

A single-tooth crossbite involves only one upper and one lower tooth (**FIGURE 6-12**). A multiple-tooth crossbite involves a combination of anterior and posterior teeth. Multiple-tooth crossbites are described by their position in the dental arch as either anterior or posterior.

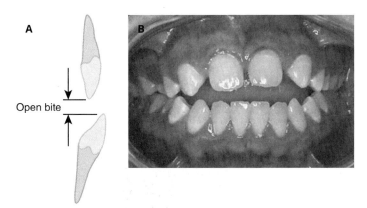
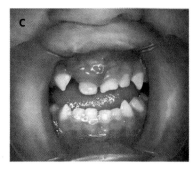
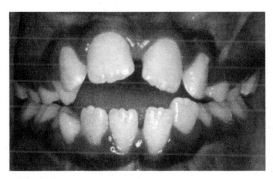
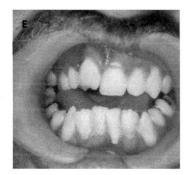

FIGURE 6-11 Anterior open bite. **(A)** The anterior teeth are not in contact. **(B)–(E)** Examples of an anterior open bite. Open bite is often attributed to tongue thrust, but little evidence exists to support that assumption. Open bite is difficult to treat and often involves orthognathic surgery in conjunction with orthodontics.

SPEECH NOTES

Open Bite

The effect of an open bite on speech depends on the size of the oral cavity. If the oral cavity size is normal, there may be no effect on speech because, again, normal speech does not require teeth (Moller, 1994). If the palatal arch is low, flat, or narrow or there is maxillary retrusion or macroglossia, it will cause oral cavity crowding during occlusion. This inhibits tongue movement for the production of sibilant phonemes. To compensate, the tongue may protrude through the open bite, causing fronting of sibilants and even lingual-alveolar sounds.

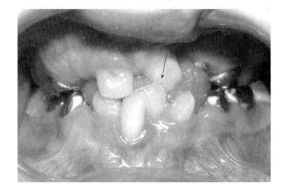

FIGURE 6-12 Single-tooth crossbite. A crossbite involving only one tooth may be referred to as a single-tooth crossbite. Often, a maxillary central or lateral incisor is involved, as in this case with the upper left central incisor being displaced lingually to the lower left central incisor (see arrow).

An anterior crossbite (also called an under-jet), characterized by the maxillary incisors positioned inside the mandibular incisors, is commonly seen in patients with dental or skeletal Class III malocclusion. An anterior crossbite may involve any or all of the anterior teeth, including the central incisors, lateral incisors, and/or canines (**FIGURE 6-13**).

A lateral crossbite (also known as a posterior crossbite) involves any combination of teeth distal (posterior) to the canines and usually occurs because the maxilla is too narrow. Posterior crossbites can be unilateral (**FIGURE 6-14**) or bilateral (**FIGURE 6-15A**). When mild, a bilateral crossbite may produce a shift of the mandible to one side, which gives the clinical appearance

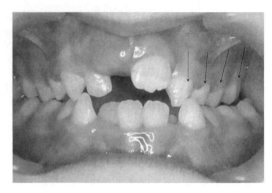

FIGURE 6-14 Unilateral posterior crossbite. The posterior teeth of the patient's maxillary left side are lingual to the mandibular teeth (see arrows). This is referred to as a posterior crossbite. It may also be called a unilateral posterior crossbite.

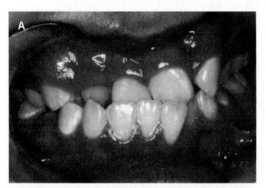

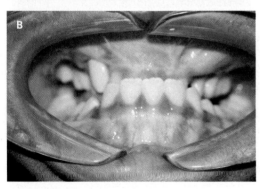

FIGURE 6-13 Anterior crossbite. An anterior crossbite is when most of the maxillary incisors are inside the mandibular incisors. **(A)** This patient has an anterior crossbite of both the maxillary incisors and right cuspid. **(B)** This patient has an anterior crossbite involving all incisors.

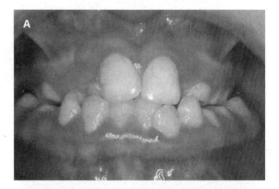

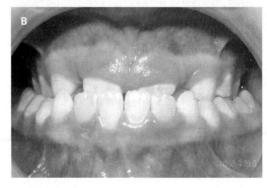

FIGURE 6-15 Bilateral crossbite. **(A)** The maxillary posterior teeth on both sides are lingual to the mandibular teeth. **(B)** When all the maxillary teeth fit inside the mandibular teeth, a total crossbite exists.

SPEECH NOTES

Crossbite

Anterior crossbite: An anterior crossbite can affect many groups of speech sounds, depending on the severity, because most sounds are produced at the front of the mouth. There may be obligatory distortions and/or compensatory errors as a result. If an anterior crossbite causes the maxillary teeth to articulate against the tongue during occlusion, it can cause fronting on sibilants and sometimes even lingual-alveolar sounds as an obligatory distortion. If the tongue moves back to compensate, the dorsum of the tongue will articulate against the palate. This diverts the airstream to each side, which results in a lateral distortion.

Lateral and complete crossbite: A lateral crossbite, and especially a complete crossbite, can cause distorted speech caused by oral cavity crowding. The speech often sounds "slushy" because of significant lateral distortion.

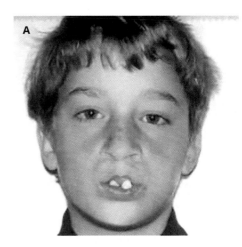

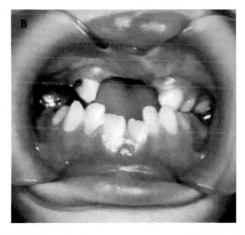

FIGURE 6-16 (A) Protruding premaxilla. **(B)** Missing maxillary incisors from excision of a protruding premaxilla. Fortunately, this procedure is not commonly done anymore.

of a unilateral crossbite. Careful examination of the patient's occlusion as the teeth first contact during closure helps to distinguish a bilateral crossbite with mandibular shift from a true unilateral crossbite.

A buccal crossbite occurs when one or more maxillary teeth are positioned buccally, such that the maxillary lingual cusps reside buccal to the mandibular cusps. The relatively rare Brodie crossbite occurs when the lingual cusps of all the maxillary posterior teeth are buccal to the mandibular teeth. Finally, a complete crossbite is when the maxilla is very narrow, and as a result, the entire maxillary arch fits inside the mandibular arch during occlusion (**FIGURE 6-15B**).

Protruding Premaxilla

Infants affected by a bilateral complete cleft of the primary palate often have a protruding premaxilla because the premaxilla is untethered by the lateral maxillary segments on both sides. In addition, the lateral segments of the maxillary are usually displaced medially so that there is no room for the premaxilla to fit within these segments. Untreated, the premaxilla remains protrusive from lack of space (**FIGURE 6-16A**). Past treatment included surgical removal of the premaxilla (**FIGURE 6-16B**), but this had major detrimental effects on midfacial growth and, of course, resulted in a lack of maxillary incisors

SPEECH NOTES

Protruding Premaxilla

A protruding premaxilla can affect bilabial competence at rest and also during speech. As a result, bilabial sounds may be produced as labiodental sounds. Although this may be visually distracting, there is usually little speech distortion as a result of this placement.

(Proffit, White, & Sarver, 2003). Fortunately, removal of the premaxilla has been abandoned in the United States and Europe but may still be done in some underdeveloped countries.

Normal Skeletal Occlusion and Skeletal Malocclusion

Occlusion refers to the way the maxillary and mandibular teeth fit together when the jaws are closed, as when biting. Malocclusion, therefore, refers to an abnormal dental relationship between the maxillary and mandibular teeth during biting.

A system that describes normal occlusion and three types of malocclusion was first described by E. H. Angle in 1899. Brilliant in its simplicity, Angle's Classification System remains in widespread use today (TABLE 6-2) (Katz, 1992; Proffit et al., 2013). With this system, the type of dental occlusion is determined by the anterior–posterior relationship between the mesiobuccal cusp of the upper molar and the buccal groove of the lower molar. Despite its utility, Angle's classification applies only to the teeth and does not account for the influence of the jaws on tooth position or facial profile.

The way the jaws (not just the teeth) come together is called the skeletal relationship. To describe this relationship, contemporary practitioners have adapted Angle's dental occlusion classification system because in most cases, the

TABLE 6-2 Angle's Classification of Occlusion and Skeletal Relationships

Classification	Example	Skeletal Classification	Diagram
Class I occlusion The mesiobuccal cusp of the upper molar occludes in the buccal groove of the lower molar. The remaining teeth are arranged upon a smoothly curving line.		Class I—Normal	
Class I malocclusion The relationship of the molars is normal, but the line of occlusion is incorrect because of malpositioned teeth, rotations, or other causes.		Class I—Normal	

Class II malocclusion
The lower molar is distally positioned relative to upper molar. The line of occlusion is not specified.

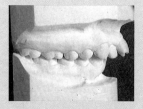

Class II— Mandibular retrusion and/ or maxillary protrusion

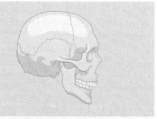

Class III malocclusion
The lower molar is mesially positioned relative to upper molar. The line of occlusion is not specified.

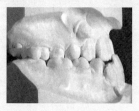

Class III— Mandibular protrusion and/ or maxillary retrusion

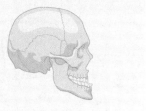

jaw (skeletal) relationship is reflected in the dental relationship.

Using Angle's Classification System to describe skeletal relationships, a Class I occlusion is when the jaws are in normal alignment with each other, regardless of abnormalities of the dentition within the arches.

In contrast, Class II malocclusion is when the mandible is small (micrognathic) or retrusive (retrognathic) or when the maxilla is too far forward (maxillary protrusion). Class II malocclusion is common in patients with Pierre Robin sequence as a result of the micrognathia.

Finally, Class III malocclusion is when the lower jaw is relatively large (prognathic) and/ or the upper jaw is relatively small (maxillary retrusion). Individuals with a cleft of the primary palate often have maxillary retrusion causing midface deficiency. Class III malocclusion is common in children with cleft lip and palate because of primary dysplasia of the maxillary bone and the possible restrictive influences from scarring after surgical correction.

The jaw relationship and the soft tissue profile of the forehead, nose, lips, and chin can be measured with a lateral skull X-ray, or cephalometric radiograph (also called a cephalogram), taken with the patient's head held in a standardized position (**FIGURE 6-17**). A cephalometric tracing is done for treatment planning (**FIGURE 6-18**).

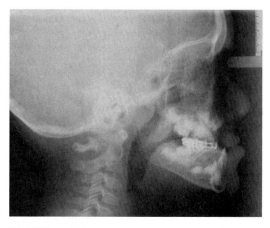

FIGURE 6-17 Cephalometric X-ray. A cephalometric X-ray is a lateral skull film made with a cephalostat, a device with ear rods and a nasal bridge rest to allow reproducible head positioning. This allows comparisons of X-rays of the patient taken at different times for use in longitudinal growth studies.

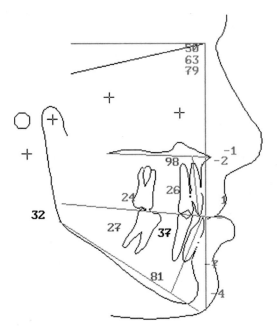

FIGURE 6-18 Cephalometric tracing. A tracing of a cephalometric X-ray is made so that measurement can be drawn without damaging the film. A set of measurements is called an analysis and is frequently named after its founder (e.g., the Steiner Analysis or the McNamara Analysis). This particular depiction is the COGS Analysis, or Cephalometric Analysis for Orthognathic Surgery, devised by Burstone. The image was generated by Dentofacial Planner.

SPEECH NOTES

Skeletal Malocclusion

Skeletal malocclusion: Malocclusion of the jaws can have a far more significant effect on speech than the dental anomalies noted previously. Depending on the type of malocclusion, the mandible (and thus the tongue) can be positioned too far behind or too far in front of the maxilla, thus affecting the relationship of the tongue tip to the alveolar ridge. The relationship between the upper and lower lip can also be affected.

Class II malocclusion: When Class II malocclusion is severe, the position of the tongue tip rests under the palate rather than the alveolar ridge (**FIGURE 6-19**). This can cause obligatory distortion of sibilants and even lingual-alveolar phonemes. The individual may compensate by backing, which is using the back of the tongue for anterior lingual sounds. In addition to affecting lingual sounds, a Class II malocclusion can interfere with lip closure, causing a lack of bilabial closure at rest and during production of most bilabial sounds. The individual may compensate by producing these sounds with a labiodental placement. This placement causes very little speech distortion, but it can be visually distracting because of abnormal lip placement.

Class III malocclusion: A Class III malocclusion includes a significant anterior crossbite because it is caused by an abnormal jaw relationship, not just abnormal dental relationship (**FIGURE 6-20**). With a Class III malocclusion, the mandible, along with the tongue, is in an anterior position relative to the alveolar ridge. This causes difficulty with production of sibilant and lingual-alveolar sounds, which require the tongue tip to be under the alveolar ridge. If the tongue remains in the normal position in the mandible while trying to produce these sounds, it will cause the perception of fronting, which is an obligatory distortion (Kummer, Strife, Grau, Creaghead, & Lee, 1989; Moller, 1994; Taher, 1997). If the tongue retracts to compensate for the anterior crowding, it will cause the dorsum of the tongue to articulate against the palate, resulting in a lateral distortion (a compensatory error). Class III malocclusion can also interfere with production of lip sounds. Labiodental (/f/, /v/) sounds may be affected because of the difficulty retracting the bottom lip far enough to articulate against the maxillary incisors. To compensate, the individual may use a reverse labiodental placement so that the upper lip articulates with the mandibular incisors (Moller, 1994). Bilabial sounds can also be difficult to produce with this Class III malocclusion. The individual may compensate by using a reverse labiodental production for these sounds as well.

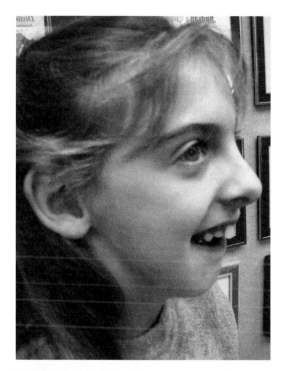

FIGURE 6-19 Class II malocclusion. Note the micrognathia.

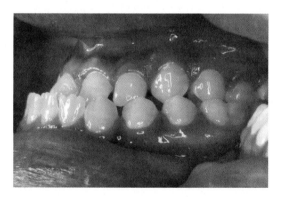

FIGURE 6-20 Class III malocclusion. Note that this includes an anterior crossbite.

Dental Development and Stages of Treatment

Treatment of dental problems in children with a cleft lip and palate is timed to follow the normal stages of dental development. Some interventions may be done to coincide with growth spurts. Others, such as combined orthodontic and orthognathic surgical treatment, may be delayed until the completion of growth (Posnick & Ricalde, 2004).

Infant Stage (0–12 Months)

Most infants are born without any erupted teeth. The infant stage, therefore, involves the eruption of the primary teeth and lasts until 12 months of age. However, natal or neonatal teeth are common in children with either a unilateral or bilateral cleft (Cabete, Gomide, & Costa, 2000). If a tooth is present at birth, a pediatric dentist should examine it to evaluate its stability in the arch. Most often, these teeth are not supernumerary, and therefore, every attempt is made to retain them when possible.

The eruption sequence for the primary teeth, as well as for the permanent teeth, is fairly predictable (**TABLE 6-3**). The lower primary incisors are usually the first teeth to erupt, at around 8 months of age. The remaining incisors are close behind, completing their eruption by 10 to 13 months of age. The canines erupt between 19 and 20 months, followed by the first molars at 16 months and, finally, the second molars by 27 to 29 months (Proffit et al., 2013). Although the sequence of eruption is predictable, there is considerable variation with regard to chronological timing. In fact, for primary teeth, a variation in eruption of 6 months on either side of the expected eruption is no cause for alarm.

Treatment for an infant with a cleft lip and palate is done in two stages: lip closure at about 3 months of age and then palate closure between 9 and 12 months of age. During the first year, clefts of the lip and alveolus, particularly bilateral clefts, require coordinated treatment between the surgeon and the dentist.

Clefts of the lip only, or incomplete clefts of the lip and alveolus, usually don't require manipulation of the alveolar segment before surgical repair. For a complete or wide unilateral

Primary Tooth	Maxillary	Mandibular
Permanent Dentitions		
Central	10 mo.	8 mo.
Lateral	11 mo.	13 mo.
Canine	19 mo.	20 mo.
Ist Molar	16 mo.	16 mo.
2nd Molar	29 mo.	27 mo.
Permanent Tooth		
Central	7.25 yr.	6.25 yr.
Lateral	8.25 yr.	7.5 yr.
Canine	11.5 yr.	10.5 yr.
Ist Premolar	10.25 yr.	10.5 yr.
2nd Premolar	11 yr.	11.25 yr.
Ist Molar	6.25 yr.	6 yr.
2nd Molar	12.5 yr.	12 yr.
3rd Molar	20 yr.	20 yr.

TABLE 6-3 Tooth Eruption for Primary and Permanent Dentition

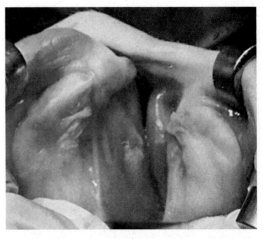

FIGURE 6-21 The occlusal view of the palate of a newborn with unilateral cleft lip and palate. The greater segment (GS) is on the left in the photograph, and the lesser segment (LS) is on the right.

cleft, however (**FIGURE 6-21**), many surgeons prefer to have the intra-alveolar gap reduced before surgical closure of the lip. Bilateral clefts of the lip and palate are particularly challenging (**FIGURE 6-22**). Not only are there two clefts, but there is often a protruding premaxillary and a narrow opening between the two lateral segments of the maxillary bone (Bartzela et al., 2010; Bitter, 2001). Treatment is usually directed at widening the opening between the lateral segments and retracting the protruding premaxilla into that space.

There are numerous ways to accomplish alignment of the alveolar segments in both unilateral and bilateral clefts of the palate. Regardless of which technique is chosen, the process is referred to as infant oral orthopedics (also known as premaxillary orthopedics or palatal orthopedics), which is the correction of deformities of bones (**FIGURE 6-23**). From least to most invasive, the techniques include taping of the lip (**FIGURE 6-24**); elastic straps over the lip and attached to a bonnet; passive molding appliances, with or without taping; lip adhesion (temporary surgical closure) before lip repair; and pin-retained active intraoral appliances (Cho, 2001; Oosterkamp et al., 2005). Each method has advantages and disadvantages (**TABLE 6-4**). The method of choice depends on the needs of the patient, the experience of the practitioners, and the overall philosophy of treatment at a particular treatment center.

Palatal orthopedic methods are controversial and remain a lively topic of debate among practitioners (Smith, Henry, & Scott, 2016). Some authors disparage any repositioning of the palatal segments, believing that these procedures

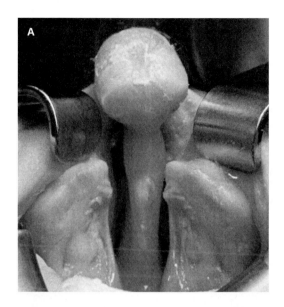

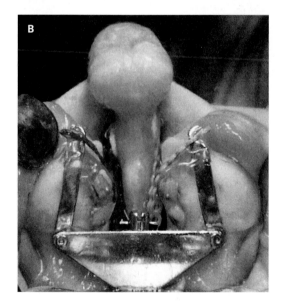

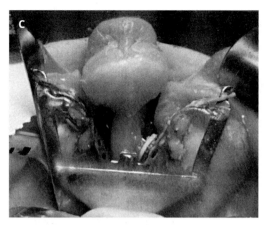

FIGURE 6-22 Premaxillary orthopedics. **(A)** The occlusal view of the palate of an infant with bilateral cleft lip and palate. The premaxillary segment is at the top middle of the photograph, and the two lateral segments are on either side, left or right and posterior to the premaxillary segment in the photograph. **(B)** A pin-retained appliance used to reposition the segments. **(C)** The maxillary segment is retracted, and the lateral segment is widened.

Keilig, Bourauel, & Jager, 2002; Chan, Hayes, Shusterman, Mulliken, & Will, 2003; Millard, Latham, Huifen, Spiro, & Morovic, 1999; Prahl, Kuijpers-Jagtman, van't Hof, & Prahl-Andersen, 2003; Prahl, Kuijpers-Jagtman, van't Hof, & Prahl-Andersen, 2005).

Because a cleft of the lip and alveolus also affects the nose, nasal alveolar molding (NAM) is often done to reposition the deformed nasal cartilage, lengthen the deficient columella, and reposition the alveolar segments (Cutting et al., 1998; Da Silveira et al., 2003). This technique involves applying pressure to the tip of the affected nostril(s) from an intraoral or extra-oral approach, using various struts of wire or acrylic (**FIGURE 6-25**). Taping of the lip is also frequently done (Grayson & Cutting, 2001; Grayson & Maull, 2004). The molding appliance is worn from early infancy for a period of several months after the lip is closed (Doruk & Kilic, 2005). Proponents of the technique report encouraging results and follow-up findings

may result in decreased midfacial growth (Berkowitz, Mejia, & Bystrik, 2004; Bongaarts, Kuijpers-Jagtman, van't Hof, & Prahl-Andersen, 2004). Hopefully, further research will clarify the appropriate application of each method (Berkowitz et al., 2005; Braumann,

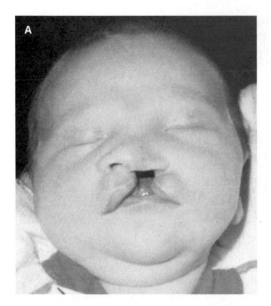

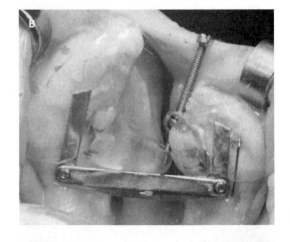

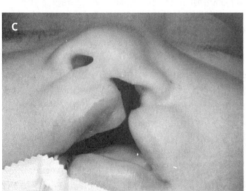

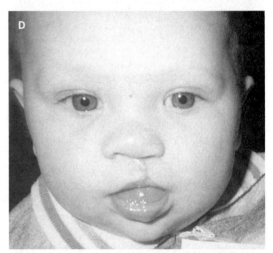

FIGURE 6-23 Pin-retained intraoral appliance. **(A)** A wide unilateral cleft lip and palate. **(B)** In cases of wide clefts, some surgeons prefer to have the width of the cleft between greater and lesser segments reduced with an appliance. **(C)** The appliance gives a closer approximation of the lip segments. **(D)** The close approximation of the segments allows for lip closure with less tension than by other means.

(Garfinkle, King, Grayson, Brecht & Cutting, 2011; Nazarian et al., 2011).

Some centers also perform primary alveolar bone grafting in the infant stage, usually with the lip repair at around 3 months. Bone formation–inducing material from the rib or the hip is placed into the cleft site to bridge the gap between the bony segments of the alveolus. The soft tissue is then repaired through a gingivoperiosteoplasty (Hathaway, Eppley, Hennon, Nelson, & Sadove, 1999; Hathaway, Eppley, Nelson, & Sadove, 1999; Millard et al., 1999). The goal of primary alveolar bone grafting is to bring the alveolar segments together to stabilize the arch and create bone for eruption of teeth near the cleft (Lee, Grayson, Cutting, Brecht, & Lin, 2004). Unfortunately, results of primary alveolar bone grafting are mixed, and secondary alveolar bone grafting may be required regardless (Millard et al., 1999; Renkielska, Wojtaszek-Slominska, & Dobke, 2005). In addition, primary alveolar

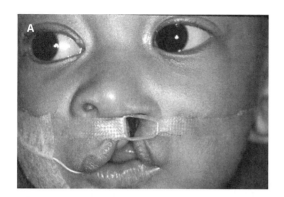

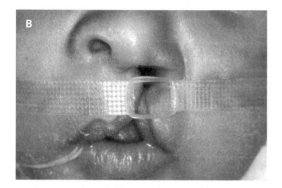

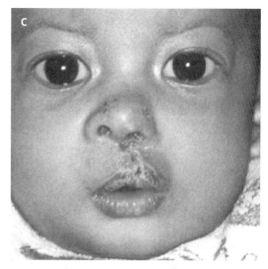

FIGURE 6-24 Taping of the lip. Narrow separations of the lip may be approximated by extraoral taping, in this case with an additional elastic, making surgical closure less difficult. **(A)** Beginning of taping. This shows separation of lip. **(B)** After a few weeks, the lip segments are approximated. **(C)** In this view, taken very shortly after lip closure, one can appreciate that there is little tension across the now joined lip segments.

TABLE 6-4 Methods of Unilateral Cleft Lip and Palate Closure

Method	Advantages	Disadvantages
Surgical only	Quick; no pre-op manipulations required.	Limited to smaller clefts; no control of segment position postoperatively.
Taping	Noninvasive; no dental impressions required.	Parent cooperation essential; skin irritation common; no control of segments.
Passive molding plates, with or without taping	Allows some repositioning of segments; serves as retainers or aids feeding.	Dental impressions required; parents' cooperation is a must; denture adhesives are often used.
Lip adhesion	Decreases size of intra-alveolar gap; allows tension-free closure.	Requires additional surgery; surgeon must perform final closure through scar tissue; no post-op segment control.
Pin-retained active appliance	Greater control of segments; effective at reducing wide clefts; allows tension-free lip closure.	Requires dental impressions and visit for placement; parent cooperation is required; there is surgical placement of the pins; long-term effects on maxillary growth are unknown.
Nasal alveolar molding (NAM)	Allows repositioning of the segments; lengthens columella.	Is very labor intensive; periodic dental impressions are required; is uncomfortable for the infant; requires significant parent cooperation to learn complex taping techniques; dental adhesives can cause skin irritation.

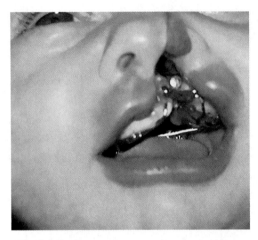

FIGURE 6-25 Extraoral nasal alveolar molding (NAM) appliance in combination with alveolar orthopedics.

bone grafting has been associated with markedly decreased growth of the midface. Centers debate about whether results vary because of differences in surgical technique and timing (Pfeifer, Grayson, & Cutting, 2002; Sachs, 2002) or the amount of gingival, nasal, and oral mucosa that is manipulated during the gingivoperiosteoplasty.

Primary Dentition (1–6 Years)

The primary dentition is usually complete by 24 to 30 months of age, with 10 teeth in the upper arch and 10 in the lower arch. Ideally, there should be spacing between all the primary teeth so there is room for the larger permanent teeth that will replace them.

Children with little or no spacing between the primary teeth are at risk for significant crowding of the permanent dentition (Ngan, Alkire, & Fields, 1999). Crowding of the primary teeth is of particular concern for children with repaired cleft lip and palate because they often have a maxilla that is smaller than normal from primary dysplasia of the

structures (DiBiase, DiBiase, Hay, & Sommerlad, 2002; Garrahy, Millett, & Ayoub, 2005).

There are several other dental abnormalities that commonly occur in children with clefts during the primary dentition stage. The lateral incisor and/or the canine may be missing because both are in the line of the cleft. Conversely, a supernumerary or ectopic tooth may be located near the cleft site. Malformations of these teeth are common (Chapple & Nunn, 2001; Maciel, Costa, & Gomide, 2005; Malanczuk, Opitz, & Retzlaff, 1999). Children with clefts are also at risk for periodontal disease localized around teeth near the cleft. Therefore, every effort should be made to establish proper oral hygiene measures at home and early management by a pedodontist (pediatric dentist) before age 2 (Chapple & Nunn, 2001; Dewinter et al., 2003; Gaggl, Schultes, Karcher, & Mossbock, 1999; Kirchberg, Treide, & Hemprich, 2004; Quirynen et al., 2003; Schultes, Gaggl, & Karcher, 1999).

Crossbites are very common in children with clefts because of the altered anatomy of the palate. With unilateral clefts, the maxilla is divided into two segments—a greater segment on the noncleft side and a lesser segment on the cleft side (see Figure 6-21). Because these segments are not joined together, they can be easily displaced by lip pressure. It is common, therefore, to find a crossbite on the lesser segment side. In bilateral clefts, there are three maxillary segments—the premaxilla and two lateral segments. Although the premaxilla is frequently protrusive, the lateral segments are often displaced medially, which results in a bilateral crossbite (see Figure 6-15A).

Children with cleft lip and palate frequently appear to have a relatively normal upper to lower skeletal (jaw) relationship in the primary dentition (**FIGURE 6-26A**). This is because, although the maxilla is smaller than normal in children with clefts, the mandible is normally small at this stage of development as well. During the adolescent growth spurt, however, the mandible increases to its normal size.

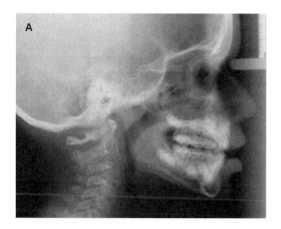

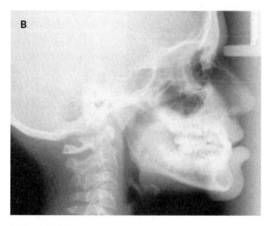

FIGURE 6-26 Normal occlusion in early dentition, which will change in adolescence. **(A)** The jaw and dental relationships are good in the early mixed dentition cephalogram of a patient with unilateral cleft lip and palate. This patient exhibits a nearly Class I occlusion, and midfacial retrusion is not obvious. **(B)** Unfortunately, because of the mandibular growth spurt of adolescence, the relationships have changed for the worse. The patient now has a dental and skeletal Class III malocclusion with underbite and underjet, manifestations of the lack of midfacial growth often seen in patients with cleft lip and palate.

As a result, the maxilla will appear to become more retrusive relative to the mandible, thereby exposing its deficiency (**FIGURE 6-26B**) (Lisson, Hanke, & Trankmann, 2004; Scheuer, Holtje, Hasund, & Pfeifer, 2001; Veleminska, Smahel, & Mullerova, 2003).

Few conditions require orthodontic intervention in the primary dentition. In children with clefts, however, significant narrowing of the maxillary segments is sometimes addressed during this time, especially if a crossbite or crowding of the primary teeth occurs. In addition, any crossbite that causes a functional shift of the mandible—that is, a reposturing of the mandible to achieve a more comfortable bite—is addressed as soon as possible. Left untreated, this posturing can cause overgrowth of one condyle (jaw joint), resulting in an asymmetry of the mandible so that the chin is deviated to the nonaffected side (Proffit et al., 2013).

Treatment for crossbite in the primary dentition involves some form of maxillary expansion. One appliance for maxillary expansion is the quad helix. This device consists of orthodontic bands on the most posterior molars and frequently on the canines (**FIGURE 6-27A**) (Kirchberg et al., 2004). The bands are connected by a palatal spring that has four loops, or helices, thus giving the quad helix its name. Some clinicians prefer not to include the helices, and the resulting W-shaped palatal spring is called a W-arch. Another appliance for maxillary expansion to correct a crossbite is the rapid palatal expander (RPE). This device consists of two or four orthodontic bands connected by a jackscrew in the middle of the palate (**FIGURE 6-27B**). Turning the screw creates the necessary force to widen the arch. The rapid palatal expander is capable of delivering very heavy forces, so it is used with caution in the primary dentition. The goal for both of these devices is to create adequate width of the maxilla.

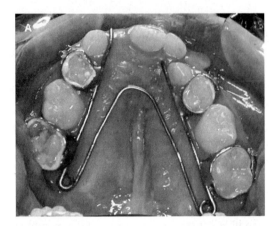

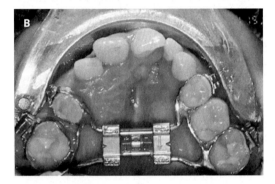

FIGURE 6-27 Appliances used for maxillary expansion. **(A)** The quad helix consists of a palatal spring that has four helices. **(B)** The rapid palatal expander (RPE) consists of a jackscrew mechanism that is activated with a key by the parents. Both appliances are versatile in that they can be modified to fit the individual needs of the patient. For instance, the quad helix actually has only two helices. The anterior helices were not used in this case because of the constricted space of the anterior palate. Both appliances are bulky and may interfere with articulation while in use.

Because children with clefts often have an anterior crossbite as well as a posterior crossbite, some clinicians correct the incisor position at this time (Sakamoto, Sakamoto, Harazaki, Isshiki, & Yamaguchi, 2002). This is rarely necessary with primary incisors, however, and is usually reserved for the permanent incisors, preferably at a stage of nearly completed root development.

Maxillary expansion can be started as early as 4 to 5 years of age with a cooperative child.

SPEECH NOTES

Maxillary Expansion Devices

Quad helix: The quad helix device can interfere with tongue tip movement and thus affect lingual-alveolar sounds temporarily while it is in place.

Rapid palatal expander (RPE): The RPE goes across the midpart of the palate. As such, it does not interfere with speech production. In fact, it can often be helpful in the correction of palatal–dorsal productions. The child is merely told to elevate the tongue tip in front of the device while avoiding tongue contact against the device.

For most children, however, it's better to wait until the permanent upper first molars erupt. Adequate expansion can then be accomplished within a few months. Following treatment, children with clefts require a fixed lingual upper arch wire to maintain the maxillary expansion. Without proper retention, the scar tissue from the repaired cleft palate can exert enough force on the maxilla to cause it to relapse back into crossbite.

In children with repaired cleft palate, maxillary expansion can correct the crossbite but often at the expense of widening a preexisting oronasal fistula. This is because widening the arch of the palate further stretches the tissue over the absent bone of the palate. Without proper bony support, palatal tissue necrosis (death of cellular tissue) may occur, causing the fistula to manifest. If this happens, the fistula can be temporarily closed with a removable acrylic obturator. Surgical repair is usually accomplished later at the time of the alveolar bone graft (Proffit et al., 2013).

Early Mixed Dentition (6–9 Years)

Mixed dentition refers to the presence of both primary and secondary teeth. The permanent lower central incisors usually erupt first, followed by the upper central incisors, lower lateral incisors, and finally, the upper lateral incisors. The permanent first molars usually erupt shortly after the lower central incisors, but it is not uncommon for them to erupt first.

The most noticeable sign that a child with a cleft of the primary palate is entering the early mixed dentition stage is the eruption of malpositioned permanent maxillary incisors. **FIGURE 6-28** shows some examples of misaligned maxillary teeth secondary to a cleft. Although unaesthetic, correcting anterior misalignment with orthodontics should be avoided at this stage of dentition for the sake of a better long-term outcome (Reisberg, 2000; Rivkin, Keith, Crawford, & Hathorn, 2000a; Rivkin, Keith, Crawford, & Hathorn, 2000b). This is because the root formation of the teeth remains incomplete

for at least 3 years after crown eruption. The pressure from orthodontic appliances at this stage can damage forming roots, resulting in roots of less than half their normal length.

During the mixed dentition stage, the appearance of crossbite increases. This is because the interosseous sutures of the maxilla begin to fuse together, thus restricting further maxillary growth. At the same time, the mandible begins its normal growth spurt. If the patient requires maxillary advancement to treat a crossbite, a reverse pull headgear (or face mask) is a nonsurgical option (**FIGURE 6-29**). The face mask is attached with labial hooks to a crossbite appliance, such as a quad helix or rapid palatal expander (Kawakami, Yagi, & Takada, 2002; Sakamoto et al., 2002). Some clinicians report success with the

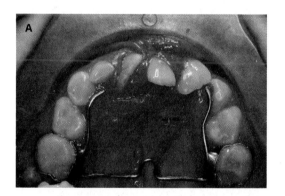
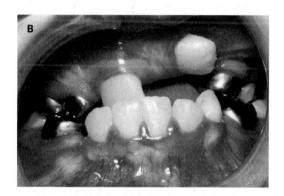
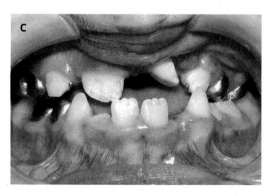
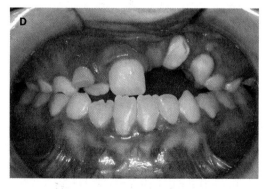

FIGURE 6-28 The erupting upper incisors are often misaligned in children who have had a unilateral or bilateral cleft. These are various examples of misaligned maxillary incisors as the result of a cleft.

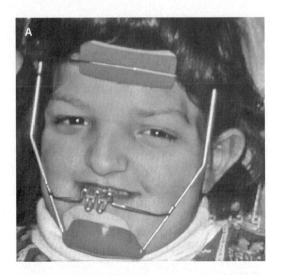

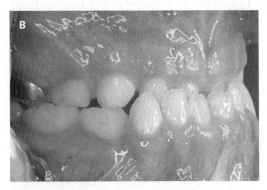

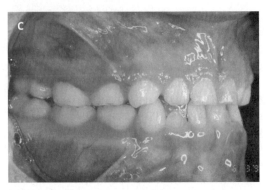

FIGURE 6-29 A patient with reverse-pull headgear. **(A)** Removable reverse-pull headgear, also known as a Delaire facial mask, can be used in cooperative children to correct midfacial retrusion. An appliance attached to the teeth engages the elastic bands on the face mask to generate an anterior force on the teeth that is transmitted to the maxilla and its surrounding interosseous sutures. **(B)** Underbite caused by maxillary deficiency, as shown in this photograph, is an indication for this device before treatment. **(C)** The correction achievable with the facial mask is readily apparent in this patient.

additional use of a chin cup appliance (Ishikawa, Kitazawa, Iwasaki, & Nakamura, 2000). Treatment is usually done before the age of 8 to take advantage of remaining maxillary growth before suture fusion begins. Face-mask treatment requires 12 to 14 hours of wear per day to show midface improvement (Ahn, Figueroa, Braun, & Polley, 1999).

Another consideration during the early mixed dentition stage is the need for a secondary alveolar bone graft to correct the deficiency of bone in the dental arch (**FIGURE 6-30**). As with a primary alveolar bone graft, a secondary alveolar bone graft is also done to introduce bone matrix–inducing material into the alveolar cleft site, but it is done during mixed dentition rather than infancy. Frequently, bone from the iliac crest

(part of the greater pelvis) is used, although other sources of bone (e.g., the tibia, cranium, anterior chin, freeze-dried cadaver bone, and artificial substitutes such as hydroxyl apatite) can also be used (Bohman, Yamashita, Baek, & Yen, 2004; Chin, Ng, Tom, & Carstens, 2005; Enemark, Jensen, & Bosch, 2001; Hughes & Revington, 2002; Kalaaji, Lilja, Elander, & Friede, 2001; Nwoku, Al Atel, Al Shlash, Oluyadi, & Ismail, 2005; Sivarajasingam, Peil, Morse, & Shepherd, 2001). When successful, the bone graft stimulates new bone formation in the cleft site to replace the missing segment of the alveolar ridge. This provides bony support for normal eruption of the permanent lateral incisor and later the canine. Without adequate bone, the erupting teeth will have a periodontal defect, which compromises not only these teeth but other adjacent teeth as well (Shashua & Omnell, 2000; Solis, Figueroa, Cohen, Polley, & Evans, 1998). The bone graft also serves to replace the missing part of the nasal floor and piriform (nasal) rim (De Riu, Lai, Congiu, & Tullio, 2004; Hynes & Earley, 2003).

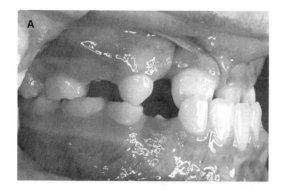

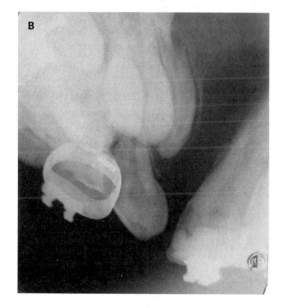

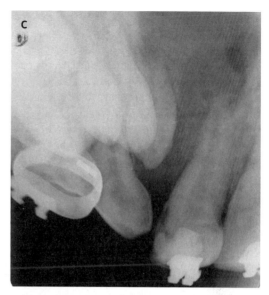

FIGURE 6-30 A patient needing an alveolar bone graft. **(A)** One can see the notching of the alveolus between the primary canine and the permanent lateral incisor. **(B)** In the occlusal radiograph, one can see the developing lateral incisor and the deficiency of alveolar bone. This is an indication for alveolar bone grafting. The anterior crossbite and narrowness of the maxilla will be corrected orthodontically prior to the bone graft. This gives the surgeon better access to the cleft and allows the lateral incisor to erupt through normal bone, thereby avoiding periodontal defects. **(C)** In this example of a larger defect, one can appreciate the deficiency of bone.

Maxillary expansion is usually required preoperatively if it hasn't already been done.

Alveolar bone grafting is usually done when the lateral incisor is beginning to reach one-half to two-thirds of normal root length (Hogan, Shand, Heggie, & Kilpatrick, 2003; Matsui, Echigo, Kimizuka, Takahashi, & Chiba, 2005; Murthy & Lehman, 2005). If the maxillary lateral incisor is missing or unusable, the bone grafting can be delayed until the maxillary canine is ready to erupt—usually between ages 11 and 13 (Da Silva Filho, Teles, Ozawa, & Filho, 2000). Some clinicians argue, however, that delaying the bone graft until the time of canine eruption creates a defect around the central incisor. More studies are needed to evaluate the long-term outcome of periodontal health as it relates to early versus late bone grafting (De Moor, De Vree, Cornelis, & De Boever, 2002; Dempf, Teltzrow, Kramer, & Hausamen, 2002; Kolbenstvedt, Aalokken, Arctander, & Johannessen, 2002; Schultze-Mosgau, Nkenke, Schlegel, Hirschfelder, & Wiltfang, 2003; Witherow, Cox, Jones, Carr, & Waterhouse, 2002).

Secondary alveolar bone grafting is highly predictable in unilateral clefts when the greater and lesser segments are stabilized properly. In these cases, there is close to a 95% success rate (Arctander, Kolbenstvedt, Aalokken,

Abyholm, & Froslie, 2005; Bajaj, Wongworawat, & Punjabi, 2003; Hynes & Earley, 2003; Kindelan & Roberts-Harry, 1999; Williams, Semb, Bearn, Shaw, & Sandy, 2003). For bilateral clefts, the success rate approaches 90% when the graft is done on one side at a time (Bohman et al., 2004; Kamakura, Yamaguchi, Kochi, Sato, & Motegi, 2003). When simultaneous grafting of both sides of a bilateral cleft is done, the success rate drops to about 70% (Mao, Ma, & Li, 2000; Shashua & Omnell, 2000).

Late Mixed Dentition (9–12 Years)

Once the permanent incisors and first molars have erupted, visible changes in the dentition may not be noticeable for another 2 to 3 years. If there is midface retrusion, however, it may become more noticeable during the late mixed dentition stage.

Maxillary expansion for alveolar bone grafting may be done during this stage (if it has not been done already) and is timed around the eruption of the maxillary canine. In addition, orthodontics can be started as soon as 1 to 3 months after the bone grafting (Vig, 1999). The incisors can finally be aligned through orthodontics because there is sufficient root formation by this time and also because the alveolar bone graft provides adequate bone to support the incisors (Cavassan Ade, de Albuquerque, & Filho, 2004; Semb & Ramstad, 1999). Also, missing teeth may be replaced by adding artificial teeth to the orthodontic appliances, at least as a temporary measure.

During this age range, some patients with maxillary retrusion are candidates for treatment through bone-anchored maxillary protraction (BAMP) (**FIGURE 6-31**). This technique has recently been introduced as an alternative to more traditional dentofacial orthopedics (De Clerck, Geerinckx, & Siciliano, 2002). The technique has been successful in the treatment of noncleft children, around ages 11 to 13, with more advancement than typical face-mask treatment at earlier ages (De Clerck & Proffit, 2005). Response to BAMP has been shown to be comparable in

children with cleft lip and palate and is a possible alternative to later osteotomies (Yatabe et al., 2017; Yen, 2011).

In addition to cleft-related issues, treatment may be needed for problems common to children without clefts during the late mixed dentition period. These problems may include space maintenance for prematurely lost primary teeth, the need to control moderate to severe crowding problems through selective tooth extraction, or correction of jaw position with dentofacial orthopedic measures, such as headgear or functional appliances. The decreased maxillary growth in children with repaired clefts must be considered when prescribing any of these treatment modalities.

There are both risks and benefits of initiating treatment in the late mixed dentition stage as opposed to waiting until later (Proffit et al., 2013). The child with a cleft is likely to require orthodontic treatment in the permanent dentition regardless, and it is well-known that tooth eruption is frequently delayed in patients with clefts (McNamara, Foley, Garvey, & Kavanagh, 1999). Also, because orthodontic treatment depends on the cooperation of the child, it is important that the child does not become "burned out" from orthodontic treatment before it is completed (Proffit et al., 2003). Therefore, every attempt should be made to delay or combine treatment whenever possible to avoid "orthodontic fatigue" (Kapp-Simon, 2004). Most clinicians try to accomplish interceptive orthodontic treatment in a short 12- to 18-month period and then give the child a rest from orthodontics until the permanent dentition completely erupts.

Adolescent Dentition (12–18 Years)

Ideally, by the time of eruption of the permanent dentition, crossbites have been corrected, alveolar bony defects are repaired, the incisors are well aligned, crowding has been managed, and the child has experienced good maxillary growth. Unfortunately, this is not always the case (Veleminska et al., 2003). For many children with clefts, the maxilla remains hypoplastic in

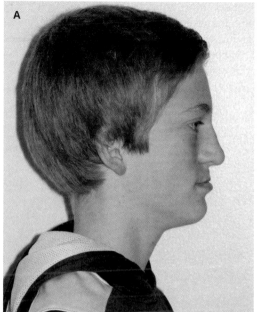

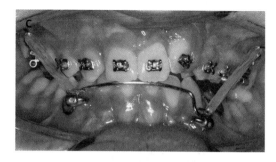

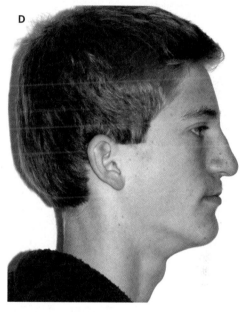

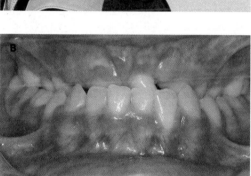

FIGURE 6-31 (A) Patient profile at age 12 years, 8 months showing midface deficiency associated with unilateral cleft lip and palate. Note lack of upper lip support and relatively protruding lower lip. **(B)** Intraoral view at age 12 years, 8 months showing characteristic anterior crossbite and Class III malocclusion associated with unilateral cleft lip and palate. **(C)** Intraoral view at age 14 years, 3 months showing complete correction of anterior crossbite. Orthodontic appliances are in place to address upper left canine impaction. A lower bite block retainer is visible too. **(D)** Patient profile at age 14 years, 3 months after 11 months of bone-anchored maxillary protraction (BAMP) treatment. Note improved upper lip and cheek bone support from maxillary protraction.

all dimensions—vertical, sagittal, and transverse (Gaggl, Schultes, & Karcher, 1999). The adolescent growth spurt may have made these deficits more noticeable because of both the mandible's relatively normal growth and the growth of the nose (Scheuer et al., 2001). The discrepancy from an underdeveloped maxilla and normal mandible often leads to either a Class III malocclusion with

deep underbite or a Class I malocclusion with anterior open bite.

If a severe anterior crossbite persists during growth, the mandibular incisors may overerupt, causing a deep underbite. Also, because the maxilla is shorter than normal, the mandible may be overclosed, further contributing to deep underbite. Conversely, in some patients with relatively normal occlusion, mandibular growth is directed inferiorly and posteriorly. This allows the teeth to remain in a more normal occlusion but results in a longer facial profile and possible open bite (Lisson et al., 2004). Fortunately, these two phenomena appear to be occurring less often now because improvements in surgical techniques have led to fewer detrimental effects on maxillary growth. Thus, although percentages vary between treatment centers, about 80% of adolescents with a repaired cleft can now be successfully treated with orthodontics alone (**FIGURE 6-32**).

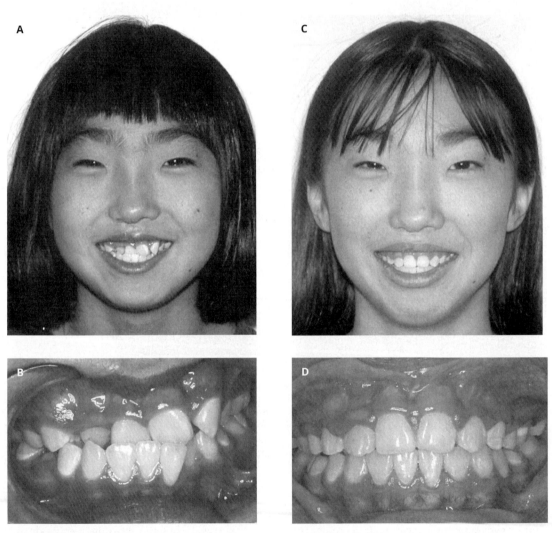

FIGURE 6-32 Adolescent treatment with orthodontics only. **(A)** This patient with right unilateral cleft lip and palate exhibits only mild midfacial retrusion. **(B)** The anterior crossbite of this patient was judged to be amenable to orthodontic treatment alone. Orthognathic surgery was not considered to be necessary. **(C)** After adolescent growth and orthodontic treatment, the facial proportions remain well balanced. **(D)** The post-treatment occlusal result was excellent. One lateral incisor was missing, the remaining lateral incisor was extracted, and the canines were substituted for the lateral incisors.

The remaining 20% or so require orthognathic surgery, in addition to orthodontics, to align the dental arches (Proffit et al., 2003). Of course, actual results vary from center to center.

Orthognathic surgery, which is surgery to move the bones of the jaws, frequently involves a maxillary Le Fort I osteotomy to reposition the maxilla anteriorly (Heliovaara, Ranta, Hukki, & Rintala, 2002) (**FIGURE 6-33**). Orthodontic treatment in preparation for surgery intentionally worsens the discrepancy between the upper and lower teeth to create sufficient space for maximum jaw

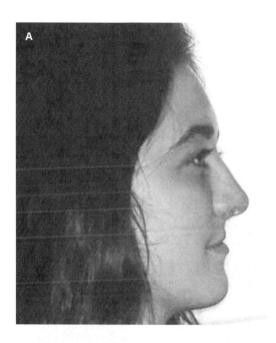

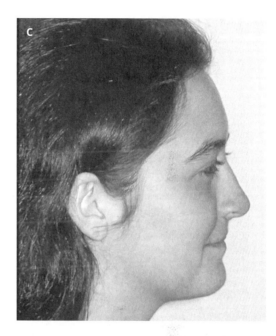

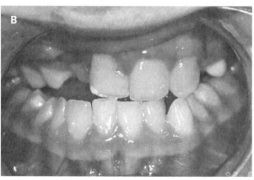

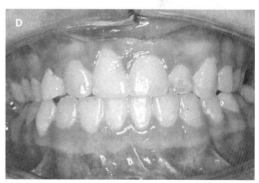

FIGURE 6-33 Adolescent dentition treatment with orthodontics and orthognathic surgery. **(A)** This patient with unilateral right cleft lip and palate needed orthodontics and orthognathic surgery to correct her moderate midfacial retrusion. **(B)** This shows her malocclusion with anterior and posterior crossbite and missing right lateral incisor. **(C)** After orthodontic preparation, she underwent a Le Fort I maxillary osteotomy to advance the upper jaw and teeth as well as malar implants to augment the cheeks. As a result, she has an improved profile and upper lip position. **(D)** Postoperative occlusion is greatly improved as well. Extraction of multiple teeth to correct her malocclusion only (without maxillary advancement surgery) would have lessened her lip support and given her an "aged" or edentulous appearance.

repositioning. (See the chapter *Surgical Management* for more information regarding orthognathic surgery.)

A relatively recent development in orthognathic surgical treatment is distraction osteogenesis (**FIGURE 6-34**). This involves making a

corticotomy (cut in bone) and then slowly distracting the cut ends apart with a mechanical device. Osteogenesis (creation of new bone) occurs between the cut ends and in time becomes normal bone, obviating the need for bone grafts (Kusnoto, Figueroa, & Polley, 2001; Swennen, Figueroa, Schierle, Polley, & Malevez, 2000). This is a very effective treatment option for many patients (Albert, 2000; Kita, Kochi, Imai, Yamada, & Yamaguchi, 2005; Molina, 2009). Rigid external distraction osteogenesis for the midface

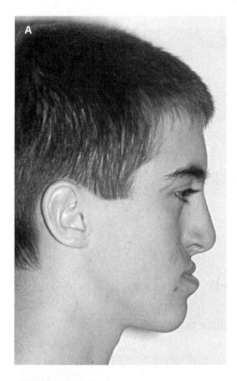

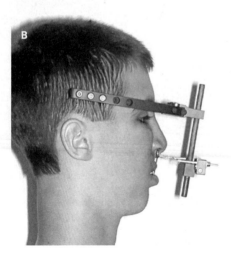

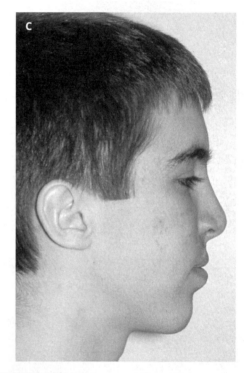

FIGURE 6-34 Rigid external distraction osteogenesis. **(A)** This patient with bilateral cleft lip and palate exhibits midfacial retrusion that is far outside the limits of conventional orthognathic surgery. **(B)** He elected to undergo the rigid external distraction procedure. Following maxillary Le Fort I osteotomy, the rigid framework is attached to the skull with scalp pins, and the maxilla is pulled forward, or "distracted," with a screw mechanism over about an 8-week period. **(C)** Following stabilization, the headframe is removed, and the improvement in facial profile can be readily seen.

SPEECH NOTES

Maxillary Distraction

The effect on speech of distraction as compared to standard surgery has recently been reviewed through a meta-study of the literature (Chanchareonsook, Samman, & Whitehill, 2006). Many studies in the review found that maxillary advancement surgery had no effect on speech or velopharyngeal status. Others reported worsening of speech only in patients with either preexisting velopharyngeal insufficiency or borderline velopharyngeal function before surgery. Although there were very few systematic comparisons between distraction and conventional osteotomy, there seemed to be no clear difference in outcome of one over the other (see the chapter *Speech Therapy* for additional information).

is commonly done (Figueroa & Polley, 1999; Figueroa, Polley, & Ko, 1999; Guyette, Polley, Figueroa, & Smith, 2001; Polley & Figueroa, 2000), although internal appliances are sometimes used (Cohen, 1999; Scolozzi, 2008). Orthodontists and surgeons work closely together to determine the final occlusion with these techniques (Motohashi & Kuroda, 1999). This field is rapidly changing with new devices and their variants being introduced at a rapid pace. At present, distraction osteogenesis is primarily being used to reduce or correct severe facial deformities that are not amenable to standard surgical techniques (Combs & Harshbarger, 2014; Figueroa, Polley, Friede, & Ko, 2004; Liou & Tsai, 2005; Mitsugi, Ito, & Alcalde, 2005; Wang et al., 2005; Yen et al., 2005; Zwahlen & Butow, 2004).

Lastly, an adolescent who has had orthodontics and orthognathic surgery is likely to require prosthodontic replacement of missing teeth. This can be accomplished with removable dental prostheses, such as dentures or partials (see the chapter *Prosthetic Management*). More commonly, it is corrected with fixed crowns and bridges or dental

implants (Moore & McCord, 2004; Reisberg, 2004). Dental implants are cylindrical pieces of titanium that can take the place of a missing tooth's root and are able to support crowns (Fukuda, Takahashi, & Iino, 2003; Isono et al., 2002). The coordinated involvement of the surgeon, orthodontist, and prosthodontist is required for a successful outcome (Kawakami, Yokozeki, Horiuchi, & Moriyama, 2004; Kearns, Perrott, Sharma, Kaban, & Vargervik, 1997; Kramer et al., 2005; Laine, Vahatalo, Peltola, Tammisalo, & Happonen, 2002; Sailer, Zembic, Jung, Hammerle, & Mattiola, 2007).

The Role of Speech Therapy

Speech-language pathologists, dental professionals, and surgeons must work closely together to correct speech problems related to abnormal dentition and/or malocclusion (Pinsky & Goldberg, 1977; Shprintzen et al., 1985; Vallino, Zuker, & Napoli, 2008). The role of the speech-language pathologist is to first determine whether the abnormal speech is related to abnormal structure or abnormal function. If the cause is abnormal structure, it is important to determine whether there are obligatory distortions or compensatory productions. Speech therapy is never appropriate for obligatory distortions related to dental or occlusal abnormalities (Shprintzen, 1991). Instead, correction of the occlusion will correct the distortion of speech without the need for speech therapy (Kummer et al., 1989; Wakumoto et al., 1996). On the other hand, if there are compensatory errors as a result of the dentition or occlusion, then speech therapy is required for correction but should be done after correction of the abnormal structure. Speech-language pathologists and dentists should coordinate their interventions to coincide with the stages of dental development as outlined in the preceding sections. Coordination of treatment timing, sequencing, and follow-up is important for the efficient use of resources and for ensuring the best overall outcome.

SUMMARY

Children with clefts or other craniofacial anomalies are at risk for dental and occlusal abnormalities. Most consonants are produced in the anterior portion of the oral cavity. Therefore, dental and occlusal abnormalities often affect speech by interfering with lip and tongue tip placement.

Because so many children with craniofacial anomalies have dental and speech problems, it is important for dental professionals and speech-language pathologists to work closely together. Interdisciplinary communication and coordination will help to determine the appropriate form of treatment needed to achieve a maximal outcome in aesthetics, mastication, and speech.

FOR REVIEW AND DISCUSSION

1. What is the dental term for baby teeth? How many baby teeth are in each arch? What is the dental term for adult teeth? How many adult teeth are in each arch?

2. With a cleft of the primary palate, which teeth are most likely to be affected? Explain why this affects primarily these two types of teeth?

3. What types of dental anomalies have the potential to affect speech? List the category of phonemes that are most likely to be affected by dental anomalies, and list other categories of phonemes that can be affected.

4. What is Angle's Classification System? Define Class I, Class II, and Class III occlusion. Which type of malocclusion is commonly seen in individuals with cleft palate only caused by Pierre Robin sequence? Which type of malocclusion is commonly seen in individuals with a cleft of the primary palate (with or without cleft of the secondary palate)? What are the factors that cause each type of malocclusion?

5. What types of compensatory articulation errors might you expect with an anterior crossbite and Class III malocclusion? What is the appropriate treatment?

6. What types of obligatory distortions might you expect with an anterior crossbite and Class III malocclusion? What is the appropriate treatment?

7. What is the purpose of infant oral orthopedics? What are some of the methods in which this can be done?

8. What is the general procedure for an alveolar bone graft? Why is it done? When is it done for primary alveolar bone grafting? When is it done for secondary alveolar bone grafting?

9. Describe the dental concerns and usual dental or orthodontic treatment during the following stages: infant stage, primary dentition (1–6 years), early mixed dentition (6–9 years), late mixed dentition (9–12 years), and adolescent dentition (12–18 years).

10. Under what circumstances is speech therapy appropriate for speech issues secondary to dental or occlusal anomalies? When is speech therapy not appropriate?

REFERENCES

Ahn, J. G., Figueroa, A. A., Braun, S., & Polley, J. W. (1999). Biomechanical considerations in distraction of the osteotomized dentomaxillary complex. *American Journal of Orthodontics & Dentofacial Orthopedics, 116*(3), 264–270.

Akcam, M. O., Evirgen, S., Uslu, O., & Toygar Memikoğlu, U. (2010). Dental anomalies in individuals with cleft lip and/or palate. *European Journal of Orthodontics, 32*(2), 207–213.

Albert, T. W. (2000). Oral and maxillofacial surgery: Considerations in cleft nasal deformities. *Facial Plastic Surgery, 16*(1), 79–84.

Aljamal, G., Hazza'a, A., & Rawashdeh, M. A. (2010). Prevalence of dental anomalies in a population of cleft lip and palate patients. *The Cleft Palate–Craniofacial Journal, 47*(4), 413–420.

Angle, E. H. (1899). Classification of malocclusion. *Dental Cosmos, 41,* 248–264, 350–357.

Arctander, K., Kolbenstvedt, A., Aalokken, T. M., Abyholm, F., & Froslie, K. F. (2005). Computed tomography of alveolar bone grafts 20 years after repair of unilateral cleft lip and palate. *Scandinavian Journal of Plastic & Reconstructive Surgery & Hand Surgery, 39*(1), 11–14.

Bajaj, A. K., Wongworawat, A. A., & Punjabi, A. (2003). Management of alveolar clefts. *Journal of Craniofacial Surgery, 14*(6), 840–846.

Bartzela, T., Katsaros, C., Shaw, W. C., Rønning, E., Rizzell, S., Bronkhorst, E. M., . . . Kuijpers-Jagtman, A. M. (2010). A longitudinal three-center study of dental arch relationship in patients with bilateral cleft lip and palate. *The Cleft Palate–Craniofacial Journal, 47*(2), 167–174.

Berkowitz, S., Duncan, R., Evans, C., Friede, H., Kuijpers-Jagtman, A. M., Prahl-Anderson, B., & Rosenstein, S. (2005). Timing of cleft palate closure should be based on the ratio of the area of the cleft to that of the palatal segments and not on age alone. *Plastic and Reconstructive Surgery, 115*(6), 1483–1499.

Berkowitz, S., Mejia, M., & Bystrik, A. (2004). A comparison of the effects of the Latham-Millard procedure with those of a conservative treatment approach for dental occlusion and facial aesthetics in unilateral and bilateral complete cleft lip and palate: Part I. Dental occlusion. *Plastic and Reconstructive Surgery, 113*(1), 1–18.

Bitter, K. (2001). Repair of bilateral clefts of lip, alveolus and palate. Part 1: A refined method for the lip-adhesion in bilateral cleft lip and palate patients. *Journal of Craniomaxillofacial Surgery, 29*(1), 39–43.

Bohman, P., Yamashita, D. D., Baek, S. H., & Yen, S. L. (2004). Stabilization of an edentulous premaxilla for an alveolar bone graft: Case report. *The Cleft Palate–Craniofacial Journal, 41*(2), 214–217.

Bongaarts, C. A., Kuijpers-Jagtman, A. M., van't Hof, M. A., & Prahl-Andersen, B. (2004). The effect of infant orthopedics on the occlusion of the deciduous dentition in children with complete unilateral cleft lip and palate (Dutchcleft). *The Cleft Palate–Craniofacial Journal, 41*(6), 633–641.

Braumann, B., Keilig, L., Bourauel, C., & Jager, A. (2002). Three-dimensional analysis of morphological changes in the maxilla of patients with cleft lip and palate. *The Cleft Palate–Craniofacial Journal, 39*(1), 1–11.

Cabete, H. F., Gomide, M. R., & Costa, B. (2000). Evaluation of primary dentition in cleft lip and palate children with and without natal/neonatal teeth. *The Cleft Palate–Craniofacial Journal, 37*(4), 406–409.

Camporesi, M., Baccetti, T., Marinelli, A., Defraia, E., & Franchi, L. (2010). Maxillary dental anomalies in children with cleft lip and palate: A controlled study. *International Journal of Paediatric Dentistry, 20*(6), 442–450.

Cavassan Ade, O., de Albuquerque, M. D., & Filho, L. C. (2004). Rapid maxillary expansion after secondary alveolar bone graft in a patient with bilateral cleft lip and palate. *The Cleft Palate–Craniofacial Journal, 41*(3), 332–339.

Chan, K. T., Hayes, C., Shusterman, S., Mulliken, J. B., & Will, L. A. (2003). The effects of active infant orthopedics on occlusal relationships in unilateral complete cleft lip and palate. *The Cleft Palate–Craniofacial Journal, 40*(5), 511–517.

Chanchareonsook, N., Samman, N., & Whitehill, T. L. (2006). The effect of cranio-maxillofacial osteotomies and distraction osteogenesis on speech and velopharyngeal status: A critical review. *The Cleft Palate–Craniofacial Journal, 43*(4), 477–487.

Chapple, J. R., & Nunn, J. H. (2001). The oral health of children with clefts of the lip, palate, or both. *The Cleft Palate–Craniofacial Journal, 38*(5), 525–528.

Chin, M., Ng, T., Tom, W. K., & Carstens, M. (2005). Repair of alveolar clefts with recombinant human bone morphogenetic protein (rhBMP-2) in patients with clefts. *Journal of Craniofacial Surgery, 16*(5), 778–789.

Cho, B. (2001). Unilateral complete cleft lip and palate repair using lip adhesion and passive alveolar molding appliance. *Journal of Craniofacial Surgery, 12*(2), 148–156.

Cohen, S. R. (1999). Midface distraction. *Seminars in Orthodontics, 5*(1), 52–58.

Combs, P. D., & Harshbarger, R. J. (2014). Le Fort I maxillary advancement using distraction osteogenesis. *Seminars in Plastic Surgery, 28*(4), 193–198.

Cutting, C., Grayson, B., Brecht, L., Santiago, P., Wood, R., & Kwon, S. (1998). Presurgical columellar elongation and primary retrograde nasal reconstruction in one-stage bilateral cleft lip and nose repair. *Plastic and Reconstructive Surgery, 101*(3), 630–639.

Da Silva Filho, O. G., Teles, S. G., Ozawa, T. O., & Filho, L. C. (2000). Secondary bone graft and eruption of the permanent canine in patients with alveolar clefts: Literature review and case report. *Angle Orthodontist, 70*(2), 174–178.

Da Silveira, A. C., Oliveira, N., Gonzalez, S., Shahani, M., Reisberg, D., Daw, J. L., Jr., & Cohen, M. (2003). Modified nasal alveolar molding appliance for management of cleft lip defect. *Journal of Craniofacial Surgery, 14*(5), 700–703.

De Clerck, H., Geerinckx, V., & Siciliano, S. (2002). The zygoma anchorage system. *Journal of Clinical Orthodontics, 36*(8), 455–459.

De Clerck, H. J., & Proffit, W. R. (2015). Growth modification of the face: A current perspective with emphasis on Class III treatment. *American Journal of Orthodontic and Dentofacial Orthopedics, 148*(1), 37–46.

De Moor, R. J., De Vree, H. M., Cornelis, C., & De Boever, J. A. (2002). Cervical root resorption in two patients with unilateral complete cleft of the lip and palate. *The Cleft Palate–Craniofacial Journal, 39*(5), 541–545.

Dempf, R., Teltzrow, T., Kramer, F. J., & Hausamen, J. E. (2002). Alveolar bone grafting in patients with complete clefts: A comparative study between secondary and tertiary bone grafting. *The Cleft Palate–Craniofacial Journal, 39*(1), 18–25.

De Riu, G., Lai, V., Congiu, M., & Tullio, A. (2004). Secondary bone grafting of alveolar cleft. *Minerva Stomatologica, 53*(10), 571–579.

Dewinter, G., Quirynen, M., Heidbuchel, K., Verdonck, A., Willems, G., & Carels, C. (2003). Dental abnormalities, bone graft quality, and periodontal conditions in patients with unilateral cleft lip and palate at different phases of orthodontic treatment. *The Cleft Palate–Craniofacial Journal, 40*(4), 343–350.

DiBiase, A. T., DiBiase, D. D., Hay, N. J., & Sommerlad, B. C. (2002). The relationship between arch dimensions and the 5-year index in the primary dentition of patients with complete UCLP. *The Cleft Palate–Craniofacial Journal, 39*(6), 635–640.

Doruk, C., & Kilic, B. (2005). Extraoral nasal molding in a newborn with unilateral cleft lip and palate: A case report. *The Cleft Palate–Craniofacial Journal, 42*(6), 699–702.

Enemark, H., Jensen, J., & Bosch, C. (2001). Mandibular bone graft material for reconstruction of alveolar cleft defects: Long-term results. *The Cleft Palate–Craniofacial Journal, 38*(2), 155–163.

Figueroa, A. A., & Polley, J. W. (1999). Management of severe cleft maxillary deficiency with distraction osteogenesis: Procedure and results. *American Journal of Orthodontic and Dentofacial Orthopedics, 115*(1), 1–12.

Figueroa, A. A., Polley, J. W., Friede, H., & Ko, E. W. (2004). Long-term skeletal stability after maxillary advancement with distraction osteogenesis using a rigid external distraction device in cleft maxillary deformities. *Plastic and Reconstructive Surgery, 114*(6), 1382–1392; discussion 1393–1394.

Figueroa, A. A., Polley, J. W., & Ko, E. W. (1999). Maxillary distraction for the management of cleft maxillary hypoplasia with a rigid external distraction system. *Seminars in Orthodontics, 5*(1), 46–51.

Fukuda, M., Takahashi, T., & Iino, M. (2003). Dentoalveolar reconstruction of a missing premaxilla using bone graft and endosteal implants. *Journal of Oral Rehabilitation, 30*(1), 87–90.

Gable, T. O., Kummer, A. W., Lee, L., Creaghead, N. A., & Moore, L. J. (1995). Premature loss of the maxillary primary incisors: Effect on speech production. *Journal of Dentistry for Children, 62*(3), 173–179.

Gaggl, A., Schultes, G., & Karcher, H. (1999). Aesthetic and functional outcome of surgical and orthodontic correction of bilateral clefts of lip, palate, and alveolus. *The Cleft Palate–Craniofacial Journal, 36*(5), 407–412.

Gaggl, A., Schultes, G., Karcher, E. L., & Mossbock, R. (1999). Periodontal disease in patients with cleft palate and patients with unilateral and bilateral clefts of lip, palate, and alveolus. *Journal of Periodontology, 70*(2), 171–178.

Garfinkle, J. S., King, T. W., Grayson, B. H., Brecht, L. E., & Cutting, C. B. (2011). A 12-year anthropometric evaluation of the nose in bilateral cleft lip-cleft palate patients following nasoalveolar molding and cutting bilateral cleft lip and nose reconstruction. *Plastic and Reconstructive Surgery, 127*(4), 1659–1667.

Garrahy, A., Millett, D. T., & Ayoub, A. F. (2005). Early assessment of dental arch development in repaired unilateral cleft lip and unilateral cleft lip and palate versus controls. *The Cleft Palate–Craniofacial Journal, 42*(4), 385–391.

Grayson, B., & Cutting, C. B. (2001). Presurgical nasoalveolar orthopedic molding in primary correction of the nose, lip, and alveolus of infants born with unilateral and bilateral clefts. *The Cleft Palate–Craniofacial Journal, 38*(3), 193–198.

Grayson, B., & Maull, D. (2004). Nasoalveolar molding for infants born with clefts of the lip, alveolus, and palate. *Clinics in Plastic Surgery, 31*(2), 149–158, vii.

Guyette, T. W., Polley, J. W., Figueroa, A., & Smith, B. E. (2001). Changes in speech following maxillary distraction osteogenesis. *The Cleft Palate–Craniofacial Journal, 38*(3), 199–205.

Hathaway, R. R., Eppley, B. L., Hennon, D. K., Nelson, C. L., & Sadove, A. M. (1999). Primary alveolar cleft bone grafting in unilateral cleft lip and palate: Arch dimensions at age 8. *Journal of Craniofacial Surgery, 10*(1), 58–67.

Hathaway, R. R., Eppley, B. L., Nelson, C. L., & Sadove, A. M. (1999). Primary alveolar cleft bone grafting in unilateral cleft lip and palate: Craniofacial form at age 8. *Journal of Craniofacial Surgery, 10*(1), 68–72.

Heliovaara, A., Ranta, R., Hukki, J., & Rintala, A. (2002). Skeletal stability of Le Fort I osteotomy in patients with isolated cleft palate and bilateral cleft lip and palate. *International Journal of Oral & Maxillofacial Surgery, 31*(4), 358–363.

Heliovaara, A., Ranta, R., & Rautio, J. (2004). Dental abnormalities in permanent dentition in children with submucous cleft palate. *Acta Odontologica Scandinavica, 62*(3), 129–131.

Hogan, L., Shand, J. M., Heggie, A. A., & Kilpatrick, N. (2003). Canine eruption into grafted alveolar clefts: A retrospective study. *Australian Dental Journal, 48*(2), 119–124.

Hughes, C. W., & Revington, P. J. (2002). The proximal tibia donor site in cleft alveolar bone grafting: Experience of 75 consecutive cases. *Journal of Craniomaxillofacial Surgery, 30*(1), 12–16; discussion 17.

Hynes, P. J., & Earley, M. J. (2003). Assessment of secondary alveolar bone grafting using a modification of the Bergland grading system. *British Journal of Plastic Surgery, 56*(7), 630–636.

Ishikawa, H., Kitazawa, S., Iwasaki, H., & Nakamura, S. (2000). Effects of maxillary protraction combined with chin-cap therapy in unilateral cleft lip and palate patients. *The Cleft Palate–Craniofacial Journal, 37*(1), 92–97.

Isono, H., Kaida, K., Hamada, Y., Kokubo, Y., Ishihara, M., Hirashita, A., & Kuwahara, Y. (2002). The reconstruction of bilateral clefts using endosseous implants after bone grafting. *American Journal of Orthodontics & Dentofacial Orthopedics, 121*(4), 403–410.

Johnson, N. C. L., & Sandy, J. R. (1999). Tooth position and speech: Is there a relationship? *The Angle Orthodontist, 69*(4), 306–310.

Kalaaji, A., Lilja, J., Elander, A., & Friede, H. (2001). Tibia as donor site for alveolar bone grafting in patients with cleft lip and palate: Long-term experience. *Scandinavian Journal of Plastic & Reconstructive Surgery & Hand Surgery, 35*(1), 35–42.

Kamakura, S., Yamaguchi, T., Kochi, S., Sato, A., & Motegi, K. (2003). Preliminary report of two-stage secondary alveolar bone grafting for patients with bilateral cleft lip and palate. *The Cleft Palate–Craniofacial Journal, 40*(5), 449–452.

Kapp-Simon, K. A. (2004). Psychological issues in cleft lip and palate. *Clinics in Plastic Surgery, 31*(2), 347–352.

Katz, M. I. (1992). Angle classification revisited 2: A modified Angle classification. *American Journal of Orthodontic and Dentofacial Orthopedics, 102*(3), 277–284.

Kawakami, M., Yagi, T., & Takada, K. (2002). Maxillary expansion and protraction in correction of midface retrusion in a complete unilateral cleft lip and palate patient. *Angle Orthodontist, 72*(4), 355–361.

Kawakami, S., Yokozeki, M., Horiuchi, S., & Moriyama, K. (2004). Oral rehabilitation of an orthodontic patient with cleft lip and palate and hypodontia using secondary bone grafting, osseo-integrated implants, and prosthetic treatment. *The Cleft Palate–Craniofacial Journal, 41*(3), 279–284.

Kearns, G., Perrott, D. H., Sharma, A., Kaban, L. B., & Vargervik, K. (1997). Placement of endosseous implants in grafted alveolar clefts. *The Cleft Palate–Craniofacial Journal, 34*(6), 520–525.

Kindelan, J., & Roberts-Harry, D. (1999). A 5-year post-operative review of secondary alveolar bone grafting in the Yorkshire region. *British Journal of Orthodontics, 26*(3), 211–217.

Kirchberg, A., Treide, A., & Hemprich, A. (2004). Investigation of caries prevalence in children with cleft lip, alveolus, and palate. *Journal of Craniomaxillofacial Surgery, 32*(4), 216–219.

Kirschner, R. E., & LaRossa, D. (2000). Cleft lip and palate. *Otolaryngologic Clinics of North America, 33*(6), 1191–1215, v–vi.

Kita, H., Kochi, S., Imai, Y., Yamada, A., & Yamaguchi, T. (2005). Rigid external distraction using skeletal anchorage to cleft maxilla united with alveolar bone grafting. *The Cleft Palate–Craniofacial Journal, 42*(3), 318–327.

Kolbenstvedt, A., Aalokken, T. M., Arctander, K., & Johannessen, S. (2002). CT appearances of unilateral cleft palate 20 years after bone graft surgery. *Acta Radiologica, 43*(6), 567–570.

Kramer, F. J., Baethge, C., Swennen, G., Bremer, B., Schwestka-Polly, R., & Dempf, R. (2005). Dental implants in patients with orofacial clefts: A long-term follow-up study. *International Journal of Oral & Maxillofacial Surgery, 34*(7), 715–721.

Kuijpers-Jagtman, A. M., Borstlap-Engels, V. M., Spauwen, P. H., & Borstlap, W. A. (2000). Team management of orofacial clefts. *Nederlands Tijdschrift voor Tandheelkunde, 107*(11), 447–451.

Kummer, A. W., Strife, J. L., Grau, W. H., Creaghead, N. A., & Lee, L. (1989). The effects of Le Fort I osteotomy with maxillary movement on articulation, resonance, and velopharyngeal function. *Cleft Palate Journal, 26*(3), 193–199; discussion 199–200.

Kusnoto, B., Figueroa, A. A., & Polley, J. W. (2001). Radiographic evaluation of bone formation in the pterygoid region after maxillary distraction with a rigid external distraction (RED) device. *Journal of Craniofacial Surgery, 12*(2), 109–117; discussion 118.

Laine, J., Vahatalo, K., Peltola, J., Tammisalo, T., & Happonen, R. P. (2002). Rehabilitation of patients with congenital unrepaired cleft palate defects using free iliac crest bone grafts and dental implants. *International Journal of Oral Maxillofacial Implants, 17*(4), 573–580.

Lee, C. T., Grayson, B. H., Cutting, C. B., Brecht, L. E., & Lin, W. Y. (2004). Prepubertal midface growth in unilateral cleft lip and palate following alveolar molding and gingivoperiosteoplasty. *The Cleft Palate–Craniofacial Journal, 41*(4), 375–380.

Liou, E. J., & Tsai, W. C. (2005). A new protocol for maxillary protraction in cleft patients: Repetitive weekly protocol of alternate rapid maxillary expansions and constrictions. *The Cleft Palate–Craniofacial Journal, 42*(2), 121–127.

Lisson, J. A., Hanke, L., & Trankmann, J. (2004). Vertical changes in patients with complete unilateral and bilateral cleft lip, alveolus and palate. *Journal of Orofacial Orthopedics, 65*(3), 246–258.

Maciel, S. P., Costa, B., & Gomide, M. R. (2005). Difference in the prevalence of enamel alterations affecting central incisors of children with complete unilateral cleft lip and palate. *The Cleft Palate–Craniofacial Journal, 42*(4), 392–395.

Malanczuk, T., Opitz, C., & Retzlaff, R. (1999). Structural changes of dental enamel in both dentitions of cleft lip and palate patients. *Journal of Orofacial Orthopedics, 60*(4), 259–268.

Mao, C., Ma, L., & Li, X. (2000). A retrospective study of bilateral alveolar bone grafting. *Chinese Medical Sciences Journal, 15*(1), 49–51.

Matsui, K., Echigo, S., Kimizuka, S., Takahashi, M., & Chiba, M. (2005). Clinical study on eruption of permanent canines after secondary alveolar bone grafting. *The Cleft Palate–Craniofacial Journal, 42*(3), 309–313.

McNamara, C. M., Foley, T. F., Garvey, M. T., & Kavanagh, P. T. (1999). Premature dental eruption: Report of case. *Journal of Dentistry for Children, 66*(1), 70–72.

Millard, D. R., Latham, R., Huifen, X., Spiro, S., & Morovic, C. (1999). Cleft lip and palate treated by presurgical orthopedics, gingivoperiosteoplasty, and lip adhesion (POPLA) compared with previous lip adhesion method: A preliminary study of serial dental casts. *Plastic and Reconstructive Surgery, 103*(6), 1630–1644.

Mitsugi, M., Ito, O., & Alcalde, R. E. (2005). Maxillary bone transportation in alveolar cleft-transport distraction osteogenesis for treatment of alveolar cleft repair. *British Journal of Plastic Surgery, 58*(5), 619–625.

Molina, F. (2009). Mandibular distraction osteogenesis: A clinical experience of the last 17 years. *Journal of Craniofacial Surgery, 20*(Suppl. 2), 1794–1800.

Moller, K. T. (1994). Dental-occlusal and other oral conditions and speech. In J. E. Bernthal & N. W. Bankson (Eds.), *Child phonology: Characteristics, assessment, and intervention with special populations* (pp. 3–28). New York, NY: Thieme Medical Publishers.

Moore, D., & McCord, J. F. (2004). Prosthetic dentistry and the unilateral cleft lip and palate patient: The last 30 years. A review of the prosthodontic literature in respect of treatment options. *European Journal of Prosthodontics & Restorative Dentistry, 12*(2), 70–74.

Motohashi, N., & Kuroda, T. (1999). A 3-D computer-aided design system applied to diagnosis and treatment planning in orthodontics and orthognathic surgery. *European Journal of Orthodontics, 21*(3), 263–274.

Mouradian, W. E., Omnell, M. L., & Williams, B. (1999). Ethics for orthodontists. *Angle Orthodontist, 69*(4), 295–299.

Murthy, A. S., & Lehman, J. A. (2005). Evaluation of alveolar bone grafting: A survey of ACPA teams. *The Cleft Palate–Craniofacial Journal, 42*(1), 99–101.

Nazarian Mobin, S. S., Karatsonyi, A., Vidar, E. N., Gamer, S., Groper, J., Hammoudeh, J. A., & Urata, M. M. (2011). Is presurgical nasoalveolar molding therapy more effective in unilateral or bilateral cleft lip-cleft palate patients? *Plastic and Reconstructive Surgery, 127*(3), 1263–1269.

Ngan, P., Alkire, R. G., & Fields, H., Jr. (1999). Management of space problems in the primary and mixed dentitions. *Journal of the American Dental Association, 130*(9), 1330–1339.

Nwoku, A. L., Al Atel, A., Al Shlash, S., Oluyadi, B. A., & Ismail, S. (2005). Retrospective analysis of secondary alveolar cleft grafts using iliac of chin bone. *Journal of Craniofacial Surgery, 16*(5), 864–868.

Oosterkamp, B. C., Van Oort, R. P., Dijkstra, P. U., Stellingsma, K., Bierman, M. W., & de Bont, L. G. (2005). Effect of an intraoral retrusion plate on maxillary arch dimensions in complete bilateral cleft lip and palate patients. *The Cleft Palate–Craniofacial Journal, 42*(3), 239–244.

Pfeifer, T. M., Grayson, B. H., & Cutting, C. B. (2002). Nasoalveolar molding and gingivoperiosteoplasty versus alveolar bone graft: An outcome analysis of costs in the treatment of unilateral cleft alveolus. *The Cleft Palate–Craniofacial Journal, 39*(1), 26–29.

Pinsky, T. M., & Goldberg, H. J. (1977). Potential for clinical cooperation between dentistry and speech pathology. *International Dental Journal, 27*(4), 363–369.

Polley, J., & Figueroa, A. (2000). Re: Maxillary distraction osteogenesis: A method with skeletal anchorage. *Journal of Craniofacial Surgery, 11*(3), 295.

Posnick, J. C., & Ricalde, P. (2004). Cleft-orthognathic surgery. *Clinics in Plastic Surgery, 31*(2), 315–330.

Prahl, C., Kuijpers-Jagtman, A. M., van't Hof, M. A., & Prahl-Andersen, B. (2003). A randomized prospective clinical trial of the effect of infant orthopedics in unilateral cleft lip and palate: Prevention of collapse of the alveolar segments (Dutchcleft). *The Cleft Palate–Craniofacial Journal, 40*(4), 337–342.

Prahl, C., Kuijpers-Jagtman, A. M., van't Hof, M. A., & Prahl-Andersen, B. (2005). Infant orthopedics in UCLP: Effect on feeding, weight, and length: A randomized clinical trial (Dutchcleft). *The Cleft Palate–Craniofacial Journal, 42*(2), 171–177.

Proffit, W. R., Fields, H. W., Jr., Sarver, D. M., & Ackerman, J. L. (2013). *Contemporary orthodontics* (5th ed.). St. Louis, MO: Elsevier Mosby.

Proffit, W. R., White, R. P., & Sarver, D. M. (2003). *Contemporary treatment of dento-facial deformity.* St. Louis, MO: Mosby.

Quirynen, M., Dewinter, G., Avontroodt, P., Heidbuchel, K., Verdonck, A., & Carels, C. (2003). A split-mouth study on periodontal and microbial parameters in children with complete unilateral cleft lip and palate. *Journal of Clinical Periodontology, 30*(1), 49–56.

Reisberg, D. J. (2000). Dental and prosthodontic care for patients with cleft or craniofacial conditions. *The Cleft Palate–Craniofacial Journal, 37*(6), 534–537.

Reisberg, D. J. (2004). Prosthetic habilitation of patients with clefts. *Clinics in Plastic Surgery, 31*(2), 353–360.

Renkielska, A., Wojtaszek-Slominska, A., & Dobke, M. (2005). Early cleft lip repair in children with unilateral complete cleft lip and palate: A case against primary alveolar repair. *Annals of Plastic Surgery, 54*(6), 595–597; discussion 598–599.

Rivkin, C. J., Keith, O., Crawford, P. J., & Hathorn, I. S. (2000a). Dental care for the patient with a cleft lip and palate. Part 1: From birth to the mixed dentition stage. *British Dental Journal, 188*(2), 78–83.

Rivkin, C. J., Keith, O., Crawford, P. J., & Hathorn, I. S. (2000b). Dental care for the patient with a cleft lip and palate. Part 2: The mixed dentition stage through to adolescence and young adulthood. *British Dental Journal, 188*(3), 131–134.

Sachs, S. A. (2002). Nasoalveolar molding and gingiv-operiosteoplasty verses alveolar bone graft: An outcome analysis of costs in the treatment of unilateral cleft alveolus. *The Cleft Palate–Craniofacial Journal, 39*(5), 570; author reply 570–571.

Sailer, I., Zembic, A., Jung, R. E., Hammerle, C. H., & Mattiola, A. (2007). Single-tooth implant reconstructions: Esthetic factors influencing the decision between titanium and zirconia abutments in anterior regions. *The European Journal of Esthetic Dentistry, 2*(3), 296–310.

Sakamoto, T., Sakamoto, S., Harazaki, M., Isshiki, Y., & Yamaguchi, H. (2002). Orthodontic treatment for jaw deformities in cleft lip and palate patients with the combined use of an external-expansion arch and a facial mask. *Bulletin of Tokyo Dental College, 43*(4), 223–229.

Scheuer, H. A., Holtje, W. J., Hasund, A., & Pfeifer, G. (2001). Prognosis of facial growth in patients with unilateral complete clefts of the lip, alveolus and palate. *Journal of Craniomaxillofacial Surgery, 29*(4), 198–204.

Schultes, G., Gaggl, A., & Karcher, H. (1999). Comparison of periodontal disease in patients with clefts of palate and patients with unilateral clefts of lip, palate, and alveolus. *The Cleft Palate–Craniofacial Journal, 36*(4), 322–327.

Schultze-Mosgau, S., Nkenke, E., Schlegel, A. K., Hirschfelder, U., & Wiltfang, J. (2003). Analysis of bone resorption after secondary alveolar cleft bone grafts before and after canine eruption in connection with orthodontic gap closure or prosthodontic treatment. *Journal of Oral & Maxillofacial Surgery, 61*(11), 1245–1248.

Scolozzi, P. (2008). Distraction osteogenesis in the management of severe maxillary hypoplasia in cleft lip and palate patients. *Journal of Craniofacial Surgery, 19*(5), 1199–1214.

Semb, G., & Ramstad, T. (1999). The influence of alveolar bone grafting on the orthodontic and prosthodontic treatment of patients with cleft lip and palate. *Dental Update, 26*(2), 60–64.

Shashua, D., & Omnell, M. L. (2000). Radiographic determination of the position of the maxillary lateral incisor in the cleft alveolus and parameters for assessing its habilitation prospects. *The Cleft Palate–Craniofacial Journal, 37*(1), 21–25.

Shprintzen, R. J. (1991). Fallibility of clinical research. *The Cleft Palate–Craniofacial Journal, 28*(2), 136–140.

Shprintzen, R. J., Siegel-Sadewitz, V. L., Amato, J., & Goldberg, R. B. (1985). Anomalies associated with cleft lip, cleft palate, or both. *American Journal of Medical Genetics, 20*(4), 585–595.

Sivarajasingam, V., Peil, G., Morse, M., & Shepherd, J. P. (2001). Secondary bone grafting of alveolar clefts: A densitometric comparison of iliac crest and tibial bone grafts. *The Cleft Palate–Craniofacial Journal, 38*(1), 11–14.

Smith, K. S., Henry, B. T., & Scott, M. A. (2016). Presurgical dentofacial orthopedic management of the cleft patient. *Oral and Maxillofacial Surgery Clinics of North America, 28*(2), 169–176.

Solis, A., Figueroa, A. A., Cohen, M., Polley, J. W., & Evans, C. A. (1998). Maxillary dental development in complete unilateral alveolar clefts. *The Cleft Palate–Craniofacial Journal, 35*(4), 320–328.

Strauss, R. P. (1998). Cleft palate and craniofacial teams in the United States and Canada: A national survey of team organization and standards of care. The American Cleft Palate–Craniofacial Association (ACPA) Team Standards Committee. *Cleft Palate–Craniofacial Journal, 35*(6), 473–480.

Strauss, R. P. (1999). The organization and delivery of craniofacial health services: The state of the art. *The Cleft Palate–Craniofacial Journal, 36*(3), 189–195.

Strong, S. M. (2002). Adolescent dentistry: Multidisciplinary treatment for the cleft lip/palate patient. *Practical Procedures & Aesthetic Dentistry, 14*(4), 333–338; quiz 340, 342.

Swennen, G., Figueroa, A. A., Schierle, H., Polley, J. W., & Malevez, C. (2000). Maxillary distraction osteogenesis: A two-dimensional mathematical model. *Journal of Craniofacial Surgery, 11*(4), 312–317.

Taher, A. (1997). Speech defect associated with Class III jaw relationship. *Plastic and Reconstructive Surgery, 99*(4), 1200.

Tannure, P. N., Oliveira, C. A., Maia, L. C., Vieira, A. R., Granjeiro, J. M., & de Castro Costa, M. (2012). Prevalence of dental anomalies in nonsyndromic individuals with cleft lip and palate: A systematic review and meta-analysis. *The Cleft Palate–Craniofacial Journal, 49*(2), 194–200.

Trost-Cardamone, J. E. (1997). Diagnosis of specific cleft palate speech error patterns for planning therapy of physical management needs. In K. R. Bzoch (Ed.), *Communicative disorders related to cleft lip and palate* (vol. 4, pp. 313–330). Austin, TX: Pro-Ed.

Turvey, T. A., Vig, K. W. L., & Fonseca, R. J. (1996). *Facial clefts and craniosynostosis: Principles and management.* Chapel Hill, NC: W. B. Saunders.

Vallino, L. D., Zuker, R., & Napoli, J. A. (2008). A study of speech, language, hearing, and dentition in children with cleft lip only. *The Cleft Palate–Craniofacial Journal, 45*(5), 485–494.

Vasan, N. (1999). Management of children with clefts of the lip or palate: An overview. *New Zealand Dental Journal, 95*(419), 14–20.

Veleminska, J., Smahel, Z., & Mullerova, Z. (2003). Facial growth and development during the pubertal period in patients with complete unilateral cleft of lip and palate. *Acta Chirurgiae Plasticae, 45*(1), 22–31.

Vig, K. W. (1999). Alveolar bone grafts: The surgical/orthodontic management of the cleft maxilla. *Annals of the Academy of Medicine, Singapore, 28*(5), 721–727.

Wakumoto, M., Isaacson, K. G., Friel, S., Suzuki, N., Gibbon, F., Nixon, F., . . . Michi K. (1996). Preliminary study of the articulatory reorganization of fricative consonants following osteotomy. *Folia Phoniatrica et Logopedica, 48*(6), 275–289.

Wang, X. X., Wang, X., Yi, B., Li, Z. L., Liang, C., & Lin, Y. (2005). Internal midface distraction in correction of severe maxillary hypoplasia secondary to cleft lip and palate. *Plastic and Reconstructive Surgery, 116*(1), 51–60.

Wangsrimongkol, T., & Jansawang, W. (2010). The assessment of treatment outcome by evaluation of dental arch relationships in cleft lip/palate. *Journal of the Medical Association of Thailand, 93*(Suppl. 4), S100–S106.

Williams, A., Semb, G., Bearn, D., Shaw, W., & Sandy, J. (2003). Prediction of outcomes of secondary alveolar bone grafting in children born with unilateral cleft lip and palate. *European Journal of Orthodontics, 25*(2), 205–211.

Witherow, H., Cox, S., Jones, E., Carr, R., & Waterhouse, N. (2002). A new scale to assess radiographic success of secondary alveolar bone grafts. *The Cleft Palate–Craniofacial Journal, 39*(3), 255–260.

Yatabe, M., Garib, D. G., Faco, R. A. S., Clerck, H., Janson, G., Nguyen, T., . . . Ruellas A. C. (2017). Bone-anchored maxillary protraction therapy in patients with unilateral complete cleft lip and palate: 3-dimensional assessment of maxillary effects. *American Journal of Orthodontic and Dentofacial Orthopedics, 152*(3), 327–335.

Yen, S. L. (2011). Protocols for late maxillary protraction in cleft lip and palate patients at Childrens Hospital Los Angeles. *Seminars in Orthodontics, 17*(2), 138–148.

Yen, S. L., Yamashita, D. D., Gross, J., Meara, J. G., Yamazaki, K., Kim, T. H., & Reinisch, J. (2005). Combining orthodontic tooth movement with distraction osteogenesis to close cleft spaces and improve maxillary arch form in cleft lip and palate patients. *American Journal of Orthodontics & Dentofacial Orthopedics, 127*(2), 224–232.

Zwahlen, R. A., & Butow, K. W. (2004). Maxillary distraction resulting in facial advancement at Le Fort III level in cleft lip and palate patients: A report of two cases. *Oral Surgery, Oral Medicine, Oral Pathology, Oral Radiology & Endodontics, 98*(5), 541–545.

CREDITS

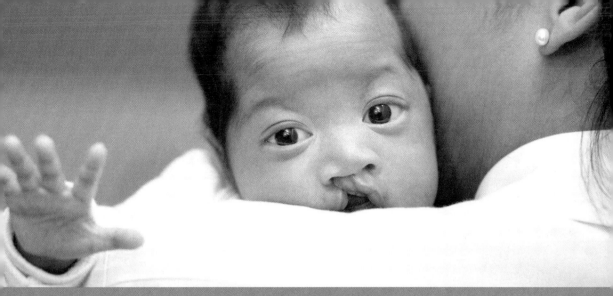

PART
2

Functional Effects of Clefts and Craniofacial Conditions

CHAPTER 7   Early Feeding Problems

CHAPTER 8   Developmental Aspects: Speech, Language, and Cognition

CHAPTER 9   Psychosocial Aspects

CHAPTER 10   Speech/Resonance Disorders and Velopharyngeal Dysfunction

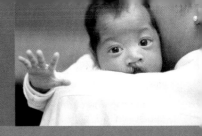

CHAPTER 7

Early Feeding Problems

With acknowledgment to Claire K. Miller for her contributions to this chapter.

CHAPTER OUTLINE

INTRODUCTION

Feeding is one of the most immediate challenges parents face following the birth of a baby born with a cleft palate. In fact, parents report that obtaining appropriate instructions about effective feeding methods is a high priority during the first few weeks (Bessell et al., 2011; Chuacharoen, Ritthagol, Hunsrisakhun, & Nilmanat, 2009; Lindberg & Berglund, 2014; Young, O'Riordan, Goldstein, & Robin, 2001). Fortunately, most feeding problems caused by a cleft can be easily resolved using certain feeding adaptations and other therapeutic interventions.

An open palate can affect an infant's ability to feed in many ways. First, it can have a profound effect on the oral-motor mechanics and the ability to generate the necessary negative intraoral pressure for effective sucking. In addition, the open palate may cause difficulty with coordination of sucking, swallowing, and respiration during feeding. Inadequate airway protection during swallowing has significant implications in regard to respiratory health (Arvedson & Brodsky, 2002; Boesch et al., 2006). Finally, parental frustration from difficulty in feeding their child can have a negative effect on the parent–infant bonding process (Johansson & Ringsberg, 2004).

Generally, the more extensive the cleft of the palate is, the greater the chance will be for significant feeding problems and poor oral intake. Because the volume of intake must be sufficient for adequate weight gain before the surgical repair of lip or palatal clefts, early identification and treatment of feeding problems must be made so that the infant can receive adequate nutrition for growth.

This chapter focuses on the disruptions in the normal feeding process that occur secondary to clefts and other craniofacial conditions. Assessment of feeding difficulties and the options for individualizing feeding modifications are discussed.

Infant Feeding and Early Development

The primary purpose of feeding is to satisfy the infant's hunger and provide adequate nourishment for normal growth and development. However, the process of feeding is also important for the infant's neuromotor development and sense of well-being (Miller, 2009).

The act of feeding serves to provide the infant with both oral-sensory and oral-motor stimulation. The nipple's tactile input to the mouth initiates the sucking reflex in neurologically intact infants. This sensory input represents the first step in initiation of the suck–swallow–breathe synchrony that is central to the infant feeding process.

Feeding is accomplished exclusively by sucking in early infancy. However, the active use of the lower jaw, cheeks, lips, and tongue during sucking provides a basis for the development of more mature feeding skills later on (Morris & Klein, 1987). These oral movements also help to develop skills for speech production.

In addition to nutrition and stimulation, the reflexive activity of both nutritive and nonnutritive sucking facilitates state regulation and helps the infant to maintain homeostasis. The infant quickly learns to use sucking for calming and self-regulation.

Finally, the activity of feeding serves as a very important part of the bonding process between the caregiver and infant. The caregiver spends time holding and cuddling the infant during the feeding process and learns to identify the infant's cues. In addition, there is mutual eye contact and vocalizations between the caregiver and infant. The behaviors of both the caregiver and infant during feeding have been shown to contribute significantly to the overall success of the feeding and even the bonding process (Black & Aboud, 2011; Meyer et al., 1994).

In summary, the infant's early experiences with feeding form the foundation for important developmental functions. Because a cleft has the potential to interrupt the normal feeding process, it can have significant implications not only for nutrition but also for other functions that are important to the infant's development (Bessell et al., 2011).

Anatomy and Physiology Relevant to Infant Feeding

The oral, pharyngeal, and laryngeal anatomy of an infant is different from that of an adult (**FIGURE 7-1**). There are differences not only in the size of the structures but also in their relative position in the cervical spine region. There are also significant variations in feeding physiology in that an infant's mode of feeding is through sucking and is dependent on an efficient suck–swallow–breathe synchrony.

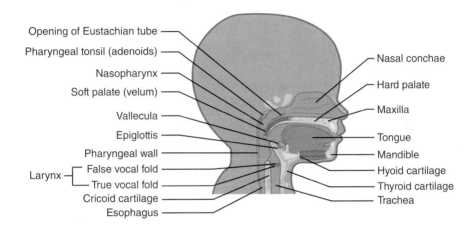

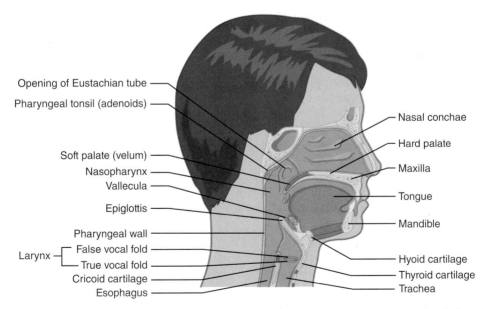

FIGURE 7-1 Anatomy of the head and neck as it relates to feeding in the infant as compared with the adult.

Anatomy Relevant to Infant Feeding

The oral cavity of a newborn infant is small, and the tongue is relatively large (although only half the size of the adult tongue). As such, the tongue completely fills the oral cavity. The infant's buccal pads (encapsulated fat masses inside the cheek) are also relatively large and stabilize the lateral walls of the oral cavity. Because the infant has not yet developed teeth, the effective vertical dimension of the oral cavity is reduced in size, causing the tongue to rest in a more anterior position than is typically seen in the adult. The tongue tip protrudes past the alveolar ridge and maintains contact with the lower lip. The temporomandibular joint does not allow much movement of jaw because of undeveloped connective tissue, causing the mouth opening to be smaller in the infant than in the adult. All these oral characteristics facilitate early suckling, characterized by extension–retraction movements of the tongue as well as the development of more mature up–down tongue movements that are characteristic of true sucking (Arvedson & Brodsky, 2002; Miller, 2009; Morris & Klein, 1987; Wolf & Glass, 1992).

The pharynx of the newborn is short so that the tongue base, velum, and pharyngeal walls are all in close approximation. The inferior border of the velum rests just in front of the epiglottis, and the velum has a large area of contact with the tongue.

The size of the infant's larynx is one-third the size of an adult's larynx. It is positioned high in the hypopharynx, residing adjacent to cervical vertebrae C-1 through C-3. In comparison, the larynx of an adult is located at the C-6 to C-7 vertebral level. The high position of the infant larynx causes the epiglottis to pass superiorly to the free margin of the soft palate and project into the nasopharynx. The epiglottis is tubular, proportionally narrow, and more vertical in the infant as compared with the adult (Myer, Cotton, & Shott, 1995). The pharyngeal anatomy is well suited for the suck–swallow–breathe synchrony.

Physiology Relevant to Infant Feeding

The infant's feeding process is dependent on smooth synchronization of sucking, swallowing, and breathing. Sucking and swallowing occur in phases generally described as the oral, pharyngeal, and esophageal stages of swallowing.

Oral Phase

The oral phase of swallowing in infants is composed of rhythmic sucking, during which the oral structures work together to stabilize the nipple, create pressure gradients for fluid flow, and control the bolus prior to transfer into the pharynx for swallowing initiation. The presence of the rooting reflex aids in the search for the nipple and the subsequent lip seal around the nipple. The sucking reflex is initiated as the tongue elevates to squeeze the nipple against the alveolar ridge and hard palate. The compression of the nipple against this bony surface creates positive pressure within the nipple and causes the release of a small amount of fluid. The infant then initiates sucking, which requires a rhythmic forward–backward motion of the tongue. The tongue is cupped around the nipple, and a depression in the center of the tongue forms a groove. As the tongue moves backward during sucking, the infant's jaw drops, thus enlarging the space in the oral cavity. This action generates negative pressure, resulting in suction and expression of fluid from the nipple into the infant's oral cavity. Therefore, both nipple compression and the generation of negative pressure are essential for normal infant sucking (**FIGURE 7-2**).

Pharyngeal Phase

The pharyngeal phase of swallowing is initiated once the fluid bolus is channeled by the tongue into the pharynx. When the liquid reaches the posterior oral cavity, the tongue base, velum, and posterior pharyngeal wall all work together to provide the pressure, or driving force, for bolus transfer through the pharynx. The velum elevates (partly because of the backward movement of the tongue),

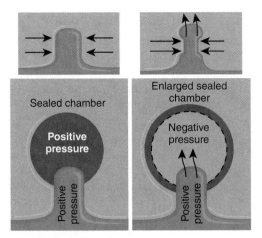

FIGURE 7-2 Comparison of positive pressure (compression) and negative pressure (suction) components during sucking.

and the velopharyngeal valve closes to completely separate the nasal cavity from the oral cavity. As the posterior aspect of the tongue moves downward and the sealed oral cavity is enlarged, negative pressure and suction are created, propelling the fluid bolus to the pharynx. The bolus diverts around the epiglottis as the pharynx fills and contracts sequentially for swallowing (Newman, Cleveland, Blickman, Hillman, & Jaramillo, 1991). During swallowing, the larynx is closed by adduction of the true and false vocal folds, the forward and medial movement of the arytenoids, and the subsequent retroversion of the epiglottis (Koenig, Davies, & Thach, 1990; Mathew, 1991).

Throughout the sucking action, the infant continues to maintain nasal breathing. To facilitate this, the epiglottis is positioned around the back of the velum, which keeps the pharynx open and allows the nasal cavity to be in direct contact with the glottis for a continuous patent airway. However, at the time of swallow initiation, vocal fold adduction occurs and respiration ceases.

Esophageal Phase

The bolus moves through the pharynx and into the esophagus, where the esophageal phase of swallowing is initiated. The upper part of the esophagus, commonly referred to as the upper esophageal sphincter (UES), is normally closed but stretches open as the bolus travels through the hypopharynx and into the esophagus. The lower esophageal sphincter (LES) relaxes to allow the bolus to enter the stomach. After each swallow occurs, the velum drops down to the base of the tongue and in front of the epiglottis, the tongue returns to an anterior position, sucking and breathing resume, and both the upper and lower esophageal sphincters maintain a closed position.

Synchrony of Sucking, Swallowing, and Respiration

Because the pharynx serves as a conduit for food as well as respiratory air, precise coordination of sucking, swallowing, and breathing is crucial to prevent aspiration (entry of material into the airway) (**FIGURE 7-3**). The suck–swallow–breathe ratio during feeding is generally considered to be 1:1:1 or 2:1:1. Some variations to this pattern occur, particularly during the initial 2 to 3 minutes of feeding, when the sucking rate is often higher (Bu'Lock, Woolridge, & Baum, 1990; Mathew, 1991; Wolf & Glass, 1992). Although additional respiratory effort is necessary to support the

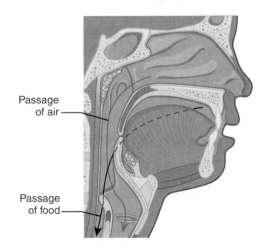

FIGURE 7-3 The pharynx as a conduit of food and air.

work of feeding, the intact infant is able to tolerate the decreased ventilation during feeding. This
may not be the case in infants presenting with
borderline respiratory reserve (Glass & Wolf,
1999; Mathew, 1988b; Mathew, Clark, Pronske,
Luna-Solarzano, & Peterson, 1985).

Changes with Growth and Maturation

The size and anatomic relationships of the oral,
pharyngeal, and laryngeal structures change significantly during the first 2 to 3 years of life (see
Figure 7-1). As a result, the process of feeding
and swallowing changes as the infant grows and
matures.

The oral cavity becomes larger, with concurrent mandibular growth and dental eruption. The
tongue begins to descend and move back into the
mouth, with the tip becoming positioned under
the alveolar ridge. This increased oral space facilitates the development of more refined oral-motor
skills for cup drinking, chewing, and speech
production.

At the same time, the pharynx elongates, and
the larynx begins its gradual descent from C-3 to
C-6, which is complete by age 3 (Sasaki, Levine,
Laitman, Phil, & Crelin, 1977). Neuromuscular maturation, in addition to increased cartilage and connective tissue, results in increased
mobility of the hyoid and larynx to elevate and
provide sphincteric closure during swallowing.
This allows maintenance of airway protection
that was previously facilitated by the proximity of
structures (Bosma, 1985).

Feeding Problems Caused by Clefts and Other Craniofacial Conditions

The feeding problems of infants who have a cleft
depend on the type of cleft (lip or palate) and
the severity of the cleft (unilateral or bilateral;
incomplete or complete).

Cleft Lip and Alveolus Only

Infants with a cleft of the primary palate (lip
and alveolus) only usually do not have significant problems with feeding, especially if the cleft
is unilateral. They may have initial problems in
achieving an adequate lip seal on the nipple to
generate effective negative pressure for sucking. With breastfeeding however, the breast tissue tends to conform to and fill in the cleft area.
When bottle feeding, the use of a soft, wide-based
nipple will close the area of the cleft and allow
suction generation. The mother can also assist
with lip closure by gently holding the upper lip
together while the baby sucks. Infants with cleft
lip and alveolus may also have initial difficulty in
latching on to the nipple. However, once the nipple is placed intraorally, the infant's tongue and
jaw movements are usually sufficient to produce
compression of the nipple against the intact part
of the alveolus and palate for effective sucking.

Cleft Palate Only

Infants with a small cleft of the velum only are
often able to feed without special modifications.
In fact, in some cases, the infant is able to occlude
the cleft with the back of the tongue during part
of the sucking movement so that negative pressure can be obtained (Glass & Wolf, 1999).

Infants with a cleft that extends through the
velum and hard palate are more likely to experience feeding difficulties (de Vries et al., 2014).
The cleft palate results in an open cavity with
oral and nasal coupling. Therefore, the infant is
unable to generate negative pressure for suction.
Infants with a complete cleft of the soft and hard
palate are usually not able to breastfeed because
of the fact that they will simply be unable to create negative pressure for suction. The use of a
supplemental nursing system, such as the Medela
Supplemental Nursing System™, may be of some
benefit in supporting breastfeeding; however,
the infant's growth and hydration status should
be closely monitored. Supplemental or exclusive
transition to bottle feeding is highly likely.

Depending on the extent of the cleft, the infant may also be unable to find a hard palatal surface for compression of the nipple. If placement cannot be achieved against an area of hard palate, the nipple will be pushed into the area of the cleft.

The open palate often results in **nasal regurgitation**, which is the reflux of fluid into the nasopharyngeal and nasal cavities. This can cause discomfort and disorganization with breathing during feeding. In addition, the open cleft allows air to continue to flow in through the nose and then the mouth during feeding. This can result in an excessive intake of air and may cause the infant to become bloated or have episodes of frequent spitting up.

The difficulty with oral feeding can cause excessive expenditure of energy, and thus calories, during feeding. In addition, nasal regurgitation must be subtracted from total intake of formula. Therefore, weight gain and adequate nutrition during the early months of infancy are primary concerns for infants with cleft palate (Glass & Wolf, 1999; Jones, 1988; Kaye et al., 2017; Redford-Badwal, Mabry, & Frassinelli, 2003). A full-term newborn infant generally needs 2 to 3 ounces of breast milk or formula per pound of body weight per day to gain weight appropriately (Butte, 2005; The Cleft Palate Foundation, 1998). Therefore, an infant who weighs 10 pounds requires between 20 and 30 ounces per day—a significant amount for an infant having feeding difficulty. As the infant gains weight, his daily intake should increase accordingly.

A final concern is for the parents. Most intact infants can complete a feeding within 20 to 30 minutes. The infant with a cleft palate usually takes much longer to feed. The lengthy feeding times caused by the feeding difficulty can be very stressful for both the infant and caretaker, thus affecting the normally pleasurable bonding experience (Carlisle, 1998; Zeytinoğlu, Davey, Crerand, Fisher, & Akyil, 2017).

Fortunately, there are several effective methods for bottle-feeding an infant with cleft palate, using special bottles and nipples. These feeding devices allow the feeder to assist with the delivery of formula or breast milk. The use of assisted feeding techniques has been shown to be effective in mitigating the above problems for infants with clefts, although continued outcomes research is needed (Bessell et al., 2011; de Vries et al., 2014; Reid, 2004; Shaw, Bannister, & Roberts, 1999).

Cleft Lip and Palate

The infant presenting with a cleft of the lip and palate generally has significant difficulty with all aspects of feeding because of the inability to achieve an anterior seal with the lips, inability to compress the nipple because of the open palate, and failure to generate negative pressure suction (Masarei et al., 2007). Significant nasopharyngeal reflux of liquid secondary to the open nasopharynx is also present. Breastfeeding is usually not possible in this group of infants. As with infants with cleft palate only, the use of assisted feeding techniques is usually necessary for successful feeding.

After the Cleft Lip and Palate Repair

Postoperative feeding recommendations following cleft lip and palate repair vary among centers and remain a controversial topic (Burianova, Kulihova, Vitkova, & Janota, 2017; Gailey, 2016; Katzel, Basile, Koltz, Marcus, & Firotto, 2009; Skinner, Arvedson, Jones, Spinner, & Rockwood, 1997). Immediate unrestricted feeding is allowed by some groups, whereas others recommend a restricted approach to facilitate good healing. For example, some centers discourage sucking following cleft lip and palate repair and recommend the use of a cup or a spoon instead. Other centers may recommend supplemental tube feeding for a period of 7–10 days. In contrast, some centers have implemented immediate, unrestricted feeding after the cleft repair without problems.

Other Craniofacial Conditions

In addition to cleft lip and palate, there are other conditions of the oral cavity, pharynx, or larynx that can cause or contribute to a feeding or swallowing problem. These conditions include micrognathia (small mandible) and macroglossia (large tongue), which can interfere with the oral-motor mechanics of feeding and swallowing. Pharyngeal stenosis (narrowing) and vascular conditions can cause compression in the esophagus or airway. A laryngeal cleft or tracheoesophageal fistula can result in aspiration during feeding secondary to miscommunication between the esophagus and trachea. Cortical or cranial nerve involvement, resulting in hypotonia, hypertonia, or generalized oral-motor dysfunction, may affect the neuromuscular coordination required for sucking and swallowing. Finally, conditions that can cause airway compromise, such as glossoptosis (posterior displacement of the tongue in the pharynx), midface retrusion, congenital heart or lung disease, or choanal atresia (congenital closure of the opening to the pharynx from the back of the nose) can interfere with the suck–swallow–breathe sequence. Many of these anomalies are seen in craniofacial syndromes or conditions.

One such condition is Pierre Robin sequence, which includes micrognathia, glossoptosis, and often a characteristic U-shaped cleft palate. Pierre Robin sequence can be isolated or part of certain syndromes, including Treacher Collins syndrome, Stickler syndrome, and velocardiofacial/22q11.2 deletion syndrome. Underdevelopment of the mandible reduces the size of the oropharyngeal area and is considered to be the primary anomaly in Pierre Robin sequence (Rathe et al., 2015). This results in the posterior and superior displacement of the tongue (glossoptosis), which interferes with the fusion of the palatal plates, resulting in cleft palate. The characteristic micrognathia and retracted tongue position of Pierre Robin sequence affect the infant's ability to compress the nipple adequately against the alveolar ridge to express breast milk or formula. In addition, the overall coordination of the suck–swallow–breathe triad may be disrupted (Lehman, Fishman, & Neiman, 1995; Miller, 2009; Shprintzen, 1992; van den Elzen, Semmekrot, Bongers, Huygen, & Marres, 2001). Glossoptosis can cause chronic airway obstruction. This may be exacerbated with the respiratory effort of feeding and can disrupt the sequential chain of suck–swallow–breathe sequences (Miller & Willging, 2007; Nassar, Marques, Trindade, & Bettiol, 2006; Shprintzen & Singer, 1992). Therefore, a patent airway must be confirmed before attempts at oral feeding (Bath & Buil, 1997). Some patients may require placement of a nasopharyngeal (NP) airway, and fortunately, oral feedings can be done with the NP tube in place (Wagener, Rayatt, Tatman, Gornall, & Slator, 2003). Finally, if the infant has the typical U-shaped cleft palate, problems with generation of negative pressure also contribute to feeding difficulty.

Despite these problems, feeding modifications can be made to help the infant with Pierre Robin sequence feed successfully (Kochel et al., 2011; Nassar et al., 2006). If medical clearance is given for oral feedings, prone (on the tummy) or side-lying (on the side) positioning may help to position the tongue anteriorly and facilitate tongue movements during feeding (Arvedson & Brodsky, 2002; Glass & Wolf, 1999; Litman et al., 2005; Park, Thoyre, Knafl, Hodges, & Nix, 2014). However, if the infant has a cleft palate, prone positioning is generally not helpful because the infant is not able to move the milk to the back of the mouth for swallowing. A standard, semi-reclined feeding position helps to minimize gravitational pull on the tongue. Side-lying positioning may be an option with use of a modified bottle. Despite these modifications, supplemental feedings are often necessary (Glass & Wolf, 1999).

Micrognathia and upper airway obstruction are treated in a variety of ways, including positioning, tracheotomy, tongue–lip adhesion, and mandibular distraction (Al-Samkari, Kane, Molter, & Vachharajani, 2010; Chigurupati &

Myall, 2005; Izadi et al., 2003; Khansa et al., 2017; Kochel et al., 2011; Mandell, Yellon, Bradley, Izadi, & Gordon, 2004; Schaefer, Stadier, & Gosain, 2004; Tibesar, Price, & Moore, 2006; Zim, 2007). Infants who undergo mandibular distraction to improve posterior airway space are unable to orally feed during the distraction procedure because their jaws are immobilized and they are unable to suck. During that time, they are usually fed through a nasogastric (NG) tube. However, once the distraction procedure is completed, oral feeding can be resumed as before.

Moebius syndrome is another condition that affects infant feeding. Moebius syndrome is a genetic disorder that involves absence or underdevelopment of the abducent nerve (VI) and the facial nerve (VII). Affected individuals have weakness or lack of movement in the lips, which limits the infant's ability to achieve and maintain an adequate seal on the nipple. In addition, there may be a chronic open-mouth posture with limited range of movement in the jaw and tongue. A high palatal vault may cause difficulty in establishing an adequate tongue–palate seal. All these conditions can have a profound effect on the oral-motor mechanics necessary for efficient sucking (Arvedson & Brodsky, 2002; Broussard & Borazjani, 2008). Excessive drooling and anterior loss of formula also commonly occur. Modified presentation of fluid is necessary for infants with Moebius syndrome because of the significantly restricted range of movement in the jaw, lips, and tongue. The use of feeder-assisted squeezing or presentation by a specialized feeding nipple or bottle is likely necessary.

Hemifacial microsomia results in various degrees of mandibular hypoplasia and facial weakness and is usually unilateral but actually can be bilateral (Caron et al., 2015; Heike et al., 2013; Strömland et al., 2007). This generally results in limitations to the range of motion in the jaw, lips, and tongue on one side. Utilization of the stronger side of the mouth during feeding while stabilizing the weaker side can reduce the feeding problems (Arvedson & Brodsky, 2002).

Feeding Modifications and Facilitation Techniques

With simple modifications, most infants with a cleft are able to feed with relative ease and obtain an adequate amount of nutrition in a reasonable amount of time. There is no single feeding method that will be successful for infants with different types of clefts or craniofacial abnormalities. Instead, the infant's performance during the initial feedings determines which feeding method and technique are most appropriate for that child (Miller, 2009; Miller, 2011; Wolf & Glass, 1992).

General feeding tips are summarized in **APPENDIX 7A**. Also, the American Cleft Palate–Craniofacial Association (ACPA) has a video and online resources for parents and caregivers on how to feed a baby with a cleft (ACPA, 2012).

Breastfeeding

Most pediatricians and healthcare providers agree that breast milk is best for the newborn infant for several reasons (Eidelman, 2012). It contains the mother's antibodies against illnesses and therefore can provide the infant with some immunity. In addition, early food allergies can be avoided through the use of breast milk. It also has been suggested that feeding with breast milk offers some protection from otitis media (Aniansson, Svensson, Becker, & Ingvarsson, 2002; Paradise, Eister, & Tan, 1994). However, opinions regarding the feasibility of breastfeeding a child with a cleft vary across centers (Alexander-Doelle, 1997; Alperovich, Frey, Shetye, Grayson & Vyas, 2017; Biancuzzo, 1998; Crossman, 1998; Darzi, Chowdri, & Bhat, 1996; Kogo et al., 1997; Mei, Morgan, & Reilly, 2009). The clinical protocol for breastfeeding infants with cleft lip, cleft palate, or cleft lip and palate developed by the Academy of Breastfeeding offers some general guidelines (Reilly et al., 2013). As with other feeding methods, the success of breastfeeding depends on the location and severity of the cleft. If the mother wishes to breastfeed her infant with a cleft, consultation with a certified lactation consultant is advisable.

In general, breastfeeding is usually not a problem for the infant who has only a cleft lip because the infant should still be able to achieve adequate suction. Even with a cleft in the lip and alveolus, the breast tends to fill the opening by molding to the shape of the oral cavity. Upright positioning while attempting breastfeeding is generally recommended. Supplemental bottle-feeding or a complete switch to the bottle may be necessary if difficulties with breastfeeding are immediately apparent.

As noted previously, breastfeeding an infant with a cleft palate is often challenging because the infant is unable to generate negative pressure for suction. This can be a particular disappointment for new mothers. If the mother of a child with cleft palate wishes to try breastfeeding, she should confer with a feeding specialist or lactation consultant who has experience feeding infants with cleft palate. Monitoring weight gain closely during a trial period of breastfeeding will provide both objective evidence regarding its feasibility and definitive information as to whether a supplementary feeding method is needed. If a trial of breastfeeding proves unsuccessful and the mother still wishes to continue breastfeeding, a supplemental nursing system may be an option (Wolf & Glass, 1992). The supplemental nursing system utilizes a reservoir that is filled with formula or milk that the mother has expressed. A thin tube, connected to the reservoir, is taped above the mother's breast and nipple (**FIGURE 7-4**). As the infant latches onto the breast for feeding, the mother supplements the breast milk with milk that is squeezed manually from the reservoir through the tube. The flow of milk needs to be simultaneous with the baby's efforts at sucking. With this method, the baby is supplemented at the breast while maintaining the important physical contact for the infant and mother. In addition, this method stimulates the breast to continue to produce and maintain the milk supply. Drawbacks to the use of supplemental nursing systems include the

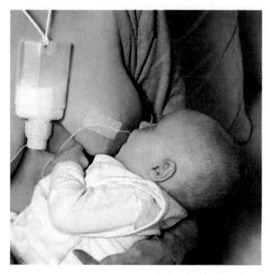

FIGURE 7-4 Breastfeeding with modifications.

potential for difficulty in maintaining the proper flow rate, though adjustable flow rate systems are available on some supplemental nursing systems. There is also the possibility that the baby will reject intraoral placement of the tube during breastfeeding.

After attempting breastfeeding with modifications, some mothers may find that using a modified bottle and/or a modified nipple is easier and more efficient. These mothers can still use breast milk, but in this case, the breast milk is given via the modified bottle or nipple. Breast milk can be expressed through the use of a breast pump, which can be purchased or rented through a local home health equipment supplier. In some cases, breast pumps are covered by insurance, but this usually requires a prescription in the baby's name and a letter from the physician describing the special circumstances that make this equipment necessary.

There are several kinds of breast pumps, including manual pumps, battery-operated pumps, and electric pumps. The electric pumps tend to be more efficient and faster than the manual pumps. As such, they allow both breasts to be pumped at the same time, thus reducing the amount of time required to express the milk.

Bottle-Feeding

There are two basic categories of feeding systems for bottle-feeding infants with cleft palate and craniofacial conditions: infant-driven and assisted delivery systems. Selection of the feeding system is dependent upon the infant's anatomy and oral sensorimotor skills.

Infant-directed or self-paced systems are designed with a one-way valve in the nipple. When the infant responds to the tactile input of the nipple with compression sucking efforts, liquid is released. The infant is able to independently modulate the flow of liquid during the feeding. Infants who demonstrate intact rooting and sucking skills are generally good candidates for infant-directed systems. Types of infant-driven systems include the Medela SpecialNeeds® Feeder, Pigeon™ nursing bottles and nipples, and Dr. Brown's® Specialty Feeding System.

In contrast, assisted delivery feeding systems involve the use of a pliable bottle and/or nipple that the feeder squeezes in synchrony with the infant's compressions on the nipple. Assisted delivery systems are appropriate for infants who have difficulty initiating and maintaining a rhythmic suck–swallow pattern during feeding. It should be noted that the force of the assistive squeeze and the squeeze duration may vary across feeders. Care must be taken to coordinate the assistive squeeze with the infant's sucking efforts and to monitor the infant's physiologic responses during feeding, including color, oxygen saturation, and respiratory rate.

Nipple Characteristics

If problems with feeding are immediately apparent, a variety of specialized nipples are available, as described in TABLE 7-1. Instructions for feeding using adapted nipples are given in **APPENDIX 7B**.

When choosing a nipple for enhancement of sucking, there are five basic nipple characteristics

---

TABLE 7-1 Commerically Available Nipples and Bottles

Nipples

- Orthodontic nipple: This style of nipple is wide based and has a fast flow rate. It can be used with a squeeze bottle for infants who show good ability to rapidly coordinate the suck–swallow–breathe sequence.
- Premature nipple: Several brands of premature nipples are available, including Similac® and Enfamil® brands. Premature nipples are typically smaller, thinner, and softer than a standard nipple, making suction easier. Clinicians should be aware that premature nipples are often designed to be fast flow as opposed to slow flow and should be used only by those infants who have demonstrated tolerance for the increased respiratory effort associated with fast fluid flow.
- Standard traditional nipple: This nipple (widely available) has a narrow base and has been shown to be effective when used in conjunction with a squeeze bottle while feeding infants who have demonstrated the ability to develop some suction independently. A slight enlargement of the nipple hole may be necessary, but caution should be taken to increase the size only slightly because the enlarged hole may result in an inappropriately fast flow rate.

Specialized Nipple and Bottle Systems

- Mead Johnson™ Cleft Lip/Palate Nurser (Mead Johnson Nutrition, Glenview, Illinois): This is a soft bottle that is easily squeezed and also has a long, soft, crosscut nipple. Other nipples will also fit onto the Mead Johnson bottle. The caregiver can help to regulate the liquid through assistive squeezing. The selection of an alternative nipple on the Mead Johnson bottle depends on the oral-motor skills of the infant (Figure 7-7).
- Bionix Controlled Flow® Baby Feeder: This feeder includes a silicone, standard shaped nipple and bottle with adjustable flow rates that range from no flow for non-nutritive sucking to the equivalent flow of a standard nipple. Flow is adjusted to the feeding capabilities of the infant.

(continues)

TABLE 7-1 Commerically Available Nipples and Bottles	*(continued)*

- Dr. Brown's Specialty Feeding System: This system includes a bottle, silicone nipple, and valve system designed for management and treatment of complex oral feeding issues. It is beneficial for infants and bottle-fed children with severe to profound difficulty in expressing fluid during sucking. A unidirectional flow valve, known as the Infant Paced Feeding Valve, is inserted into the base of the Dr. Brown's silicone nipple. This allows the infant to use spontaneous tongue and jaw movements during sucking. The feeder does not need to assist with flow. This bottle is fully vented to create a positive pressure flow, reducing air intake during feeding (Figure 7-8).
- Medela SpecialNeeds Feeder (formerly Haberman™ and Mini Haberman™ Feeders): This specialized nipple and bottle system is designed to allow the release of milk through the infant's compressions alone, without the need for suction. There is a soft nipple reservoir that is filled with breast milk or formula. The nipple has a one-way valve that limits the intake of air. It also prevents rapid fluid flow because it opens only when the infant sucks. In addition, the nipple has raised markings that indicate the position of the slit valve in the infant's mouth; the longer the raised mark, the greater the flow. To adjust the rate of flow, the feeder is turned so that the required line (zero flow, medium flow, maximum flow) points toward the baby's nose. Light finger pressure can be applied on the nipple to assist with fluid delivery in synchrony with sucking compression efforts if needed. The Mini-SpecialNeeds Feeder is a smaller version of the feeder that is designed for smaller or premature babies with cleft palate or other special feeding problems (Figure 7-9).
- Medela SoftCup® Feeder and Bottle: The SoftCup Feeder is designed to be used with the Medela 80 mL polypropylene bottle. Other bottles can be used, but some leakage may occur in the collar area. The SoftCup Feeder does not require the infant to actively suck because fluid is delivered via a small, flexible, cuplike reservoir. The feeder controls the flow rate (Figure 7-10).
- Pigeon Nipple (Respironics): The Pigeon nipple has a firm side that is placed against the gumline and palate and a soft side that is placed on the tongue. The nipple has a one-way valve that works with compression, enabling the infant to express milk through a suckling motion. The Pigeon nipple comes in two sizes: small size for slow flow and larger size for fast flow. The Pigeon nipple and valve can be used with any type of bottle; however, the one-way valve is designed for use with the Pigeon nipple only (see Figure 7-6).

to consider: pliability, shape, length, hole type, and hole size (Mathew, 1988a; Miller, 2011). TABLE 7-2 compares the characteristics of commonly used nipples. The type of nipple chosen should be based on the type of cleft and the baby's oral-motor/feeding skills as determined by the initial feeding evaluation.

Pliability

A soft, wide-based nipple will help to close the area of the cleft and allow suction generation (**FIGURE 7-5**). The nipple must be pliable enough to release breast milk or formula, with limited compression and suction by the infant. At the same time, the nipple must be firm enough to provide an appropriate degree of proprioceptive input to stimulate sucking. A soft nipple tends to have a higher flow rate than a firmer nipple and thus requires less compression effort and suction. The degree of

pliability must match the infant's strength of sucking and provide an appropriate flow rate to allow the baby to coordinate the suck–swallow–breathe sequence. Nipples designed for premature infants ("preemie" nipples) or the specialized Pigeon nipple (**FIGURE 7-6**) may be used for infants with cleft palate because they are very soft and pliable.

Shape

The shape of the nipple must facilitate adequate contact between the nipple and the tongue for compression. The shape also should enhance the oral-motor patterns desired during sucking (Wolf & Glass, 1992). Nipple shapes basically fall into two categories: traditional nipples and orthodontic nipples. The traditional nipple has a straight configuration, which gradually tapers to a flared base. The orthodontic nipple has a broad, flat bulb-type end that flares to a large, wide base.

Nipple Type	Pliability	Flow Rate	Shape	Hole Type
SpecialNeeds Feeder	Soft	Feeder regulated	Long	Slit
Mead Johnson	Soft	Feeder regulated	Long, thin	Crosscut
Orthodontic	Soft	Fast	Broad, flat	Hole on top surface of tip
Dr. Brown's	Soft	Slow to fast infant directed	Traditional	Hole, Y-Cut
Premature	Soft	Medium and fast	Traditional	Hole and crosscut
Traditional	Medium	Low	Traditional	Hole and crosscut, several holes

TABLE 7-2 **Characteristics of Commonly Used Nipples**

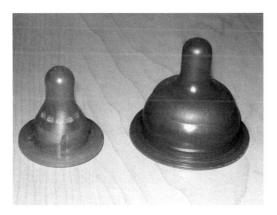

FIGURE 7-5 Basic categories of nipples: Round cross-section and broad, flat cross-section.

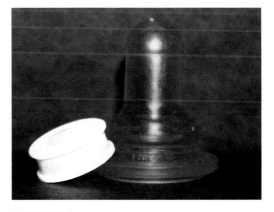

FIGURE 7-6 Pigeon nipple.

This style is perhaps best known as the NUK® nipple; however, many manufacturers, including Gerber and Playtex, now make nipples shaped similarly to the original NUK style. These nipples are generally advantageous for infants with cleft lip and alveolus because they may conform to the cleft and reduce air leakage while sucking.

Length

The length of the nipple should be based on what is needed to provide adequate contact between the nipple and tongue. Nipple length can vary substantially with regard to the type of base and the distance from the tip to the base, especially for those nipples that have tapered bases. The strength of the infant's suck, the degree of lip closure around the nipple, and the control the feeder provides to maintain the nipple position are other factors that should be considered.

Hole Type

Nipple hole types include round; Y-cut; or crosscut, which is an "X" configuration. The type of nipple hole affects the flow rate (Mathew, 1990;

Pados, Park, Thoyre, Estrem & Nix, 2015). Nipple flow rates have been found to vary widely between different brands and types of nipples regardless of the hole type.

Hole Size

The size of the nipple hole also affects the flow rate. The size can vary widely across different styles of nipples. A nipple with a traditional hole should have an opening that is large enough so that when the bottle is held upside down, the liquid drips out but does not run out rapidly. A standard nipple can be enlarged or slit to increase the fluid flow rate; however, the increased flow may cause the infant to have difficulty with coordination of swallowing and breathing.

Flexible Bottles and Assisted Fluid Delivery

Specialized bottle and nipple systems are commercially available for infants with cleft palate. Instructions for feeding using specialized bottle systems are described in Appendix 7B.

The Mead Johnson Cleft Lip/Palate Nurser (**FIGURE 7-7**) is a flexible bottle that allows the feeder to express the milk as needed by squeezing the bottle. This helps the infant to conserve energy and reduce calorie expenditure during feeding. This nurser comes with a specialized nipple, but other nipples can be used with this flexible bottle. Dr. Brown's Specialty Feeding System (**FIGURE 7-8**) has a vent system so that air enters the bottle collar and is routed through the internal vent to the end of the bottle, thus bypassing the milk. This reduces colic and burping. The Medela SpecialNeeds Feeder has a one-way valve for infant-directed flow but can also be used as an assisted delivery system when needed. The soft, flexible nipple reservoir allows feeder-assisted delivery of the milk (**FIGURE 7-9**). Finally, the Medela SoftCup Feeder (**FIGURE 7-10**) is often used when transitioning the infant from the bottle to the cup.

Even use of a simple plastic bottle liner in conjunction with a variety of nipples can be

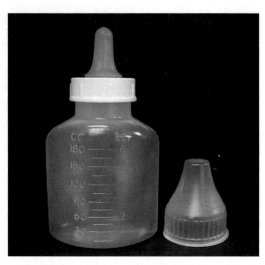

FIGURE 7-7 Mead Johnson Cleft Lip/Palate Nurser.

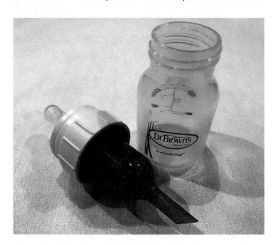

FIGURE 7-8 Dr. Brown's Specialty Feeding System.

effective for providing assistance with breast milk or formula flow. The feeder can apply intermittent pressure to the liner to push fluid out as the infant compresses the nipple (Barone & Tallman, 1998). Pushing the air out of the liner before the feeding reduces excess intake of air.

Regardless of the device used, the pressure applied to a squeeze bottle, plastic liner, or nipple reservoir must be in rhythm with the infant's suck and swallow efforts to ensure that the infant does not become discoordinated with the

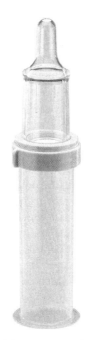

FIGURE 7-9 Medela SpecialNeeds Feeder.

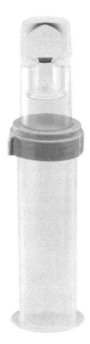

FIGURE 7-10 Medela SoftCup Feeder. This can be used as an alternative during the transitional period between a bottle and cup.

suck–swallow–breathe synchrony. An inappropriately rapid rate or continuous squeezing will result in an increased rate of swallowing, which will decrease available breathing time. This may cause the infant to have problems maintaining an appropriate respiratory rate and could cause aspiration into the airway.

Positioning the Infant

Placing the infant in a horizontal position during feeding is a common mistake. This position increases the potential for nasal regurgitation, coughing, and sneezing. In addition, there may be flooding of the eustachian tube and reflux into the middle ear, causing middle ear effusion. A semi-upright position (of at least 60°) is usually best for feeding because it facilitates control of jaw, cheek, lip, and tongue movements for sucking and swallowing coordination (Morris & Klein, 1987) (**FIGURE 7-11**). This position also allows gravity to assist with swallowing and helps to prevent nasal regurgitation (Wolf & Glass, 1992). The baby's head should be supported in a neutral anterior–posterior alignment with the shoulders symmetric and forward, trunk in midline, and hips flexed. The use of a bottle with an angled neck provides a downward flow of milk and simplifies feeding the infant in upright positioning.

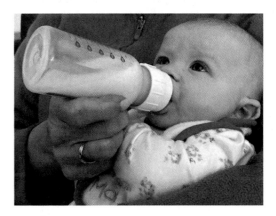

FIGURE 7-11 Appropriate feeding position.

Positioning the Nipple

Finding the optimal intraoral position for the nipple is critical for feeding success. The difference in nipple placement of only a few millimeters can affect feeding success (Clarren, Anderson, & Wolf, 1987). It is important to position the nipple under the bone of the palate to provide a base for nipple compression. Using the right nipple size and shape, based on the infant's cleft, facilitates proper intraoral positioning.

Pacing Intake

The feeder should carefully pace the flow rate during feeding by providing fluid in rhythm with the infant's sucking compressions (Law-Morstatt, Judd, Snyder, Baier, & Dhanireddy, 2003). Flow can be regulated by tilting the nipple slightly upward or partially removing the nipple from the oral cavity. The feeder should modify the pace when there are signs of stress, including eye widening, changes in facial expression, a decrease in alertness, or subtle avoidance of feeding. If the infant begins feeding rapidly and then shows signs of swallowing disorganization, such as coughing or choking, the feeder should slow the pace of fluid presentation. If the infant begins to slow down or stop sucking during the feeding, it suggests that the infant has tired and needs a pause before continuing feeding. The infant may show signs of excessive air intake and need a pause in feeding to allow burping. Although the feeder must be able to deliver enough nutrition before the infant becomes tired, allowing enough time to facilitate safe feeding is vital to feeding success. Consulting a dietitian about the use of a higher calorie formula preparation with a lower volume intake requirement will allow the infant to spend less time feeding and to use a slower pace of intake while still ingesting an adequate amount of calories for growth (Butte, 2005; Kovar, 1997).

Altering Liquid Viscosity

In cases where there is poor timing of airway protection with swallowing, a change in the fluid viscosity (thickness) should be considered to slow the speed of bolus transit, which can facilitate airway protection. Recommendations for altering liquid viscosity must be discussed and cleared with the medical team prior to implementation because of the potential medical and nutritional implications associated with intake of thickening agents. Depending on the thickening agent used (e.g., starch-based, gum-based, or gel-based thickeners or natural foods, such as baby rice cereal, pureed fruit, or yogurt), nutritional effects may occur. For example, the use of thickened liquid traps free-flowing water, which changes the nutrient density of formula and milk and introduces the potential for nutrient load toxicity. In addition, if rice cereal is used as the thickening agent, it is possible that the infant may ingest more than the recommended amount of some nutrients, such as iron. Finally, gel-based thickener has been associated with the onset of necrotizing entercolitis in infants (serious intestinal illness).

Oral Facilitation Strategies

As a result of an oral-motor/feeding assessment, oral facilitation techniques, such as gentle jaw and cheek support, may be recommended to increase the infant's oral control during feeding (Hwang, Lin, Coster, Bigsby, & Vergara, 2010). The type of bottle used can support the use of certain strategies to increase oral control. For example, the use of a small-diameter bottle, such as the infant Volu-Feed® Disposable Nurser (60 mL capacity), allows the feeder to use hand and finger positioning to facilitate support to the jaw and cheeks during feeding (Miller, 2011; Morris & Klein, 1987).

Preventing Excessive Air Intake

Because the infant with a cleft palate takes in an increased amount of air during feeding, the feeder may need to increase the frequency of burping. As a general rule of thumb, the infant should be burped after every ounce to prevent the discomfort associated with the intake of air that inevitably occurs with each feeding.

CASE REPORT

Appropriate Positioning and Placement

Lydia was born with Pierre Robin sequence with the characteristic micrognathia; glossoptosis; and a wide, U-shaped cleft palate. The potential for upper airway obstruction secondary to the posterior placement of her tongue was analyzed by continuous oxygen saturation monitoring and a formal sleep study. The results of the sleep study were within normal limits, and oxygen saturation levels were maintained except during her initial attempts at oral feedings. Lydia was described as being a poor feeder with little spontaneous sucking compression effort, frequent gasping, and oxygen desaturations. Lydia's intake during oral feeding attempts was minimal (5–10 mL) before she would completely "shut down" and fall asleep, usually 10 minutes into the feeding.

A speech pathology oral-motor/feeding consultation was requested. The results of the evaluation indicated normal oral reflexes with appropriate rooting as well as the ability to initiate and sustain a rhythmical nonnutritive sucking pattern. The mother explained that she had tried numerous nipples and bottles without success, including two types of cleft palate nipple and bottle systems.

Observation was then made of the mother as she demonstrated the methods she had been using to feed her baby. She positioned Lydia in a semi-reclined, cradled position as she offered her a standard nipple, which had been slit to assist with a faster milk delivery. Upon presentation of the nipple, Lydia made a few tentative sucking attempts as the milk rapidly flowed from the nipple. She coughed, sputtered, and pulled away from the nipple. An oxygen desaturation event was documented. The mother attempted to place the nipple intraorally again and had difficulty placing the nipple onto the tongue body. She continued with these attempts, but the baby continued with the same pattern of resistance and intermittent oxygen desaturations. Lydia then fell asleep after struggling to achieve intake of only 10 mL. The remainder of the feeding was presented via oral gavage (a means to deliver breast milk or formula directly to the stomach through a nasogastric [NG] tube).

During the next feeding time, the speech-language pathologist implemented several interventional techniques. First, Lydia was placed in a more upright position as opposed to the semi-reclined cradle position. This helped Lydia avoid further posterior displacement of her tongue during her efforts at feeding and reduced nasal regurgitation into the nasal cavity. Nonnutritive oral stimulation was provided with Lydia in the upright position to help increase her alertness and to stimulate nonnutritive oral movements. The Medela SpecialNeeds Feeder was then presented intraorally, with positioning of the nipple slit valve to zero flow. The longer size of this nipple made placement onto the tongue easier. In addition, the lack of liquid flow from the nipple before active sucking allowed Lydia to become accustomed to the presence of the nipple without being overwhelmed by formula.

Once Lydia began to demonstrate sucking compressions, a gentle assistive squeeze was given to deliver a small amount of formula in synchrony with her sucking attempts. Lydia was able to successfully transfer the small amounts of formula without any clinical signs of swallowing dysfunction. A cycle of approximately eight assistive squeezes was completed before Lydia showed some disorganization by pulling away from the nipple. After a brief pause, additional feeding trials revealed that Lydia could handle approximately five sequences of assistive squeezes for completion of suck–swallow before requiring a pause for breathing. Repetition of the cycles with pause intervals was done for approximately 15–20 minutes, resulting in an intake of approximately 30 mL.

Over a 3-week time period, the volume of Lydia's oral intake gradually increased with the use of intermittent assistive squeezing and pause intervals during feedings. Eventually the transition to complete oral feedings was accomplished with maintenance of appropriate oxygen saturation levels.

Managing Nasal Regurgitation

Infants with a cleft palate often experience nasal regurgitation. When this occurs, the feeder should stop and allow the infant time to cough or sneeze to clear the nasal passage. If nasal regurgitation occurs frequently during feeding, the caregiver should ensure that the infant is in an upright position that allows gravity to assist with downward flow of liquid. If coughing occurs frequently in conjunction with the nasal regurgitation, the feeder should consider using a slower flow nipple. Also, slowing the presentation of fluid helps to reduce the nasal regurgitation.

Consistency of Feeding Method

Consistency in how the baby is fed contributes to overall feeding success. The baby should be fed in the same position, with the same nipple and bottle, and with the same technique during each feeding. The feeder must learn how to easily position the baby, how much of an assistive squeeze is required, how long to keep feeding, how often to burp the baby, and how to read the baby's cues related to feeding. If several different nipples and bottles are intermittently tried and varying positions and different rates of assistive squeezing by a range of feeders are used, it is almost certain that feeding confusion and a poor feeding outcome will result. Fortunately, normal maturation and increased feeding experience of the infant and caregiver help to gradually improve the feeding process in spite of variations in method that may occur.

Use of Feeding Obturators

A feeding obturator is a prosthetic appliance that can be used in the first few months of life to assist the infant with cleft palate in feeding (refer to **FIGURE 7-12**). It is retained in the crevices of the cleft and provides a partial seal between the mouth and the nasal cavity. The obturator keeps the tongue from resting inside the cleft and provides a solid surface so that the tongue can achieve compression of the nipple against the plate (Masarei et al., 2007). Obturators do not improve the generation of negative pressure, however (Choi, Kleinheinz, Joos, & Komposch, 1991). A pediatric dentist or prosthodontist is the professional who can construct the feeding appliance and check it frequently so that it can be modified periodically as the child grows.

There are differing views regarding the use of feeding obturators for infants with cleft palate (Choi et al., 1991; Crossman, 1998; Delgado,

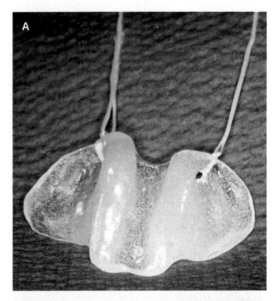

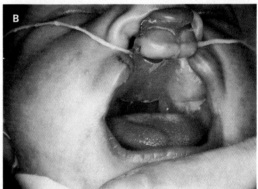

FIGURE 7-12 (A) Infant feeding obturators. **(B)** The infant feeding obturator is in place and provides a separation of the nasal cavity from the oral cavity to eliminate regurgitation of liquids into the nose. The appliance also keeps the tongue from resting inside the cleft and provides a solid surface for the tongue to achieve compression of the nipple to express the milk.

Schaaf, & Emrich, 1992; Hanson, Cook, & Ahmad, 2016; Kochel et al., 2011; Kogo et al., 1997; Masarci et al., 2007; Osuji, 1995; Savion & Huband, 2005; Sultana, Rahman, Nessa, & Alam, 2011). Some craniofacial centers use feeding obturators routinely, believing that the appliance improves the ability of the infant to compress the nipple (Crossman, 1998), which can lead to better weight gain (Balluff & Udin, 1986).

Most craniofacial centers do not routinely use these appliances because they feel that with modifications of the nipple or bottle, correct positioning, and appropriate feeding techniques, the obturator simply is not necessary. In fact, research has shown no significant difference in feeding abilities for infants fitted with a maxillary plate compared to those without a plate (Glenny et al., 2004). In addition, there are certain disadvantages to using an obturator, including the expense and need for periodic replacement to accommodate growth. Retention of the obturator can be challenging because the infant has no teeth to stabilize it. Finally, there can be irritation of the oral tissues, and the obturator can cause hygiene concerns.

Oral Hygiene

With all infants, it is important to maintain good oral hygiene. Although the mouths of infants tend to be self-cleaning, it is particularly important to attend to oral hygiene if the infant has a cleft. This is because the open cleft allows fluid to enter the cleft area and nose, even with an upright feeding position. The fluid can mix with mucous secretions from the mouth and nose and form a hard crust, which can become infected, causing irritation and soreness.

For good oral hygiene, the caregiver should cleanse the cleft and surrounding areas following feedings. This can be done by gently wiping the mucous membrane in the oral cavity using a washcloth; a small piece of gauze; or a Toothette®, which is soft and spongy. These can be moistened with plain water or water with hydrogen peroxide. Although the caregiver should be careful not to cause discomfort or injury during the cleansing process, she should remember that the cleft is not a wound and therefore will not be sore to touch during gentle cleansing.

Transitioning to a Cup

Most infants are ready to transition to the cup by 8 or 9 months of age, although some show readiness as early as 6 to 8 months of age. The initial response to the cup is generally sucking, with tongue protrusion and loss of liquid from the mouth. The infant's oral skills for cup drinking gradually increase so that she is able to take one or two sip swallows as the caregiver holds the cup. It is often beneficial to use a slightly thickened liquid to slow the liquid flow during early cup training.

There are many cup options for weaning the infant from a bottle to a cup. Selecting a cup that does not promote continued sucking is important. A small open cup without a spout, straw, or in-dwelling valve is generally the best option for transitioning away from sucking and toward true cup-drinking skills. Using the Medela SoftCup Feeder is an alternative during the transitional period (see Figure 7-10). Milk or breast milk is delivered through a narrow, flexible cup reservoir, facilitating development of oral skills for handling small amounts of liquid from a cup.

Most surgeons recommend weaning the infant from the bottle before palate repair because sucking may cause a breakdown of the repair. Therefore, weaning an infant with cleft palate from bottle to cup drinking should be done sometime before 9 or 10 months of age, which is the typical time for the palate repair.

Introduction of Solid Foods

Solid foods can be introduced to the baby with an unrepaired cleft palate at the same time as with any infant. The timing of solid food introduction is usually dependent on the preferences of the pediatrician and parent. Usually, rice cereals and strained foods are presented around 6 months of age. The baby will respond to the spoon-feedings at first by suckling. This may result in food being pushed into the nasal cavity. As the baby becomes more skilled in eating and begins to use more mature tongue patterns, this occurs less often. Mixing the pureed fruit with the cereal provides a degree of thickness that can reduce the tendency for nasal reflux.

The feeder can assist with the transition to solids by using appropriate positioning, small boluses, and a slow pace and by alternating food with liquid to assist with clearance. The slow rate of presentation is particularly important because it allows the baby to gradually learn how to direct the food around the area of the cleft. The feeder should watch the baby for cues to know when to present the next bite. The baby's cues include leaning forward or opening the mouth in anticipation of the spoon. Placing the spoon onto the baby's tongue encourages the baby to close her lips on the spoon and stimulates active tongue movements to transfer the food for swallowing. This is especially important following the surgery for cleft lip repair. Rapid spoon-feeding or presentation of large spoonfuls can cause more frequent nasal regurgitation as well as disorganized swallowing.

The transition to more textured foods, including easily dissolvable and later bite-sized, easy-to-manage table foods, can also be introduced in the same sequence as for other children. Foods should initially be offered with the baby seated in an upright position to reduce nasal regurgitation. When developmentally appropriate, the baby should be provided with guided opportunities to practice finger feeding. This can be done with small pieces of crunchy, dissolvable solid foods (e.g., toddler crackers and cookies) or soft, easy-to-manage food items (e.g., bite-sized pieces of soft fruits, shredded cheese, or pasta pieces). This helps to develop independence with self-feeding, gives the baby practice with the tongue movements around the cleft, and increases the efficiency of skills needed for mastication. If food is observed in the nose or becomes lodged in the cleft, it should be removed gently with either a finger or a swab. Foods that are acidic or spicy should be avoided because the lining of the nose is particularly sensitive to this kind of food. As the baby's oral-motor skills become more proficient, the baby will learn to efficiently manage transfer of solids for swallowing.

Assessment and Management of Complex Feeding Problems

Weight gain of infants with demonstrated feeding problems should be monitored closely by the pediatrician. If there is any evidence of inadequate weight gain, the pediatrician may consider the need for further assessment of feeding. In addition, some infants present with complex feeding problems that are not easily resolved with simple modifications.

Signs of significant feeding dysfunction or airway protection problems include the inability to establish and maintain a coordinated suck–swallow–breathe sequence, coughing or choking, color change during or after feeding, increased respiratory rate, and oxygen desaturations during feedings (Weir, McMahon, Barry, Masters, & Chang, 2009). The infant with significant feeding problems may respond to feeding attempts by arching or refusing to accept the nipple. If the infant has these clinical signs or takes 45 minutes or longer to feed, with clearly increased effort and relatively little intake, then a clinical oral-motor/feeding evaluation and/or instrumental swallowing examination is indicated.

Clinical Assessment

A clinical assessment of feeding should be performed by a feeding specialist (e.g., a qualified speech-language pathologist or occupational therapist). In addition, imaging studies of swallowing should be considered to assess the infant's ability to safely feed and to determine the effect of compensatory strategies on the infant's feeding performance. By assessing the infant's structures, specific oral-motor strengths and weaknesses, and responsiveness to compensatory strategies, the clinician may be able to determine an effective way to maximize the child's ability to feed orally. The ultimate goal is to find and implement a feeding method for the infant that results in adequate nutrition and weight gain, while facilitating the suck–swallow–breathe synchrony for safe and efficient feeding.

Videofluoroscopic Swallowing Study

A videofluoroscopic swallowing study (VFSS), also referred to as a modified barium swallow (MBS), is generally performed by a radiologist and a speech-language pathologist. Barium contrast is added to liquids and solids to enable visualization of the swallowing process under fluoroscopy. The use of standardized liquid barium viscosities, such as the Varibar® products, is recommended to ensure study validity. The videofluoroscopic study allows an overall view of the oral, pharyngeal, and esophageal phases of swallowing as well as the interactions between the phases.

Swallowing function, as well as the infant's ability to maintain airway protection during swallowing, is carefully assessed through the videofluoroscopy study. The degree of nasopharyngeal reflux and the occurrence of penetration or aspiration during swallowing can be documented. The infant's protective reaction to aspirated material can also be assessed. Compensatory strategies, such as positional adaptations, different nipples, and pacing of presentations, can be tested to determine their effect on improving the feeding process (Arvedson & Brodsky, 2002; Newman et al., 1991). Disadvantages of the videofluoroscopic study include radiation to the infant and the feeder during the study, the use of barium contrast with unfamiliar taste, and the fact that the swallows viewed represent a relatively small sample of feeding overall.

Fiberoptic Endoscopic Evaluation of Swallowing

Pediatric fiberoptic endoscopic evaluation of swallowing (FEES) involves the transnasal passage of an endoscope to the pharynx for viewing of the pharyngeal and laryngeal structures (Willging, 1995). The focus of this study is on assessing the integrity of airway protection during swallowing. FEES also provides information regarding sensory threshold in the pharynx and larynx (Aviv et al., 1998; Willging & Thompson, 2005). Advantages of the FEES procedure include the ability to clearly visualize pharyngeal and laryngeal structures as well as the spontaneous swallowing of secretions. Feeding can be assessed using the infant's customary bottle and nipple and the usual formula.

Small amounts (< 1 mL) of green food coloring or liquid AquADEKs™ (multivitamin and mineral supplement) are added to enhance visualization of the bolus during the study. Compensatory swallowing strategies can be tried during the FEES study without the time limitations of fluoroscopy. Disadvantages include the temporary loss of view that occurs as the velopharyngeal valve closes around the scope during the swallow. This is generally not a problem with single swallows because the structures quickly return to their resting position, thus restoring the view. This is a disadvantage when viewing rapid chain swallowing sequences, which are characteristic of early infancy, because the view is obscured with more frequency.

Interdisciplinary Feeding Team Evaluation

In severe cases of feeding/swallowing dysfunction, an evaluation by a team of feeding specialists is indicated. Typically, an interdisciplinary feeding team consists of a core group of medical professionals that may include a gastroenterologist, nutritionist, nurse, speech-language pathologist, occupational therapist, behavioral psychologist, otolaryngologist, pulmonologist, and consulting radiologist. The composition of interdisciplinary feeding teams varies among centers (Lefton-Greif & Arvedson, 1997; Miller et al., 2001; Rudolph, 1994). With the coordinated assessment of these specialists, management and long-term planning for treatment of complicated feeding problems can be accomplished.

Alternative Feeding Methods for Severe Cases

When the feeding problem is not easily resolved with modifications of the nipple or bottle, supplemental feeding through an orogastric tube or a nasogastric tube (NG tube) (both of which deliver nutrition directly to the stomach) may be required. Even with the tube in place, treatment can be done to improve oral-motor function for feeding, as appropriate. If the feeding problems persist for a period of time and cannot be adequately resolved with other measures, gastrostomy tube (G-tube) feeding may be considered. A G-tube is inserted in the stomach through a surgical procedure and may remain in place for an extended period of time. This is particularly indicated if the infant presents with abnormal oral reflexes or shows poor ability to coordinate airway protection with swallowing during a videofluoroscopic or endoscopic swallowing study. The tube is removed if and when the infant shows signs of considerable progress with oral feeding skill development and oral intake volume (Rudolph, 1994).

SUMMARY

Feeding problems are common in patients with clefts, particularly an open cleft palate and craniofacial syndromes. Whatever feeding method is chosen, it is important that the feeding process be relatively easy and efficient. Overall, the feeding method should allow the infant to receive an adequate amount of intake for nutrition and weight gain. The feeding method should be efficient enough so that the infant can conserve energy and not require a lengthy feeding time. Consistency of the nipple, the bottle, and the feeder's method is important for early success.

The feeding system should allow the infant to experience some sucking to support and encourage normal oral-motor skill development. The option chosen should be relatively inexpensive and readily available.

Finally, it is important that the feeding process is a pleasurable experience for both the infant and the caregiver. It should not be forgotten that the time spent in feeding serves as an important part of the bonding process as well as the foundation for early sensorimotor and developmental experiences.

FOR REVIEW AND DISCUSSION

1. Describe the normal swallowing process and how it changes with growth.

2. What are reasons that cleft palate causes feeding difficulty? Why is there less of a problem with cleft lip?

3. What are some reasons that breastfeeding is particularly difficult for a baby with cleft palate? How would you counsel the mother about alternative feeding methods?

4. Describe different types of bottles that are commercially available for infants with cleft palate.

5. What is the difference between an infant-driven and assisted delivery feeding systems?

6. What factors should be considered when selecting nipple shape, length, and pliability?

7. Discuss some feeding facilitation techniques that may be helpful for a child with feeding difficulties.

8. What are the reasons that an upright feeding position is preferable to a supine position?

9. How would you counsel the caregiver to deal with oral hygiene for the infant with a cleft?

REFERENCES

Alexander-Doelle, A. (1997). Breastfeeding and cleft palates. *AWHONN Lifelines, 1*(4), 27.

Alperovich, M., Frey, J. D. Shetye, P. R., Grayson, B. H., & Vyas, R. M. (2017). Breast milk feeding rates in patients with cleft lip and palate at a North American craniofacial center. *The Cleft Palate–Craniofacial Journal, 54*(3), 334–337.

Al-Samkari, H. T., Kane, A. A., Molter, D. W., & Vachharajani, A. (2010). Neonatal outcomes of Pierre Robin sequence: An institutional experience. *Clinical Pediatrics, 49*(12), 1117–1122.

American Cleft Palate–Craniofacial Association (ACPA). (2012). Feeding your baby. Retrieved from http://www.cleftline.org/parents-individuals /feeding-your-baby/

Aniansson, G., Svensson, H., Becker, M., & Ingvarsson, L. (2002). Otitis media and feeding with breast milk of children with cleft palate. *Scandinavian Journal of Plastic and Reconstructive Surgery, 36*, 9–15.

Arvedson, J., & Brodsky, L. (Eds.). (2002). *Pediatric swallowing and feeding: Assessment and management* (2nd ed.). San Diego, CA: Singular Publishing Group.

Aviv, J. E., Kim, T., Thomson, J. E., Sunshine, S., Kaplan, S., & Close, L. G. (1998). Fiberoptic endoscopic evaluation of swallowing with sensory testing (FEESST) in healthy controls. *Dysphagia, 13*(2), 87–92.

Balluff, M. A., & Udin, R. D. (1986). Using a feeding appliance to aid the infant with a cleft palate. *Ear, Nose & Throat Journal, 65*(7), 316–320.

Barone, C. M., & Tallman, L. L. (1998). Modification of Playtex nurser for cleft palate patients. *Journal of Craniofacial Surgery, 9*(3), 271–274.

Bath, A. P., & Buil, P. D. (1997). Management of upper airway obstruction in Pierre Robin sequence. *Journal of Laryngology and Otology, 111*(12), 1155–1157.

Bessell, A., Hooper, L., Shaw, W. C., Reilly, S., Reid, J., & Glenny, A. M. (2011). Feeding interventions for growth and development in infants with cleft lip, cleft palate, or cleft lip and palate (Review). *Cochrane Database of Systematic Reviews, 2*(CD003315). doi:10.1002/14651858.CD003315.pub3

Biancuzzo, M. (1998). Clinical focus on clefts: Yes! Infants with clefts can breastfeed. *AWHONN Lifelines, 2*(4), 45–49.

Black, M. M., & Aboud, F. E. (2011). Responsive feeding is embedded in a theoretical framework of responsive parenting. *Journal of Nutrition, 141*(3), 490–494.

Boesch, R. P., Daines, C., Willging, J. P., Kaul, A., Cohen, A. P., Wood, R. E., & Amin, R. S. (2006). Advances in the diagnosis and management of chronic pulmonary aspiration in children. *European Respiratory Journal, 24*(4), 847–861.

Bosma, J. D. (1985). Postnatal ontogeny of performances of the pharynx, larynx, and mouth. *American Review of Respiratory Disorders, 131*, S10–S15.

Broussard, A. B., & Borazjani, J. G. (2008). The faces of Moebius syndrome: Recognition and anticipatory guidance. *The American Journal of Maternal/Child Nursing, 33*(5), 272–278.

Bu'Lock, F., Woolridge, M. W., & Baum, J. D. (1990). Development of co-ordination of sucking, swallowing and breathing: Ultrasound study of term and preterm infants. *Developmental Medicine & Child Neurology, 32*(8), 669–678.

Burianova, I., Kulihova, K., Vitkova, V., & Janota, J. (2017). Breastfeeding after early repair of cleft lip in newborns with cleft lip or cleft lip and palate in a baby-friendly designated hospital. *Journal of Human Lactation, 33*(3), 504–508.

Butte, N. F. (2005). Energy requirements of infants. *Public Health Nutrition, 8*(7a), 953–967.

Carlisle, D. (1998). Feeding babies with cleft lip and palate. *Nursing Times, 94*(4), 59–60.

Caron, C. J., Pluijmers, B. I., Joosten, K. F., Mathijssen, I. M., van der Schroeff, M. P., Dunaway, D. J., . . . Koudstaal, M. J. (2015). Feeding difficulties in craniofacial microsomia: A systematic review. *International Journal of Oral and Maxillofacial Surgery, 44*(6), 732–737.

Chigurupati, R., & Myall, R. (2005). Airway management in babies with micrognathia: The case against early distraction. *Journal of Oral and Maxillofacial Surgery, 63*, 1209–1215.

Choi, B. H., Kleinheinz, J., Joos, U., & Komposch, G. (1991). Sucking efficiency of early orthopaedic plate and teats in infants with cleft lip and palate. *International Journal of Oral and Maxillofacial Surgery, 20*(3), 167–169.

Chuacharoen, R., Ritthagol, W., Hunsrisakhun, J., & Nilmanat, K. (2009). Felt needs of parents who have a 0–3-month-old child with a cleft lip and palate. *The Cleft Palate–Craniofacial Journal, 46*(3), 252–257.

Clarren, S. K., Anderson, B., & Wolf, L. S. (1987). Feeding infants with cleft lip, cleft palate, or cleft lip and palate. *Cleft Palate Journal, 24*(3), 244–249.

The Cleft Palate Foundation. (1998). *Feeding an infant with a cleft*. Chapel Hill, NC: Author.

Crossman, K. (1998). Breastfeeding a baby with a cleft palate: A case report. *Journal of Human Lactation, 14*(1), 47–50.

Darzi, M. A., Chowdri, N. A., & Bhat, A. N. (1996). Breast feeding or spoon feeding after cleft lip repair: A prospective, randomised study. *British Journal of Plastic Surgery, 49*(1), 24–26.

Delgado, A. A., Schaaf, N. G., & Emrich, L. (1992). Trends in prosthodontic treatment of cleft palate patients at one institution: A twenty-one year review. *The Cleft Palate–Craniofacial Journal, 29*(5), 425–428.

de Vries, I. A., Breugem, C. C., van der Heul, A. M., Eijkemans, M. J., Kon, M., & Mink van der Molen, A. B. (2014). Prevalence of feeding disorders in children with cleft palate only: A retrospective study. *Clinical Oral Investigations, 18*(5), 1507–1515.

Eidelman, A. I. (2012). Breastfeeding and the use of human milk: An analysis of the American Academy of Pediatrics 2012 Breastfeeding Policy Statement. *Breastfeeding Medicine, 7*(5), 323–324.

Gailey, D. G. (2016). Feeding infants with cleft and the postoperative cleft management. *Oral and Maxillofacial Surgery Clinics of North America, 28*, 153–159.

Glass, R. P., & Wolf, L. S. (1999). Feeding management of infants with cleft lip and palate and micrognathia. *Infants and Young Children, 12*(1), 70–81.

Glenny, A. M., Hooper, L., Shaw, W. C., Reilly, S., Kasem, S., & Reid, J. (2004). Feeding interventions for growth and development in infants with cleft lip, cleft palate or cleft lip and palate. *Cochrane Database of Systematic Reviews, 3*(CD003315). doi:10.1002/14651858.CD003315.pub3

Hanson, P. A., Cook, N. B., & Ahmad, O. (2016). Fabrication of a feeding obturator for infants. *The Cleft Palate–Craniofacial Journal, 53*(2), 240–244.

Heike, C. L., Hing, A. V., Aspinall, C. A., Bartlett, S. P., Birgfeld, C. B., Drake, A. F., . . . Luquetti, D. V. (2013). Clinical care in craniofacial microsomia: A review of current management recommendations and opportunities to advance research. *American Journal of Medical Genetics Part C: Seminars in Medical Genetics, 163C*(4), 271–282.

Hwang, Y., Lin, C., Coster, W., Bigsby, R., & Vergara, E. (2010). Effectiveness of cheek and jaw support to improve feeding performance of preterm infants. *The American Journal of Occupational Therapy, 64*(6), 886–894.

Izadi, K., Yellon, R., Mandell, D., Smith, M., Song, S., Bidic, S., & Bradley, J. (2003). Correction of upper airway obstruction in the newborn with internal mandibular distraction osteogenesis. *Journal of Craniofacial Surgery, 14*(4), 493–499.

Johansson, B., & Ringsberg, K. C. (2004). Parents' experiences of having a child with cleft lip and palate. *Journal of Advanced Nursing, 47*(2), 165–173.

Jones, W. B. (1988). Weight gain and feeding in the neonate with cleft: A three-center study. *Cleft Palate Journal, 25*(4), 379–384.

Katzel, E., Basile, P., Koltz, P., Marcus, J., & Firotto, J. (2009). Current surgical practices in cleft care: Cleft palate repair techniques and postoperative care. *Plastic and Reconstructive Surgery, 124*(3), 899–906.

Kaye, A., Thaete, K., Snell, A., Chesser, C., Goldak, C., & Huff, H. (2017). Initial nutritional assessment of infants with cleft lip and/or palate: Interventions and return to birth weight. *The Cleft Palate–Craniofacial Journal, 54*(2), 127–136.

Khansa, I., Hall, C., Madhoun, L., Splaingard, M., Baylis, A., Kirschner, R., & Pearson, G. (2017). Airway and feeding outcomes of mandibular distraction, tongue-lip adhesion, and conservative management in Pierre Robin sequence: A prospective study. *Plastic and Reconstructive Surgery, 139*(4), 975e–983e.

Kochel, J., Meyer-Marcotty, P., Wirbelauer, J., Böohm, H., Kochel, M., Thomas, W., . . . Stellzig-Eisenhauer, A. (2011). Treatment modalities of infants with upper airway obstruction: Review of the literature and presentation of novel orthopedic appliances. *The Cleft Palate–Craniofacial Journal, 48*(1), 44–55.

Koenig, J. S., Davies, A. M., & Thach, B. T. (1990). Coordination of breathing, sucking, and swallowing during bottle feedings in human infants. *Journal of Applied Physiology, 69*, 1623–1629.

Kogo, M., Okada, G., Ishii, S., Shikata, M., Iida, S., & Matsuya, T. (1997). Breast feeding for cleft lip and palate patients, using the Hotz-type plate. *The Cleft Palate–Craniofacial Journal, 34*(4), 351–353.

Kovar, A. J. (1997). Nutrition assessment and management in pediatric dysphagia. *Seminars in Speech and Language, 18*(1), 39–49.

Law-Morstatt, L., Judd, D. M., Snyder, P., Baier, R. J., & Dhanireddy, R. (2003). Pacing as a treatment strategy for transitional sucking patterns. *Journal of Perinatology, 23*, 483–488.

Lefton-Greif, M. A., & Arvedson, J. C. (1997). Pediatric feeding/swallowing teams. *Seminars in Speech and Language, 18*(1), 5–11; quiz 12.

Lehman, J. A., Fishman, J. R., & Neiman, G. S. (1995). Treatment of cleft palate associated with Robin sequence: Appraisal of risk factors. *The Cleft Palate–Craniofacial Journal, 32*(1), 25–29.

Lindberg, N., & Berglund A. (2014). Mothers' experiences of feeding babies born with cleft lip and palate. *Scandinavian Journal of Caring Sciences, 28,* 66–73.

Litman, R. S., Wake, N., Chan, L. M., McDonough, J. M., Sin, S., Mahboubi, S., & Arens, R. (2005). Effect of lateral positioning on upper airway size and morphology in sedated children. *Anesthesiology, 103*(3), 484–488.

Mandell, D., Yellon, R., Bradley, J., Izadi, K., & Gordon, C. (2004). Mandibular distraction for micrognathia and severe upper airway obstruction. *Archives of Otolaryngology-Head & Neck Surgery, 130*(3), 344–348.

Masarei, A. G., Sell, D., Habel, A., Mars, M., Sommerlad, B. C., & Wade, A. (2007). The nature of feeding infants with unrepaired cleft lip and/or palate compared with healthy noncleft infants. *The Cleft Palate–Craniofacial Journal, 44*(3), 321–328.

Mathew, O. P. (1988a). Nipple units for newborn infants: A functional comparison. *Pediatrics, 81*(5), 688–691.

Mathew, O. P. (1988b). Respiratory control during nipple feeding in preterm infants. *Pediatric Pulmonology, 5*(4), 220–224.

Mathew, O. P. (1990). Determinants of milk flow through nipple units: Role of hole size and nipple thickness. *American Journal of Diseases of Children, 144*(2), 222–224.

Mathew, O. P. (1991). Science of bottle feeding. *Journal of Pediatrics, 119*(4), 511–519.

Mathew, O. P., Clark, M. L., Pronske, M. L., Luna-Solarzano, H. G., & Peterson, M. D. (1985). Breathing pattern and ventilation during oral feeding in term newborn infants. *Journal of Pediatrics, 106*(5), 810–813.

Mei, C., Morgan, A., & Reilly, S. (2009). Benchmarking clinical practice against best evidence: An example from breastfeeding infants with cleft lip and/or palate. *Evidence-Based Communication Assessment and Intervention, 3*(1), 48–66.

Meyer, E. C., Coll, C. T., Lester, B. M., Boukydis, C. F., McDonough, S. M., & Oh, W. (1994). Family-based intervention improves maternal psychological well-being and feeding interaction of preterm infants. *Pediatrics, 93*(2), 241–246.

Miller, C., Burklow, K., Santoro, K., Kirby, E., Mason, D., & Rudolph, C. (2001). An interdisciplinary team approach to the management of pediatric feeding and swallowing disorders. *Children's Health Care, 30*(3), 201–218.

Miller, C. K. (2009). Updates on pediatric feeding and swallowing problems. *Current Opinion in Otolaryngology & Head & Neck Surgery, 17*(3), 194–199.

Miller, C. K. (2011). Feeding issues and interventions in infants and children with clefts and craniofacial syndromes. *Seminars in Speech and Language, 32*(2), 115–126.

Miller, C. K., & Willging, J. P. (2007). The implications of upper-airway obstruction on successful infant feeding. *Seminars in Speech and Language, 28*(3), 190–203.

Morris, S. E., & Klein, M. D. (1987). *Prefeeding skills: A comprehensive resource for feeding development.* Tucson, AZ: Therapy Skill Builders.

Myer, C. M., Cotton, R. T., & Shott, S. R. (1995). *The pediatric airway: An interdisciplinary approach.* Philadelphia, PA: J. B. Lippincott.

Nassar, E., Marques, I. L., Trindade, A. S., & Bettiol, H. (2006). Feeding-facilitating techniques for the nursing infant with Robin sequence. *The Cleft Palate–Craniofacial Journal, 43*(1), 55–60.

Newman, L. A., Cleveland, R. H., Blickman, J. G., Hillman, R. E., & Jaramillo, D. (1991). Videofluoroscopic analysis of the infant swallow. *Investigative Radiology, 26*(10), 870–873.

Osuji, O. O. (1995). Preparation of feeding obturators for infants with cleft lip and palate. *Journal of Clinical Pediatric Dentistry, 19*(3), 211–214.

Pados, B. F., Park, J., Thoyre, S. M., Estrem, H., & Nix, W. B. (2015). Milk flow rates from bottle nipples used for feeding infants who are hospitalized. *American Journal of Speech Pathology, 24,* 671–679.

Paradise, J., Eister, B., & Tan, L. (1994). Evidence in infants with cleft palate that breast milk protects against otitis media. *Pediatrics, 94*(6), 853–860.

Park, J., Thoyre, S., Knafl, G. J., Hodges, E. A., & Nix, W. B. (2014). Efficacy of semielevated side-lying positioning during bottle-feeding of very preterm infants: A pilot study. *The Journal of Perinatal & Neonatal Nursing, 28*(1), 69–79.

Rathe, M., Rayyan, M., Schoenaers, J., Dormaar, J. T., Breuls, M., Verdonck, A., . . . Hens, G. (2015). Pierre Robin sequence: Management of respiratory and feeding complications during the first year of life in a tertiary referral centre. *International Journal of Pediatric Otorhinolaryngology, 79*(8), 1206–1212.

Redford-Badwal, D. A., Mabry, K., & Frassinelli, J. D. (2003). Impact of cleft lip and/or palate on nutritional health and oral-motor development. *Dental Clinics of North America, 47*(2), 305–317.

Reid, J. (2004). A review of feeding interventions for infants with cleft palate. *The Cleft Palate–Craniofacial Journal, 41*(3), 268–278.

Reilly, S., Reid, J., Skeat, J., Cahir, P., Mei, C., Bunik, M., & the Academy of Breastfeeding Medicine, M. (2013). ABM Clinical Protocol #17: Guidelines for breastfeeding infants with cleft lip, cleft palate, or cleft lip and palate, revised 2013. *Breastfeeding Medicine, 8*(4), 349–353.

Rudolph, C. D. (1994). Feeding disorders in infants and children. *Journal of Pediatrics, 125*(6, Pt. 2), S116–S124.

Sasaki, C. T., Levine, P. A., Laitman, J. T., Phil, M., & Crelin, E. S. (1977). Postnatal descent of the epiglottis in man. *Archives of Otolaryngology, 103*, 169–171.

Savion, L., & Huband, M. (2005). A feeding obturator for a preterm baby with Pierre Robin sequence. *Journal of Prosthetic Dentistry, 93*(2), 197–200.

Schaefer, R., Stadier, J., & Gosain, A. (2004). To distract or not distract: An algorithm for airway management in isolated Pierre Robin sequence. *Plastic and Reconstructive Surgery, 113*(4), 1113–1125.

Shaw, W., Bannister, R., & Roberts, C. (1999). Assisted feeding is more reliable for infants with clefts: A randomized trial. *The Cleft Palate–Craniofacial Journal, 36*(3), 262–268.

Shprintzen, R. J. (1992). The implications of the diagnosis of Robin sequence. *The Cleft Palate–Craniofacial Journal, 29*(3), 205–209.

Shprintzen, R. J., & Singer, L. (1992). Upper airway obstruction and the Robin sequence. *International Anesthesiology Clinics of North America, 30*(4), 109–114.

Skinner, J., Arvedson, J. C., Jones, G., Spinner, C., & Rockwood, C. (1997). Post-operative feeding strategies for infants with cleft lip. *International Journal of Pediatric Otorhinolaryngology, 42*, 169–178.

Strömland, K., Miller, M., Sjögreen, L., Johansson, M., Joelsson, B., Billstedt, E., . . . Granström, G. (2007). Oculo-auriculo-vertebral spectrum: Associated anomalies, functional deficits, and possible developmental risk factors. *American Journal of Medical Genetics Part A, 143A*, 1317–1325.

Sultana, A., Rahman, M. M., Nessa, J., & Alam, M. S. (2011). A feeding aid prosthesis for a preterm baby with cleft lip and palate. *Mymensingh Medical Journal, 20*(1), 22–27.

Tibesar, R. J., Price, D. L., & Moore, E. J. (2006). Mandibular distraction osteogenesis to relieve Pierre Robin upper airway obstruction. *American Journal of Otolaryngology–Head and Neck Surgery, 27*, 436–439.

van den Elzen, A., Semmekrot, B., Bongers, E., Huygen, P., & Marres, H. (2001). Diagnosis and treatment of Pierre Robin sequence: Results of a retrospective clinical study and review of literature. *European Journal of Pediatrics, 160*, 47–53.

Wagener, S., Rayatt, S. S., Tatman, A. J., Gornall, P., & Slator, R. (2003). Management of infants with Pierre Robin sequence. *The Cleft Palate–Craniofacial Journal, 40*(2), 180–185.

Weir, K., McMahon, S., Barry, L., Masters, I. B., & Chang, A. B. (2009). Clinical signs and symptoms of aspiration and dysphagia in children. *European Respiratory Journal, 33*, 604–611.

Willging, J. P. (1995). Endoscopic evaluation of swallowing in children. *International Journal of Pediatric Otorhinolaryngology, 32*(Suppl.), S107–S108.

Willging, J. P., & Thompson, D. M. (2005). Pediatric FEESST: Fiberoptic endoscopic evaluation of swallowing with sensory testing. *Current Gastroenterology Reports, 7*(3), 240–243.

Wolf, L. S., & Glass, R. P. (1992). *Feeding and swallowing disorders in infancy: Assessment and management.* Tucson, AZ: Therapy Skill Builders.

Young, J., O'Riordan, M., Goldstein, J., & Robin, N. (2001). What information do parents of newborns with cleft lip, palate, or both want to know? *The Cleft Palate–Craniofacial Journal, 38*(1), 55–58.

Zeytinoğlu, S., Davey, M. P., Crerand, C., Fisher, K., & Akyil, Y. (2017). Experiences of couples caring for a child born with cleft lip and/or palate: Impact of the timing of diagnosis. *Journal of Family and Marital Therapy, 43*(1), 82–99.

Zim, S. (2007). Treatment of upper airway obstruction in infants with micrognathia using mandibular distraction osteogenesis. *Facial Plastic Surgery, 23*(2), 107–112.

CREDITS

Part/Chapter opener photo: © PeopleImages/Getty Images

All photos courtesy of the Cleft and Craniofacial Center at Cincinnati Children's Hospital Medical Center.

General Feeding Tips for Parents

With acknowledgment to Claire K. Miller for her contributions to this appendix.

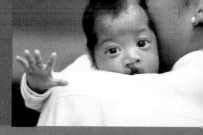

Relax

Most parents report feeling anxious about learning how to feed their baby with a cleft but find the problems to be fewer than expected and easy to overcome when using the right type of nipple, bottle, and technique.

Feeding Equipment and Methods

A particular method of feeding is usually recommended shortly after birth by a nurse, speech-language pathologist, or occupational therapist. Try to use the adapted nipples, bottles, and feeding methods that are recommended, and be sure not to hesitate to call the nurse or speech-language pathologist if any questions arise about how to use the equipment.

Using Appropriate Positioning

Feeding a baby with cleft palate in an upright position as opposed to the traditional cradle or reclined position reduces the amount of liquid that can escape up into the nose during feeding. Try using a pillow or small foam wedge to support the baby against you in an upright position.

Dealing with Nasal Regurgitation

If milk does have a tendency to come from the baby's nose even while using an upright position, the flow of the liquid may be too fast. Try using a nipple with a slower flow rate, such as one with a smaller crosscut or slit.

Feeding Refusal

- The baby may seem to be refusing to breast- or bottle-feed. Try to problem-solve what might be happening by considering the length of time between feedings. If the feedings are too close together, the baby may not be hungry enough to be motivated to feed.
- Consider the size of the nipple hole and whether the baby is working too hard to extract the fluid. This is a common problem. Explore using a nipple that either has a faster

flow rate or that is flexible enough to allow assistive squeezing if necessary.

- If breastfeeding, the baby may be overwhelmed with the initial milk letdown during feeding and demonstrate avoidance. Experiment with hand-expressing some milk before beginning to breastfeed.
- Experiment with the temperature of the formula if bottle-feeding. Although not proven by research, many infants seem to prefer warm formula as opposed to room temperature.
- Try to be consistent with the method being used for feeding. Train others who may be feeding the baby to use the same positioning, the same feeding equipment, and the same type of strategies you use when feeding your baby. For example, demonstrate how to use assistive squeezing or how often you give the baby breaks for resting or burping during a feeding.

Managing Air Intake during Feeding

Babies with clefts will tend to swallow some extra air while feeding. After intake of every ounce (or so), giving the baby a pause from feeding and a chance to burp may help to alleviate discomfort associated with excessive air intake.

Persistent Oral Feeding Problems

Most feeding problems can be easily resolved. If your baby continues to have trouble feeding and you are concerned, consult your pediatrician for a referral to a speech-language pathologist or occupational therapist experienced with the special feeding issues associated with cleft lip/palate or other craniofacial conditions.

CREDITS

Appendix opener photo: PeopleImages/Getty Images

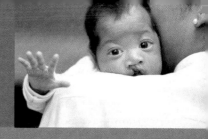

Feeding Infants with Clefts Using Adapted Nipples and Bottles

With acknowledgment to Claire K. Miller for her contributions to this appendix.

Bottle Feeding Using the Mead Johnson Lip/Cleft Palate Nurser

- Position baby in a semi-upright position in your lap. Hold the Mead Johnson bottle in your right hand, using your left arm/hand to support the baby's head and shoulders.
- The Mead Johnson nipple or nipple of choice (Pigeon nipple, standard nipple, orthodontic nipple, etc.) can be used with the Mead Johnson flexible bottle.
- Use the nipple to touch the corner of the baby's lip to help stimulate mouth opening. When the baby's mouth opens, take care to place the nipple onto the body of the tongue, not in the space in front of the tongue.
- If the baby has a cleft lip and palate, allow the baby to try sucking the nipple first before beginning to provide a gentle assistive squeeze of the bottle.
- Begin with one gentle squeeze of the bottle, watching the baby's reaction.

- Try to squeeze in a rhythmic manner in time to the baby's sucking.
- Avoid using a continuous squeezing motion because this will overwhelm the baby.
- Use regular squeezing at the beginning of the feeding when the baby is eating vigorously; slow the rate toward the middle and end of the feeding when the baby's sucking rate slows down.

Bottle Feeding Using the Medela SpecialNeeds Feeder

- The Medela SpecialNeeds Feeder has several parts: bottle, nipple, disc, collar, and valve membrane.
- Begin assembling the feeder by pressing the valve membrane onto the upper side of the disc (the stud should go through the center hole).
- Fill the bottle compartment with breast milk or formula. Put the valve membrane into the nipple, and then use the collar to put

all the parts together onto the bottle. Squeeze the nipple compartment while the feeder is upright. Then, turn the feeder upside down, releasing the nipple compartment. This allows the formula to enter the nipple reservoir.

- Position the baby in a semi-upright position on your lap, holding the bottle in one hand and supporting the baby with your other arm/hand.
- Begin by lining up the shortest line (zero flow) on the nipple reservoir with the baby's nose.
- Touch the nipple to the corner of the baby's mouth, and when the mouth opens, gently advance the nipple onto the baby's tongue.
- Try to position the nipple under any intact part of the palate.
- Allow the baby some time to begin sucking.
- The nipple will release fluid as the baby compresses it with sucking.
- Based on the baby's sucking efforts, rotate the nipple until the medium line (medium flow) or longest line (maximum flow) is under the baby's nose—determine flow rate based upon baby's response.
- If needed, you may compress the reservoir to give extra assistance with fluid expression every second or third suck.

Bottle Feeding Using the Pigeon Nipple

- The Pigeon nipple has a Y-shaped opening. Rub a soft, clean cloth over the opening to loosen it before using.
- Use the nipple with a flexible bottle, such as the Mead Johnson.
- Find the "V" in the base of the nipple. This is the air vent that should be placed on the top of the nipple, under the infant's nose while feeding.
- Position the nipple on the infant's tongue. The infant's sucking motion will activate the flow.

Bottle Feeding Using the Bionix Controlled Flow Baby Feeder

- The Bionex Controlled Flow Baby Feeder has six parts: 60 mL feeding bottle, clear silicone nipple, blue ring cap, green flow adjuster, purple silicone seal, and a yellow five-hole flow restrictor.
- The yellow five-hole restrictor is screwed onto the bottle, and the purple silicone seal is pressed onto the yellow restrictor.
- The green flow adjustor is then placed over the purple seal and snapped onto the yellow flow restrictor so that the number "0" is viewable through the window on the green flow adjuster.
- The Bionix nipple is placed inside the blue ring cap to create the nipple assembly.
- The nipple assembly is then screwed onto the green flow adjustor.
- The channel inside the nipple should be guided into the green flow adjustor by gently pulling up on the nipple to help align it into the green flow adjustor.
- Once aligned, squeeze the nipple and push down, inserting the channel into the raised component of the green flow adjuster.
- Unscrew the completed feeder assembly to fill the bottle with the formula of choice.
- Reassemble the feeder assembly on the bottle, and begin with the flow adjustment set at "0" flow to establish nonnutritive sucking. Adjust the flow setting (1–5), depending on the feeding ability of the baby.

Bottle Feeding Using the Dr. Brown's Specialty Feeding System

- The Dr. Brown's Specialty Feeding System is manufactured as a fully assembled, ready-to-use system. The fully assembled system comes with either a 4 oz (120 mL) or 8 oz

(240 mL) bottle system with an internal vent system, including an insert and a reservoir. The specialty feeding system will not function without the insert, reservoir, and infant-paced feeding valve.

- A Dr. Brown's standard silicone Level 1 nipple and the unidirectional Infant-Paced Feeding Valve come with the standard assembly.
- All levels of the Dr. Brown's standard neck nipples (Preemie Flow™, Levels 1–4, and Y-Cut) can be used with the Infant-Paced Feeding Valve. The selection of the nipple is dependent on the infant's oral-motor skills and feeding ability. For example, an infant may be able to move from a Level 1 nipple (slow flow) to higher nipple levels (faster flow rates) as feeding skills develop.
- Fill the bottle with the desired amount of formula; do not fill the bottle above the "fill line warning."
- Insert plastic valve into the base of the nipple, making sure the valve is fully secured, flush with the nipple.
- Insert the nipple into the nipple collar.
- Make sure the nipple is fully seated.
- Snap the reservoir fully onto the insert.
- Place the reservoir into the bottle, making sure that the insert makes full contact with the top of the bottle.
- Place the nipple collar loosely on the bottle and then tighten. If the specialty feeding system is leaking, check the tightness of the collar and the assembly of the insert and the reservoir.

- Mixing and shaking formula in the bottle is not recommended because it may cause the internal vent system to separate and the bottle to leak.

Feeding with the Medela SoftCup Feeder

- The SoftCup Feeder has a silicone reservoir, disc, valve membrane, and collar.
- The valve should be pressed onto the upper side of the disc so that the stud goes completely through the center hole.
- Slip the reservoir into the collar.
- Put the assembled valve into the reservoir, making sure that the valve and the high rim of the disc are facing the inside of the reservoir.
- Place the reservoir over the bottle, and tighten the collar to make a good seal.
- Hold the feeder upright and squeeze below the pads of the reservoir.
- Keep squeezing and tip the feeder upside down.
- Release the pads and some fluid will flow into the reservoir; repeat until almost filled.
- Position the baby and present the soft cup to the lips; the baby's mouth will slightly open.
- Present small amounts of the fluid, allowing time for the baby to transfer and swallow each small amount given.

CREDITS

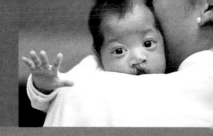

CHAPTER 8

Developmental Aspects: Speech, Language, and Cognition

CHAPTER OUTLINE

INTRODUCTION

Children born with a cleft palate will be behind their unaffected peers in the acquisition of some early developmental phonemes (e.g., plosives) because these phonemes are impossible to produce with an unrepaired cleft palate. This delay persists, at least until the palate is repaired and often for some time later. If the child has velopharyngeal insufficiency (VPI) after the palate has been repaired, speech development will be further delayed and abnormal speech with compensatory productions may develop.

Speech problems secondary to VPI have been well documented in the literature. There is a good understanding of how abnormal structure and function of the velopharyngeal valve can affect speech, frequently causing obligatory distortions and compensatory errors (Kummer, 2011; Trost-Cardamone, 1997). The association between clefts and language and/or cognitive development is less clear. Of course, significant difficulties with speech production may cause expressive language skills to appear delayed because of the difficulty with speech production. However, there may be subtle factors that affect other aspects of development in patients with cleft palate.

In contrast to children with nonsyndromic clefts, there is good evidence that children with certain craniofacial syndromes are at risk for not only speech disorders but also for language and cognitive problems. This risk is because of associated brain anomalies and neurological dysfunction that can be features of craniofacial syndromes.

This chapter outlines what is known about the development of children with clefts and craniofacial conditions, particularly in the area of language. It is hoped that the reader will learn to be attentive to all aspects of development, including language and learning, when evaluating a child from one of these populations. Developmental delays are particularly important to recognize and remediate during the critical period of brain development for the child to reach his full potential.

Prerequisites for Normal Development

Unlike other primates, humans have the innate ability to learn to communicate through spoken language. The ability to learn is the key factor and is dependent on the individual's cognition. (Cognition is the ability to engage in conscious intellectual activities that are important for learning.) Although cognition is important for language learning, the development of language further enhances the development of cognitive skills (Dowling, 2004). In fact, language is a tool for thought and problem solving.

Speech, language, and cognitive development are dependent on some basic prerequisites, including brain structure and function, environmental stimulation, hearing, motivation, and attention skills. Normal anatomy and physiology of the speech mechanism are also important for expressive language and speech production. When one considers the basic prerequisites for speech development and language learning, it is easy to understand why some children have difficulty developing these skills.

This section describes these basic prerequisites for speech and language learning and how these prerequisites may be affected by the occurrence of a cleft or craniofacial condition.

Brain Structure and Function

The brain determines an individual's intelligence, which includes the ability to perceive, comprehend, assimilate, analyze, categorize, imitate, and learn. When intelligence is significantly below normal, there are usually generalized delays that affect function in all aspects of development, including language and speech. Intelligence and cognitive function are totally dependent on the structure of the brain and the function of the central nervous system. Therefore, normal brain structure and function are necessary requirements for the development of both speech and language.

Relatively recent research suggests that individuals with clefts may also have structural differences in the brain and are at risk for brain abnormalities. Using magnetic resonance imaging (MRI) technology, Nopoulos and colleagues found structural abnormalities in the brain morphology of men with nonsyndromic clefts of the lip and/or palate (Nopoulos et al., 2001; Nopoulos et al., 2005; Nopoulos, Berg, Canady, et al., 2002; Nopoulos, Berg, Van Demark, et al., 2002; Richman & Nopoulos, 2009; Weinberg et al., 2013). Their findings included midline anomalies, enlarged regions of the cerebrum, decreased volumes of the posterior cerebrum and cerebellum, and abnormalities in the frontal lobe. In addition, Rosen and colleagues (Rosen et al., 2011) discovered brain abnormalities in 6.3% of fetuses with cleft lip and/or palate through prenatal MRI imaging. These reports suggest that there may be a relationship between facial development and brain development.

Neurologic dysfunction is a particular risk for children with cleft palate only (CPO), especially those who have other congenital anomalies (Broder, Richman, & Matheson, 1998; Richman, 1980; Richman, Eliason, & Lindgren, 1988; Strauss & Broder, 1993). This increased risk is because of the fact that isolated cleft palate often occurs as part of a syndrome that includes neurologic dysfunction and low intelligence as phenotypic features. In fact, there are many craniofacial syndromes that include a form of neurological dysfunction as a phenotypic feature, including Apert syndrome, Opitz syndrome, CHARGE syndrome, Down syndrome, Cornelia de Lange syndrome, fetal alcohol syndrome, fetal hydantoin, velocardiofacial/22q11.2 deletion syndrome (VCFS/22q deletion syndrome) and Williams syndrome (Shprintzen et al., 1978; Shprintzen, 1998).

Intellectual impairment and language disorder are common phenotypic features of VCFS/22q deletion syndrome (also known as DiGeorge syndrome) (D'Antonio, Scherer, Miller, Kalbfleisch, & Bartley, 2001; Persson et al., 2006; Scherer, D'Antonio, & Kalbfleisch, 1999; Scherer, D'Antonio, & Rodgers, 2001). It is, therefore, not surprising that significant brain abnormalities have been found with this syndrome, including reduced brain volume of both white and gray matter (Eliez, Antonarakis, Morris, Dahoun, & Reiss, 2001; Eliez, Schmitt, White, & Reiss, 2000; Eliez, Blasey, et al., 2001; Kates et al., 2001; van Amelsvoort et al., 2004), cerebellar hypoplasia (Devriendt, Van Thienen, Swillen, & Fryns, 1996; Lynch et al., 1995; van Amelsvoort et al., 2004; Yamagishi, 2002), larger corpus callosum area (Antshel, Conchelos, Lanzetta, Fremont, & Kates, 2005), and Chiari malformation (Hultman et al., 2000). These findings certainly have implications for cognitive, social, and language development in the VCFS/22q deletion syndrome population.

Some syndromes and conditions do not have cognitive or neurological dysfunction as typical phenotypic features but have the potential for causing impairment in intellectual or neurological function. For example, in craniofrontonasal dysplasia, intellect is generally normal unless there are also midline defects of the brain. In Crouzon syndrome, cognition is also typically within normal limits. However, hydrocephalus with increased intracranial pressure may occur, and if left untreated, it can have a permanent effect on intelligence and cognitive function.

Environmental Stimulation

Environmental stimulation and environmental experience are important factors in language development. Just as is the case with adults learning a foreign language, children learning their first language need to be constantly exposed to language for efficient learning to take place. In addition, they must have experiences with the environment before words about the environment are meaningful to them. Therefore, children who live in a language-rich environment are likely to develop language skills faster and have a more extensive vocabulary than children with little language stimulation. Language learning is easier under the age of 5, during the period of critical brain development (Dowling, 2004). Consequently, stimulation during this period of time is particularly important. The difficulty with speech and language learning after the critical period is particularly evident in the children with clefts who are adopted internationally in that the younger the child is when adopted, the faster and easier new speech and language skills are developed (Scherer, Baker, Kaiser, & Frey, 2016).

Children with a cleft or craniofacial condition are usually not different from other children in the amount of stimulation that they receive from their environment (Chapman & Hardin, 1991). In some cases, children with a cleft or craniofacial condition may actually have an advantage over their unaffected peers. This is because some parents are so concerned about the potential effect of the anomalies on their child's development that they become particularly diligent in providing speech and language stimulation. Affected children may have another advantage in that they often qualify for enrollment in an early intervention program, most of which are geared toward the development of cognitive and language skills.

Although some affected children may have some advantages in early stimulation, others are not as fortunate. Children with significant anomalies and serious medical conditions undergo several surgical procedures and frequent hospitalizations in the early years. Unfortunately, a hospital room is usually not a language-rich environment. Additionally, the severely affected child may have less opportunity to interact with others because of a compromised medical condition, and there may be social isolation caused by the child's appearance.

Hearing and Vision

It is through sensory perception that we learn about the world around us and develop a method for communicating with each other. Both speech and language learning is done through the use of hearing and vision.

Children with cleft palate are at high risk for chronic middle ear effusion and conductive hearing loss from eustachian tube malfunction. Hearing loss is suspected to be a primary reason that children with clefts often score lower on verbal performance measures than their noncleft peers

in the early years (Broen, Devers, Doyle, Prouty, & Moller, 1998; Jocelyn, Penko, & Rode, 1996; Kritzinger, Louw, & Hugo, 1996; Lamb, Wilson, & Leeper, 1973). Additional support for hearing loss as a factor in early measures of intelligence comes from the studies that show that differences in intelligence disappear with age or with the insertion of pressure-equalizing (PE) tubes (Paradise, 1998).

Children with craniofacial syndromes are even more likely to have conductive and/orsensorineural hearing loss because hearing loss is a phenotypic feature of many syndromes. For example, a primary phenotypic feature of Waardenburg syndrome is congenital sensorineural hearing loss that is usually severe and bilateral. Sensorineural hearing loss can also be found in hemifacial microsomia (also known as Goldenhar syndrome, facio–auriculo–vertebral malformation sequence, and oculo–auriculo–vertebral dysplasia), CHARGE syndrome, Stickler syndrome, Treacher Collins syndrome, and others.

A severe hearing loss or deafness affects the child's ability to perceive and thus imitate speech sounds. A child with a severe hearing impairment has difficulty learning all aspects of language. Even resonance is affected by the inability to monitor and therefore modulate velopharyngeal function. Overall, verbal communication is extremely difficult, if not impossible, to acquire without adequate hearing.

Some craniofacial syndromes affect the eyes and thus vision. Although the need for adequate hearing for speech and language development is obvious, vision is also important. We learn speech by watching faces. We learn meaning by watching expressions and body gestures. Vision is particularly important for learning the meaning of spoken words.

Motivation

The next prerequisite for language development is motivation. Although many new skills can be learned passively, a skill will be acquired much more rapidly if there is a need and desire to learn the skill. This general principle certainly holds true for language learning (Syal & Finlay, 2011).

In most cases, young children are motivated to talk because it is the best way to communicate. However, if a caregiver or an older sibling anticipates the child's needs and wants, there is little reason to learn to talk. This is particularly true for children under the age of 2 when gestures are an effective method for communicating needs. It is only when the child wants to communicate something more than the "here and now" that this gestural system is no longer effective. With an increase in the need to communicate, there is a corresponding increase in the motivation to communicate and the development of verbal language.

For the most part, children with a history of cleft are no different from their unaffected peers in communicating their needs through gestures during the first year (Long & Dalston, 1982a). During the second year, the child begins to use verbal language and discontinues the use of gestures because verbal language is usually a more effective form of communication.

One problem is that some parents of children with clefts tend to overprotect their child, especially during times of surgery or medical appointments. In doing so, they may respond to the child's requests without requiring verbal communication from the child. Although this is understandable at times, persistent overprotection reduces the child's need to communicate verbally, and this can have a detrimental effect on the child's expressive language development.

Another issue with motivation occurs if the child has difficulty with speech sound production. When speech intelligibility is poor, verbal language may be an ineffective means of communication (Grunwell & Russell, 1988). Therefore, the child may be motivated to revert back to using gestures, at least to augment speech. If intelligibility continues to be poor as the child gets older, it can cause the child to be less assertive when engaging in conversational skills compared with others (Chapman, Graham, Gooch, & Visconti, 1998; Frederickson, Chapman, & Hardin-Jones, 2006).

Attention

Another prerequisite for language learning is the ability to attend to the environment and particularly to the verbal communication of others. **Attention deficit-hyperactivity disorder (ADHD)** refers to a cluster of behavioral characteristics that involves impaired attention, impulsivity, distractibility, and hyperactivity.

The percentage of children estimated to have ADHD has changed over time and can vary by how it is measured. For example, in the *Diagnostic and Statistical Manual of Mental Disorders, Fifth Edition* (DSM-5), of the American Psychiatric Association (APA), it was estimated that 5% of children are diagnosed with ADHD (APA, 2013). In contrast, the Centers for Disease Control and Prevention (CDC) estimates that approximately 11% of children, ages 4–17 years of age (about 6.4 million in the United States), have been diagnosed with ADHD, based on a parent survey from 2011–2012 (CDC, n.d.a; CDC, n.d.b). The CDC report also notes that the percentage of children diagnosed with ADHD has increased over time—from 7.8% in 2003, to 9.5% in 2007, to 11.0% in 2011–2012. ADHD is five to nine times more prevalent in boys than in girls (Lecendreux, Konofal, & Faraone, 2010).

When a child has a significant attention deficit, distractibility, and a high activity level, the stimulation from the environment may not be adequately perceived or processed, and language learning is affected as a result. In addition, the child with ADHD is less likely to participate in language-enriching activities, such as reading, listening to a story, or playing a game. Children with ADHD are often diagnosed with learning disabilities (Cantwell & Baker, 1991; Cherkes-Julkowski, 1998; Sidoti, Marsh, Marty-Grames, & Noetzel, 1996; Tirosh, Berger, Cohn-Ophir, Davidovitch, & Cohen, 1998) and language disorders (Cantwell & Baker, 1991; Cherkes-Julkowski, 1998; Damico, Damico, & Armstrong, 1999; Fergusson & Horwood, 1992; Love & Thompson, 1988; Purvis & Tannock, 1997; Tirosh et al., 1998; Tirosh & Cohen, 1998). One study found that 30% of children with speech and language impairments also had ADHD (Beitchman, Hood, Rochon, & Peterson, 1989).

Although ADHD is usually diagnosed in children with no identified neurological lesion, the same characteristics are commonly seen in individuals with documented brain damage or neurological deficits (Max et al., 1998; Niemann, Ruff, & Kramer, 1996). Children with craniofacial syndromes that include neurological dysfunction are at significant risk for difficulties with attention and concentration. As an example, attention deficits and difficulty with concentration are typical problems with VCFS/22q deletion syndrome (Heineman-de Boer, Van Haelst, Cordia-de Haan, & Beemer, 1999; Swillen et al., 1997; Swillen et al., 1999).

Vocal Tract Anatomy and Physiology

There are many physical prerequisites that are important for speech production. There must be structural integrity of the entire vocal tract. In addition, physiology must be normal for respiration, phonation, velopharyngeal function, articulation, and neurological function. Clefts and craniofacial conditions may include a variety of structural abnormalities, including dental malocclusion and velopharyngeal insufficiency. The effects of these abnormalities on speech are covered in the other chapters.

Development in Children with Clefts and Craniofacial Syndromes

The literature on the developmental status of children with clefts and craniofacial anomalies is often contradictory and difficult to interpret. This is partly because these populations of children are very heterogeneous. They can differ not only in the type and severity of the cleft or craniofacial condition but also with respect to other medical conditions, such as chronic middle ear effusion and hearing loss, the number of hospitalizations, the type and effectiveness of the surgical repairs, parental attitudes and involvement, and even environmental factors. Children with clefts and craniofacial anomalies may show deficits when compared to a peer group but still score well within the normal range (Hardin-Jones & Chapman, 2011). Finally, deficits that are noted early in development may no longer be noted in later years. Therefore, it is very difficult to determine the characteristics of "typical" development for children affected by clefts.

Language and Cognitive Development

Several authors have reported that children with nonsyndromic clefts show some early deficits in prelinguistic skills during the first 3 years of life (Fox, Lynch, & Brookshire, 1978; Hentges et al., 2011; Kapp-Simon & Krueckeberg, 2000; Neiman & Savage, 1997; Scherer, Williams, & Proctor-Williams, 2008; Snyder & Scherer, 2004; Speltz et al., 2000). In addition, some studies have found that children with clefts have lower scores in verbal performance than nonverbal performance on standardized tests (Broen et al., 1998; Lamb et al., 1973). In contrast, other studies have found no verbal–nonverbal differences in the cleft population (Leeper, Pannbacker, & Roginski, 1980; McWilliams & Matthews, 1979). One study showed no differences in comprehension compared to unaffected peers (Long & Dalston, 1983). Some studies have reported that children with clefts have immature syntactic development, short utterance length, and overall delays in expressive language compared with their unaffected peers (Whitcomb, Ochsner, & Wayte, 1976). Others have found the linguistic abilities of children with repaired clefts to be within the normal range. One study found that children with clefts who demonstrate compensatory articulation productions had a higher frequency of language delays than those without compensatory productions (Pamplona, Ysunza, Gonzalez, Ramirez, & Patino, 2000).

Considering the cognitive development of children with nonsyndromic clefts, there are a few studies that show that children with clefts are at risk for minor delays in cognitive development when compared to their unaffected peers, particularly in the early years (Hardin-Jones & Chapman, 2011; Kapp-Simon & Krueckeberg, 2000; Neiman & Savage, 1997; Snyder & Scherer, 2004; Speltz et al., 2000). This is consistent with the studies on language development. There is also some research to show that children with clefts have a higher rate of reading disability than their peers (Broder et al., 1998; Chapman, 2011; Richman et al., 1988).

Although children with nonsyndromic clefts may be at risk for early delays in both language and cognitive development, these delays seem to disappear with time (Broen et al., 1998; Collett, Leroux, & Speltz, 2010; Jocelyn et al., 1996; Neiman & Savage, 1997; Richman & Nopoulos, 2009; Shames & Rubin, 1979). This may be because of the cleft palate repair, the resolution of middle ear disease that can cause fluctuant hearing loss, and/or the correction of velopharyngeal insufficiency that can affect expressive language development.

The prognosis for normal language and cognition is not as good for children with isolated cleft palate compared to children with cleft lip or cleft lip and palate (Broder et al., 1998; Richman et al., 1988; Strauss & Broder, 1993). For example, the phenotypic characteristics of VCFS/22q deletion syndrome include cleft or submucous cleft of the velum only and language and learning disorders (Glaser et al., 2002; Kok & Solman, 1995; Motzkin, Marion, Goldberg, Shprintzen, & Saenger, 1993; Scherer et al., 1999; Shprintzen, 1998; Shprintzen et al., 1978; Swillen et al., 1999; Vantrappen et al., 1999). McWilliams and Matthews (1979) found that in a population of 108 children with isolated cleft palate and other anomalies, 51% had a full-scale IQ of 89 or below, and 37% had IQs of 69 or below. Children with a craniofacial syndrome are also more likely to exhibit other characteristics that can affect language and cognitive development, including sensorineural hearing loss, attention deficits, frequent hospitalizations, and social isolation (Mossey, Little, Munger, Dixon, & Shaw, 2009).

Speech Sound Development

Early sound production, in the form of cooing and babbling, is an important part of normal speech development. By associating the physical movement of sound production with the auditory results through a tactile–kinesthetic–auditory feedback loop, infants are able to learn to produce sounds volitionally. Infants with cleft palate, however, have an inadequate sound production mechanism and also frequently have hearing deficits. With these factors alone, they are at risk for delays in speech sound development, even after the palate has been repaired (Jones, Chapman, & Hardin-Jones, 2003; O'Gara & Logemann, 1988).

Infants with an unrepaired cleft palate usually begin to babble around the age of 6 months, just like their unaffected peers. However, unlike their peers, they are not able to impound oral airflow for plosives. Therefore, their babbling sounds are restricted to nasal phonemes (/m/, /n/) only, at least until the palate has been repaired. Infants with an open cleft palate may even vocalize less than their unaffected peers (Harding & Grunwell, 1996; Kummer, 2011; Long & Dalston, 1982b; O'Gara & Logemann, 1988). They may also begin to use glottal stops for plosives rather than developing the typical babbling pattern (Chapman, 1991; Smith & Kuehn, 2007).

The open palate can also affect the infant's place of articulation. Unaffected infants use anterior sounds in prespeech productions (Roug,

Landberg, & Lundberg, 1989; Smith & Oller, 1981; Stoel-Gammon, 1985). In contrast, infants with clefts, regardless of type, babble with a predominant use of posterior consonants, particularly glottal stops and velars (Hardin-Jones, Chapman, & Schulte, 2003; Lohmander-Agerskov, Soderpalm, Friede, Persson, & Lilja, 1994; Russell, 1991; Willadsen & Albrechtsen, 2006).

Once the palate is repaired, most children have adequate structure for speech sound production. However, even if the palate is repaired by 9–10 months, the child will have missed the developmental stage where plosives are usually produced and practiced through normal babbling. As a result, some of these infants continue to show deficits in the production of certain early developmental sounds for some time after the palate has been repaired (Estrem & Broen, 1989; Hardin, 1991; Jones et al., 2003; O'Gara, Logemann, & Rademaker, 1994). Within the first few years, however, glottal productions gradually decrease and oral productions increase. As a result, the speech of those with a successful palate repair may gradually become similar to noncleft peers' speech by the age of 4 or 5 (Chapman, 1993; Chapman & Hardin, 1992; O'Gara & Logemann, 1988; O'Gara et al., 1994).

How quickly children with repaired clefts are able to acquire oral sounds naturally and catch up with their unaffected peers after the palate repair has been a subject of several investigations. One factor that may affect the acquisition of articulation skills is the age of palate repair. Many authors have suggested that children who undergo early palate repair demonstrate better overall speech than those with a later repair (Dorf & Curtin, 1990; Grobbelaar, Hudson, Fernandes, & Lentin, 1995; McWilliams, Morris, & Shelton, 1990; O'Gara & Logemann, 1988; Peterson-Falzone, 1996). Considering the critical period for brain development for speech sound production (Dowling, 2004), it makes sense that the longer the palate remains unrepaired, the harder it is to correct the child's speech. Another factor is regular otologic care, which can prevent hearing loss and help mitigate the risk for delayed speech development. A final

factor is access to early intervention. Through early intervention, speech-language pathologists can do a great deal to lessen the effects of the cleft on developing communication skills (Hardin-Jones, Chapman, & Scherer, 2006). This is most effective if the parents are trained in methods of speech (and language) stimulation so that they can work with the child on a daily basis at home.

If the child has significant velopharyngeal insufficiency (short velum or velar defect) following palate repair, it will limit the oral consonants that can be produced. As the child's expressive language increases, a wider range of consonants are needed for intelligibility. In this situation, many children with velopharyngeal insufficiency either decrease their language output by shortening utterance length or increase their consonant repertoire by developing compensatory articulation productions where articulation is primarily produced in the pharynx or larynx. Harding and Grunwell (1996) reported that around 30 months of age, the pharyngeal fricative (a compensatory production) became prevalent in the speech of their patients with persistent velopharyngeal insufficiency after palate repair. This is because at this point in speech development, there is a need for a fricative–plosive contrast. If a normal fricative cannot be produced because of a lack of intraoral air pressure, the pharyngeal fricative will be produced instead. Once acquired and habituated, compensatory productions usually persist, even after the velopharyngeal insufficiency has been corrected.

Although compensatory productions can usually be corrected with speech therapy, delays in correcting the structure can have a serious effect on the time it takes to remediate the errors. Just as the ability to learn a new language after the age of 6 years is decreased—and after puberty is almost impossible without retaining an accent—the ability to correct faulty speech patterns is also reduced as the child passes the critical period for brain development and speech/language learning (Dowling, 2004).

Finally, children with craniofacial syndromes often have symptoms of childhood apraxia of speech (CAS). For example, children with VCFS/22q deletion syndrome can have mild to severe apraxia, in addition to obligatory and compensatory productions from velopharyngeal insufficiency (Kummer, Lee, Stutz, Maroney, & Brandt, 2007).

SUMMARY

Based on existing research, it appears that children with nonsyndromic clefts are at risk for mild delays in language development during the first 3 years of life. These delays may be secondary and the result of fluctuating conductive hearing loss and/or velopharyngeal insufficiency (McWilliams et al., 1990; Mossey et al., 2009). Fortunately, language development seems to improve with early intervention and time so that ultimately these children catch up with their noncleft peers.

The risk for developmental delay is greatest for children with a known craniofacial syndrome or those with history of cleft palate only (which is often indicative of a syndrome). The language deficits found in many craniofacial syndromes have more complex etiologies than those found in the noncleft population. Therefore, these children should be carefully evaluated at an early age so that intervention can be initiated as soon as possible if needed.

In considering speech sound development, children with an unrepaired cleft palate necessarily acquire speech sounds differently than their unaffected peers. Even though the prognosis for normal speech development is fairly good once the palate has been repaired, the child remains at risk for persistent compensatory articulation errors and abnormal resonance caused by malocclusion and velopharyngeal insufficiency. Therefore, speech and resonance, in addition to language, should be carefully monitored throughout the preschool and early school years.

FOR REVIEW AND DISCUSSION

1. What populations of children with clefts are at particular risk for developmental delays? Why is this?

2. What recent evidence could explain the language disorders and neurological dysfunction in children with VCFS/22q deletion syndrome?

3. Why do you think some children with craniofacial conditions actually receive more language stimulation than unaffected children? Why do some affected children receive less language stimulation than the norm?

4. Why do children with cleft palate seem delayed in language development in the early years but catch up by the time they are in school? What do you think could be done to mitigate these initial delays?

5. What is the effect of an open palate on speech sound acquisition? Why do children still demonstrate abnormal speech after the palate has been repaired?

6. How would you explain to a physician that early palate repair is better for speech development and ultimate speech outcomes than later palate repair?

7. Describe how you would counsel the parent of an infant with cleft palate about speech and language stimulation. In addition to regular stimulation techniques, what additional instructions would you give to the parent of a child with a cleft? What should be a focus of stimulation after the palate repair?

REFERENCES

American Psychiatric Association (APA). (2013). *Diagnostic and Statistical Manual of Mental Disorders* (5th ed.). Washington, DC: American Psychiatric Association.

Antshel, K., Conchelos, J., Lanzetta, G., Fremont, W., & Kates, W. R. (2005). Behavioral and corpus callosum morphology relationships in velocardiofacial syndrome (22q11.2 deletion syndrome). *Psychiatry Research, 138,* 235–245.

Beitchman, J. H., Hood, J., Rochon, J., & Peterson, M. (1989). Empirical classification of speech/language impairments in children: II. Behavioral characteristics. *Journal of the American Academy of Child and Adolescent Psychiatry, 28,* 118–123.

Broder, H. L., Richman, L. C., & Matheson, P. B. (1998). Learning disability, school achievement, and grade retention among children with cleft: A two-center study. *The Cleft Palate–Craniofacial Journal, 35*(2), 127–131.

Broen, P. A., Devers, M. C., Doyle, S. S., Prouty, J. M., & Moller, K. T. (1998). Acquisition of linguistic and cognitive skills by children with cleft palate. *Journal of Speech, Language, and Hearing Research, 41*(3), 676–687.

Cantwell, D. P., & Baker, L. (1991). Association between attention deficit-hyperactivity disorder and learning disorders. *Journal of Learning Disabilities, 24*(2), 88–95.

Centers for Disease Control and Prevention (CDC). (n.d.a). Attention-deficit/hyperactivity disorder (ADHD): Data and statistics. Retrieved from https://www.cdcgov/ncbddd/adhd/data.html#ref

Centers for Disease Control and Prevention (CDC). (n.d.b). Attention-deficit/hyperactivity disorder (ADHD). Key findings: Trends in the Parent-Report of Health Care Provider-Diagnosis and Medication Treatment for ADHD: United States, 2003–2011. Retrieved from https://www.cdc.gov/ncbddd/adhd/features/key-findings-adhd72013.html

Chapman, K. L. (1991). Vocalizations of toddlers with cleft lip and palate. *The Cleft Palate–Craniofacial Journal, 28*(2), 172–178.

Chapman, K. L. (1993). Phonologic processes in children with cleft palate. *The Cleft Palate–Craniofacial Journal, 30*(1), 64–72.

Chapman, K. L. (2011). The relationship between early reading skills and speech and language performance in young children with cleft lip and palate. *The Cleft Palate–Craniofacial Journal, 48*(3), 301–311.

Chapman, K. L., Graham, K. T., Gooch, J., & Visconti, C. (1998). Conversational skills of preschool and school-age children with cleft lip and palate. *The Cleft Palate–Craniofacial Journal, 35*(6), 503–516.

Chapman, K. L., & Hardin, M. A. (1991). Language input of mothers interacting with their young children with cleft lip and palate. *The Cleft Palate–Craniofacial Journal, 28*(1), 78–85; discussion 85–86.

Chapman, K. L., & Hardin, M. A. (1992). Phonetic and phonological skills of two-year-olds with cleft palate. *The Cleft Palate–Craniofacial Journal, 29*(5), 435–443.

Cherkes-Julkowski, M. (1998). Learning disability, attention-deficit disorder, and language impairment as outcomes of prematurity: A longitudinal descriptive study. *Journal of Learning Disabilities, 31*(3), 294–306.

Collett, B. R., Leroux, B., & Speltz, M. L. (2010). Language and early reading among children with orofacial clefts. *The Cleft Palate–Craniofacial Journal, 47*(3), 284–292.

Damico, J. S., Damico, S. K., & Armstrong, M. B. (1999). Attention-deficit hyperactivity disorder and communication disorders: Issues and clinical practices. *Child and Adolescent Psychiatric Clinics of North America, 8*(1), 37–60.

D'Antonio, L. L., Scherer, N. J., Miller, L. L., Kalbfleisch, J. H., & Bartley, J. A. (2001). Analysis of speech characteristics in children with velocardiofacial syndrome (VCFS) and children with phenotypic overlap without VCFS. *The Cleft Palate–Craniofacial Journal, 38*(5), 455–467.

Devriendt, K., Van Thienen, M., Swillen, A., & Fryns, J. (1996). Cerebellar hypoplasia in a patient with velocardiofacial syndrome. *Developmental Medicine and Neurology, 38,* 945–949.

Dorf, D. S., & Curtin, J. W. (1990). Early cleft repair and speech outcome: A ten-year experience. In J. Bardach & H. L. Morris (Eds.), *Multidisciplinary management of cleft lip and palate* (pp. 341–348). Philadelphia, PA: W. B. Saunders.

Dowling, J. E. (2004). *The great brain debate: Nature or nurture?* Washington, DC: Joseph Henry Press.

Eliez, S., Antonarakis, S. E., Morris, M. A., Dahoun, S. P., & Reiss, A. L. (2001). Parental origin of the deletion 22q11.2 and brain development in velocardiofacial syndrome: A preliminary study. *Archives of General Psychiatry, 58,* 64–68.

Eliez, S., Blasey, C. M., Schmitt, E. J., White, C. D., Hu, D., & Reiss, A. L. (2001). Velocardiofacial syndrome: Are structural changes in the temporal and mesial temporal regions related to schizophrenia? *American Journal of Psychiatry, 158,* 447–453.

Eliez, S., Schmitt, J. E., White, C. D., & Reiss, A. L. (2000). Children and adolescents with velocardiofacial syndrome. *American Journal of Psychiatry, 157,* 409–415.

Estrem, T., & Broen, P. A. (1989). Early speech production of children with cleft palate. *Journal of Speech and Hearing Research, 32*(1), 12–23.

Fergusson, D. M., & Horwood, L. J. (1992). Attention deficit and reading achievement. *Journal of Child Psychology and Psychiatry and Allied Disciplines, 33*(2), 375–385.

Fox, D., Lynch, J., & Brookshire, B. (1978). Selected developmental factors of cleft palate children between two and thirty-three months of age. *Cleft Palate Journal, 15*(3), 239–245.

Frederickson, M. S., Chapman, K. L., & Hardin-Jones, M. (2006). Conversational skills of children with cleft lip and palate: A replication and extension. *The Cleft Palate–Craniofacial Journal, 43*(2), 179–188.

Glaser, B., Mumme, D. L., Blasey, C., Morris, M. A., Dahoun, S. P., Antonarakis, S. E., . . . Eliez, S. (2002). Language skills in children with velocardiofacial syndrome (deletion 22q11.2). *Journal of Pediatrics, 140*(6), 753–758.

Grobbelaar, A. O., Hudson, D. A., Fernandes, D. B., & Lentin, R. (1995). Speech results after repair of the cleft soft palate. *Plastic and Reconstructive Surgery, 95*(7), 1150–1154.

Grunwell, P., & Russell, V. J. (1988). Phonological development in children with cleft palate. *Clinical Linguistics and Phonetics, 2,* 75–95.

Hardin, M. A. (1991). Cleft palate: Intervention. *Clinics in Communication Disorders, 1*(3), 12–18.

Harding, A., & Grunwell, P. (1996). Characteristics of cleft palate speech. *European Journal of Disorders of Communication, 31,* 331–357.

Hardin-Jones, M., & Chapman, K. L. (2011). Cognitive and language issues associated with cleft lip and palate. *Seminars in Speech and Language, 32*(2), 127–140.

Hardin-Jones, M., Chapman, K., & Scherer, N. J. (2006, June 13). Early intervention in children with cleft palate. *The ASHA Leader, 11*(8), 8–9, 32.

Hardin-Jones, M., Chapman, K. L., & Schulte, J. (2003). The impact of cleft type on early vocal development in babies with cleft palate. *The Cleft Palate–Craniofacial Journal, 40*(5), 453–459.

Heineman-de Boer, J. A., Van Haelst, M. J., Cordia-de Haan, M., & Beemer, F. A. (1999). Behavior problems and personality aspects of 40 children with velocardiofacial syndrome. *Genetic Counseling, 10*(1), 89–93.

Hentges, F., Hill, J., Bishop, D. V., Goodacre, T., Moss, T., & Murray, L. (2011). The effect of cleft lip on cognitive development in school-aged children: A paradigm for examining sensitive period effects. *Journal of Child Psychology and Psychiatry, 52*(6), 704–712.

Hultman, C. S., Riski, J. E., Cohen, S. R., Burstein, F. D., Boydston, W. R., Hudgins, R. J., . . . Simms, C. (2000). Chiari malformation, cervical spine anomalies, and neurologic deficits in velocardiofacial syndrome. *Plastic and Reconstructive Surgery, 106*(1), 16–24.

Jocelyn, L. J., Penko, M. A., & Rode, H. L. (1996). Cognition, communication, and hearing in young children with cleft lip and palate and in control children: A longitudinal study. *Pediatrics, 97*(4), 529–534.

Jones, C. E., Chapman, K. L., & Hardin-Jones, M. A. (2003). Speech development of children with cleft palate before and after palatal surgery. *The Cleft Palate–Craniofacial Journal, 40*(1), 19–31.

Kapp-Simon, K. A., & Krueckeberg, S. (2000). Mental development in infants with cleft lip and/or palate. *The Cleft Palate–Craniofacial Journal, 37*(1), 65–70.

Kates, W. R., Burnette, C. P., Jabs, E. W., Rutberg, J., Murphy, A. M., Grados, M., . . . Pearlson, G. D. (2001). Regional cortical white matter reductions in velocardiofacial syndrome: A volumetric MRI analysis. *Biological Psychiatry, 49*(8), 677–684.

Kok, L. L., & Solman, R. T. (1995). Velocardiofacial syndrome: Learning difficulties and intervention. *Journal of Medical Genetics, 32*(8), 612–618.

Kritzinger, A., Louw, B., & Hugo, R. (1996). Early communication functioning of infants with cleft lip and palate. *South African Journal of Communication Disorders, 43,* 77–84.

Kummer, A. W. (2011). Disorders of resonance and airflow secondary to cleft palate and/or velopharyngeal dysfunction. *Seminars in Speech and Language, 32*(2), 141–149.

Kummer, A. W., Lee, L., Stutz, L., Maroney, A., & Brandt, J. W. (2007). The prevalence of apraxic characteristics in patients with velocardiofacial syndrome as compared to other populations. *The Cleft Palate–Craniofacial Journal, 44*(2), 175–181.

Lamb, M., Wilson, F., & Leeper, H. (1973). The intellectual function of cleft palate children compared on the basis of cleft type and sex. *Cleft Palate Journal, 10,* 367.

Lecendreux, M., Konofal, E., & Faraone, S. V. (2010). Prevalence of attention deficit hyperactivity disorder and associated features among children in France. *Journal of Attention Disorders, 15*(6), 516–524.

Leeper, H. A., Jr., Pannbacker, M., & Roginski, J. (1980). Oral language characteristics of adult cleft-palate speakers compared on the basis of cleft type and sex. *Journal of Communication Disorders, 13*(2), 133–146.

Lohmander-Agerskov, A., Soderpalm, E., Friede, H., Persson, E. C., & Lilja, J. (1994). Pre-speech in children with cleft lip and palate or cleft palate only: Phonetic analysis related to morphologic and functional factors. *The Cleft Palate–Craniofacial Journal, 31*(4), 271–279.

Long, N. V., & Dalston, R. M. (1982a). Gestural communication in twelve-month-old cleft lip and palate children. *Cleft Palate Journal, 19*(1), 57–61.

Long, N. V., & Dalston, R. M. (1982b). Paired gestural and vocal behavior in one-year-old cleft lip and palate children. *Journal of Speech and Hearing Disorders, 47*(4), 403–406.

Long, N. V., & Dalston, R. M. (1983). Comprehension abilities of one-year-old infants with cleft lip and palate. *Cleft Palate Journal, 20*(4), 303–306.

Love, A. J., & Thompson, M. G. (1988). Language disorders and attention deficit disorders in young children referred for psychiatric services: Analysis of prevalence and a conceptual synthesis. *American Journal of Orthopsychiatry, 58*(1), 52–64.

Lynch, D. R., McDonald-McGinn, D. M., Zackai, E. H., Emanuel, B. S., Driscoll, D. A., Whitaker, L. A., & Fischbeck, K. H. (1995). Cerebellar atrophy in a patient with velocardiofacial syndrome. *Journal of Medical Genetics, 32*(7), 561–563.

Max, J. E., Arndt, S., Castillo, C. S., Bokura, H., Robin, D. A., Lindgren, S. D., . . . Mattheis, P. J. (1998). Attention-deficit hyperactivity symptomatology after traumatic brain injury: A prospective study. *Journal of the American Academy of Child Adolescent Psychiatry, 37*(8), 841–847.

McWilliams, B. J., & Matthews, H. P. (1979). A comparison of intelligence and social maturity in children with unilateral complete clefts and those with isolated cleft palates. *Cleft Palate Journal, 16,* 363.

McWilliams, B. J., Morris, H. L., & Shelton, R. L. (1990). Language disorders. In B. J. McWilliams, H. L. Morris, & R. L. Shelton (Eds.), *Cleft palate speech* (vol. 2, pp. 236–246). Philadelphia, PA: B. C. Decker.

Mossey, P. A., Little, J., Munger, R. G., Dixon, M. J., & Shaw, W. C. (2009). Cleft lip and palate. *Lancet, 374*(9703), 1773–1785.

Motzkin, B., Marion, R., Goldberg, R., Shprintzen, R., & Saenger, P. (1993). Variable phenotypes in velocardiofacial syndrome with chromosomal deletion. *Journal of Pediatrics, 123*(3), 406–410.

Neiman, G. S., & Savage, H. E. (1997). Development of infants and toddlers with clefts from birth to three years of age. *The Cleft Palate–Craniofacial Journal, 34*(3), 218–225.

Niemann, H., Ruff, R. M., & Kramer, J. H. (1996). An attempt towards differentiating attentional deficits in traumatic brain injury. *Neuropsychological Review, 6*(1), 11–46.

Nopoulos, P., Berg, S., Canady, J., Richman, L., Van Demark, D., & Andreasen, N. C. (2002). Structural brain abnormalities in adult males with clefts of the lip and/or palate. *Genetics in Medicine, 4*(1), 1–9.

Nopoulos, P., Berg, S., Van Demark, D., Richman, L., Canady, J., & Andreasen, N. C. (2001). Increased incidence of a midline brain anomaly in patients with nonsyndromic clefts of the lip and/or palate. *Journal of Neuroimaging, 11*(4), 418–424.

Nopoulos, P., Berg, S., Van Demark, D., Richman, L., Canady, J., & Andreasen, N. C. (2002). Cognitive dysfunction in adult males with nonsyndromic clefts of the lip and/or palate. *Neuropsychologia, 40*(12), 2178–2184.

Nopoulos, P., Choe, L., Berg, S., Van Demark, D., Canady, J., & Richman, L. (2005). Ventral frontal cortex morphology in adult males with isolated orofacial clefts: Relationship to abnormalities in social function. *The Cleft Palate–Craniofacial Journal, 42*(2), 138–144.

O'Gara, M. M., & Logemann, J. A. (1988). Phonetic analyses of the speech development of babies with cleft palate. *Cleft Palate Journal, 25*(2), 122–134.

O'Gara, M. M., Logemann, J. A., & Rademaker, A. W. (1994). Phonetic features by babies with unilateral cleft lip and palate. *The Cleft Palate–Craniofacial Journal, 31*(6), 446–451.

Pamplona, M. C., Ysunza, A., Gonzalez, M., Ramirez, E., & Patino, C. (2000). Linguistic development in cleft palate patients with and without compensatory articulation disorder. *International Journal of Pediatric Otorhinolaryngology, 54*(2–3), 81–89.

Paradise, J. L. (1998). Otitis media and child development: Should we worry? *Pediatric Infectious Disease Journal, 17*(11), 1076–1083; discussion 1099–1100.

Persson, C., Niklasson, L., Oskarsdottir, S., Johansson, S., Jonsson, R., & Soderpalm, E. (2006). Language skills in 5–8-year-old children with 22q11 deletion syndrome. *International Journal of Language and Communication Disorders, 41*(3), 313–333.

Peterson-Falzone, S. J. (1996). The relationship between timing of cleft palate surgery and speech outcome: What have we learned, and where do we stand in the 1990s? *Seminars in Orthodontics, 2*(3), 185–191.

Purvis, K. L., & Tannock, R. (1997). Language abilities in children with attention deficit hyperactivity disorder, reading disabilities, and normal controls. *Journal of Abnormal Child Psychology, 25*(2), 133–144.

Richman, L. C. (1980). Cognitive patterns and learning disabilities of cleft palate children with verbal deficits. *Journal of Speech and Hearing Research, 23*(2), 447–456.

Richman, L. C., Eliason, M. J., & Lindgren, S. D. (1988). Reading disability in children with clefts. *Cleft Palate Journal, 25*(1), 21–25.

Richman, L. C., & Nopoulos, P. (2009). Neuropsychological and neuroimaging aspects of cleft lip and palate. In J. E. Losee & R. E. Kirschner (Eds.), *Comprehensive cleft care* (pp. 991–1000). New York, NY: McGraw-Hill.

Rosen, H., Chiou, G. J., Stoler, J. M., Mulliken, J. B., Tarui, T., Meara, J. G., & Estroff, J. A. (2011). Magnetic resonance imaging for detection of brain abnormalities in fetuses with cleft lip and/or cleft palate. *The Cleft Palate–Craniofacial Journal, 48*(5), 619–622.

Roug, L., Landberg, L., & Lundberg, L. J. (1989). Phonetic development in early infancy: A study of four Swedish children during the first eighteen months of life. *Journal of Child Language, 16*(1), 19–40.

Russell, V. J. (1991). *Speech development in children with cleft lip and palate.* (Unpublished doctoral dissertation). Leicester Polytechnic, Leicester, UK.

Scherer, N. J., Baker, S., Kaiser, A., & Frey, J. R. (2016). Longitudinal comparison of the speech and language performance of United States-born and internationally adopted toddlers with cleft lip and palate: A pilot study. *The Cleft Palate–Craniofacial Journal.*

Retrieved from https://www.ncbi.nlm.nih.gov/pubmed/27723377

Scherer, N. J., D'Antonio, L. L., & Kalbfleisch, J. H. (1999). Early speech and language development in children with velocardiofacial syndrome. *American Journal of Medical Genetics, 88*(6), 714–723.

Scherer, N. J., D'Antonio, L. L., & Rodgers, J. R. (2001). Profiles of communication disorder in children with velocardiofacial syndrome: Comparison to children with Down syndrome. *Genetics in Medicine, 3*(1), 72–78.

Scherer, N. J., Williams, A. L., & Proctor-Williams, K. (2008). Early and later vocalization skills in children with and without cleft palate. *International Journal of Pediatric Otorhinolaryngology, 72*(6), 827–840.

Shames, C., & Rubin, H. (1979). Psycholinguistic measures of language and speech. In K. R. Bzoch (Ed.), *Communicative disorders related to cleft lip and palate* (p. 202). Boston, MA: Little, Brown.

Shprintzen, R. J. (1998). Complex craniofacial disorders. In S. E. Gerber (Ed.), *Etiology and prevention of communicative disorders* (vol. 2, pp. 147–199). San Diego, CA: Singular Publishing Group.

Shprintzen, R. J., Goldberg, R. B., Lewin, M. L., Sidoti, E. J., Berkman, M. D., Argamaso, R. V., & Young, D. (1978). A new syndrome involving cleft palate, cardiac anomalies, typical facies, and learning disabilities: Velocardiofacial syndrome. *Cleft Palate Journal, 15*(1), 56–62.

Sidoti, E. J., Jr., Marsh, J. L., Marty-Grames, L., & Noetzel, M. J. (1996). Long-term studies of metopic synostosis: Frequency of cognitive impairment and behavioral disturbances. *Plastic and Reconstructive Surgery, 97*(2), 276–281.

Smith, B. E., & Kuehn, D. P. (2007). Speech evaluation of velopharyngeal dysfunction. *The Journal of Craniofacial Surgery, 18*(2), 251–261.

Smith, B. L., & Oller, D. K. (1981). A comparative study of premeaningful vocalizations produced by normally developing and Down's syndrome infants. *Journal of Speech and Hearing Disorders, 46*(1), 46–51.

Snyder, L. E., & Scherer, N. (2004). The development of symbolic play and language in toddlers with cleft palate. *American Journal of Speech-Language Pathology, 13*(1), 66–80.

Speltz, M. L., Endriga, M. C., Hill, S., Maris, C. L., Jones, K., & Omnell, M. L. (2000). Cognitive and psychomotor development of infants with orofacial clefts. *Journal of Pediatric Psychology, 25*(3), 185–190.

Stoel-Gammon, C. (1985). Phonetic inventories, 15–24 months: A longitudinal study. *Journal of Speech & Hearing Research, 28*(4), 505–512.

Strauss, R. P., & Broder, H. (1993). Children with cleft lip/palate and mental retardation: A subpopulation of cleft-craniofacial team patients. *The Cleft Palate–Craniofacial Journal, 30*(6), 548–556.

Swillen, A., Devriendt, K., Legius, E., Eyskens, B., Dumoulin, M., Gewillig, M., & Fryns, J. P. (1997). Intelligence and psychosocial adjustment in velo-cardiofacial syndrome: A study of 37 children and adolescents with VCFS. *Journal of Medical Genetics, 34*(6), 453–458.

Swillen, A., Devriendt, K., Legius, E., Prinzie, P., Vogels, A., Ghesquière, P., & Fryns, J. P. (1999). The behavioural phenotype in velo-cardio-facial syndrome (VCFS): From infancy to adolescence. *Genetic Counseling, 10*(1), 79–88.

Syal, S., & Finlay, B. L. (2011). Thinking outside the cortex: Social motivation in the evolution and development of language. *Developmental Science, 14*(2), 417–430.

Tirosh, E., Berger, J., Cohen-Ophir, M., Davidovitch, M., & Cohen, A. (1998). Learning disabilities with and without attention-deficit hyperactivity disorder: Parents' and teachers' perspectives. *Journal of Child Neurology, 13*(6), 270–276.

Tirosh, E., & Cohen, A. (1998). Language deficit with attention-deficit disorder: A prevalent comorbidity. *Journal of Child Neurology, 13*(10), 493–497.

Trost-Cardamone, J. E. (1997). Diagnosis of specific cleft palate speech error patterns for planning therapy of physical management needs. In K. R. Bzoch (Ed.), *Communicative disorders related to cleft lip and palate* (vol. 4, pp. 313–330). Austin, TX: Pro-Ed.

van Amelsvoort, T., Daly, E., Henry, J., Robertson, D., Ng, V., Owen, M., . . . Murphy, D. G. (2004). Brain anatomy in adults with velocardiofacial syndrome with and without schizophrenia: Preliminary results of a structural magnetic resonance imaging study. *Archives of General Psychiatry, 61,* 1085–1096.

Vantrappen, G., Devriendt, K., Swillen, A., Rommel, N., Vogels, A., Eyskens, B., . . . Fryns, J. P. (1999). Presenting symptoms and clinical features in 130 patients with the velocardiofacial syndrome: The Leuven experience. *Genetic Counseling, 10*(1), 3–9.

Weinberg, S. M., Parsons, T. E., Fogel, M. R., Walter, C. P., Conrad, A. L., & Nopoulos, P. (2013). Corpus callosum shape is altered in individuals with non-syndromic cleft lip and palate. *American Journal of Medical Genetics, Part A, 161a*(5), 1002–1007.

Whitcomb, L., Ochsner, G., & Wayte, R. (1976). A comparison of expressive language skills of cleft-palate and non-cleft-palate children: A preliminary investigation. *Journal of the Oklahoma Speech and Hearing Association, 3,* 25–28.

Willadsen, E., & Albrechtsen, H. (2006). Phonetic description of babbling in Danish toddlers born with and without unilateral cleft lip and palate. *The Cleft Palate–Craniofacial Journal, 43*(2), 189–200.

Yamagishi, H. (2002). The 22q11.2 deletion syndrome. *The Keio Journal of Medicine, 52*(2), 77–88.

CREDITS

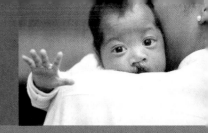

CHAPTER 9

Psychosocial Aspects

With acknowledgment to Patricia K. Marik and Janet R. Schultz for their contributions to this chapter.

CHAPTER OUTLINE

INTRODUCTION

When a baby is born, the infant is not just born to his parents. The child is born into a family, a social network, and society. These layers of context into which the child is born are also forces that affect the child's development. At the same time, the child brings into the world her genetic endowment and the characteristics developed during intrauterine life. Among these are temperament, certain instinctual behaviors, and physical appearance.

For some children, one characteristic is a cleft lip and/or palate or other craniofacial condition. The child's genetic contribution interacts with the complex context into which he is born so that the developing individual is both affected by and affecting that environment.

Family Issues

At the birth of any child, the lives of the parents and other family members are changed forever. This is especially true when the child is born with a cleft or other craniofacial condition. There is always an initial shock when parents learn that the child is not what they expected. The parents may struggle with initial issues of attachment. A time of adjustment follows. Finally, the family settles in with the reality of dealing with a child with a chronic medical condition.

Initial Shock and Adjustment

The birth of a child is typically a very happy event. Parents' first questions almost always include "Is the baby alright?" When a baby is born with a cleft lip, there is immediate knowledge of the cleft and, therefore, distress. When an infant is born with a cleft of the velum or a submucous cleft, however, hours (or longer) may elapse before the parents are informed that there is a problem.

For most families, the birth of a child with a cleft is a stressful event in their lives. Parents often experience both shock and sadness and describe the experience as traumatic (Habersaat Peter, & Borghini, 2009). There may be a period of mourning for the anticipated child and then adjustment to the child that they actually have (van Staden & Gerhardt, 1995). Strong feelings of love, protectiveness, and excitement often conflict with other feelings of hurt, fear, disappointment, betrayal, resentment, and guilt (Coy, Speltz, & Jones, 2002; Despars et al., 2011).

Resolution of the emotional aspects of the birth is complicated by a whirlwind of medical concerns that characterize early infancy for the child with a cleft or craniofacial condition. Although parents are given information about the cause and future treatment, many parents report that they did not receive the information that they most wanted at that time (Young, O'Riordan, Goldstein, & Robin, 2001).

During the first few weeks, parents must deal with particular challenges because of the cleft or condition, including those related to feeding. Because feeding an infant with cleft palate requires additional time, parents lose some of their restorative time, such as relaxing, sleeping, and engaging in favorite activities (Winston, Dunbar, Reed, & Francis-Connolly, 2010). There is also the emotional challenge of feeling less than confident and competent about feeding. Finally, parents may find themselves emotionally supporting grandparents or other relatives instead of receiving the necessary support themselves. Some parents face accusations or perceived accusations about the reason for the cleft from various family members or medical personnel.

Parents of infants with visible differences are likely to experience the staring of children, and even other adults, when they take their babies out in public. The more visible the anomaly is to the public, the more stressful the situation is for the parents (Rosenberg, Kapp-Simon, Starr, Cradock, & Speltz, 2011). These experiences may serve to confirm the fears of the child's social rejection, which tend to rise rapidly in the minds of parents at their first contact with the baby (Barr, Thibeault, Muntz, & de Serres, 2007). Therefore, parents need to learn how to cope with staring and how to talk to other people about the baby's cleft.

There are some reports that mothers of babies with clefts may be less interactive with their infants than mothers of babies without anomalies (Habersaat et al., 2013). On the other hand, the additional challenges of the cleft may actually help parents to create strong, protective bonds to their babies. One study found that babies with cleft lip and palate (CLP) were more securely attached to their parents than those who had cleft palate only (CPO) (Coy et al., 2002). Another study showed that mothers and babies with clefts are bonded similarly to nonaffected baby–parent dyads (Habersaat et al., 2013).

Mothers of babies with clefts report higher levels of stress than mothers of unaffected babies (Pope, Tillman, & Snyder, 2005). Some report a higher degree of marital conflict, although there is little evidence that the divorce rate is higher in these families. About 10% of parents reported that their marriage was adversely affected, whereas a quarter to a third reported that the birth of a child with a cleft brought the parents closer together.

The level of the parents' stress has been found to correlate with the child's adjustment later in life (Pope et al., 2005). Therefore, intervening with parents who are experiencing considerable stress may help to prevent adjustment problems for the child later on. Possible interventions can include peer support (connections with other parents of children with clefts), spiritual support from clergy, or more formal mental health support from a psychotherapist or psychologist.

When the parents have other children, this causes additional challenges during the early adjustment period. Parents may find it difficult to explain to siblings that the baby looks different and has some challenges while trying to reassure them that the doctors are going to fix the problem. The parents also have to balance the time required for taking care of the baby with the needs of the other children. This is particularly difficult if the baby requires a long time to feed, has frequent ear infections, is scheduled for many medical visits, or has surgery. There is not much research on nonaffected siblings, but a qualitative study suggests that issues of jealousy and resentment as well as feelings of protectiveness and closeness occur just as in siblings without medical issues (Stock, Stoneman, Cunniffe, & Rumsey, 2016).

Fortunately, the negative feelings and adjustment problems tend to subside fairly rapidly after the first few months without impairing the parent–child relationship on a long-term basis (Habersaat et al., 2013) or the quality of life of the parents (Kramer, Baethge, Sinikovic, & Schliephake, 2007). One reason for this relatively rapid resolution is the "fixable" quality of clefts. In addition, family support has been found to be a significant factor in the parents' overall adjustment to the child with a cleft, whereas having a low level of social support is a predictor of depression in mothers of children with clefts (Baker, Owens, Stern, & Willmot, 2009; Sank, Berk, Cooper, & Marazita, 2003). Other factors that affect the parents' adjustment include the extent and visibility of the cleft and each parent's coping style and level of education (Sank et al., 2003). Overall, negative outcomes are not frequent or severe in most families, especially those who have strong social supports (Baker et al., 2009). It has been pointed out that fathers are not often included in this kind of research, however. It appears though that fathers experience many of the same concerns as mothers but may receive less support and may not feel free to express their emotions publicly (Stock & Rumsey, 2015).

During the early months, it is very important that parents receive sufficient information and support from healthcare professionals (generally nurses or pediatricians). New parents need to have someone with whom they can talk who is positive, encouraging, and able to answer their questions. Many parents want contact with other parents who have been through the same experiences (Kerr & McIntosh, 2000). Parents seem less

TABLE 9-1 **Resources for Parents**
AboutFace
http://www.aboutface.ca
American Cleft Palate–Craniofacial Association (ACPA)
http://acpa-cpf.org
Children's Craniofacial Association
https://ccakids.org
FACES: The National Craniofacial Association
http://www.faces-cranio.org/home.html
Parents Helping Parents (PHP)
http://www.php.com
Smile Train
https://www.smiletrain.org

afraid to show their vulnerability to sympathetic veterans of the process and may voice more of their fears and questions with them.

Many hospitals help parents of newborns with clefts link with other parents so that they can compare experiences and solutions to problems. A common activity is sharing pictures, which the newer parents often use as a peek into the future of their own child. The Internet has also become a resource for medical and parenting information. Some sites that specifically focus on cleft palate or other craniofacial conditions can be found in TABLE 9-1.

Cleft Palate as a Chronic Medical Condition

Parents of a child with a cleft or craniofacial condition spend a lot of time taking their child to medical appointments. This can pose practical challenges, including difficulty with transportation, time away from work (which can threaten their employment), time away from their other children, and a strain on their financial resources. The visits can be stressful because they remind them of their baby's "difference," and they may hear more bad news. In some ways, these visits may feel like an evaluation of their efficacy

as parents, particularly when feeding has been a major challenge and the physician is charting the infant's growth. It is very important to parents that healthcare professionals are supportive of them and relate to their child as a person, not as an assortment of physical problems.

The first surgery is a stressful and frightening time for family members. Having a helpless baby taken from their arms for surgery reawakens the sad, frightened, and protective feelings that may have quieted since the birth. For many of the normal challenges of growing up, parents and grandparents have the ability to "make it all better" for their children. When surgery is required, however, the parents and other family members are confronted with their powerlessness to fix the baby's problems. Instead, they have to trust the surgeon and all other professionals involved, often leaving them feeling out of control. There is always a bit of concern that something might go wrong and that the baby could die as a result of their decision regarding the surgery. The stress level and emotional response of the parents are influenced not only by the nature and severity of the child's condition but also specific treatment procedures (Sischo, Clouston, Phillips, & Broder, 2016). After the surgery for a cleft lip repair, parents often report a mixed experience because the child looks different than the baby they had before. Making decisions about subsequent surgeries is a mix of knowledge, emotions, and risk/benefit analysis. The decision as to whether surgery is worth the risk only becomes more complicated as the child grows older and the emphasis of surgery is more on appearance than function.

Parents play a unique role in helping their child through the surgeries that no health professional can assume. It is therefore important that they receive practical advice from professionals about staying with the infant during the entire hospitalization, preparing siblings for the event and the baby's changed appearance, and caring for the baby after surgery. This advice can increase a parent's sense of being able to contribute to the child's well-being. For the baby, having a parent or other familiar adult available during the entire hospital stay is important for security and comfort (Redsell & Glazebrook, 2010).

Even when there are positive relationships between healthcare professionals and parents, some aspects of dealing with the medical system can be overwhelming for parents and continue to be problematic for years. For example, dealing with paperwork, insurance authorization, and bills can cause frustration and anger. This can lead to misdirected anger toward professionals and even to noncompliance of the medical regimen.

The intensity of concerns about the child's cleft and the associated stresses usually diminish over time, with resurgent peaks at times of surgery, social rejection, or the child's own distress. Parents often experience some fatigue during the whole process and are eager for everything to be done. Disagreement between the parents regarding medical decisions is not unusual. As the child grows older, this disagreement can even be between parents and the child, especially during the teen years. Parental fears may be reawakened when the teenager or adult child moves into a serious relationship, where reproductive and hence genetic issues are important. On the whole however, most families of children with craniofacial conditions function in the normative range (Crerand et al., 2015).

When the parent also has a cleft, there is an added dimension to the relationship. It usually answers the question as to the cause of the child's cleft. Although the parent is in an unusually good position to be knowledgeable about the cleft and understanding of the child's feelings, there is also the risk that the parent's unresolved negative feelings may color her response to the challenges facing the child. Sometimes parents make decisions that reflect an attempt to "get it right this time." Factors that can affect how a parent with a cleft copes with having a child with a cleft include the prenatal diagnosis, her perception of the severity of the cleft, and the feeling of guilt or blame that can be exacerbated by the feelings of

other family members (Stock & Rumsey, 2015). It is particularly important to help the parent see differences between his situation and that of the child's. An important consideration is the advancement of surgical techniques since the parent's own repair.

Although having a child with a cleft is stressful, there is no evidence that it leads to a higher frequency of psychiatric symptoms in parents (Dabit et al., 2014; Grollemund et al., 2010). Having a positive attitude and strong support system can greatly reduce the stress. Also, using coping strategies that involve approaching rather than avoiding the issues (i.e., seeking support, active problem-solving, logical analysis, etc.) is particularly helpful to parents (Baker et al., 2009). Poverty and the presence of several other children were noted to increase parental stress.

School Issues

Once the child enters school, there are additional challenges. Many people, including teachers, underestimate the abilities and intelligence of individuals who have facial anomalies or abnormal speech. Some children with clefts or other craniofacial conditions actually do have learning issues, even though they have normal intelligence. Perhaps the greatest concerns for affected children are difficulties with social interactions, periodic teasing or even bullying, and a relatively negative self-concept.

Knowledge and Expectation of Teachers

Teachers have reported that they do not know much about CLP (like most of the population) and what they think they know may be incorrect (Finnegan, 1982). As a group, teachers have also been found to underestimate the intelligence of children with a cleft, especially when either appearance or speech is significantly impaired. As such, they may expect less from the children who look different from those who appear "normal" (Richman & Eliason, 1982). Underestimates of the abilities of these children can actually cause lower performance and less positive evaluations of their academic performance. In fact, several studies have found that children with clefts do not achieve the level that would be predicted by their intelligence alone (Broder, Richman, & Matheson, 1998; Millard & Richman, 2001).

Learning Ability and School Performance

Children with CLP and CPO have consistently shown lower academic achievement scores than nonaffected peers (Persson, Becker, & Svenson, 2012; Wehby, Collet, Barron, Romitti, & Ansley, 2015; Wehby et al., 2014). Despite these findings, children and teenagers with a nonsyndromic CLP have overall intelligence that is in the average range, as measured by formal IQ tests (Millard & Richman, 2001; Persson, Becker, & Svenson, 2008). Lower academic performance may be because of the lower expectations, as previously noted. However, these children generally score lower on test sections that require verbal skills, especially oral responses, than on performance-based sections.

In contrast to children with CLP, children with CPO, which is often associated with various craniofacial syndromes, tend to score lower on intelligence tests than unaffected peers (Persson et al., 2008). They also score lower in academic achievement than norms or matched controls (Bell et al., 2016; Wehby et al., 2015). Many children with CPO have specific learning disabilities. It has been found that a significant number of children with CPO have reading problems that persist throughout the grade school years (Richman, Ryan, Wilgenbusch, & Millard, 2004). In addition, children with CPO have more speech and language disorders than those with CLP or nonaffected peers (Broen, Devers, Doyle, Prouty, & Moller, 1998; Roberts, Mathias, & Wheaton, 2012).

Certainly, children who have speech problems often lack self-confidence in reading aloud, which may influence the teachers' evaluation of their abilities. Children with CLP who have reading disabilities have been shown to have specific deficits in rapid naming and verbal expression. Their problem does not appear to be phonemic awareness, despite some early attempts to link reading problems to articulation difficulties (Richman & Ryan, 2003).

Several craniofacial syndromes are associate with cognitive dysfunction, including velocardiofacial/22q11.2 deletion syndrome (VCFS/22q deletion syndrome). Children with VCFS/22q deletion syndrome often have a learning disability or intellectual impairment that can range from very mild to severe (Fuerst, Dool, & Rourke, 1995; Furniss, Biswas, Gumber, & Singh, 2011; Simon et al., 2002). Academic achievement in the primary grades may be higher than in later grades, where abstract thinking is more important than memorization. Other syndromes associated with cognitive impairment and learning disabilities include Smith–Lemli–Opitz syndrome (Kelley & Hennekam, 2000), fetal alcohol syndrome, and fetal alcohol spectrum disorder (Sokol, Delaney-Black, & Nordstrom, 2003). Other syndromes, such as Treacher Collins syndrome and hemifacial microsomia, are not associated with problems in cognitive function (Speltz et al., 2017).

Cognitive deficits have been found in some specific craniosynostosis syndromes. One study found that, as a group, children with craniosynostosis scored in the average range of intelligence with a mean IQ of 95 (DaCosta et al., 2006). However, there was a significant difference between those children with a syndromic presentation (mean IQ of 83) and those who were not diagnosed with a syndrome (mean IQ of 104). Craniosynostosis syndromes associated with cognitive dysfunction include Apert, Crouzon, and Muenke syndromes. Children with Crouzon syndrome usually have normal cognitive function (deJong, Maliepaard, Bannink, Raat, & Mathijssen, 2012).

Social Interaction

In the early years of a child's life, the negative social implications of the cleft are primarily experienced by the parents. They are the ones who note the stares or answer the questions about the child's condition. By the preschool years, however, the child starts to be asked directly about what happened to her lip. Sometimes the question comes from well-meaning adults who believe the child's scar to be from a fall or a minor accident. Other times, it comes from curious peers who notice a difference in the child's appearance. Although preschool children prefer attractive children as friends, they are rarely cruel or tease their peers. They notice differences in appearance, speech, and behavior, but unless the differences interfere with play, they are not generally important in relationships. One advantage of enrolling an affected child in preschool or daycare is the opportunity to build social skills and confidence at a time when teasing and rudeness are rare.

By school age, a significant number of children with a cleft or craniofacial condition do not have as many friendships as other children their age (Tobiasen & Speltz, 1996). This appears to be a result of several factors. First, affected children, especially girls, seem to be more socially inhibited than their peers. They are sometimes reluctant to initiate friendships and may have difficulty maintaining friendships. In addition, the lack of friends may be because of communication challenges associated with hearing impairment and/or speech difficulties. Finally, concerns about appearance may be a contributor to the lack of friends.

In a now-classic experiment, Joyce Tobiasen (1988, 1989) showed pictures of children to second- through fourth-graders. Some of the children in the unretouched photos had no cleft, some had a repaired unilateral cleft, and some had a repaired bilateral cleft. The viewers rated the pictured children on personal qualities. Children rated those with a bilateral cleft as having fewer positive attributes than those with a unilateral cleft, and both cleft groups fared worse than the children without a visible cleft. The younger viewers were harsher in their ratings than the somewhat older ones. A later study of photos of children with facial scars found that peers rate them as less intelligent, less attractive, and less likely to be identified as a potential friend (Nabors, Lehmkuhl, & Warm, 2004). A Swiss study further substantiated those findings using digitally altered photos. Nonaffected children and teens rated those children depicted with a facial difference to have fewer positive and more negative characteristics than those without. The participants also felt they would be less likely to befriend the persons with facial differences. The strength of findings diminished with age of the raters (Masnari, Schiestl, Weibel, Wuttke, & Landolt, 2013). Similarly, children with hemifacial microsomia were found to have lower social competence and less peer acceptance, especially if eye anomalies were present (Dufton et al., 2011). One study found that a common reason people with clefts or craniofacial syndromes choose to have surgery is the hope of reducing stigmatization from appearance (Bemmels et al., 2013).

Although the degree of facial impairment is strongly correlated with perceptions of attractiveness and social desirability, the social relationships of an individual child cannot be accurately predicted on the basis of facial attractiveness alone (Feragen, Kvalem, Rumsey, & Borge, 2010; Shute, McCarthy, & Roberts, 2007). The child's temperament, family support, social skills, personal experiences, and coping strategies also make a difference.

Older children and teenagers tend to have increasing concerns about interpersonal relationships. In particular, children with a craniofacial condition tend to have over-inhibition and shyness that continue into adolescence. Slifer and his colleagues videotaped interactions of children, ages 8 to 15, with and without clefts and found that children with clefts responded less often to questions from peers and made fewer choices during interactions (Slifer et al., 2004). Those children with clefts who rated themselves as more socially acceptable were more likely to look their peers in the face. In another study, teachers rated social competence and peer acceptance lower for children with cleft than the children's parents (Dufton et al., 2011). It is not clear whether teachers have a more realistic or negative lens or perhaps they see a different sample of behavior.

Problems with social skills may be because of the conversational experiences of those growing up with facial and speech differences, and/or these problems may be attributable to neuropsychological differences of individuals with clefts (Berger & Dalton, 2011). The latter theory is suggested by the findings of Nopoulos and colleagues (2005). These researchers found that, compared to a control group, men with nonsyndromic clefts had morphologic abnormalities in the part of the brain known to govern social functioning, as noted through magnetic resonance imaging (MRI). They also reported that the larger the abnormality, the more problems in socializing.

How these differences may relate to romantic outcomes is not yet known. Although the frequency of dating relationships among young people with a cleft relative to their peers has not been studied, it appears that teens with a cleft show more self-doubts and have lower expectations for relationships than their peers. One study showed that girls who were dissatisfied with their facial appearance had more negative psychosocial outcomes, which was not found in boys (Shapiro, Waljee, Ranganathan, Buchman, & Warschausky, 2015). Although appearance may affect a girl's self-confidence, the relative societal importance of physical attractiveness for females may play a role in this finding. This pattern continues into adulthood with women reporting greater concern about their appearance than men (Sinko et al., 2005). Both men and women express more concerns about appearance than unaffected adults and report that their facial appearance has worked against them socially (Hamlet & Harcourt, 2015; Hutchinson,

Wellman, Noe, & Kahn, 2011; Sarwer et al., 1999). It is interesting to note that ratings of facial esthetics by surgeons tend to be higher than those of nonprofessionals, who see a greater need for surgery to improve appearance of other adults with facial differences (Foo, Sampson, Roberts, Jamieson, & David, 2013).

Teasing

Children with clefts are probably teased more often than their unaffected peers (Broder, Smith, & Strauss, 2001). Teasing seems to be influenced by the child's physical appearance and speech differences because children tend to report less teasing after surgeries that address those problems. Children with craniofacial anomalies who have lower academic achievement report being teased more often than normally achieving affected children (Feragen, Saervold, Aukner, & Stock, 2017). Other factors that affect teasing are the child's personality, social standing, and response to teasing. Children who laugh off teasing or respond in kind appear to be teased less than those who respond with distress or helpless anger. The use of humor or attributing teasing to a flaw in the person who does the teasing is protective of the child's self-esteem.

The likelihood of teasing is also affected by the response of adults in the child's environment, especially at school. If the adults help the child to present information to other children about the cleft and the various surgeries, it can reduce teasing and elicit empathy, especially among children in lower grades. Teasing is also reduced when school officials take an active role in demonstrating that respect for all students is expected. On the other hand, when teasing is viewed as an inevitable behavior of children, teasing is more likely to continue or increase.

By high school, teasing tends to diminish or takes on a friendlier tone for children with craniofacial conditions. There is a greater understanding of clefts and a greater acceptance of differences at this age. When unpleasant teasing continues, however, it can take on a cruel edge and even a group rejection that may result in social withdrawal. Some social scientists see this kind of teasing as having the same power and domination quality as more general "bullying." Hunt and colleagues (2006) found that almost two-thirds of teenagers and young adults reported being teased or bullied, with several reporting physical bullying more frequently than typical peers. Bullying is associated with depression, anxiety, and fear of negative evaluation (Storch et al., 2003). It has been found that the experience of being teased affects children more negatively than the cleft per se (Hunt et al., 2006). Teasing and bullying represent societal problems, although the effect is felt by individuals. Changing the norms for children's behavior would be an intervention that matches the problem more closely than surgery.

Self-Perception

Children with clefts have consistently been found to have a more negative self-concept when compared to their unaffected peers (Slifer et al., 2003; Sousa, Devare, & Ghanshani, 2009). They see themselves as less acceptable to their peers, less socially competent, less satisfied with their facial appearance, and more often sad or angry than their peers. Children can develop a negative concept of self-worth over time. Broder and Strauss (1989) found that children with CLP scored lower with regard to self-concept than those with an "invisible" CPO, but children with any type of cleft rated themselves lower than unaffected children. Higher levels of acceptance of the cleft were associated with better self-concepts. In school-age children with clefts, greater physical attractiveness correlated with better overall adjustment (Pillemer & Cook, 1989). In one study, 10-year-olds reported lower self-esteem associated with the luminance and redness of their cleft surgery scar (Millar et al., 2013). A study of older teens and young adults found that satisfaction with appearance was related to adjustment but

also that these older individuals were more satisfied than their younger counterparts (Thomas, Turner, Rumsey, Dowell, & Sandy, 1997).

Concerns regarding physical appearance affect the self-perception of individuals with clefts or craniofacial conditions across the life span. Women report greater feelings of self-consciousness and negative self-perception than their male counterparts (Clifford, Crocker, & Pope, 1972). As can be expected, adults with a cleft lip are less satisfied with facial appearance than those with CPO, whereas adults with cleft palate are more displeased with their speech than those with cleft lip only. More dissatisfaction with their mouth, teeth, lips, voice, and speech was expressed by both cleft groups than by the control group of adults with no history of cleft (Clifford et al., 1972).

Societal Issues

Humans are naturally social beings who require human interaction, communication, and acceptance by others. Individuals with clefts or craniofacial anomalies are often hindered in their communication by speech and hearing difficulties. In addition, they can be viewed more negatively by others because of their appearance and speech.

Physical Attractiveness

One of the forces at work for a child with a cleft is society's response to facial difference. Physical attractiveness, especially facial beauty, is an area that has been well researched, with findings that are among the most reliable and robust in the psychological literature. There is some evidence that mouth shape is especially important across cultures, even though the specific standards for beauty may differ. Dental differences certainly carry meaning for adults, although this is less clear in the case of children.

Within a culture, there is considerable consensus about general characteristics of attractiveness.

This consensus develops early. By preschool age, children know the standards of beauty that the adults hold and share those values.

More important than the consensual nature of cultural standards of beauty are the meanings associated with being considered either attractive or unattractive. In a nutshell, beauty is equated with goodness. Attractive people are rated as smarter, kinder, friendlier, and more likely to be a good friend than those who are less attractive. Ethnologists have found that characteristics in babies, such as a round head, large eyes, and short and narrow features are rated as "cute" (witness how most people respond to pandas) and elicit caregiving behaviors from adults. Infants considered to be highly attractive tend to be rated as more likable, smarter, and less problematic. The significance of these ratings and beliefs lie in their power to shape the behavior and attitudes of people, directly and indirectly. These in turn become part of the feedback loop that shapes how an individual behaves and views himself.

Physical attractiveness is important across the life span. Preschoolers prefer attractive children as their friends. The social power of attractiveness continues to increase until the early grade school years and then tends to hold steady until adolescence. Teachers also have more favorable expectations of attractive children than unattractive children. Teachers may respond differentially to more physically attractive children, and as a group, the grades of attractive children are often higher than those of less attractive peers (Gordon, Crosnoe, & Wu, 2013). Attractive teens are more likely to be elected to school office than other youth and, as no surprise to most people, date more frequently and have a higher number of partners. Even being seen with attractive people increases a person's social desirability. Physical attractiveness affects the likelihood of being hired for a job, even when public contact is not a major factor. It may also influence job performance evaluations.

The power of physical attractiveness appears to hold in middle and older age as well, but this is less well established. People sometimes hope that this influence only holds at first impression, but research suggests that this is not the case (Ambady & Rosenthal, 1993; Hosoda, Stone-Romero, & Coats, 2003). Less attractive adults have slower rates of being hired, earning promotions, and getting raises (Hosoda et al., 2003). In one survey, almost 40% of adults with craniofacial anomalies believed that their condition affected them in the workplace (Sarwer et al., 1999). Although physical attractiveness is only one of many variables contributing to the social responses to a person, it is a powerful force indeed.

Speech Quality

The quality of a person's speech is a factor rather similar to physical attractiveness. Speech quality affects the social judgments of others, which in turn shapes behaviors and attitudes of both the speaker and the listener. Poor speech, especially hypernasality, appears to be associated with the assumption that the speaker has negative social characteristics (Havstam, Laakso, Lohmander, & Ringsberg, 2011; Lee, Gibbon, & Spivey, 2017; Watterson, Mancini, Brancamp, & Lewis, 2013). Children are less likely to initiate conversations with those with impaired speech, and children and adults associate speech problems of both children and adults with undesirable personal characteristics. Although cultural differences exist in these stereotypes, listeners often believe that people with speech disorders are more likely to be emotionally disturbed (Bebout & Bradford, 1992) or mentally deficient. Third, a person's satisfaction with her speech, similar to satisfaction with appearance, is often more important than what others think. One study found that affected children's satisfaction with their speech was positively correlated with their psychological adjustment and well-being but was not consistent with ratings by speech-language pathologists (Feragen et al., 2017).

It also appears that speech quality and facial appearance interact with each other in determining how a person is perceived by others. Facial attractiveness may not change ratings of speech quality, but impaired speech seems to lower ratings of physical attractiveness of the speaker. Hypernasality appears to be particularly unattractive to listeners so that ratings of social desirability of a speaker decrease steadily as hypernasality increases. The combination of facial appearance and hypernasality contributed to "a lack of perceived competence" in individuals with cleft palate and velopharyngeal insufficiency. One study found that unaffected children rated speech samples of children with clefts as indicating that they were more likely to be ugly than speakers with typical intelligibility (Lee et al., 2017).

Hearing Impairment

Having a hearing impairment can add to the social judgments that people make. Many children with clefts have some degree of hearing impairment, which may vary with the frequency of recurrent ear infections. Negative stereotypes exist of people who have hearing impairments, with or without visible hearing aids. More importantly, however, hearing is central to many aspects of social interactions among members of the general population (Fujiki, Brinton, & Clarke, 2002; Moeller, 2007). Children often avoid wearing hearing aids out of concern for their social desirability. In some respects, these children cannot win because both hearing impairment and hearing aids have a negative social value.

When an individual misunderstands even subtle nuances in a conversation, it shapes the next phase of interaction. If the person is perceived as not understanding some of the communication, he can be viewed as annoying or frustrating. With repetition, interactions may be avoided. This is another example of the importance of the social feedback loop.

Stigma

The concept of stigma is a common thread unifying all three areas described above. Stigma is a factor that is different from cultural standards and results in discrediting and objectifying an individual. In the case of persons with craniofacial anomalies, they are evaluated in a negative fashion because of their difference from the cultural standards of beauty, speech, hearing, and/or social interactions. Stigma diminishes a person's social acceptability, which negatively affects self-esteem (Masnari, Schiestl, Rössler, et al., 2013).

Another effect of stigma is the reduction or blocking of social and economic opportunities. The effect of stigmatization may be felt in the absence of negative intent, as when people stare out of curiosity, ignorance, or sympathy. Essentially, it is a problem of people being defined by their stigma and coming to anticipate stigmatization as well. They then may behave accordingly, as if stigmatized, regardless of the behavior or attitudes of the other people involved in interactions. People with facial anomalies are particularly vulnerable to stigma. In a survey of parents and teens with facial differences, mostly congenital facial anomalies, it was found that stigmatizing experiences occur regularly for at least one-third of them, sometimes on a weekly basis (Strauss et al., 2007).

Behavior and Psychiatric Issues

Children with clefts or other craniofacial anomalies are subjected to multiple surgeries and therapies that are not experienced by their unaffected peers. These can cause stress for the child and behavioral issues that require professional intervention. For individuals with certain syndromes, there is also a risk of psychiatric disorders that tend to manifest in adolescence and adulthood. Finally, having a cleft or other craniofacial condition may affect overall quality of life.

Behavioral Issues Related to Medical Care

As discussed earlier in this chapter, having to undergo major medical procedures is generally stressful and often difficult for family members and patients. For some, the experience is traumatizing, and for others, it is an inevitable event to be faced in a matter-of-fact manner. Multiple surgeries may have a cumulative effect as well.

Psychological interventions can help children with clefts with their concerns related to their treatment. Most children dread even relatively minor procedures, such as injections or having dental caries filled. For a small proportion of children, however, multiple surgeries or medical procedures can contribute to the development of significant anxiety and distress (see Case Report: Brian's Story). Teaching children coping skills can help to reduce both the distress associated with a procedure and the time it takes to carry it out. It is also helpful if the psychologist or other support professional is present for some of the procedures to coach the child in coping during the procedure.

When children have to wear devices, such as a distraction device or reverse face mask, the treatment is very visible and can take considerable time. These children and their families often benefit from coaching on how to prepare peers, answer questions, and deal with the inconvenience or discomfort.

Pediatric psychologists can also help children and families with adherence to various treatment recommendations. For example, for children who suck their thumbs past early childhood, a psychologist can help parents develop ways to break this difficult habit through increased awareness and a reward system (Friman & Leibowitz, 1990). Parents are taught to avoid power struggles while focusing on times when the child is not sucking her thumb. Similarly, children with clefts often have very poor dental hygiene that prevents needed, and even desired, orthodontia. They avoid brushing because looking in the mirror while brushing teeth forces the child to confront the presence of an undesirable difference in appearance. A psychologist can improve the child's adherence to brushing recommendations while addressing the underlying concerns

expressed through poor hygiene (Philippot, Lenoir, D'Hoore, & Bercy, 2005).

Psychiatric and Psychological Concerns

The rates of diagnosed psychiatric disorders for children and teens with clefts appears no different than those of the general population. In addition, research has consistently failed to provide evidence of a personality type in individuals with clefts. The biggest risk for affected individuals appears to be for social competence problems, including those relating to development of friendships and participation in organizations (Murray et al., 2010).

Although there is no known link between nonsyndromic facial anomalies and psychiatric disorders, coping with the added stress and stigmatization may raise the risk of depression or anxiety (Kapp-Simon, Simon, & Kristovich, 1992; Pope & Snyder, 2005). In one study of 4- to 9-year-old children with orofacial clefts, nearly a quarter of the children screened positive for separation anxiety (Tyler, Wehby, Robbins, & Damiano, 2013). Having speech or feeding problems doubles a child's risk. There have been some reports that suggest attentional problems in children with clefts (Richman et al., 2004). Other research has not supported these findings (Klatt, Schultz, Lee, & Saal, 2002; Speltz, Morton, Goodell, & Clarren, 1993). In fact, it has become more evident that airway problems and obstructive sleep apnea (OSA), which are common in children with cleft, may be a cause for poor attention (Ferini-Strambi et al., 2003).

Although children with nonsyndromic clefts are at no increased risk for psychiatric disorders, psychiatric disorders have been associated with some craniofacial syndromes. The syndrome with the greatest frequency of schizophrenia or mood disorders is VCFS/22q deletion syndrome, with some estimates reaching as high as 40% (Murphy, Jones, & Owen, 1999; Papolos et al., 1996; Shprintzen, Goldberg, Golding-Kushner, & Marion, 1992). Shprintzen's 2008 summary of VCFS/22q deletion syndrome indicated that, although many affected persons do not develop psychiatric problems, the risk for developing a serious disorder with VCFS/22q deletion syndrome is increased 25 times that of the general population. Symptoms typically reach clinical levels in late adolescence or early adulthood.

Quality of Life

A psychosocial outcome that is coming into widespread use across many pediatric conditions is quality of life. Quality of life (QOL) is defined by the World Health Organization as "individuals' perceptions of their position in life in the context of culture and value systems in which they live and in relation to their goals, expectations, standards and concerns." QOL is inherently subjective and therefore cannot be observed by others (Bonomi, Patrick, Bushnell, & Martin, 2000). Health-related QOL (HRQOL) describes "QOL as it relates to disease or treatments people experience" (Bonami et al., 2000).

The effect of clefts and other craniofacial conditions on HRQOL remains an area of much research. One study found differences in oral HRQOL, including in the domains of functional well-being (problems eating, difficulty saying certain words, and keeping teeth clean) and social–emotional well-being compared to controls (Ward et al., 2013). Oral HRQOL, especially related to social well-being, may worsen in

adolescence. Although some studies have found a similar negative effect of cleft on HRQOL (Kortelainen et al., 2016), others have not found a difference in HRQOL between individuals with clefts and controls (Pisula, Lukowska, & Fudalej, 2014). It is possible that the effect of craniofacial conditions on HRQOL or QOL in general may be affected by additional factors, such as stigmatization, attractiveness, and temperament of the individual. Surgery may also have a positive effect on HRQOL, especially as reported by adolescents (Broder, Wilson-Genderson, & Sischo, 2017).

One condition-specific QOL measure for pediatric patients with velopharyngeal insufficiency is the Velopharyngeal insufficiency Effects on Life Outcomes (VELO) instrument. The VELO includes a questionnaire for both parents and children, ages 8 and older. It has been shown to have concurrent validity, test-retest reliability, and responsiveness to change in QOL with treatment (Skirko et al., 2013).

Taking all of this into consideration, it is important that professionals working with individuals with clefts and other craniofacial conditions be aware of the possible negative effect of these conditions on QOL. Individuals who are struggling significantly with low QOL may benefit from additional intervention by a behavioral health specialist, ideally one who is well versed in working with individuals with craniofacial conditions and their families.

CASE REPORT

Brian's Story

Brian was a 9-year-old boy with a bilateral cleft lip and palate. His surgical repairs had been without complications, and he was able to go home at the expected time after each surgery. He was an honor student at a private school, which was considered to be one of the more rigorous in the area. He had friends and had not experienced teasing since second grade. His family was close-knit and generally supportive, except for a typical sibling rivalry with a sister. Brian had interacted well with his healthcare providers. His family was careful to adhere to recommendations and reliably attended scheduled appointments.

(continues)

CASE REPORT

Brian's Story *(continued)*

Unfortunately, Brian became highly anxious at the thought of the hospital after undergoing a bone graft, which he found to be painful at the donor site. The smell of bubble gum, which had been used as a spray on the mask before surgery, brought distress, regardless of the circumstances. A few months later, Brian required ventilation tube reinsertion. Although this was a minor outpatient procedure, Brian's anxiety about the hospital led to nausea and vomiting. He began to have episodes of fearfulness accompanied by cold hands and nausea.

The usual route from Brian's house to his grandmother's passed near the children's hospital. Brian developed nausea as they neared the hospital, and on several occasions, the driver had to pull over to the curb so Brian could vomit. They began driving a more convoluted, lengthy route that avoided the hospital area, which eliminated his vomiting. Brian expressed his appreciation for avoiding the hospital but realized it was "stupid" to react so strongly "to nothing." When coming for a craniofacial team appointment at the hospital, he vomited twice, once about four blocks from the hospital and once in the parking lot. Although Brian knew that there was no surgery planned for that day, that fact did nothing to curb his feelings.

Brian was referred to the craniofacial team psychologist to address his symptoms. His family was supportive and hopeful that intervention would lead to greater comfort for Brian and shorter and more pleasant car travel for all. Brian agreed to come to sessions "to get over this," even though the psychologist's office was at the hospital.

At the first visit, the psychologist took a detailed history of Brian's symptoms. She then had Brian monitor his thoughts and feelings throughout the week. From the results, it was evident that Brian had become classically conditioned to this response to the hospital. Brian's therapy sessions often included his mother, who enlisted the cooperation of Brian's sister and father to carry out home assignments.

Brian was treated with a combination of systematic desensitization and methods to improve and broaden his coping strategies. One of the strategies was for Brian to talk about his fears, concerns, and desires for surgery and then role-play talking to his surgeon about questions and preferences. Then, his mother made an appointment for him to talk to the plastic surgeon with whom the psychologist had previously spoken and prepared. Empowering Brian to be an active participant in his care allowed Brian some sense of control. In three sessions, Brian was able to attend therapy without nausea, and in eight sessions he was able to visit the surgical floors without anxiety. His family resumed more direct driving routes without difficulty, and Brian managed his next surgery two years later without relapse.

SUMMARY

A child born with a cleft or other craniofacial condition does not necessarily develop a major psychopathology as a result (Christensen & Mortensen, 2002). In fact, many individuals with craniofacial conditions are amazingly resilient because of a variety of factors (Mani, Carlsson, & Marcusson, 2010; Strauss, 2001). However, having a facial difference and dealing with speech issues complicate life and present challenges that children without medical problems generally do not face. These challenges are not restricted to the child but extend to the family of the child as well. In fact, early in the child's development, the majority of the psychological "fallout" of the cleft is on the family rather than on the child. Later, the challenges to the individual seem most often to be related to school achievement and peer relationships. People with clefts appear to be particularly at risk for diminished social interaction and social competence.

Because of the prevalence of increased levels of stress and psychosocial problems in children with clefts and in their families, cleft palate/craniofacial teams should include a psychologist as a member or at least available on a referral basis. The American Cleft Palate–Craniofacial Association (ACPA) has made access to a mental health professional, as well as regular assessment of psychological and social needs of patients and family, a part of the standards for approval of cleft palate teams. The psychologist can be helpful in addressing the behaviors and attitudes of the child and family that can interfere with an optimal treatment outcome.

FOR REVIEW AND DISCUSSION

1. What are factors that contribute to the shock of having a baby with a cleft? What are some factors that help parents to adjust? What can healthcare professionals do to lessen the immediate shock and distress?

2. Why is cleft palate a "chronic" medical condition? How does this affect the parents? How does it affect the child?

3. What are some issues that a child with a cleft may experience in school? What are some ways that parents and healthcare providers can lessen these issues? How would you suggest that the child deal with teasing?

4. What are factors that affect self-perception of individuals with a cleft? How do you explain the fact that some children with significant malformations are better adjusted than other children with minor differences?

5. How does physical attractiveness affect an individual's ability to fit into society? What is a common perception of individuals with speech problems regarding intelligence? Why do you think this occurs?

REFERENCES

Ambady, N., & Rosenthal, R. (1993). Half a minute: Predicting teacher evaluations from thin slices of nonverbal behavior and physical attractiveness. *Journal of Personality and Social Psychology, 64,* 431–441.

Baker, S. R., Owens, J., Stern, M., & Willmot, D. (2009). Coping strategies and social support in the family impact of cleft lip and palate and parents' adjustment and psychological distress. *The Cleft Palate–Craniofacial Journal, 46,* 229–236.

Barr, L., Thibeault, S. L., Muntz, H., & de Serres, L. (2007). Quality of life in children with velopharyngeal insufficiency. *Archives of Otolaryngology–Head and Neck Surgery, 133,* 224–229.

Bebout, L., & Bradford, A. (1992). Cross-cultural attitudes toward speech disorders. *Journal of Speech and Hearing Research, 35,* 45–52.

Bell, J. C., Raynes-Greenow, C., Turner, R., Bower, C., Dodson, A., Nicholls, W., & Nassar, N. (2016). School-performance for children with cleft lip and palate: A population-based study. *Child: Care, Health and Development, 43,* 222–231.

Bemmels, H., Biesecker, B., Schmidt, J. L., Krokosky, A., Guidotti, R., & Sutton, E. J. (2013). Psychological and social factors in undergoing reconstructive surgery among individuals with craniofacial conditions: An exploratory study. *The Cleft Palate–Craniofacial Journal, 50,* 158–167.

Berger, Z. E., & Dalton, L. J. (2011). Coping with a cleft II: Factors associated with psychosocial adjustment of adolescents with a cleft lip and palate and their parents. *The Cleft Palate–Craniofacial Journal, 48,* 82–90.

Bonomi, A. E., Patrick, D. L., Bushnell, D. M., & Martin, M. (2000). Validation of the United States' version of the World Health Organization Quality of Life (WHOQOL) instrument. *Journal of Clinical Epidemiology, 53,* 1–12.

Broder, H., Richman, L. C., & Matheson, P. B. (1998). Learning disabilities, school achievement, and grade retention among children with clefts: A two-center study. *The Cleft Palate–Craniofacial Journal, 35,* 127–131.

Broder, H., Smith, F. B., & Strauss, R. (2001). Developing a behavior rating scale for comparing teachers' ratings of children with and without craniofacial anomalies. *The Cleft Palate–Craniofacial Journal, 38*(6), 560–565.

Broder, H., & Strauss, R. (1989). Self-concept of early primary school-age children with visible or invisible defects. *Cleft Palate Journal, 26*(2), 114–117.

Broder, H. L., Wilson-Genderson, M., & Sischo, L. (2017). Oral health-related quality of life in youth receiving cleft-related surgery: Self-report and proxy ratings. *Quality of Life Research, 26,* 859–867.

Broen, P. A., Devers, M. C., Doyle, S. S., Prouty, J. M., & Moller, K. T. (1998). Acquisition of linguistic and cognitive skills by children with cleft palate. *Journal of Speech, Language, and Hearing Research, 41,* 676–687.

Christensen, K., & Mortensen, P. B. (2002). Facial clefting and psychiatric diseases: A follow-up of the Danish 1936–1987 Facial Cleft cohort. *The Cleft Palate–Craniofacial Journal, 39*(4), 392–396.

Clifford, E., Crocker, E. C., & Pope, B. A. (1972). Psychological findings in the adulthood of 98 cleft palate children. *Journal of Plastic and Reconstructive Surgery, 50,* 234.

Coy, K., Speltz, M. L., & Jones, K. (2002). Facial appearance and attachment in infants with orofacial clefts: A replication. *The Cleft Palate–Craniofacial Journal, 39,* 66–72.

Crerand, C. E., Rosenberg, J., Magee, L., Stein, M. B., Wilson-Genderson, M., & Broder, H. L. (2015). Parent-reported family functioning among children with cleft lip/palate. *The Cleft Palate–Craniofacial Journal, 52,* 651–659.

Dabit, J. Y., Romitti, P. R., Makelarski, J. A., Tyler, M., Damiano, P. C., Druschel, C. M., . . . Burnett, W. B. (2014). Examination of mental health status and aggravation level among mothers with isolated oral clefts. *The Cleft Palate–Craniofacial Journal, 51,* e80–e87.

DaCosta, A. C., Walters, I., Savarirayan, R., Anderson, V. A., Wrennall, J. A., & Meara, J. G. (2006). Intellectual outcomes in children and adolescents with syndromic and nonsyndromic craniosynostosis. *Plastic & Reconstructive Surgery, 118,* 175–181.

deJong, T., Maliepaard, M., Bannink, N., Raat, H., & Mathijssen, I. M. (2012). Health-related problems and quality of life in patients with syndromic and complex craniosynostosis. *Children's Nervous System, 28*(6), 879–882.

Despars, J., Peter, C., Borghini, A., Pierrehumbert, B., Habersaat, S., Müller-Nix, C., . . . Hohlfeld, J. (2011). Impact of a cleft lip and/or palate on maternal stress and attachment representations. *The Cleft Palate–Craniofacial Journal, 48,* 419–424.

Dufton, L. M., Speltz, M. L., Kelly, J. P., Leroux, B., Collett, B. R., & Werler, M. M. (2011). Psychosocial outcomes in children with hemifacial microsomia. *Journal of Pediatric Psychology, 36,* 794–805.

Feragen, K. B., Kvalem, I. L., Rumsey, N., & Borge, A. I. H. (2010). Adolescents with and without a facial difference: The role of friendships and social acceptance in perceptions of appearance and emotional resilience. *Body Image, 7,* 271–279.

Feragen, K. B., Saervold, T. K., Aukner, R., & Stock, N. M. (2017). Speech, language, and reading in 10-year-olds with cleft: Associations with teasing, satisfaction with speech, and psychological adjustment. *The Cleft Palate–Craniofacial Journal, 54,* 153–165.

Ferini-Strambi, L., Baietto, C., DiGioia, M. R., Castaldi, P., Castronovo, C., Zucconi, M., & Cappa, S. F. (2003). Cognitive dysfunction in patients with obstructive sleep apnea (OSA): Partial reversibility after continuous positive airway pressure (CPAP). *Brain Research Bulletin, 6,* 87–92.

Finnegan, D. E. (1982). General and special educators' basic information and experience with cleft palate. *Cleft Palate Journal, 19,* 222–229.

Foo, P., Sampson, W., Roberts, R., Jamieson, L., & David, D. (2013). Facial aesthetics and perceived need for further treatment among adults with repaired cleft as assessed by cleft team professionals and laypersons. *European Journal of Orthodontics, 35,* 341–346.

Friman, P. C., & Leibowitz, J. M. (1990). An effective and acceptable treatment alternative for chronic thumb- and finger-sucking. *Journal of Pediatric Psychology, 15,* 57–65.

Fuerst, K. B., Dool, C. B., & Rourke, B. P. (1995). Velocardiofacial syndrome. In B. P. Rourke (Ed.), *Syndrome of nonverbal learning disabilities: Neurodevelopmental manifestations* (pp. 119–137). New York, NY: Guilford Press.

Fujiki, M., Brinton, B., & Clarke, D. (2002). Emotion regulation in children with specific language impairment. *Language, Speech, and Hearing Services in Schools, 33,* 102–111.

Furniss, F., Biswas, A. B., Gumber, R., & Singh, N. (2011). Cognitive phenotype of velocardiofacial syndrome: A review. *Research in Developmental Disabilities, 32,* 2206–2213.

Gordon, R. A., Crosnoe, R., & Wu, X. (2013). *Physical attractiveness and the accumulation of social and human capital in adolescence and young adulthood: Assets and distractions.* New York, NY: Wiley.

Grollemund, B., Galliani, E., Soupre, V., Vazquez, M. P., Guedeney, A., & Danion, A. (2010). The impact of cleft lip and palate on the parent-child relationships. *Archives de Pediatric, 17,* 1380–1385.

Habersaat, S., Monnier, M., Peter, C., Bolomey, L., Borghini, A., Despars, J., . . . Hohlfeld, J. (2013). Early mother-child interaction and later quality of attachment in infants with an orofacial cleft compared to infants without cleft. *The Cleft Palate–Craniofacial Journal, 50,* 704–712.

Habersaat, S., Peter, C., & Borghini, A. (2009). Effet du stress sur l'évolution des représentations parentales au cours des 12 premiers mois de vie d'un enfant né avec une fente faciale. *Neuropsychiatrie de l'Enfance et de l'Adolescence, 57,* 199–205.

Hamlet, C., & Harcourt, D. (2015). Older adults' experiences of living with cleft lip and palate: A qualitative study exploring aging and appearance. *Cleft Palate–Craniofacial Journal, 52,* e32–e40.

Havstam, C., Laakso, K., Lohmander, A., & Ringsberg, K. C. (2011). Taking charge of communication: Adults' descriptions of growing up with a cleft-related speech impairment. *The Cleft Palate–Craniofacial Journal, 48,* 717–726.

Hosoda, M., Stone-Romero, E. F., & Coats, G. (2003). The effects of physical attractiveness on job-related outcomes: A meta-analysis of experimental studies. *Personnel Psychology, 56,* 431–462.

Hunt, O., Burden, D., Hepper, P., Stevenson, M., Johnson, C. (2006). Self-reports of psychosocial functioning among children and young adults with cleft lip and palate. *The Cleft Palate–Craniofacial Journal, 43,* 598–605.

Hutchinson, K., Wellman, M. A., Noe, D. A., & Kahn, A. (2011). The psychosocial effects of cleft lip and palate in non-Anglo populations: A cross-cultural meta-analysis. *The Cleft Palate–Craniofacial Journal, 48,* 497–509.

Kapp-Simon, K. A., Simon, D. J., & Kristovich, S. (1992). Self-perception, social skills, adjustment and inhibition in young adolescents with craniofacial anomalies. *The Cleft Palate–Craniofacial Journal, 29,* 352–356.

Kelley, R. I., & Hennekam, R. C. M. (2000). Smith-Lemli-Opitz syndrome. *Journal of Medical Genetics, 37,* 321–355.

Kerr, S. M., & McIntosh, J. B. (2000). Coping when a child has a disability: Exploring the impact of parent-to-parent support. *Child: Care, Health and Development, 26,* 309–322.

Klatt, R., Schultz, J., Lee, L., & Saal, H. (2002). Parent and teacher concerns of school age children with isolated cleft lip or cleft palate. Annual Conference of National Society of Genetics Counselors, Phoenix, Arizona.

Kortelainen, T., Tolvanen, M., Luoto, A., Ylikontiola, L. P., Sandor, G. K., & Lahti, S. (2016). Comparison of oral health-related quality of life among schoolchildren with and without cleft lip and/or palate. *The Cleft Palate–Craniofacial Journal, 53,* e172–e176.

Kramer, F-J., Baethge, C., Sinikovic, H., & Schliephake, H. (2007). An analysis of quality of life in 130 families having small children with cleft lip/palate using the Impact on Family Scale. *International Journal of Oral and Maxillofacial Surgery, 36,* 1146–1152.

Lee, A., Gibbon, F. E., & Spivey, K. (2017). Children's attitudes toward peers with unintelligible speech associated with cleft lip and/or palate. *The Cleft Palate–Craniofacial Journal, 54,* 262–268.

Mani, M., Carlsson, M., & Marcusson, A. (2010). Quality of life varies with gender and age among adults treated for unilateral cleft lip and palate. *The Cleft Palate–Craniofacial Journal, 47,* 491–498.

Masnari, O., Schiestl, C., Rössler, J., Gütlein, S. K., Neuhaus, K., Weibel, L., . . . Landolt, M. A. (2013). Stigmatization predicts psychological adjustment and quality of life in children and adolescents with a facial difference. *Journal of Pediatric Psychology, 38,* 162–172.

Masnari, O., Schiestl, C., Weibel, I., Wuttke, F., & Landolt, M. A. (2013). How children with facial differences are perceived by non-affected children and adolescents: Perceiver effects on stereotypical attitudes. *Body Image, 10,* 515–523.

Millar, K., Bell, A., Bowman, A., Brown, D., Lo, T., Siebert, P., . . . Ayoub, A. (2013). Psychological status as a function of residual scarring and facial asymmetry after surgical repair of cleft lip and palate. *The Cleft Palate–Craniofacial Journal, 50,* 150–157.

Millard, T., & Richman, L. C. (2001). Different cleft conditions, facial appearance, and speech: Relationship to psychological variables. *The Cleft Palate–Craniofacial Journal, 38,* 68–75.

Moeller, M. P. (2007). Current state of knowledge: Psychosocial development in children with hearing impairment. *Ear and Hearing, 28,* 729–739.

Murphy, K. C., Jones, L. A., & Owen, M. J. (1999). High rates of schizophrenia in adults with velo-cardio-facial syndrome. *Archives of General Psychiatry, 56,* 940–945.

Murray, L., Arteche, A., Bingley, C., Hentges, F., Bishop, D. V., Dalton, L., . . . Hill, J. (2010). The effect of cleft lip on socio-emotional functioning in school-aged children. *Journal of Child Psychology and Psychiatry, and Allied Disciplines, 51,* 94–103.

Nabors, L. A., Lehmkuhl, H. D., & Warm, J. S. (2004). Children's acceptance ratings of a child with a facial scar: The impact of positive scripts. *Early Education and Development, 15,* 79–92.

Nopoulos, P., Choe, L., Berg, S., Van Demark, D., Canady, J., & Richman L. (2005). Ventral frontal cortex morphology in adult males with isolated orofacial clefts: Relationship to abnormalities in social function. *The Cleft Palate–Craniofacial Journal, 42,* 138–144.

Papolos, D. F., Faedda, G. L., Veit, S., Goldberg, R., Morrow, B., Kucherlapati, R., & Shprintzen, R. J. (1996). Bipolar spectrum disorders in patients diagnosed with velo-cardio-facial syndrome: Does a hemizygous deletion of chromosome 22q11 result in affective disorder? *American Journal of Psychiatry, 153,* 1541–1547.

Persson, M., Becker, M., & Svensson, H. (2008). General intellectual capacity of young men with cleft lip with or without cleft palate and cleft palate alone. *Scandinavian Journal of Plastic and Reconstructive Surgery and Hand Surgery, 42,* 14–16.

Persson, M., Becker, M., & Svensson, H. (2012). Academic achievement in individuals with cleft: A population-based register study. *The Cleft Palate–Craniofacial Journal, 49,* 153–159.

Philippot, P., Lenoir, N., D'Hoore, W., & Bercy, P. (2005). Improving patients' compliance with the treatment of periodontitis: A controlled study of behavioural intervention. *Journal of Clinical Periodontology, 32,* 653–658.

Pillemer, F. G., & Cook, K. V. (1989). The psychosocial adjustment of pediatric craniofacial patients after surgery. *Cleft Palate Journal, 26,* 201–207.

Pisula, E., Lukowska, E., & Fudalej, P. S. (2014). Self-esteem, coping styles and quality of life in Polish adolescents and young adults with unilateral cleft lip and palate. *The Cleft Palate–Craniofacial Journal, 51,* 290–299.

Pope, A. W., & Snyder, H. T. (2005). Psychosocial adjustment in children and adolescents with a craniofacial anomaly: Age and sex patterns. *The Cleft Palate–Craniofacial Journal, 42,* 349–354.

Pope, A. W., Tillman, K., & Snyder, H. T. (2005). Parenting stress in infancy and psychosocial adjustment in toddlerhood: A longitudinal study of children with craniofacial anomalies. *The Cleft Palate–Craniofacial Journal, 42,* 556–559.

Redsell, S., & Glazebrook, C. (2010). Finding a voice: The development of children's healthcare. In S. Redsell & A. Hastings (Eds.), *Listening to children and young people in healthcare consultations.* Abingdon Oxon: Radcliffe Publishing.

Richman, L. C., & Eliason, M. (1982). Psychological characteristics of children with cleft lip and palate: Intellectual, achievement, behavioral, and personality variables. *Cleft Palate Journal, 19,* 249.

Richman, L. C., & Ryan, S. M. (2003). Do the reading disabilities of children with cleft fit into current models of developmental dyslexia? *The Cleft Palate–Craniofacial Journal, 40,* 154–157.

Richman, L. G., Ryan, S., Wilgenbusch, T., & Millard, T. (2004). Overdiagnosis and medication for attention-deficit hyperactivity disorder in children with cleft: Diagnostic examination and follow-up. *The Cleft Palate–Craniofacial Journal, 41,* 351–354.

Roberts, R., Mathias, J. L., & Wheaton, P. (2012). Cognitive functioning in children and adults with non-syndromal cleft lip and/or palate: A meta-analysis. *Journal of Pediatric Psychology, 37,* 786–797.

Rosenberg, J. M., Kapp-Simon, K. A., Starr, J. R., Cradock, M., & Speltz, M. L. (2011). Mothers' and fathers' reports of stress in families of infants with and without single-suture craniosynostosis. *The Cleft Palate–Craniofacial Journal, 48,* 509–518.

Sank, J., Berk, N. W., Cooper, M. E., & Marazita, M. I. (2003). Perceived social support of mothers of children with clefts. *The Cleft Palate–Craniofacial Journal, 40*(2), 165–171.

Sarwer, D. B., Bartlett, S. P., Whitaker, L. A., Paige, K. T., Pertschuk, M. J., & Wadden, T. A. (1999). Adult psychological functioning of individuals born with craniofacial anomalies. *Plastic and Reconstructive Surgery, 103,* 412–418.

Shapiro, D. N., Waljee, J., Ranganathan, K., Buchman, S., & Warschausky, S. (2015). Gender and satisfaction with appearance in children with craniofacial anomalies. *Plastic and Reconstructive Surgery, 136,* 789e–795e.

Shprintzen, R. J. (2008). Velo-cardio-facial syndrome: 30 years of study. *Developmental Disabilities Research Review, 14,* 3–10.

Shprintzen, R. J., Goldberg, R., Golding-Kushner, K. J., & Marion, R. W. (1992). Late-onset psychosis in the velo-cardio-facial syndrome. *American Journal of Medical Genetics, 42,* 141–142.

Shute, R., McCarthy, K. R., & Roberts, R. (2007). Predictors of social competence in young adolescents with craniofacial anomalies. *International Journal of Clinical and Health Psychology, 7,* 595–613.

Simon, T. J., Bearden, C. E., Moss, E. M., McDonald-McGinn, D., Zackai, E., & Wang, P. P. (2002). Cognitive development in VCFS. *Progress in Pediatric Cardiology, 15,* 109–117.

Sinko, K., Jagsch, R., Prechtl, V., Watzinger, F., Hollmann, K., & Baumann A. (2005). Evaluation of esthetic, functional, and quality-of-life outcome in adult cleft lip and palate patients. *The Cleft Palate–Craniofacial Journal, 42,* 355–361.

Sischo, L., Clouston, S. A. P., Phillips, C., & Broder, H. L. (2016). Caregiver responses to early cleft palate care: A mixed method approach. *Health Psychology, 35,* 474–482.

Skirko, J. R., Weaver, E. M., Perkins, J. A., Kinter, S., Eblen, L. K., & Sie, K. C. Y. (2013). Validity and responsiveness of VELO: A velopharyngeal insufficiency quality of life measure. *Otolaryngology–Head and Neck Surgery, 149*(2), 304–311.

Slifer, K. J., Amari, A., Diver, T., Hilley, L., Beek, M., Kane, A., & McDonnell, S. (2004). Social interaction patterns of children and adolescents with and without oral clefts during a videotaped analogue social encounter. *The Cleft Palate–Craniofacial Journal, 41,* 175–184.

Slifer, K. J., Beek, M., Amari, A., Diver, T., Hilley, L., Kane, A., & McDonnell, S. (2003). Self-concept and satisfaction with physical appearance in youth with and without oral clefts. *Children's Health Care, 32,* 81–101.

Sokol, R. J., Delaney-Black, V., & Nordstrom, B. (2003). Fetal alcohol spectrum disorder. *JAMA, 290*(22), 2996–2999.

Sousa, A. D., Devare, S., & Ghanshani, J. (2009). Psychological issues in cleft lip and palate. *Journal of Indian Association of Pediatric Surgeons, 14,* 55–58.

Speltz, M. L., Morton, K., Goodell, E. W., & Clarren, S. K. (1993). Psychological functioning of children with craniofacial anomalies and their mothers: Follow-up from late infancy to school entry. *The Cleft Palate–Craniofacial Journal, 30,* 482–489.

Speltz, M. L., Wallace, E. R., Collett, B. R., Heike, C. L., Luquetti, D. V., & Werler, M. M. (2017). Intelligence and academic achievement of adolescents with craniofacial macrosomia. *Plastic and Reconstructive Surgery, 140,* 571–580.

Stock, N. M., & Rumsey, N. (2015). Parenting a child with a cleft: The father's perspective. *The Cleft Palate–Craniofacial Journal, 52,* 31–43.

Stock, N. M., Stoneman, K., Cunniffe, C., & Rumsey, N. (2016). The psychosocial impact of cleft lip and/or palate on unaffected siblings. *The Cleft Palate–Craniofacial Journal, 53*(6), 670–682.

Storch, S. A., Bravata, E. A., Storch, J. B., Johnson, J. A., Roth, D. A., & Roberti, J. W. (2003). Psychosocial adjustment in early adulthood: The role of childhood teasing and father support. *Child Study Journal, 33,* 153–163.

Strauss, R. P. (2001). "Only skin deep": Health, resilience, and craniofacial care. *The Cleft Palate–Craniofacial Journal, 38,* 226–230.

Strauss, R. P., Ramsey, B. L., Edwards, T. C., Topolski, T. D., Kapp-Simon, K. A., Thomas, C. R., . . . Patrick, D. L. (2007). Stigma experiences in youth with facial differences: A multi-site study of adolescents and their mothers. *Orthodontics and Craniofacial Research, 10,* 96–103.

Thomas, P. S., Turner, S. R., Rumsey, N., Dowell, T., & Sandy, J. R. (1997). Satisfaction with facial appearance among subjects affected by a cleft. *The Cleft Palate–Craniofacial Journal, 34,* 226–231.

Tobiasen, J. M. (1988). Psychosocial outcome of craniofacial surgery in children: Discussion. *Plastic and Reconstructive Surgery, 82,* 745–746.

Tobiasen, J. M. (1989). Scaling facial impairment. *Cleft Palate Journal, 26,* 249–254.

Tobiasen, J., & Speltz, M. (1996). Cleft palate: A psychosocial developmental prospective. In S. Berkowitz (Ed.), *Cleft lip and palate: Perspectives in management* (vol. II, pp. 15–23). Singular Publishing Group: San Diego.

Tyler, M. C., Wehby, G. L., Robbins, J. M., & Damiano, P. C. (2013). Separation anxiety in children ages 4 through 9 with oral clefts. *The Cleft Palate–Craniofacial Journal, 50,* 520–527.

Van Staden, F., & Gerhardt, C. (1995). Mothers of children with facial cleft deformities: Reactions and effects. *South American Journal of Psychology, 25*(1), 39–46.

Ward, J. A., Vig, K. W. L., Firestone, A. R., Mercado, A., da Fonseca, M., & Johnston, W. (2013). Oral health-related quality of life in children with orofacial clefts. *The Cleft Palate–Craniofacial Journal, 50,* 174–181.

Watterson, T., Mancini, M. C., Brancamp, T. U., & Lewis, K. E. (2013). Relationship between the perception of hypernasality and social judgments in school-aged children. *Cleft Palate–Craniofacial Journal, 50,* 498–502.

Wehby, G. L., Collett, B. R., Barron, S., Romitti, P., & Ansley, T. (2015). Children with oral clefts are at greater risk for persistent low achievement in school than classmates. *Archives of Disease in Childhood, 100,* 1148–1154.

Wehby, G. L., Collet, B., Barron, S., Romitti, P. A., Ansley, T. N., & Speltz, M. (2014). Academic achievement of children and adolescents with oral clefts. *Pediatrics, 133,* 785–792.

Winston, K. A., Dunbar, S. B., Reed, C. N., & Francis-Connolly, E. (2010). Mothering occupations when parenting children with feeding concerns: A mixed method study. *Canadian Journal of Occupational Therapy, 77,* 181–189.

Young, J. L., O'Riordan, M., Goldstein, J. A., & Robin, N. H. (2001). What information do parents of newborns with cleft lip, palate, or both want to know? *The Cleft Palate–Craniofacial Journal, 38,* 55–58.

CREDITS

CHAPTER 10

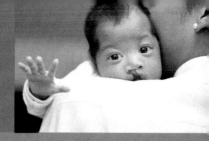

Speech/Resonance Disorders and Velopharyngeal Dysfunction

CHAPTER OUTLINE

INTRODUCTION

Speech production requires both airflow and sound. Sound from vocal fold vibration is needed for voiced consonants and all vowels. Airflow is needed for consonants, particular plosives, fricatives, and affricates.

During normal speech production, sound is generated by the vocal folds. As the sound travels upward through the cavities of the vocal tract, its resonance quality is changed by the cavities of the vocal tract (pharynx, oral cavity, and nasal cavity).

It is important that both sound energy and airflow within the vocal tract are directed through the pharynx without obstruction. Once through the pharynx, the velopharyngeal valve plays a key role in directing the sound and airflow into the appropriate cavity (nasal or oral) for each speech sound.

Velopharyngeal dysfunction can have a significant effect on speech and resonance. It can cause hypernasality (a resonance disorder) and nasal emission of the airstream. When there is significant nasal emission caused by a large velopharyngeal opening, several other speech characteristics can occur as a result of inadequate oral airflow and air pressure for consonants.

In addition to hypernasality, there are other resonance disorders that occur in individuals with clefts or other craniofacial conditions. Differential diagnosis of the type of resonance disorder is imperative to determine appropriate recommendations and necessary referrals across disciplines.

The purpose of this chapter is to acquaint the reader with the speech characteristics of velopharyngeal dysfunction and the various types and causes of velopharyngeal dysfunction. In addition, different types of resonance disorders are described.

Voice, Resonance, and Airflow

Voice is the sound that is generated by vocal fold vibration and is emitted through the mouth or nose during speech and singing. The voice is produced through the act of phonation, also known as voicing, which is the production of sound through vocal fold vibration.

To initiate phonation, the vocal folds close through muscular forces. Expiratory air causes a buildup of subglottic air pressure that forces the vocal folds apart. The high-velocity airflow produces a lowered pressure within the glottis (space between the vocal folds), which then brings the lower edges of the vocal folds back together. The elasticity of the tissue then brings the upper edge of the vocal folds together. This completes one vibratory cycle of the vocal folds (Titze, 2000). The vibration of the vocal folds (caused by rapid cycles of opening and closing) causes oscillation of the airstream, thus producing the sound of voicing.

The intensity (loudness) of the voice is determined by the degree of subglottal air pressure during phonation. With an increase in air pressure, there is also an increase in airflow. This causes the vocal fold edges to have greater lateral displacement, which increases the amplitude of the sound pressure wave and thus the intensity of the sound.

All objects have a frequency or set of frequencies with which they naturally vibrate when set in motion. The vocal folds are no exception. In response to the driving force of subglottic air pressure, the natural frequency (pitch) of this vibration is a function of the length, thickness, and elasticity of the vocal folds. The strongest and slowest vibration of the vocal folds is known as the fundamental frequency, which is the lowest frequency of a periodic waveform. The faster vibrations that occur simultaneously are called overtones or harmonics. These component frequencies are whole number multiples of the fundamental frequency.

As the sound travels upward from the vocal folds, it is modified by the natural resonance of the cavities of the vocal tract. By definition, resonance refers to the tendency of a system to vibrate (oscillate) with a larger amplitude at certain frequencies than at others. Therefore, as the complex phonated sound goes through a cavity, it is filtered by the cavity's natural resonance, resulting in selective enhancement of certain formant frequencies as opposed to others. This interaction between phonation and resonance has been called the source–filter model of speech production, where the vocal folds are the source and the vocal tract is the filter.

The frequencies that are enhanced through resonance depend on the size and shape of the resonating cavity. As a rule of thumb (and of physics), when a complex sound passes through a relatively short or small cavity, the higher frequencies in that sound will be enhanced. If that same complex sound passes through a longer or larger cavity, the lower frequencies in that sound will be enhanced.

The effect of cavity size on resonance can be illustrated several ways. For example, if you blow across a bottle that is half full, you will hear a certain pitch. If you pour out some of the liquid and blow again, the pitch will be perceived as lower, despite the same sound source. This is because as the bottle is emptied, the resonating cavity becomes bigger, thus enhancing more of the lower formant frequencies. The same principle applies to wind instruments. A longer chamber results in perception of a lower sound than a shorter chamber. Therefore, resonance for speech is directly related to the size and shape of the resonating cavities of the vocal tract (pharyngeal cavity, oral cavity, and nasal cavity) (Kummer, 2011a). Smaller cavities of the vocal tract enhance higher frequencies, whereas larger cavities enhance lower frequencies and result in a richer sound.

When considering the effects of vocal fold vibration and vocal cavity size on pitch and resonance, it is easy to understand why the voice of a child is perceived as higher than the voice of an adult. In comparison, a child has a smaller larynx than an adult and thus a faster vocal fold vibration rate, plus higher harmonics. In addition, the pharynx is shorter, and the oral cavity is smaller. Therefore, more of the higher harmonics are enhanced during speech as compared to an adult with a larger pharyngeal and oral cavity. In addition, it has been shown that adult males and females differ not only in the length and thickness of the vocal folds but also with respect to oral and pharyngeal cavity sizes. These differences affect the resonant frequencies that influence the overall perception of voice quality and pitch (Ikeda, Matsuzaki, & Aomatsu, 2001). Overall, both phonation and resonance combine to provide the unique qualities of each individual's voice.

During connected speech, normal speakers use prosody, which is a combination of changes in frequency, intensity, rate, and stress. The variation of pitch is used for emphasis, to express emotions, to ask a question, to differentiate meaning, and for many other functions. These pitch changes occur as a result of changes in vocal fold length and mass and alterations in pharyngeal cavity size. For example, for higher pitches, the vocal folds are lengthened and tensed, with decreased mass. In addition, the larynx raises, which shortens the pharynx, and the lateral pharyngeal walls contract, which narrows the pharynx (Ikeda et al., 2001). The decrease in the size of the pharynx further enhances the higher frequencies produced by the vocal folds.

Although there is sound energy in the oral cavity for all oral sounds, there are subtle differences in resonance between various voiced phonemes. Because the larynx, pharynx, mandible, tongue, and velum are all interconnected by the hyoid muscle group, the height of the velum and the configuration of the pharynx are affected by tongue position during the production of different speech phonemes (Tom, Titze, Hoffman, & Story, 2001). As a result, movement of the tongue or velum can alter the size and shape of the pharynx and/or oral cavity, thus altering the resonance (Hiiemae & Palmer, 2003).

Resonance is a component of all voiced phonemes, but it is particularly important for vowels. In fact, it can be said that vowels are "resonance sounds" because they are produced by manipulating the resonance in the oral cavity. The acoustic properties of each distinct vowel are determined by the position of the tongue, mandible, and lips, which affects the size and shape of the oral cavity. Altering the position of one of these structures changes the selective enhancement of the formant frequencies and thus changes the vowel.

Despite the fact that vowels are generally considered oral sounds, normal speech is characterized by a slight degree of nasal resonance on each vowel. This can be shown through nasometry (see the chapter *Nasometry*). A high vowel, such as /i/, consistently has more nasal resonance than a low vowel, such as /ɑ/. A working theory is that the velum is like a heavy curtain. As such, some sound is transmitted through the velum during vowel production (Gildersleeve-Neumann & Dalston, 2001). In addition, there may be relatively more nasal resonance on high vowels as compared to low vowels because with a high tongue position there is more oral impedance and more oral pressure (Jones, 2005). Both of these factors can result in more transpalatal transmission of the sound. Regardless, further research is needed in this area.

Finally, it is important to discuss the role of airflow for speech. As noted above, subglottic air pressure is important for the production of voiced sounds. However, half of the plosives, fricatives, and affricates are voiceless and therefore produced with the glottis open. Once the airflow is released from the glottis, it courses superiorly through the pharynx and then is directed into the oral cavity by the velopharyngeal valve. When the intraoral airflow is blocked or restricted by the articulators (tongue, teeth, and lips), the dynamic pressure is turned into static pressure, which is then released for production of these sounds (Kummer, 2011a).

FIGURE 10-1 shows a schema of how both sound and airflow are necessary for speech production. Sound from the vocal folds is altered by the resonance of the cavities in the vocal tract. It is important for the production of voiced consonants and vowels. If there is velopharyngeal dysfunction, however, there will be hypernasality (a resonance disorder) on these sounds.

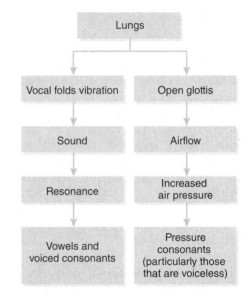

FIGURE 10-1 Schema to illustrate sound and airflow during speech production.

In contrast, airflow without sound is used for voiceless consonants. If there is velopharyngeal dysfunction, the airflow will be released through the nasal cavity, causing nasal air emission.

Resonance Disorders

A **resonance disorder** is characterized by abnormal transmission of sound energy through the oral, nasal, and/or pharyngeal cavities of the vocal tract during speech production (Kummer, 2011a). This causes the perception of what some people generally call "nasality." Resonance disorders include hypernasality (too much sound in the nasal cavity), hyponasality (too little sound in the nasal cavity), cul-de-sac resonance (blocked sound in one of the cavities), or a mixture of these types. Causes of resonance disorders include dysfunction of the velopharyngeal valve, an opening or fistula in the palate, obstruction in one or more of the vocal cavities, and even misarticulation (Smith & Kuehn, 2007). Anything that disrupts the transmission of sound in the cavities of the vocal tract will cause abnormal resonance.

Resonance disorders, particularly hypernasality, are often labeled as "voice disorders." This is an inappropriate categorization because resonance disorders are not laryngeal in origin. Therefore, most specialists consider resonance disorders to be distinct from voice disorders (Riski & Verdolini, 1999).

Hypernasality

Hypernasality is a resonance disorder that occurs when there is abnormal nasal resonance during the production of oral sounds. This is caused by abnormal coupling (sharing of acoustic energy) of the oral and nasal cavities during speech. Hypernasality is often described as "nasal," muffled, or characterized by mumbling. It is associated with very low volume from the reduction of oral acoustic energy in combination with damping (absorption of sound energy) as the sound goes through the pharynx and turbinates (Bernthal & Beukelman, 1977; Buder, 2005). In addition to the video samples with this text, there are audio samples of various degrees of hypernasality in children, men, and women on the website of the American Cleft Palate–Craniofacial Association (ACPA, n.d.).

Because hypernasality is caused by abnormal resonance of sound (as opposed to airflow), it is always associated with voiced, rather than voiceless, speech sounds (Cassassolles et al., 1995). Hypernasality is particularly perceptible on vowels because they are voiced, relatively long in duration, and typically not substituted with a different placement. Hypernasality is more noted on high vowels than low vowels (Lee, Wang, & Fu, 2009). This is because of the high tongue position, which reduces oral resonance space and causes partial impedance of sound coming through the oral cavity. The relatively narrow space as a result of the high tongue position also causes an increase in sound pressure, which can result in increased transmission of sound through the velum (Awan, Omlor, & Watts, 2011; Gildersleeve-Neumann & Dalston, 2001).

When there is moderate to severe hypernasality, it is common to note nasalization of oral phonemes, where oral plosives sound more like their nasal cognates (e.g., m/b, n/d, and ŋ/g). This makes sense because the only difference between these cognates is the closure of the velopharyngeal valve. In addition, nasal sounds may be used as a compensatory strategy for other phonemes, including voiceless sounds (e.g., n/s). Therefore, with moderate to severe hypernasality, the speech may consist primarily of nasal sounds (/m/, /n/, and /ŋ/). Hypernasality on vowels and nasalization of consonants often increase with utterance length, speed, or phonemic complexity because of the additional demands on the velopharyngeal mechanism.

The most common cause of hypernasality is a relatively large velopharyngeal opening secondary to velopharyngeal insufficiency (Kummer, Briggs, & Lee, 2003; Kummer, Curtis, Wiggs, Lee, & Strife, 1992). (Velopharyngeal insufficiency and its causes will be further described later in this chapter.) Other causes of hypernasality include a large oronasal fistula (**FIGURE 10-2**) or a very thin velum caused by a submucous cleft. Finally, hypernasality can be phoneme specific because of nasal articulation of certain oral sounds (e.g., ŋ/1, ŋ/ɚ).

Hypernasality should not be confused with a nasal twang, which has been described as a characteristic of certain dialects. This quality has been found to occur with pharyngeal area narrowing and vocal tract shortening (Story, Titze, &

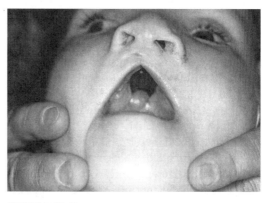

FIGURE 10-2 A very large palatal fistula that would cause significant hypernasality.

Hoffman, 2001; Titze, Bergan, Hunter, & Story, 2003; Yanagisawa, Estill, Mambrino, & Talkin, 1991; Yanagisawa, Kmucha, & Estill, 1990). It may also be related to the high posterior tongue position on certain vowels as is common with a Southern dialect.

Hyponasality and Denasality

Hyponasality occurs when there is a reduction in normal nasal resonance during speech caused by obstruction in the nasopharynx or nasal cavity. The overall perceptual feature is that the individual sounds "stuffed up." The term denasality typically refers to abnormal resonance caused by total upper airway obstruction. Because it is impossible to know whether there is total blockage of the nasal cavity through a perceptual assessment alone, the term "hyponasality" is more commonly used.

Hyponasality particularly affects the production of the nasal consonants (/m/, /n/, /ŋ/). To imitate hyponasality, close your nose while you are saying sentences loaded with nasal sounds. When nasal resonance is reduced, the nasal consonants sound similar to their oral phoneme cognates (e.g., b/m, d/n, g/ŋ). Hyponasality can also affect the quality of vowels if it is severe because all vowels, particularly high vowels, have some nasal resonance.

The cause of hyponasality is almost always obstruction somewhere in the nasopharynx or nasal cavity. Upper airway obstruction can cause symptoms other than hyponasality, including a chronic open mouth posture, mouth breathing, loud snoring, and even obstructive sleep apnea (OSA). It has even been shown that nasal obstruction can reduce lip closing force (Sabashi et al., 2011).

Common causes of hyponasality in the general population include allergic rhinitis, the common cold, and adenoid hypertrophy (Scott, Moldan, Tibesar, Lander, & Sidman, 2011). In addition to these common causes, individuals with clefts or craniofacial conditions, often have hyponasality caused by congenital structural abnormalities that obstruct the upper airway (Adil, Huntley, Choudhary, & Carr, 2011). Obstructive anomalies

include a deviated septum (particularly with unilateral clefts), choanal stenosis or atresia, a stenotic naris, or maxillary retrusion that restricts the pharyngeal and nasal cavity space. Hyponasality can be an unwanted complication of surgery for correction of velopharyngeal incompetence, which narrows or reduces the size of the nasopharyngeal space (de Serres et al., 1999; Hall, Golding-Kushner, Argamaso, & Strauch, 1991; Witt, 2009). When hyponasality is noted, it is important to rule out obstructive sleep apnea, which is very common in individuals with clefts or other craniofacial conditions (Maclean, Waters, Fitzsimons, Hayward, & Fitzgerald, 2009; Muntz, Wilson, Park, Smith, & Grimmer, 2008; Robison & Otteson, 2011a).

Because the cause of hyponasality is almost always obstruction somewhere in the nasal cavity or pharynx (unless it is caused by apraxia), treatment involves either medical or surgical intervention. Therefore, referral to an otolaryngologist would be appropriate.

Cul-de-Sac Resonance

Cul-de-sac resonance occurs when the acoustic energy enters a cavity of the vocal tract but is blocked from exiting at the cavity's normal outlet. The sound is therefore trapped in this blind pouch, and some of the sound is absorbed by the soft tissues. As a result, the speech is perceived as muffled and low in volume. Like hyponasality, cul-de-sac resonance is caused by obstruction, but in this case the place of obstruction is at the cavity's exit point rather than at the entrance or within the nasal cavity.

There are three types of cul-de-sac resonance, depending on the location of the blockage (Kummer, 2011a). All are defined by blockage at the cavity's exit point.

Oral cul-de-sac resonance occurs when the sound is partially blocked from exiting the oral cavity during speech. This can occur as a result of microstomia (a small mouth opening). It is also what is heard with mumbling or speaking without opening the mouth normally. To imitate oral cul-de-sac resonance, say oral sentences with a very small mouth opening.

Nasal cul-de-sac resonance occurs when the sound is partially blocked from exiting the nasal cavity during speech. This is most noticeable when there is a combination of velopharyngeal incompetence (which would otherwise cause hypernasality) and a blockage in the anterior part of the nose. Nasal cul-de-sac resonance is commonly found in individuals who have a combination of velopharyngeal incompetence and a blockage at or near the exit of the nasal cavity. Nasal blockage can occur as a result of a deviated septum, which is commonly caused by a unilateral cleft of the primary palate. It can also be caused by a stenotic naris, which sometimes occurs due to scarring after the cleft lip repair. Nasal cul-de-sac resonance can be simulated by imitating hypernasality while closing the nose.

Pharyngeal cul-de-sac resonance occurs when the sound is blocked from exiting the oropharynx during speech. This is typically caused by large tonsils that block the oropharyngeal opening (Kummer, Billmire, & Myer, 1993; Shprintzen, Sher, & Croft, 1987). As with other types of cul-de-sac resonance, this blockage causes speech to be low in volume and muffled in quality. Pharyngeal cul-de-sac resonance has been described in the literature as "potato-in-the-mouth" speech (Finkelstein, Bar-Ziv, Nachmani, Berger, & Ophir, 1993). This is actually a great description because a speaker with a potato in the mouth is likely to have these same muffled speech characteristics! Although enlarged tonsils are the most common cause of pharyngeal cul-de-sac resonance, it can also occur because of scar tissue or other forms of obstruction on the pharyngeal wall of the hypopharynx or oropharynx (**FIGURE 10-3**). To imitate pharyngeal cul-de-sac resonance, produce oral sentences with your closed fist over your mouth.

Cul-de-sac resonance is always caused by a structural abnormality that blocks one of the resonating cavities. Therefore, this type of resonance disorder cannot be corrected with speech therapy. Instead, correction requires medical or surgical intervention. As with obstruction causing hyponasality, referral to an otolaryngologist would be appropriate.

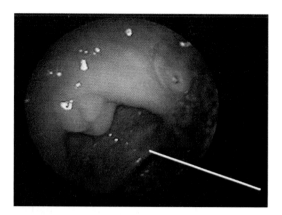

FIGURE 10-3 Scar band on the posterior pharyngeal wall. This can impede the transmission of sound energy through the pharynx, thus causing cul-de-sac resonance.

Mixed Resonance

Mixed resonance is any combination of hypernasality (with or without nasal emission), hyponasality, and cul-de-sac resonance. Although hypernasality and hyponasality cannot occur simultaneously, they can occur at different times in the connected speech of the same speaker. Therefore, there can be hypernasality on oral sounds and hyponasality on nasal sounds.

Mixed resonance is common in individuals with apraxia. If the individual has difficulty coordinating anterior articulation with velopharyngeal articulation, there may be inappropriate upward movement of the velum on nasal sounds and downward movement of the velum on oral sounds (Ogar et al., 2006). In connected speech, there is usually more hypernasality than hyponasality because moving the velum up for closure is harder than keeping it in the rest position.

Mixed resonance can also be caused by a combination of velopharyngeal incompetence and blockage in the pharynx. For example, there can be a short velum causing inadequate velopharyngeal closure on oral sounds and also enlarged adenoids that block the sound from entering the nasal cavity on nasal sounds.

In addition to mixed resonance, some individuals demonstrate hyponasality and nasal emission, which has the same cause as hypernasality.

Again, this does not occur simultaneously but rather on different speech sounds. A common cause for this combination is enlarged, yet irregular, adenoid tissue. During the production of oral sounds, the velum closes against the adenoid pad, but a tight velopharyngeal seal cannot be obtained because of the irregular tissue. As a result, there is nasal emission on oral sounds. On the other hand, when the velum goes down for the production of nasal sounds, the adenoid pad is large enough that it obstructs the transmission of sound into the nasal cavity, thus causing hyponasality.

Effect of Surgery on Resonance

A discussion of resonance would not be complete without a mention of how resonance can change as a result of surgical alteration of the structures. In some cases, adenoidectomy can improve hyponasality if there was obstruction. In other cases, it can make speech worse by causing velopharyngeal incompetence with hypernasality (and nasal emission), which can only be corrected with surgery. Tonsillectomy can eliminate cul-de-sac resonance by removing the blockage at the entrance of the oral cavity. Surgery to correct hypernasality (e.g., pharyngeal flap or sphincter pharyngoplasty) can be unsuccessful, resulting in residual hypernasality, or it can cause hyponasality from overcorrection (see the chapter *Surgical Management*). In addition, if the pharyngeal flap or sphincter (surgery for hypernasality) is placed too low in the pharynx, it can effectively shorten the resonating tube, causing an unwanted change in resonance (Smith & Kuehn, 2007). In summary, anything that changes the length or shape of the resonating cavities can affect the quality of resonance.

Treatment of Resonance Disorders

It is important to emphasize again that resonance disorders are *almost always* caused by structural anomalies and, therefore, resonance disorders *almost always* require medical or surgical intervention. Hypernasality is usually caused by a structural or neurophysiological disorder that interferes with the function of the velopharyngeal valve. This can be corrected or improved only with surgery or a prosthetic device (if surgery is not an option). Hyponasality and cul-de-sac resonance are usually caused by a blockage in one or more of the cavities of the vocal tract. Again, this is treated with medical or surgical intervention.

The *only* time that speech therapy is indicated for a resonance disorder is when the abnormal resonance is phoneme specific because of faulty articulation placement. This may include the use of a nasal sound consistently for an oral sound or an abnormally high tongue position during production of vowels. This can even be noted after surgical intervention because of the preoperative development of compensatory productions. Correction of the structure should be done first, and then speech therapy can be effective in correction of abnormal function that developed as a compensatory strategy.

Types of Velopharyngeal Dysfunction

Normal velopharyngeal function requires normal structure (anatomy), normal movement (neurophysiology), and normal function (which is learned) (**FIGURE 10-4A**). Velopharyngeal dysfunction (VPD) occurs when there is an abnormality in any one of these three components during speech production (**FIGURE 10-4B**). Velopharyngeal dysfunction is a broad term that encompasses all disorders where the velopharyngeal valve does not close consistently and completely during the production of oral sounds (D'Antonio, Muntz, Province, & Marsh, 1988; Folkins, 1988; Glade & Deal, 2016; Jones, 1991; Loney & Bloem, 1987; Marsh, 1991; Morris, 1992; Netsell, 1988; Penfold, 1997; Witt, 2009; Witt et al., 1997).

Unfortunately, the literature has been full of inconsistencies in the use of terminology for disorders of the velopharyngeal valve. Some authors and clinicians use the common terms

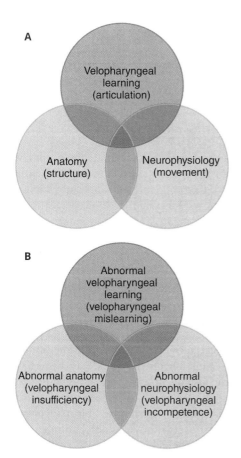

FIGURE 10-4 (A) Components of normal velopharyngeal function. **(B)** Components of velopharyngeal dysfunction.

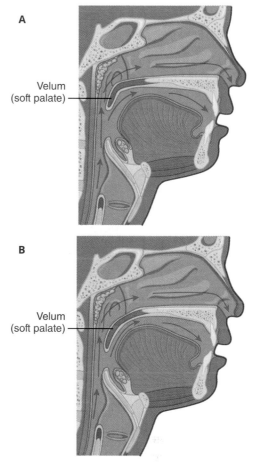

FIGURE 10-5 (A) Velopharyngeal insufficiency. In this case, the velum is too short to achieve velopharyngeal closure during speech. **(B)** Velopharyngeal incompetence. In this case, the velum does not move well enough to achieve velopharyngeal closure during speech.

velopharyngeal inadequacy, velopharyngeal impairment, velopharyngeal insufficiency, velopharyngeal incompetence, and velopharyngeal dysfunction interchangeably, whereas others use these terms in a specific way to suggest the type of VPD based on etiology (Kummer, 2011b; Loney & Bloem, 1987; Trost, 1981; Trost-Cardamone, 1989). Specificity in terminology is important because each of these categories of velopharyngeal dysfunction has a different underlying cause that has an effect on appropriate treatment. Therefore, the terminology proposed by Trost-Cardamone is used in this text and is as follows:

The term velopharyngeal insufficiency is used to describe an anatomical or structural defect that prevents adequate velopharyngeal closure. Velopharyngeal insufficiency is the most common type of VPD because it includes a short or defective velum, which is often associated with cleft palate (**FIGURE 10-5A**). Velopharyngeal incompetence is used to refer to a neurophysiological disorder that results in poor movement of the velopharyngeal structures (**FIGURE 10-5B**).

VPI (for velopharyngeal insufficiency/incompetence) is used for disorders that are medically based and therefore require physical management. Hence, VPI is not a condition that can be corrected with speech therapy. It should be noted that with either form of VPI, there is usually complete velopharyngeal closure with swallowing. This is because with a swallow, the velum does not move independently as it does for speech. Instead, it is elevated by the upward movement of the back of the tongue. In addition, the entire length of the velum (down to the uvula) is elevated and closes against the pharyngeal wall. With speech, the effective length of the velum ends at the point of levator elevation.

In contrast to VPI (regardless of type), velopharyngeal mislearning is an articulation disorder that includes the substitution of certain nasal or pharyngeal sounds, which are produced with an open velopharyngeal valve, for oral sounds, for which the valve should be closed. Velopharyngeal mislearning may be secondary to VPI as evidenced by the development of compensatory productions. However, it sometimes occurs in children with no history of VPI. Regardless, velopharyngeal mislearning is corrected by speech therapy rather than surgery.

Effects of Velopharyngeal Insufficiency/ Incompetence on Speech

Dysfunction of the velopharyngeal valve from either abnormal structure (velopharyngeal insufficiency) or abnormal neurophysiology (velopharyngeal incompetence) can affect speech in a variety of ways. Depending on the size of the opening, speech may be characterized by any or all of the following disorders: hypernasality, nasal air emission, obligatory distortions and/ or compensatory errors, and even dysphonia. The following sections further describe how VPI affects speech. (Mislearning is discussed in another section.)

Hypernasality

Hypernasality has already been described in the section on resonance disorders and, therefore, will not be repeated here. The following sections describe the other effects of VPI on speech.

Nasal Air Emission

Nasal emission of the airstream occurs when there is an attempt to build up intraoral air pressure for the production of consonants while there is a leak in the system (velopharyngeal valve or oronasal fistula). As a result, some of the airflow is released through the nose, causing a disruption in the aerodynamic process of speech. Nasal emission occurs on pressure-sensitive phonemes (plosives, fricatives, and affricates). It is most noticed on voiceless phonemes because they are associated with more airflow than their voiced counterparts, where the adduction of the vocal folds attenuates the airflow somewhat. Nasal emission often occurs with hypernasality but can also occur with normal resonance.

There are four basic types of nasal emission: inaudible nasal emission, audible nasal emission, nasal rustle (also known as nasal turbulence), and phoneme-specific nasal emission (PSNE). The type of nasal emission has to do with the relative size of the opening (which affects the acoustic properties of both nasal airflow and resonance) and its cause (e.g., abnormal structure or abnormal function).

Inaudible nasal emission occurs with a large opening. Although there is a significant loss of airflow through the opening, this type of nasal emission is inaudible because there is very little impedance to the flow. In addition, a large opening causes hypernasality, which masks the sound of nasal emission. Although the nasal emission is not audible, there is evidence that it is there because it causes several secondary characteristics. For example, the loss of airflow through the nose causes the oral consonants to be weak in intensity and pressure or seem to be omitted totally. In fact, there is a direct inverse relationship between nasal emission and oral airflow in that the greater the nasal emission, the weaker the consonants will be. In addition to weak consonants, utterance length is often shortened because of the need to take more frequent breaths to replenish the airflow. This causes connected speech to seem choppy. It has been shown that individuals with a large velopharyngeal opening attempt to increase airflow rate during consonant production. As a result, they may produce respiratory volumes that are twice that of normal speakers (Huber & Stathopoulos, 2003). This additional effort can often be noted as a nasal grimace.

A nasal grimace is characterized by muscle contractions just above the nasal bridge and/or at the side of the nose (**FIGURE 10-6**). Just as muscle contractions can be noted in the face when a person is trying to lift something heavy, the nasal grimace seems to be an overflow muscle reaction that occurs with extreme effort to achieve velopharyngeal closure. Once velopharyngeal function is corrected, the nasal grimace during speech usually disappears spontaneously.

Audible nasal emission is the second form of nasal emission. It occurs when there is a mid-sized velopharyngeal opening. The airflow is more audible than with a larger opening because there is greater resistance to the flow, causing a friction sound. In addition, there is less pronounced hypernasality to mask the sound of nasal emission. There may still be some of the secondary characteristics of a large velopharyngeal opening as noted previously.

Nasal rustle has been historically called nasal turbulence. This may be a misnomer in that there is no research that confirms that the sound source is turbulence of airflow as was postulated in the past. Instead, it has been correlated with bubbling of secretions above a small velopharyngeal opening. Despite its size, a small opening can actually cause more speech distortion than an opening that is a little larger. This is because the airflow accelerates as it goes through a small opening, which means the pressure of the airflow decreases because of its inverse relationship to velocity. As the airflow is released, however, it causes very audible bubbling of the nasal secretions (Kummer et al., 1992; Kummer et al., 2003; Mason & Grandstaff, 1971). The bubbling of a nasal rustle can be seen easily through nasopharyngoscopy (a nasal endoscopic procedure; also known as nasendoscopy or video nasendoscopy) and can be seen even through videofluoroscopy (a radiological procedure) as bubbling of the barium. Because the nasal rustle is caused by bubbling of secretions, nasal congestion can make this distortion even more noticeable. When it occurs, a nasal rustle can be very loud. As such, it can mask the sound of the consonants, thus affecting not only the quality of speech but also the intelligibility.

A nasal rustle tends to be somewhat inconsistent during speech. Because it is caused by a small velopharyngeal opening, closure can be achieved in short utterances or with additional effort. However, with an increase in utterance length, speed, phonemic complexity, or even fatigue, the nasal rustle often becomes more consistent. This is why nasal rustle cannot be corrected with speech therapy. The gains that are made in the therapy room are usually not maintained outside of structured therapy sessions.

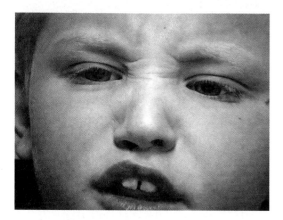

FIGURE 10-6 Nasal grimace during speech. Note the contraction above and at the side of the nose. This is caused by the extra effort of trying to achieve velopharyngeal closure.

Finally, PSNE is a type of nasal emission that occurs only on certain pressure-sensitive sounds. As such, it is the result of faulty articulation in the pharynx rather than caused by VPI. PSNE most commonly occurs on the /s/ but can occur on all sibilant sounds (/s/, /z/, /ʃ/, /ʒ/, /ʧ/, /ʤ/).

Obligatory Distortions and Compensatory Errors

When there are structural anomalies within the vocal tract (e.g., dental or occlusal anomalies, an oronasal fistula, or velopharyngeal insufficiency), the individual's speech may be characterized by obligatory distortions and/or compensatory errors (Trost-Cardamone, 1990). Obligatory distortions, sometimes called passive speech characteristics (Harding & Grunwell, 1996; Harding & Grunwell, 1998), occur when the articulation placement is normal but an abnormality of the structure causes distortion of speech sounds. In contrast, compensatory errors, sometimes called active speech characteristics (Harding & Grunwell, 1996; Harding & Grunwell, 1998), are misarticulations that occur in response to abnormal structure.

A distinction between obligatory distortions and compensatory errors is important because obligatory distortions are purely the result of abnormal structure and, therefore, require surgical or prosthetic intervention only. In contrast, compensatory characteristics are under the patient's control and can therefore be corrected with speech therapy, preferably after the structure is corrected.

Obligatory distortions secondary to significant VPI or a large oronasal fistula include hypernasality and nasal emission (despite normal placement). Additional obligatory distortions caused by a fairly large opening include weak or omitted consonants, short utterance length from the loss of airflow through the nose, and nasalization of voiced plosives.

There are several compensatory articulation productions that children use to compensate for a loss of airflow through the nose. As a general rule, compensatory productions are produced with the same manner (e.g., plosive, fricative, affricate) but an altered placement. The place of production depends on whether the nasal emission is caused by VPI or a large oronasal fistula.

Compensatory Productions for VPI

When there is VPI, the compensatory productions are all produced in the pharynx where there is airflow. After production, the airflow continues to flow superiorly through the velopharyngeal opening and is then released through the nose. Compensatory productions for VPI include both plosives and fricatives. Affricates are typically substituted by pharyngeal fricatives, however, because they are too difficult to produce in the pharynx. Compensatory productions for VPI are outlined in **TABLE 10-1**,

TABLE 10-1 **Typical Compensatory Productions for VPI**		
Place of Production in the Pharynx	Plosives	Fricatives[a]
Glottis	Glottal stop	Glottal fricative /h/
Oropharynx	Pharyngeal plosive	Pharyngeal fricative
Nasopharynx	None	Posterior nasal fricative, nasal snort, nasal sniff

[a]Note that affricates are usually too difficult to produce in the pharynx.

and the plosive and fricative sounds are further described as follows:

- A glottal stop, also known as a glottal plosive, is a voiced plosive that is produced by adduction of the vocal folds, a buildup of subglottic air pressure, and then sudden separation of the vocal folds to release the airflow (**FIGURE 10-7**). This results in a grunt-type sound. A glottal stop is often produced in normal speech for a /t/ sound when followed by an /n/ sound (e.g., "mitten," "button," "Clinton," etc.). Glottal stops are often substituted for plosive sounds, but they may also be substituted for fricatives and affricates, especially if the child has not yet developed the fricative manner in his or her phonemic repertoire. Glottal stops can be co-articulated with other plosives (Bispo et al., 2011; Trost-Cardamone, 1997). For example, the child can produce a /b/ sound with the lips and co-articulate that with a glottal stop. Glottal stops can be seen as increased laryngeal activity in the throat area.

- A glottal fricative, the /h/ sound, is often substituted for oral fricatives when there is VPI because it is produced well below the level of the velopharyngeal leak (Harding & Grunwell, 1998; Proctor, Shadle, & Iskarous, 2010).

- Breathiness is a vocal quality where the vocal folds are held farther apart than normal so that a larger volume of air escapes between them. A breathy vocal quality can be used as a compensatory strategy for VPI because it can mask the perception of hypernasality, which depends on voicing.

- A pharyngeal plosive, also known as a pharyngeal stop, is produced by moving the back of the tongue in a posterior direction to articulate against the posterior pharyngeal wall, thus taking advantage of the airflow in the pharynx (**FIGURE 10-8**). An increase in pharyngeal activity can often be noted by observing the throat when this sound is produced. Because of the difficulty of producing this phoneme, there is often a longer duration between the consonant and the following vowel than is typically noted with other

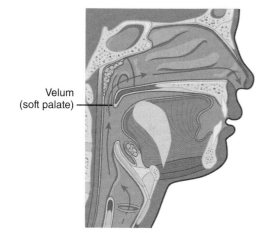

FIGURE 10-7 Placement of a glottal stop with a co-articulated /t/.

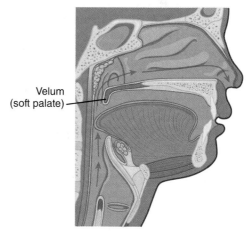

FIGURE 10-8 Placement of a pharyngeal plosive.

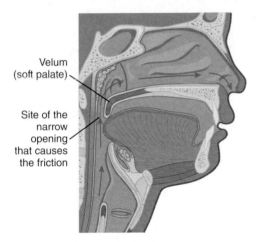

FIGURE 10-9 Placement of a pharyngeal fricative.

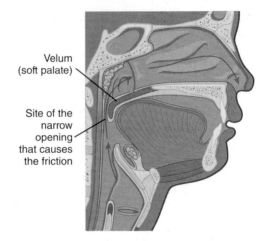

FIGURE 10-10 Placement of a posterior nasal fricative.

consonant placements. Although it can be substituted for other consonants, a pharyngeal plosive is typically substituted for velar plosives (/k/, /g/).

- A pharyngeal fricative is produced by retracting the back of the tongue so that it approximates, but does not touch, the pharyngeal wall (**FIGURE 10-9**). The fricative sound is produced as the airflow is forced through the narrow opening that is created between the back of the tongue and pharyngeal wall. As with the other pharyngeal compensatory productions, an increase in pharyngeal activity can be noted in the throat area during production. Pharyngeal fricatives are usually substituted for sibilant sounds.
- A posterior nasal fricative is produced by elevating the back of the tongue so that it articulates against the velum, just like an /ŋ/ placement. As the air flows upward through the pharynx, the back of the tongue blocks the entrance into the oral cavity. Therefore, the air is forced through the closed velopharyngeal valve, causing a small opening (**FIGURE 10-10**). This production results in a very audible nasal emission (Trost, 1981), called a nasal rustle (also known as turbulence). The posterior nasal fricative may be used as a substitution for

any of the pressure-sensitive phonemes, but it is typically used for sibilants and is always voiceless.

- A nasal snort is produced by a forcible emission of air through the nose that results in a noisy, sneeze-like sound. The nasal snort is typically associated with the production of /s/ blends. It often occurs concurrently with a nasal grimace.
- A nasal sniff is an uncommon compensatory articulation production, but it does occur in some cases. It is produced by a forcible inspiration through the nose, and therefore, it is the opposite of nasal emission. The nasal sniff is usually substituted for sibilant sounds, particularly the /s/. Because of the difficulty in coordinating the inspiration of the nasal sniff and expiration for other sounds, the nasal sniff typically occurs only in the final word position rather than in all word positions.

Compensatory Productions for an Oronasal Fistula

When there is a large oronasal fistula, the compensatory productions are all produced behind the fistula before the airflow is lost. Compensatory productions for a large fistula are outlined in

TABLE 10-2, and the plosive and fricative sounds are further described as follows:

- A palatal–dorsal plosive (also known as a mid-dorsum palatal stop) is produced with the dorsum of the tongue against the mid-portion of the hard palate (Trost, 1981) (**FIGURE 10-11**). This production is often substituted for lingual-alveolar sounds (/t/, /d/), particularly if the fistula is in the area of the alveolus. Because the place of production is between that for lingual-alveolars and velars, the boundaries for distinguishing the two placements are lost, and the acoustic product sounds like a cross between the two placements. A dorsal production is also used to close the fistula with the tongue during production of anterior sounds, particularly bilabial plosives (/p/, /b/).
- A palatal–dorsal fricative is produced with the dorsum of the tongue under the mid-portion of the hard palate. It is often used as a substitution for sibilant sounds. (A palatal–dorsal placement is also a compensatory production for anterior oral cavity crowding that occurs with dental malocclusion.)
- A velar plosive (/k/, /g/) is produced behind the hard palate. Therefore, if there is a large oronasal fistula in the hard palate, the velar placement allows the individual to impound the airflow behind the fistula before the airflow is lost through it (Trost-Cardamone, 1997). The airflow is then released and flows over the fistula rather than into it. In some cases, velar plosives are actually co-articulated (produced at the same time) with the intended lingual-alveolar sounds (Gibbon, Ellis, & Crampin, 2004).
- A velar fricative is produced with the back of the tongue slightly elevated so that it is in the same position as a /j/ (as in "yellow") (**FIGURE 10-12**). It is produced by forcing air through the narrow passage that is created between the back of the tongue and velum. It is typically substituted for sibilants.

TABLE 10-2 Typical Compensatory Productions for an Oronasal Fistula

Place of Production	Plosives	Fricatives/ Affricates
Hard palate	Palatal–dorsal plosive	Palatal–dorsal fricative/ affricate
Velum	Velar plosive (/k/ or /g/)	Velar fricative/ affricate

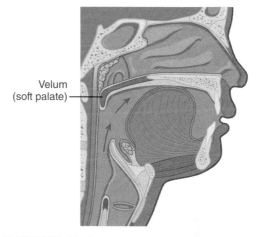

FIGURE 10-11 Placement of a palatal–dorsal production (mid-dorsum palatal stop).

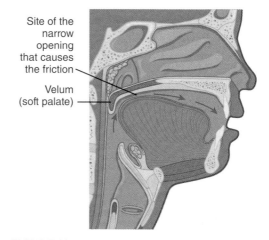

FIGURE 10-12 Placement of a velar fricative.

Dysphonia

Dysphonia is characterized by breathiness, hoarseness, low intensity, and/or glottal fry during phonation. Low volume and other dysphonic characteristics can further decrease the intelligibility of the speech in children with VPI.

Children with VPI or other craniofacial conditions have an increased risk for dysphonia for several reasons (D'Antonio et al., 1988; McWilliams, Lavorato, & Bluestone, 1973; Robison & Otteson, 2011b). One common finding is a hyperfunctional voice disorder in individuals with mildly impaired velopharyngeal valving. This is because when there is increased respiratory and muscular effort to close the velopharyngeal port, it can also result in hyperadduction of the vocal folds. Chronic hyperadduction can cause thickening and edema of the vocal folds, which ultimately leads to the formation of vocal nodules (**FIGURE 10-13**). Vocal nodules are small callus-like masses that typically occur symmetrically on both vocal folds as a result of chronic abuse, misuse, or overuse of the folds. Speech therapy to increase oral airflow when there is VPI is not only ineffective, but it can also cause or exacerbate vocal fold pathology.

Other causes of dysphonia in these populations include congenital laryngeal anomalies, which are more common in individuals with congenital craniofacial syndromes. Dysphonia can even be secondary to complications from long-term tracheostomy (e.g., tracheal stenosis). As previously noted, breathiness may occur as a compensatory strategy to mask the hypernasality and nasal emission.

Effect of Gap Size on the Characteristics of Speech

The severity of VPI can vary from a very small pinhole-sized opening to a very large opening that includes the entire velopharyngeal port. However, the size of the velopharyngeal opening does not correlate well with the severity of the

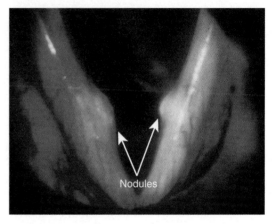

FIGURE 10-13 Bilateral vocal nodules as seen through endoscopy.

speech disorder and the effect on intelligibility (Jones, 2005). This lack of correlation is caused by several factors, including the separate effects of gap size on acoustics (resonance) versus aerodynamics (airflow), the consistency of closure, the confounding effects of compensatory articulation productions, and the co-occurrence of dysphonia.

The size of the velopharyngeal opening affects the perception of sound and airflow differently. This is illustrated in **TABLE 10-3**. There is actually an inverse relationship between audible hypernasality and audible nasal emission, as can be seen in **FIGURE 10-14**.

With a large velopharyngeal opening, air and sound go through the opening without much resistance. The movement of air is unobstructed, and therefore, nasal emission is not very audible. Although the nasal emission is inaudible, it causes consonants to be weak and utterances to be short. Compensatory productions are common because of the lack of oral airflow. The most notable characteristic of speech with a large opening is hypernasality.

With a midsized velopharyngeal opening, there is less hypernasality and more audible nasal emission. This is because with a smaller opening, there is more resistance to the flow of air as it goes through the valve. Also, there is more intraoral

TABLE 10-3 Perceptual Characteristics of Speech as a Prediction of Velopharyngeal Gap Size	
Perceptual Characteristics	**Relative Gap Size**
Severe hypernasality Inaudible nasal emission Weak consonants Short utterance length Compensatory productions	⬭
Moderate hypernasality Audible nasal emission Slightly weak consonants May be compensatory productions	⬭
Mild hypernasality Audible nasal emission	⬭
Nasal emission/rustle	⬭

airflow, so consonants are stronger and utterance length is less affected.

Small velopharyngeal openings are typically characterized by normal speech production and resonance. However, a small opening can cause inconsistent nasal emission. This is often in the form of a nasal rustle, which is a loud and distracting bubbly sound (Kummer et al., 1992; Kummer et al., 2003). The nasal rustle can be loud enough to mask the oral sound that is being articulated, which also affects the intelligibility of speech. Therefore, the speech quality from a small opening may be judged to be more severely affected than the speech quality from a midsized opening.

Although small velopharyngeal openings can cause a very audible form of nasal emission, the nasal emission/rustle is usually somewhat inconsistent. This is because with a little effort, closure can usually be achieved. However, just as it is difficult to carry a 50-pound weight for long, it is difficult for these individuals to continue to exert enough effort to maintain closure

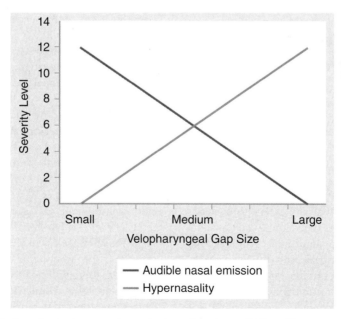

FIGURE 10-14 Prediction of velopharyngeal gap size based on the audibility of hypernasality versus nasal emission.

for a prolonged period of time. Closure may be complete for single words or short utterances but may break down with the motoric demands of connected speech. Parents often report that the child's speech is best at the beginning of the day but becomes noticeably worse as the day goes on or when the child is tired.

The use of compensatory productions has a definite effect on the perception of severity. If they are still used after surgical correction of velopharyngeal function, there will still be nasal emission and possibly hypernasality, despite a normally functioning valve.

The quality of phonation is a final factor that affects judgments of severity. The use of a breathy voice may reduce the perception of nasal emission and hypernasality. In addition, increased vocal effort may temporarily increase velopharyngeal function and decrease gap size for improved resonance (McHenry, 1997). On the other hand, low volume and other dysphonic characteristics, such as hoarseness and glottal fry, can have a negative effect on judgments of severity and intelligibility.

Causes of Velopharyngeal Dysfunction

There are many noncleft causes of velopharyngeal insufficiency, velopharyngeal incompetence, and velopharyngeal mislearning (Kummer, Marshall, & Wilson, 2015). They are listed and explained as follows:

Velopharyngeal Insufficiency

Velopharyngeal insufficiency refers to a structural defect that causes the velum to be too short or too irregular to obtain a tight closure against the posterior pharyngeal wall during speech. There are many causes of discrepancies between the length of the velum and the needed length for firm velopharyngeal contact. The following is a list of some of these causes.

Cleft Palate

Velopharyngeal insufficiency occurs most commonly from cleft palate. Although surgeons attempt to achieve as much velar length during the cleft palate repair as possible, 20% to 30% of patients with a history of cleft palate demonstrate velopharyngeal insufficiency following the cleft repair (Naran, Ford, & Losee, 2017).

Velopharyngeal insufficiency following cleft palate repair is often because the velum is congenitally short (see Figure 10-5A). The velum may also be abnormally short or thin because of the absent aponeurosis and hypoplasia of the levator veli palatini and musculus uvulae muscles (Dickson, 1972). Finally, despite best attempts, the insertion point of the levator muscles may be inadequate following surgery as well. In some cases, a midline irregularity or deficiency at the posterior border of the velar eminence can be seen through nasopharyngoscopy as the cause of a velopharyngeal gap.

Submucous Cleft Palate

Although many individuals with submucous cleft have normal speech, there is a higher risk for velopharyngeal insufficiency in this population compared to unaffected individuals (Gosain & Hettinger, 2009; McWilliams, 1991). Velopharyngeal insufficiency can occur because of a small notch in the midline of the posterior border of the velum, hypoplasticity of the muscles, or anterior orientation of the levator veli palatini muscles. If the submucous cleft extends through the velum and hard palate, the levator veli palatini muscle will insert into the hard palate as if there had been an overt cleft palate (refer to Figure 3-18 in the chapter *Clefts of the Lip and Palate*). This renders these muscles useless in elevating the velum for speech. If the submucous cleft includes a zona pellucida, there will be little, if any, underlying muscle, and the velum will be very thin. This causes an abnormal amount of sound to go through the velum to the nasal cavity. As such, an individual with a zona pellucida may have hypernasal speech despite having normal velopharyngeal closure.

Deep Pharynx

Because the posterior pharyngeal wall sits just anterior to the cervical spine, abnormal curvature of the cervical spine or cranial base anomalies (as seen in some craniosynostosis syndromes) can increase the anterior–posterior dimensions of the pharynx (Haapanen, Heliovaara, & Ranta, 1991; Leveau-Geffroy, Perrin, Khonsari, & Mercier, 2011) (**FIGURE 10-15**). Therefore, the velum may be unable to reach the posterior pharyngeal wall because of the depth of the pharynx. This can be suspected through an intraoral examination but can be confirmed only through an X-ray.

Adenoid Atrophy

In the early years, most children actually have veloadenoidal closure because the adenoids are in the place of normal velar contact. Adenoid tissue is most prominent in very young children but begins to slowly atrophy around the age of 6. With the onset of puberty, there can be significant, and sometimes sudden, atrophy of the adenoid tissue, causing an increase in the distance

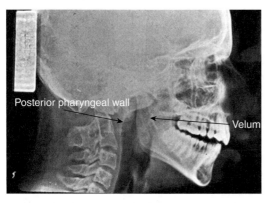

FIGURE 10-15 Deep pharynx caused by the posterior position of the cervical spine.

between the velum and posterior pharyngeal wall (Shapiro, 1980). If the velum is normal, it stretches to accommodate the difference in the depth of the pharynx; thus, normal velopharyngeal closure is maintained.

Children with a repaired cleft palate or a submucous cleft may demonstrate normal resonance and velopharyngeal function during the preschool and early school years. However, they may experience gradual deterioration in velopharyngeal closure as they reach adolescence. This is because the velum may not be capable of stretching sufficiently to accommodate the difference in pharyngeal depth with the involution of the adenoid tissue (Mason & Warren, 1980; Morris, Wroblewski, Brown, & Van Demark, 1990; Shapiro, 1980; Siegel-Sadewitz & Shprintzen, 1986). When this occurs, parents often report that their child has begun to mumble, does not speak loud enough, or has become "lazy" with speech.

Adenoidectomy

A well-known and well-documented risk of an adenoidectomy is postoperative velopharyngeal insufficiency (Andreassen, Leeper, & MacRae, 1991; Croft, Shprintzen, & Ruben, 1981; Donnelly, 1994; Fernandes, Grobbelaar, Hudson, & Lentin, 1996; Kummer, Myer, Smith, & Shott, 1993; Maryn, Van Lierde, De Bodt, & Van Cauwenberge, 2004; Parton & Jones, 1998; Ren, Isberg, & Henningsson, 1995; Robinson, 1992; Saunders, Hartley, Sell, & Sommerlad, 2004; Seid, 1990; Stewart, Ahmad, Razzell, & Watson, 2002; Witzel, Rich, Margar-Bacal, & Cox, 1986). This is because young children with a prominent adenoid pad usually achieve veloadenoidal closure rather than velopharyngeal closure (**FIGURE 10-16**). Removal of the adenoids results in a deeper nasopharynx and a greater distance for the velum to stretch to achieve closure.

Hypernasality or nasal emission following adenoidectomy can occur in individuals with no velar defect. However, this is typically short

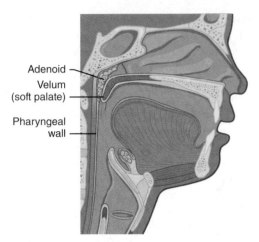

Adenoid
Velum
(soft palate)
Pharyngeal
wall

FIGURE 10-16 Position of the adenoid in the pharynx. The adenoid pad can help with closure. In many young children, there is veloadenoidal closure rather than velopharyngeal closure.

lived, lasting from a few hours to as long as 6 to 8 weeks. Certain compensations occur in the velopharyngeal mechanism to adapt to the changes in the pharyngeal dimension. These compensations include an increase in velar mobility, an increase in velar height during closure, an increase in velar stretch, and increased movement of the pharyngeal walls (Neiman & Simpson, 1975). Therefore, in most cases, the speech returns to normal once these adaptations are made.

The risk for permanent velopharyngeal insufficiency following adenoidectomy has been estimated to be between 1:1500 and 1:3000 (Donnelly, 1994; Stewart et al., 2002). The biggest risk factor is a history of cleft palate. Despite a repaired cleft palate, the child may have tenuous velopharyngeal closure preoperatively, scarring of the velum, and a lack of muscle reserve to stretch postoperatively (Parton & Jones, 1998). Presence of a submucous cleft palate is also a major risk factor for similar reasons. In fact, children with velopharyngeal insufficiency following adenoidectomy are often found through nasopharyngoscopy to have an occult submucous cleft after the fact

(Parton & Jones, 1998; Saunders et al., 2004; Schmaman, Jordaan, & Jammine, 1998). Other risk factors include a family history of cleft palate or hypernasality, sucking difficulties as an infant, and oral-motor dysfunction or other neuromuscular problems.

Adenoidectomy is usually contraindicated for children with a history of cleft palate, submucous cleft, or other risk factors. However, if the child has upper airway obstruction or a blocked eustachian tube from adenoid hypertrophy, a conservative superior half adenoidectomy can be performed (Finkelstein, Wexler, Nachmani, & Ophir, 2002). With this procedure, the airway obstruction is relieved while maintaining enough tissue inferiorly for the velum to continue to close against the adenoid pad for speech. (It should be noted that, as with other causes of velopharyngeal insufficiency, post-adenoidectomy velopharyngeal insufficiency cannot be corrected with speech therapy because it is caused by a structural defect.)

Irregular Adenoids

Although it is not commonly recognized, irregular adenoids can occasionally cause velopharyngeal insufficiency (Ren, Isberg, & Henningsson, 1995). If the adenoid pad has indentations in the surface, this can make it impossible for the velum to obtain a tight seal against it (**FIGURE 10-17A** and **10-17B**). Adenoidal protrusions can also affect closure by causing a lateral gap on one or both sides (**FIGURE 10-17C**). Irregular adenoids typically cause a small velopharyngeal (actually veloadenoidal) opening. This results in audible nasal emission (often a nasal rustle) but rarely hypernasality because of its size (Kummer et al., 2003). In fact, there may be hyponasality if the adenoid tissue is large. Ironically, irregularity of adenoid tissue commonly occurs after an adenoidectomy. This is because, unlike with tonsillectomy, the capsule deep to the adenoid pad is left in place during the surgery because it protects the underlying bone of the skull base. Therefore, irregular regrowth of the adenoid tissue can occur over time.

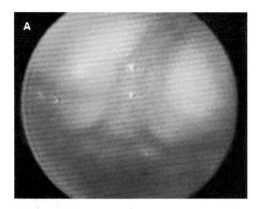

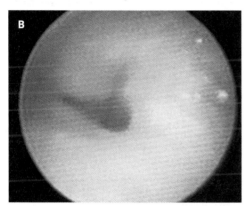

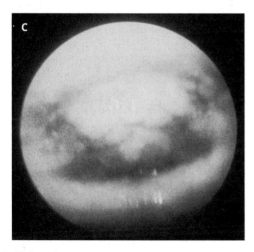

FIGURE 10-17 Irregular adenoids. **(A)** A deep cleft in the surface of the adenoid pad. **(B)** As a result of adenoid irregularity, the velum is unable to achieve a tight seal against the adenoid, resulting in nasal air emission. **(C)** A protrusive adenoid pad, which will cause a leak on each side during velar closure.

Hypertrophic Tonsils

The (faucial) tonsils are located in the oral cavity between the anterior and posterior faucial pillars. As such, they usually do not affect velopharyngeal function because they are well below and anterior to the velopharyngeal valve. On rare occasions, however, hypertrophic tonsils can cause mechanical interference with the function of the velopharyngeal valve and also affect resonance.

As tonsils become hypertrophic, they can expand anteriorly, medially, or posteriorly. If they expand posteriorly, they can often be seen through nasopharyngoscopy in the oropharynx and even in the nasopharynx. Tonsils that are in the pharynx can affect the medial movement of the lateral pharyngeal walls during speech by pushing against the posterior faucial pillars. When a tonsil is so large that its upper pole projects into the pharynx, it can also become positioned between the velum and posterior pharyngeal wall, thus preventing the velum from achieving an adequate velopharyngeal seal during speech (Abdel-Aziz, 2012; Finkelstein, Nachmani, & Ophir, 1994; Henningsson & Isberg, 1988; Kummer, Billmire, et al., 1993; MacKenzie-Stepner, Witzel, Stringer, & Laskin, 1987; Maryn, Van Lierde, De Bodt, & Van Cauwenberge, 2004; Shprintzen, Sher, & Croft, 1987) (**FIGURE 10-18**). This can result in a small velopharyngeal gap, causing nasal emission. In addition, the tonsil in the pharynx can also obstruct sound transmission into both the oral and nasal cavities, causing a mixture of hyponasality and cul-de-sac resonance. If one tonsil is much larger than the other, it will often push the velum upward on that side. Because of the pulling and stretching of the velum on that side, the uvula will deviate and appear to point toward the large tonsil.

If the tonsils expand medially, they will not affect velopharyngeal function. However, as noted previously, they can cause a pharyngeal cul-de-sac resonance by blocking the sound from entering the oral cavity. Tonsils that expand anteriorly may affect oral resonance and can also cause difficulty with articulation of posterior sounds,

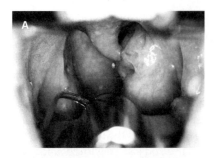

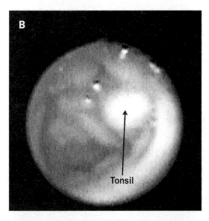

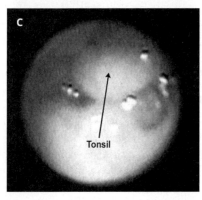

FIGURE 10-18 Intrusive tonsil in the pharynx. **(A)** Large tonsil on the right side of the photo (patient's left). The uvula can be seen to deviate toward the large tonsil, which indicates that it is pushing on the posterior faucial pillar and intruding into the pharynx. **(B)** The same tonsil in the pharynx as seen through nasopharyngoscopy. **(C)** The tonsil can be seen between the velum and posterior pharyngeal wall during velopharyngeal closure. Because there is not a tight seal, a small opening can be seen just to the left of the tonsil. There is a bubble in this area as a result of the nasal air emission.

particularly velars (/k/, /g/) (Henningsson & Isberg, 1988).

Otolaryngologists commonly perform tonsillectomies for chronic tonsillitis and/or airway obstruction. If there are speech and resonance issues secondary to hypertrophic tonsils, the primary care physician and otolaryngologist should be made aware of this. A recommendation for tonsillectomy to correct these issues would be appropriate.

Tonsillectomy

Because the tonsils reside in the oral cavity, tonsillectomy is highly unlikely to cause problems with speech. There are very rare exceptions, however. First, significant scarring of the posterior faucial pillar postoperatively can affect lateral pharyngeal wall movement. This is a particular concern for individuals who are prone to forming keloids, which is excessive scar tissue formed during healing. In addition, lesions of branches of the vagus and glossopharyngeal nerves can affect velopharyngeal function (Haapanen, Ignatius, Rihkanen, & Ertama, 1994).

Maxillary Advancement

Class III malocclusion with midface retrusion is particularly common in patients with a cleft lip and palate, but it can also occur in individuals without a history of cleft. These patients can benefit from maxillary advancement, which is done through either orthognathic surgery (surgery that involves the bones of the maxilla and mandible) or distraction osteogenesis (a method of gradually lengthening a bone) (see the chapter *Surgical Management* for more information). The purpose of maxillary advancement is to correct midface deficiency in order to normalize the occlusion and the facial profile.

Maxillary advancement can result in many positive changes for the patient. There is typically a dramatic improvement in facial profile and overall aesthetics as a result of this surgery. In addition, the normalization of occlusion often results in elimination of obligatory speech distortions, particularly on sibilant sounds, without intervening

CASE REPORT

Hypertrophic Tonsils

Ellen was a 9-year-old child with a history of normal speech and language development. She had never had speech therapy. Her parents reported that over the past 2 years, her speech had gradually become nasal and hard to understand. The parents reported that Ellen had also begun to snore loudly at night.

Upon examination, Ellen was found to have an open mouth posture with an anterior tongue position at rest. An evaluation of speech revealed normal articulation but nasal emission during the production of pressure-sensitive phonemes. Resonance was characterized by hyponasality and a cul-de-sac quality.

An intraoral examination revealed a hypertrophic tonsil on the right side. It extended medially beyond the point of the midline of the oropharynx. The left tonsil was of normal size. A nasopharyngoscopy assessment showed the tonsil to be in the nasopharynx and between the velum and posterior pharyngeal wall during velopharyngeal closure. Because of the interference of the tonsil, there was a small velopharyngeal opening on either side of the tonsil, resulting in nasal emission. The large tonsil in the pharynx interfered with the transmission of sound energy into the nasal cavity, thus causing hyponasality on nasal sounds. The size of the tonsil also blocked the sound energy from entering the oral cavity, thus causing cul-de-sac resonance on oral sounds.

Given these findings, the obvious treatment was a tonsillectomy. Once this was done, resonance returned to normal, and nasal emission was no longer noted. Ellen was able to maintain a closed mouth posture, and snoring was no longer noted at night.

speech therapy (Guyette, Polley, Figueroa, & Smith, 2001; Kummer, Strife, Grau, Creaghead, & Lee, 1989; Lee, Whitehill, Ciocca, & Samman, 2002; Maegawa, Sells, & David, 1998; Mason, Turvey, & Warren, 1980; McCarthy, Coccaro, & Schwartz, 1979; Trindade, Yamashita, Suguimoto, Mazzottini, & Trindade, 2003; Vallino, 1990; Ward, McAuliffe, Holmes, Lynham, & Monsour, 2002). Finally, by increasing the nasal cavity space, maxillary advancement can reduce or eliminate nasal obstruction or hyponasality, which is common in these patients (Jakobsone, Stenvik, & Espeland, 2011; Pourdanesh, Sharifi, Mohebbi, & Jamilian, 2012).

Although maxillary advancement results in many benefits for the patient, moving the maxilla forward also moves the velum forward. This can therefore cause the development or worsening of velopharyngeal insufficiency (Haapanen, Kalland, Heliovaara, Hukki, & Ranta, 1997; Heliovaara, Hukki, Ranta, & Haapanen, 2004; Heliovaara, Ranta, Hukki, & Haapanen, 2002; Janulewicz et al., 2004; Kummer et al., 1989; Maegawa et al., 1998; Mason et al., 1980; Niemeyer, Gomes Ade, Fukushiro, & Genaro, 2005; Okazaki et al., 1993;

Satoh et al., 2004). The effect on the velopharyngeal valve can even occur when maxillary advancement is done gradually with distraction (Chanchareonsook, Whitehill, & Samman, 2007; Guyette et al., 2001; Ko, Figueroa, Guyette, Polley, & Law, 1999; Nohara, Tachimura, & Wada, 2006; Satoh et al., 2004; Trindade et al., 2003).

Although the exact risk of velopharyngeal insufficiency following maxillary advancement is not known, it is not a common occurrence in individuals with no history of cleft palate or velar abnormality. In these cases, the velopharyngeal mechanism adapts to the changes through velar stretch (Kummer et al., 1989). Those at greatest risk following maxillary advancement are the individuals who can usually benefit the most from the procedure, such as patients with cleft lip and palate (Haapanen et al., 1997; Janulewicz et al., 2004; Kummer et al., 1989; Maegawa et al., 1998; Mason et al., 1980; McCarthy et al., 1979; Okazaki et al., 1993). The risk appears to be somewhat related to scarring of the velum (which limits velar stretch), tenuous closure preoperatively, and the amount of advancement (Maegawa et al., 1998; Phillips, Klaiman, Delorey, & MacDonald,

2005). If speech and velopharyngeal function deteriorate after maxillary advancement, secondary surgery for velopharyngeal insufficiency is recommended.

Treatment of Oral, Nasal, and Pharyngeal Cavity Tumors

Oral, nasal, and pharyngeal cavity tumors occur in both children and adults. In children, the most common tumor is a hemangioma, which is a congenital anomaly in which a proliferation of blood vessels results in a large mass. In adults, malignant tumors of the oral cavity are more commonly seen.

When a tumor or growth interferes with function or becomes life threatening, it is usually treated by resection (surgical removal). Resections of areas of the oral cavity can affect the integrity of the separation of the nasal and oral cavities and the function of the velopharyngeal valve (Bodin, Lind, & Arnander, 1994; Brown, Zuydam, Jones, Rogers, & Vaughan, 1997; Myers & Aramany, 1977; Yoshida, Michi, Yamashita, & Ohno, 1993). This is particularly a concern if tissue is taken from the hard palate, velum, or pharyngeal walls.

The use of radiation for oral or pharyngeal tumors can also affect the function of the velopharyngeal valve. Radiation can cause shrinkage of not just the tumor but also the adjacent structures, including the velum and pharyngeal walls. When this occurs, surgical correction is usually not possible because of the tissue damage. Therefore, prosthetic intervention is often used (see the chapter *Surgical Management*).

Velopharyngeal Incompetence

Velopharyngeal incompetence refers to a neurophysiological disorder that results in poor movement of the velopharyngeal structures. Velopharyngeal incompetence is characterized by poor elevation and inadequate "knee action" of the velum during speech (see Figure 10-5B). On lateral videofluoroscopy, the velum often appears to be below the level of the hard palate during speech, and the velar eminence (high point of the velum as it bends) is not significant. Lateral pharyngeal wall motion may also be very poor so that there is minimal medial movement to assist with closure.

Velopharyngeal incompetence can be caused by traumatic brain injury, cerebral palsy, cerebral vascular accident (CVA), a neuromuscular disease (e.g., muscular dystrophy, myasthenia gravis, myotonic dystrophy, and neurofibromatosis), or cranial nerve damage. Velopharyngeal incompetence is often associated with hypotonia, dysarthria, and apraxia of speech. The causes and associations of velopharyngeal incompetence are further discussed as follows.

Hypotonia

Hypotonia is a state of low muscle tonicity and sometimes reduced muscle strength. It is caused by diseases or disorders of the brain that affect motor neuron control or muscle strength. Generalized hypotonia can impair the strength and consistency of movement of the entire velopharyngeal valve, including the pharyngeal walls. Hypotonia affecting velopharyngeal function is a common characteristic of velocardiofacial/22q11.2 deletion syndrome.

Dysarthria

Dysarthria is an oral-motor disorder that can affect the subsystems of speech, including respiration, phonation, resonance, and articulation. It is characterized by abnormalities of strength, range of motion, speed, accuracy, and tonicity of the speech muscles due to central and/or peripheral nervous system impairment. Velopharyngeal incompetence causes many of the speech characteristics that are typical of dysarthria, including hypernasality, weak or omitted consonants, short utterance length, and decreased volume (Netsell, 1969; Vijayalakshmi & Reddy, 2006; Yorkston, Beukelman, & Traynor, 1988).

CASE REPORT

Hypernasality Secondary to Dysarthria

Brandon was a 20-year-old college student when he had a cerebral hemorrhage secondary to an arterial venous malformation (AVM). This affected his speech, swallowing, the movement of the right side of his body, his walking, and vision. Fortunately, there was no cognitive loss.

Almost a year after the stroke, Brandon was referred to our VPI Clinic for evaluation of velopharyngeal incompetence. He had been using a palatal lift (a prosthetic device), which was helpful, but he was interested in a more permanent solution.

At the time of the evaluation, Brandon was found to have normal articulation placement, but characteristics of dysarthria, including severe hypernasality, nasal emission that caused weak consonants and short utterance length, and slow rate. He complained about the extreme effort that speech required.

Nasopharyngoscopy showed inconsistent velar elevation, with occasional touch closure of the velum against the posterior pharyngeal wall at midline. The velum was noted to tire easily, however, and drop down inappropriately. There was also poor lateral pharyngeal wall motion.

Because Brandon no longer wanted to use a palatal lift, surgical intervention (specifically a pharyngeal flap) was offered as an option. Brandon was told that the goals of the surgery would be to improve the quality and clarity of speech, while decreasing his effort with speech. Brandon was counseled that although improvement could be expected, this would not result in normal speech. He was also informed of the potential risks of the surgery, including the possibility of airway obstruction and even sleep apnea. After weighing the potential risks and benefits, Brandon and his family decide to pursue the surgery.

Brandon was seen for a reassessment 6 weeks after placement of the pharyngeal flap. At that time, he demonstrated significantly improved speech. The hypernasality was reduced to a mild degree, and the nasal air emission was only slight. Of most significance was the increase in oral pressure and thus speech sound clarity and intensity. Because Brandon no longer needed to take frequent breaths to replenish lost airflow from nasal emission, his utterance length was much longer. In fact, he was able to count to 23 on one breath rather than to 4 as he had preoperatively.

Although the pharyngeal flap did not result in a total correction of speech, it did result in significant improvement in the quality and clarity of speech. It also made speech less effortful. Brandon and his family were very pleased with the result.

Apraxia of Speech

Apraxia of speech, called childhood apraxia of speech (CAS) when it affects speech development in children, is a motor speech disorder that causes difficulty executing, combining, and sequencing oral movements for speech. In addition to affecting the oral articulators (lips, tongue, and jaws), it can also affect the function of the velopharyngeal valve and voiced/voiceless contrasts (Bradley, 1997; Sealey & Giddens, 2010; Trost-Cardamone, 1989).

Apraxia makes it difficult for some affected individuals to coordinate oral articulation with velopharyngeal movement, especially in connected speech. As such, the velum may stay down inappropriately for oral sounds (causing hypernasality) and go up inappropriately for nasal sounds (causing hyponasality). The speaker may produce both correct and incorrect productions of each phoneme, even within a single utterance. The timing of velopharyngeal closure may also be affected so that closure does not occur until after the initiation of phonation, when it is too late (Warren, Dalston, & Mayo, 1993; Warren, Dalston, Trier, & Holder, 1985).

All errors, including those from velopharyngeal incompetence, tend to increase in severity with an increase in utterance length and phonemic complexity. With longer utterances, the velum may appear to pulse up and down erratically when viewed through nasopharyngoscopy. It may even stay down in a resting position because of difficulty coordinating velopharyngeal closure with anterior articulation of oral sounds. Therefore, although there will be mixed resonance with apraxia, the predominant feature, particularly in longer utterances, is hypernasality.

Velar Paralysis or Paresis

Individuals with either congenital or acquired lower motor neuron damage may demonstrate specific velopharyngeal paralysis or paresis (partial loss of movement or weakness) of the velum or pharyngeal musculature (Rousseaux, Lesoin, & Quint, 1987). This can occur with involvement of the glossopharyngeal nerve (CN IX), the vagus nerve (CN X), or the hypoglossal nerve (CN XII). The paralysis or paresis is usually unilateral and occurs on the ipsilateral side of the pharynx and velum and can occur in the absence of other oral-motor deficits.

A unilateral velar paralysis or paresis typically causes a unilateral velopharyngeal opening on the affected side. When this is observed from an intraoral perspective, the velum can be seen to droop on the affected side during phonation. On the other hand, the uvula will be noted to deviate to the unaffected side (Manasco, 2017). Unilateral paralysis or paresis of the velum is commonly observed in individuals with hemifacial microsomia (Tan & Chen, 2009).

Stress Incompetence and Velar Fatigue

Playing a wind instrument requires more intraoral air pressure and therefore more velopharyngeal strength and stamina than speech. Because of this, velopharyngeal incompetence sometimes occurs in musicians when playing wind instruments, even though they have no characteristics of velopharyngeal incompetence in speech (Bennett & Hoit, 2013; Conley, Beecher, & Marks, 1995; Evans, Driscoll, & Ackermann, 2011; Gordon, Astrachan, & Yanagisawa, 1994; Malick, Moon, & Canady, 2007; Raol, Diercks, Hersh, & Hartnick, 2015; Shanks, 1990). For professional musicians or students who wish to become professionals, this is more than a minor inconvenience. Stress velopharyngeal incompetence has also been noted with singers, particularly those with less experience. The opening that often occurs with stress incompetence can be small. However, this results in a loud nasal rustle, which is certainly unwanted when playing music.

Stress incompetence is evaluated through nasopharyngoscopy to determine the location of the opening and possible cause. Depending on the size, location, and cause of the opening, a prosthetic device (particularly a palatal lift) can be used. For a more permanent correction, surgical correction can be considered. If velar fatigue begins to occur during speech or if there is a gradual onset of hypernasality, the person should be monitored over a period of time because these symptoms may indicate the onset of a progressive neurological disorder.

Velopharyngeal Mislearning

Velopharyngeal mislearning is an articulation disorder (just like w/l, w/r, t/k, etc.) that includes the substitution of certain nasal or pharyngeal sounds for oral sounds. This placement results in an open velopharyngeal valve, causing nasal emission or hypernasality during the production of those particular speech sounds. Although the speech characteristics may sound just like those of individuals with velopharyngeal insufficiency or incompetence, individuals with velopharyngeal mislearning are not candidates for surgical or prosthetic intervention. Instead, speech therapy is successful in correcting these functional speech characteristics

(Kummer, 2011b). It is critically important to make a differential diagnosis between misarticulations caused by mislearning alone versus those caused by VPI so that the patient receives the appropriate treatment.

Compensatory Productions

Compensatory productions from VPI are a form of learned misarticulations. These compensatory productions continue after surgical correction of the VPI because the individual's articulation pattern has usually become habituated by the time this surgery is done. In addition, hypernasality and nasal emission may continue to persist until the patient learns to actually use the new structures. Because changing the structure does not change function, speech therapy is usually required to change those abnormal speech patterns once the structural defects have been corrected.

Other Learned Misarticulations

Learned misarticulations that are produced with the velopharyngeal valve open can occur in children with normal structures. These misarticulations will cause phoneme-specific nasal emission or phoneme-specific hypernasality on the misarticulated consonants (Kummer, 2011b).

Phoneme-specific nasal emission (PSNE) occurs when the individual uses a pharyngeal fricative or posterior nasal fricative as a substitution for oral fricatives (and sometimes affricates). As a result of the pharyngeal placement, nasal emission occurs on these misarticulated phonemes. PSNE occurs on sibilant sounds, particularly /s/ and /z/.

Phoneme-specific hypernasality occurs when the individual consistently substitutes a nasal sound for an oral sound (e.g., ŋ/l, ŋ/ɚ, ŋ/r). Phoneme-specific hypernasality can also occur on vowels, particularly high vowels, if the back of the tongue is too high during production (Falk & Kopp, 1968; Gibbon, Smeaton-Ewins, & Crampin,

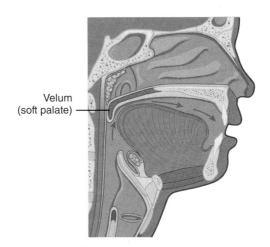

Velum
(soft palate)

FIGURE 10-19 High posterior tongue position, which can cause the perception of hypernasality on vowels.

2005) (**FIGURE 10-19**). Resonance is perceived as hypernasal on the high vowels from the increase in oral impedance (Karnell, Schultz, & Canady, 2001) and the increase in transpalatal transmission of the sound (Gildersleeve-Neumann & Dalston, 2001).

Abnormal Resonance from Hearing Loss or Deafness

Velopharyngeal function and modulation of resonance are learned through hearing, imitation, and auditory feedback. Because there is no visual or tactile–kinesthetic feedback for velopharyngeal movement, individuals with severe hearing impairment or deafness typically demonstrate abnormal resonance that can be a mixture of hypernasality, hyponasality, and cul-de-sac resonance (Abdullah, 1988; Baudonck, Van Lierde, D'Haeseleer, & Dhooge, 2015; Fletcher & Daly, 1976; Hassan et al., 2012; Subtelny, Whitehead, & Samar, 1992; Ysunza & Vazquez, 1993). Cochlear implants hold promise for not only increasing understanding of speech but also improving the resonance of oral speakers in the future.

SUMMARY

Both sound and airflow are important for normal speech production. Velopharyngeal dysfunction can affect the normal flow of sound and airflow during speech. Velopharyngeal dysfunction can be caused by abnormal structure (velopharyngeal insufficiency), abnormal neurophysiology (velopharyngeal incompetence), and even abnormal speech sound learning (velopharyngeal mislearning).

Velopharyngeal dysfunction, particularly both forms of VPI, can cause hypernasality and/or nasal emission. Inadequate oral airflow as a result of nasal emission can cause consonants to be weak in intensity and pressure. It can also cause the need to take frequent breaths during speech. Finally, compensatory productions (which are produced in the pharynx) may be used to compensate for the lack of adequate airflow for consonants.

Resonance disorders include hypernasality, hyponasality, cul-de-sac resonance, and mixed resonance. All are common in individuals with clefts or other craniofacial conditions. Although resonance disorders and VPI are not directly treated by the speech-language pathologist, it is important to make a differential diagnosis based on the speech characteristics and to determine the probable cause. This information is used to ensure that the individual receives appropriate treatment.

Speech therapy is never appropriate for the treatment of characteristics of VPI or for resonance disorders caused by abnormal structure. Instead, surgery or prosthetic management is indicated. Speech therapy is appropriate, however, for correction of compensatory errors secondary to VPI after the physical correction. In addition, speech therapy is appropriate for correction of phoneme-specific nasal emission or phoneme-specific hypernasality from abnormal articulation placement.

FOR REVIEW AND DISCUSSION

1. How does a resonating cavity affect sound? Discuss factors relating to the vocal tract that can alter resonance. Why is resonance primarily associated with vowels rather than consonants?

2. What is the role of airflow in the production of speech? What speech sounds are particularly dependent on airflow?

3. Define velopharyngeal dysfunction, velopharyngeal insufficiency, velopharyngeal incompetence, and velopharyngeal mislearning. How are they similar? How are they different? Why is it important to make a distinction between these types of velopharyngeal dysfunction?

4. Describe the difference between hypernasality and nasal emission during speech.

   What other speech characteristics can occur with significant nasal emission and why? Try to imitate these characteristics.

5. What is the difference between an obligatory distortion and a compensatory articulation error? Give examples of each. How are each treated?

6. What are some of the causes of dysphonia in children with either a history of cleft palate or other craniofacial conditions?

7. How does the size of the velopharyngeal opening affect speech characteristics? Why do you think it is important to understand this relationship?

8. Why is nasal emission inconsistent when there is a small velopharyngeal opening?

Why do you think this cannot be treated with speech therapy?

9. List some of the causes of velopharyngeal insufficiency, velopharyngeal incompetence, and velopharyngeal mislearning.

10. Describe the basic characteristics of hyponasality, hypernasality, cul-de-sac resonance, and mixed resonance. What are the possible causes of each? Try to imitate each type of abnormal resonance.

REFERENCES

Abdel-Aziz, M. (2012). Hypertrophied tonsils impair velopharyngeal function after palatoplasty. *The Laryngoscope, 122*(3), 528–532.

Abdullah, S. (1988). A study of the results of speech language and hearing assessment of three groups of repaired cleft palate children and adults. *Annals of the Academy of Medicine of Singapore, 17*(3), 388–391.

Adil, E., Huntley, C., Choudhary, A., & Carr, M. (2011). Congenital nasal obstruction: Clinical and radiologic review. *European Journal of Pediatrics, 171*(4), 641–650.

American Cleft Palate–Craniofacial Association (ACPA). (n.d.). Retrieved from http://acpa-cpf.org/education/speech-samples/.

Andreassen, M. L., Leeper, H. A., & MacRae, D. L. (1991). Changes in vocal resonance and nasalization following adenoidectomy in normal children: Preliminary findings. *Journal of Otolaryngology, 20*(4), 237–242.

Awan, S. N., Omlor, K., & Watts, C. R. (2011). Effects of computer system and vowel loading on measures of nasalance. *Journal of Speech Language Hearing Research, 54*(5), 1284–1294.

Baudonck, N., Van Lierde, K., D'Haeseleer, E., & Dhooge, I. (2015). Nasalance and nasality in children with cochlear implants and children with hearing aids. *International Journal of Pediatric Otorhinolaryngology, 79*(4), 541–545.

Bennett, K., & Hoit, J. D. (2013). Stress velopharyngeal incompetence (SVPI) in collegiate trombone players. *The Cleft Palate–Craniofacial Journal, 50*(4), 338–393.

Bernthal, J. E., & Beukelman, D. R. (1977). The effect of changes in velopharyngeal orifice area on vowel intensity. *Cleft Palate Journal, 14*(1), 63–77.

Bispo, N. H., Whitaker, M. E., Aferri, H. C., Neves, J. D., Dutka Jde, C., & Pegoraro-Krook, M. I. (2011). Speech therapy for compensatory articulations and velopharyngeal function: A case report. *Journal of Applied Oral Science, 19*(6), 679–684.

Bodin, I. K., Lind, M. G., & Arnander, C. (1994). Free radial forearm flap reconstruction in surgery of the oral cavity and pharynx: Surgical complications, impairment of speech and swallowing. *Clinics in Otolaryngology, 19*(1), 28–34.

Bradley, D. P. (1997). Congenital and acquired velopharyngeal inadequacy. In K. R. Bzoch (Ed.), *Communicative disorders related to cleft lip and palate* (vol. 4, pp. 223–243). Austin, TX: Pro-Ed.

Brown, J. S., Zuydam, A. C., Jones, D. C., Rogers, S. N., & Vaughan, E. D. (1997). Functional outcome in soft palate reconstruction using a radial forearm free flap in conjunction with a superiorly based pharyngeal flap. *Head & Neck, 19*(6), 524–534.

Buder, E. H. (2005). The acoustics of nasality: Steps towards a bridge to source literature. *Perspectives on Speech Science and Orofacial Disorders, 15*(1), 9–14.

Cassassolles, S., Paulus, C., Ajacques, J. C., Berger-Vachon, C., Laurent, M., & Perrin, E. (1995). Acoustic characterization of velar insufficiency in young children. *Revue de Stomatologie et de Chirurgie Maxillofaciale, 96*(1), 13–20.

Chanchareonsook, N., Whitehill, T. L., & Samman, N. (2007). Speech outcome and velopharyngeal function in cleft palate: Comparison of Le Fort I maxillary osteotomy and distraction osteogenesis: Early results. *The Cleft Palate–Craniofacial Journal, 44*(1), 23–32.

Conley, S. F., Beecher, R. B., & Marks, S. (1995). Stress velopharyngeal incompetence in an adolescent trumpet player. *Annals of Otology, Rhinology and Laryngology, 104*(9, Pt. 1), 715–717.

Croft, C. B., Shprintzen, R. J., & Ruben, R. J. (1981). Hypernasal speech following adenotonsillectomy. *Otolaryngology-Head & Neck Surgery, 89*(2), 179–188.

D'Antonio, L. L., Muntz, H. R., Province, M. A., & Marsh, J. L. (1988). Laryngeal/voice findings in patients with velopharyngeal dysfunction. *Laryngoscope, 98*(4), 432–438.

de Serres, L. M., Deleyiannis, F. W., Eblen, L. E., Gruss, J. S., Richardson, M. A., & Sie, K. C. (1999). Results with sphincter pharyngoplasty and pharyngeal flap. *International Journal of Pediatric Otorhinolaryngology, 48*(1), 17–25.

Dickson, D. R. (1972). Normal and cleft palate anatomy. *Cleft Palate Journal, 9,* 280–293.

Donnelly, M. J. (1994). Hypernasality following adenoid removal. *Irish Journal of Medical Science, 163*(5), 225–227.

Evans, A., Driscoll, T., & Ackermann, B. (2011). Prevalence of velopharyngeal insufficiency in woodwind and brass students. *Occupational Medicine Journal (London), 61*(7), 480–482.

Falk, M. L., & Kopp, G. A. (1968). Tongue position and hypernasality in cleft palate speech. *Cleft Palate Journal, 5*(3), 228–237.

Fernandes, D. B., Grobbelaar, A. O., Hudson, D. A., & Lentin, R. (1996). Velopharyngeal incompetence after adenotonsillectomy in noncleft patients. *British Journal of Oral and Maxillofacial Surgery, 34*(5), 364–367.

Finkelstein, Y., Bar-Ziv, J., Nachmani, A., Berger, G., & Ophir, D. (1993). Peritonsillar abscess as a cause of transient velopharyngeal insufficiency. *The Cleft Palate–Craniofacial Journal, 30*(4), 421–428.

Finkelstein, Y., Nachmani, A., & Ophir, D. (1994). The functional role of the tonsils in speech. *Archives of Otolaryngology-Head & Neck Surgery, 120*(8), 846–851.

Finkelstein, Y., Wexler, D. B., Nachmani, A., & Ophir, D. (2002). Endoscopic partial adenoidectomy for children with submucous cleft palate. *The Cleft Palate–Craniofacial Journal, 39*(5), 479–486.

Fletcher, S. G., & Daly, D. A. (1976). Nasalance in utterances of hearing-impaired speakers. *Journal of Communication Disorders, 9*(1), 63–73.

Folkins, J. W. (1988). Velopharyngeal nomenclature: Incompetence, inadequacy, insufficiency, and dysfunction. *Cleft Palate Journal, 25*(4), 413–416.

Gibbon, F., Smeaton-Ewins, P., & Crampin, L. (2005). Tongue-palate contact during selected vowels in children with cleft palate. *Folia Phoniatrica Logopaedica, 57*(4), 181–192.

Gibbon, F. E., Ellis, L., & Crampin, L. (2004). Articulatory placement for /t/, /d/, /k/ and /g/ targets in school age children with speech disorders associated with cleft palate. *Clinical Linguistic and Phonetics, 18*(6–8), 391–404.

Gildersleeve-Neumann, C. E., & Dalston, R. M. (2001). Nasalance scores in noncleft individuals: Why not zero? *The Cleft Palate–Craniofacial Journal, 38*(2), 106–111.

Glade, R. S., & Deal, R. (2016). Diagnosis and management of velopharyngeal dysfunction. *Oral and Maxillofacial Surgery Clinics of North America, 28*(2), 181–188.

Gordon, N. A., Astrachan, D., & Yanagisawa, E. (1994). Videoendoscopic diagnosis and correction of velopharyngeal stress incompetence in a bassoonist. *Annals of Otology, Rhinology and Laryngology, 103*(8, Pt. 1), 595–600.

Gosain, A. K., & Hettinger, P. C. (2009). Submucous cleft palate. In J. E. Lossee & R. E. Kirschner (Eds.), *Comprehensive cleft care* (pp. 361–369). New York, NY: McGraw-Hill.

Guyette, T. W., Polley, J. W., Figueroa, A., & Smith, B. E. (2001). Changes in speech following maxillary distraction osteogenesis. *The Cleft Palate–Craniofacial Journal, 38*(3), 199–205.

Haapanen, M. L., Heliovaara, A., & Ranta, R. (1991). Hypernasality and the nasopharyngeal space. A cephalometric study. *Journal of Craniomaxillofacial Surgery, 19*(2), 77–80.

Haapanen, M. L., Ignatius, J., Rihkanen, H., & Ertama, L. (1994). Velopharyngeal insufficiency following palatine tonsillectomy. *European Archives of Oto-Rhino-Laryngology, 251*(3), 186–189.

Haapanen, M. L., Kalland, M., Heliovaara, A., Hukki, J., & Ranta, R. (1997). Velopharyngeal function in cleft patients undergoing maxillary advancement. *Folia Phoniatrica et Logopedica, 49*(1), 42–47.

Hall, C. D., Golding-Kushner, K. J., Argamaso, R. V., & Strauch, B. (1991). Pharyngeal flap surgery in adults. *The Cleft Palate–Craniofacial Journal, 28*(2), 179–182; discussion 182–183.

Harding, A., & Grunwell, P. (1996). Characteristics of cleft palate speech. *European Journal of Disorders of Communication, 31*(4), 331–357.

Harding, A., & Grunwell, P. (1998). Active versus passive cleft-type speech characteristics. *International Journal of Language and Communication Disorders, 33*(3), 329–352.

Hassan, S. M., Malki, K. H., Mesallam, T. A., Farahat, M., Bukhari, M., & Murry, T. (2012). The effect of cochlear implantation on nasalance of speech in postlingually hearing-impaired adults. *Journal of Voice, 26*(5), 669.e18–669.e22.

Heliovaara, A., Hukki, J., Ranta, R., & Haapanen, M. L. (2004). Cephalometric pharyngeal changes after Le Fort I osteotomy in different types of clefts. *Scandinavian Journal of Plastic and Reconstructive Surgery and Hand Surgery, 38*(1), 5–10.

Heliovaara, A., Ranta, R., Hukki, J., & Haapanen, M. L. (2002). Cephalometric pharyngeal changes after Le Fort I osteotomy in patients with unilateral cleft lip and palate. *Acta Odontologica Scandinavica, 60*(3), 141–145.

Henningsson, G., & Isberg, A. (1988). Influence of tonsils on velopharyngeal movements in children with craniofacial anomalies and hypernasality. *American Journal of Orthodontics and Dentofacial Orthopedics, 94*(3), 253–261.

Hiiemae, K. M., & Palmer, J. B. (2003). Tongue movements in feeding and speech. *Critical Reviews in Oral Biology & Medicine, 14*(6), 413–429.

Huber, J. E., & Stathopoulos, E. T. (2003). Respiratory and laryngeal responses to an oral air pressure bleed during speech. *Journal of Speech Language Hearing Research, 46*(5), 1207–1220.

Ikeda, T., Matsuzaki, Y., & Aomatsu, T. (2001). A numerical analysis of phonation using a two-dimensional flexible channel model of the vocal folds. *Journal of Biomechanical Engineering, 123*(6), 571–579.

Jakobsone, G., Stenvik, A., & Espeland, L. (2011). The effect of maxillary advancement and impaction on the upper airway after bimaxillary surgery to correct Class III malocclusion. *American Journal of Orthodontics and Dentofacial Orthopedics, 139*(4 Suppl.), e369–e376.

Janulewicz, J., Costello, B. J., Buckley, M. J., Ford, M. D., Close, R., & Gassner, R. (2004). The effects of Le Fort I osteotomies on velopharyngeal and speech functions in cleft palate patients. *Journal of Oral and Maxillofacial Surgery, 62*(3), 308–314.

Jones, D. L. (1991). Velopharyngeal function and dysfunction. *Clinics in Communication Disorders, 1*(3), 19–25.

Jones, D. L. (2005). Perceptual aspects of nasality. *Perspectives on Speech Science and Orofacial Disorders, 15*(1), 9–14.

Karnell, M. P., Schultz, K., & Canady, J. (2001). Investigations of a pressure-sensitive theory of marginal velopharyngeal inadequacy. *The Cleft Palate-Craniofacial Journal, 38*(4), 346–357.

Ko, E. W., Figueroa, A. A., Guyette, T. W., Polley, J. W., & Law, W. R. (1999). Velopharyngeal changes after maxillary advancement in cleft patients with distraction osteogenesis using a rigid external distraction device: A 1-year cephalometric follow-up. *Journal of Craniofacial Surgery, 10*(4), 312–320; discussion 321–322.

Kummer, A. W. (2011a). Disorders of resonance and airflow secondary to cleft palate and/or velopharyngeal dysfunction. *Seminars in Speech and Language, 32*(2), 141–149.

Kummer, A. W. (2011b). Types and causes of velopharyngeal dysfunction. *Seminars in Speech and Language, 32*(2), 150–158.

Kummer, A. W., Billmire, D. A., & Myer, C. M., III. (1993). Hypertrophic tonsils: The effect on resonance and velopharyngeal closure. *Plastic and Reconstructive Surgery, 91*(4), 608–611.

Kummer, A. W., Briggs, M., & Lee, L. (2003). The relationship between the characteristics of speech and velopharyngeal gap size. *The Cleft Palate-Craniofacial Journal, 40*(6), 590–596.

Kummer, A. W., Curtis, C., Wiggs, M., Lee, L., & Strife, J. L. (1992). Comparison of velopharyngeal gap size in patients with hypernasality, hypernasality and nasal emission, or nasal turbulence (rustle) as the primary speech characteristic. *The Cleft Palate-Craniofacial Journal, 29*(2), 152–156.

Kummer, A. W., Marshall, J., & Wilson, M. (2015). Non-cleft causes of velopharyngeal dysfunction: Implications for treatment. *International Journal of Pediatric Otorhinolaryngology, 79*(3), 286–295.

Kummer, A. W., Myer, C. M. L., Smith, M. E., & Shott, S. R. (1993). Changes in nasal resonance secondary to adenotonsillectomy. *American Journal of Otolaryngology, 14*(4), 285–290.

Kummer, A. W., Strife, J. L., Grau, W. H., Creaghead, N. A., & Lee, L. (1989). The effects of Le Fort I osteotomy with maxillary movement on articulation, resonance, and velopharyngeal function. *Cleft Palate Journal, 26*(3), 193–199.

Lee, A. S., Whitehill, T. L., Ciocca, V., & Samman, N. (2002). Acoustic and perceptual analysis of the sibilant sound /s/ before and after orthognathic surgery. *Journal of Oral and Maxillofacial Surgery, 60*(4), 364–372; discussion 364–372.

Lee, G. S., Wang, C. P., & Fu, S. (2009). Evaluation of hypernasality in vowels using voice low tone to high tone ratio. *The Cleft Palate-Craniofacial Journal, 46*(1), 47–52.

Leveau-Geffroy, S., Perrin, J. P., Khonsari, R. H., & Mercier, J. (2011). Cephalometric study of the velo-cardiofacial syndrome: Impact of dysmorphosis on phonation. *Revue de Stomatologie et de Chirurgie Maxillofaciale, 112*(1), 11–15.

Loney, R. W., & Bloem, T. J. (1987). Velopharyngeal dysfunction: Recommendations for use of nomenclature. *Cleft Palate Journal, 24*(4), 334–335.

MacKenzie-Stepner, K., Witzel, M. A., Stringer, D. A., & Laskin, R. (1987). Velopharyngeal insufficiency due to hypertrophic tonsils. A report of two cases. *International Journal of Pediatric Otorhinolaryngology, 14*(1), 57–63.

Maclean, J. E., Waters, K., Fitzsimons, D., Hayward, P., & Fitzgerald, D. A. (2009). Screening for obstructive sleep apnea in preschool children with cleft palate. *The Cleft Palate–Craniofacial Journal, 46*(2), 117–123.

Maegawa, J., Sells, R. K., & David, D. J. (1998). Speech changes after maxillary advancement in 40 cleft lip and palate patients. *Journal of Craniofacial Surgery, 9*(2), 177–182; discussion 183–184.

Malick, D., Moon, J., & Canady, J. (2007). Stress velopharyngeal incompetence: Prevalence, treatment, and management practices. *The Cleft Palate–Craniofacial Journal, 44*(4), 424–433.

Manasco, M. H. (2017). Motor speech disorders: The dysarthrias. In *Introduction to neurogenic communication disorders* (2nd ed., pp. 220–221). Burlington, MA: Jones & Bartlett Learning.

Marsh, J. L. (1991). Cleft palate and velopharyngeal dysfunction. *Clinics in Communication Disorders, 1*(3), 29–34.

Maryn, Y., Van Lierde, K., De Bodt, M., & Van Cauwenberge, P. (2004). The effects of adenoidectomy and tonsillectomy on speech and nasal resonance. *Folia Phoniatrica Logopaedica, 56*(3), 182–191.

Mason, R., Turvey, T. A., & Warren, D. W. (1980). Speech considerations with maxillary advancement procedures. *Journal of Oral Surgery, 38*(10), 752–758.

Mason, R. M., & Grandstaff, H. L. (1971). Evaluating the velopharyngeal mechanism in hypernasal speakers. *Language, Speech, and Hearing Services in the Schools, 2*(4), 53–61.

Mason, R. M., & Warren, D. W. (1980). Adenoid involution and developing hypernasality in cleft palate. *Journal of Speech and Hearing Disorders, 45*(4), 469–480.

McCarthy, J. G., Coccaro, P. J., & Schwartz, M. D. (1979). Velopharyngeal function following maxillary advancement. *Plastic and Reconstructive Surgery, 64*(2), 180–189.

McHenry, M. A. (1997). The effect of increased vocal effort on estimated velopharyngeal orifice area. *American Journal of Speech-Language Pathology, 6*(4), 55–61.

McWilliams, B. J. (1991). Submucous clefts of the palate: How likely are they to be symptomatic? *The Cleft Palate–Craniofacial Journal, 28*(3), 247–249; discussion 250–251.

McWilliams, B. J., Lavorato, A. S., & Bluestone, C. D. (1973). Vocal cord abnormalities in children with velopharyngeal valving problems. *Laryngoscope, 83,* 1745.

Morris, H. L. (1992). Some questions and answers about velopharyngeal dysfunction during speech. *American Journal of Speech-Language Pathology, 1*(3), 26–28.

Morris, H. L., Wroblewski, S. K., Brown, C. K., & Van Demark, D. R. (1990). Velarpharyngeal status in cleft palate patients with expected adenoidal involution. *Annals of Otology, Rhinology, and Laryngology, 99*(6, Pt. 1), 432–437.

Muntz, H., Wilson, M., Park, A., Smith, M., & Grimmer, J. F. (2008). Sleep disordered breathing and obstructive sleep apnea in the cleft population. *The Laryngoscope, 118*(2), 348–353.

Myers, E. N., & Aramany, M. A. (1977). Rehabilitation of the oral cavity following resection of the hard and soft palate. *Transactions of the American Academy of Ophthalmology and Otolaryngology, 84*(5), 941–951.

Naran, S., Ford, M., & Losee, J. E. (2017). What's new in cleft palate and velopharyngeal dysfunction management? *Plastic and Reconstructive Surgery, 139*(6), 1343e–1355e.

Neiman, G. S., & Simpson, R. K. (1975). A roentgen-cephalometric investigation of the effect of adenoid removal upon selected measures of velopharyngeal function. *Cleft Palate Journal, 12,* 377–389.

Netsell, R. (1969). Evaluation of velopharyngeal function in dysarthria. *Journal of Speech and Hearing Disorders, 34*(2), 113–122.

Netsell, R. (1988). Velopharyngeal dysfunction. In D. Yoder & R. Kent (Eds.), *Decision-making in speech-language pathology* (pp. 150–151). Toronto: B. C. Decker.

Niemeyer, T. C., Gomes Ade, O., Fukushiro, A. P., & Genaro, K. F. (2005). Speech resonance in orthognathic surgery in subjects with cleft lip and palate. *Journal of Applied Oral Science, 13*(3), 232–236.

Nohara, K., Tachimura, T., & Wada, T. (2006). Prediction of deterioration of velopharyngeal function associated with maxillary advancement using electromyography of levator veli palatini muscle. *The Cleft Palate–Craniofacial Journal, 43*(2), 174–178.

Ogar, J., Willock, S., Baldo, J., Wilkins, D., Ludy, C., & Dronkers, N. (2006). Clinical and anatomical correlates of apraxia of speech. *Brain and Language, 97*(3), 343–350.

Okazaki, K., Satoh, K., Kato, M., Iwanami, M., Ohokubo, F., & Kobayashi, K. (1993). Speech and velopharyngeal function following maxillary advancement in patients with cleft lip and palate. *Annals of Plastic Surgery, 30*(4), 304–311.

Parton, M. J., & Jones, A. S. (1998). Hypernasality following adenoidectomy: A significant and avoidable complication. *Clinical Otolaryngology, 23*(1), 18–19.

Penfold, C. N. (1997). Management of velopharyngeal dysfunction. *British Journal of Oral and Maxillofacial Surgery, 35*(6), 454.

Phillips, J. H., Klaiman, P., Delorey, R., & MacDonald, D. B. (2005). Predictors of velopharyngeal insufficiency in cleft palate orthognathic surgery. *Plastic Reconstructive Surgery, 115*(3), 681–686.

Pourdanesh, F., Sharifi, R., Mohebbi, A., & Jamilian, A. (2012). Effects of maxillary advancement and impact on nasal airway function. *International Journal of Oral and Maxillofacial Surgery, 41*(11), 1350–1352.

Proctor, M. I., Shadle, C. H., & Iskarous, K. (2010). Pharyngeal articulation in the production of voiced and voiceless fricatives. *Journal of the Acoustical Society of America, 127*(3), 1507–1518.

Raol, N., Diercks, G., Hersh, C., & Hartnick, C. J. (2015). Stress velopharyngeal incompetence: Two case reports and options for diagnosis and management. *International Journal of Otorhinolaryngology, 79*, 2456–2459.

Ren, Y. F., Isberg, A., & Henningsson, G. (1995). Velopharyngeal incompetence and persistent hypernasality after adenoidectomy in children without palatal defect. *The Cleft Palate–Craniofacial Journal, 32*(6), 476–482.

Riski, J. E., & Verdolini, K. (1999). Is hypernasality a voice disorder? *ASHA, 41*(1), 10–11.

Robinson, J. H. (1992). Association between adenoidectomy, velopharyngeal incompetence, and submucous cleft. *The Cleft Palate–Craniofacial Journal, 29*(4), 385.

Robison, J. G., & Otteson, T. D. (2011a). Increased prevalence of obstructive sleep apnea in patients with cleft palate. *Archives of Otolaryngology-Head & Neck Surgery, 137*(3), 269–274.

Robison, J. G., & Otteson, T. D. (2011b). Prevalence of hoarseness in the cleft palate population. *Archives of Otolaryngology-Head & Neck Surgery, 137*(1), 74–77.

Rousseaux, M., Lesoin, F., & Quint, S. (1987). Unilateral pseudobulbar syndrome with limited capsulothalamic infarction. *European Neurology, 27*(4), 227–230.

Sabashi, K., Washino, K., Saitoh, I., Yamasaki, Y., Kawabata, A., Mukai, Y., & Kitai, N. (2011). Nasal obstruction causes a decrease in lip-closing force. *Angle Orthodontist, 81*(5), 750–753.

Satoh, K., Nagata, J., Shomura, K., Wada, T., Tachimura, T., Fukuda, J., & Shiba, R. (2004). Morphological evaluation of changes in velopharyngeal function following maxillary distraction in patients with repaired cleft palate during mixed dentition. *The Cleft Palate–Craniofacial Journal, 41*(4), 355–363.

Saunders, N. C., Hartley, B. E., Sell, D., & Sommerlad, B. (2004). Velopharyngeal insufficiency following adenoidectomy. *Clinical Otolaryngology & Allied Sciences, 29*(6), 686–688.

Schmaman, L., Jordaan, H., & Jammine, G. H. (1998). Risk factors for permanent hypernasality after adenoidectomy. *South African Medical Journal, 88*(3), 266–269.

Scott, A. R., Moldan, M. M., Tibesar, R. J., Lander, T. A., & Sidman, J. D. (2011). A theoretical cause of nasal obstruction in patients with repaired cleft palate. *American Journal of Rhinology and Allergy, 25*(1), 58–60.

Sealey, L. R., & Giddens, C. L. (2010). Aerodynamic indices of velopharyngeal function in childhood apraxia of speech. *Clinical Linguistics & Phonetics, 24*(6), 417–430.

Seid, A. B. (1990). Velopharyngeal insufficiency versus adenoidectomy for obstructive apnea: A quandary. *Cleft Palate Journal, 27*(2), 200–202.

Shanks, J. C. (1990). Velopharyngeal incompetence manifested initially in playing a musical instrument. *Journal of Voice, 4*(2), 169–171.

Shapiro, R. S. (1980). Velopharyngeal insufficiency starting at puberty without adenoidectomy. *International Journal of Pediatric Otorhinolaryngology, 2*(3), 255–260.

Shprintzen, R. J., Sher, A. E., & Croft, C. B. (1987). Hypernasal speech caused by tonsillar hypertrophy. *International Journal of Pediatric Otorhinolaryngology, 14*(1), 45–56.

Siegel-Sadewitz, V. L., & Shprintzen, R. J. (1986). Changes in velopharyngeal valving with age. *International Journal of Pediatric Otorhinolaryngology, 11*(2), 171–182.

Smith, B. E., & Kuehn, D. P. (2007). Speech evaluation of velopharyngeal dysfunction. *The Journal of Craniofacial Surgery, 18*(2), 251–261.

Stewart, K. J., Ahmad, R. E., Razzell, R. E., & Watson, A. C. H. (2002). Altered speech following adenoidectomy: A 20-year experience. *British Journal of Plastic Surgery, 55,* 469–473.

Story, B. H., Titze, I. R., & Hoffman, E. A. (2001). The relationship of vocal tract shape to three voice qualities. *Journal of the Acoustical Society of America, 109*(4), 1651–1667.

Subtelny, J. D., Whitehead, R. L., & Samar, V. J. (1992). Spectral study of deviant resonance in the speech of women who are deaf. *Journal of Speech & Hearing Research, 35*(3), 574–579.

Tan, Y. C., & Chen, P. K. (2009). Hemipalatal hypoplasia. *The Journal of Craniofacial Surgery, 20*(4), 1150–1153.

Titze, I. R. (2000). *Principles of voice production* (2nd ed.). Iowa City, IA: National Center for Voice and Speech.

Titze, I. R., Bergan, C. C., Hunter, E. J., & Story, B. (2003). Source and filter adjustments affecting the perception of the vocal qualities twang and yawn. *Logopedics, Phoniatrics, Vocology, 28*(4), 147–155.

Tom, K., Titze, I. R., Hoffman, E. A., & Story, B. H. (2001). Three-dimensional vocal tract imaging and formant structure: Varying vocal register, pitch, and loudness. *Journal of the Acoustical Society of America, 109*(2), 742–747.

Trindade, I. E., Yamashita, R. P., Suguimoto, R. M., Mazzottini, R., & Trindade, A. S., Jr. (2003). Effects of orthognathic surgery on speech and breathing of subjects with cleft lip and palate: Acoustic and aerodynamic assessment. *The Cleft Palate–Craniofacial Journal, 40*(1), 54–64.

Trost, J. E. (1981). Articulatory additions to the classical description of the speech of persons with cleft palate. *Cleft Palate Journal, 18*(3), 193–203.

Trost-Cardamone, J. E. (1989). Coming to terms with VPI: A response to Loney and Bloem. *Cleft Palate Journal, 26*(1), 68–70.

Trost-Cardamone, J. E. (1990). Speech in the first year of life: A perspective on early acquisition. In D. E. Kernahan & S. W. Rosenstein (Eds.), *Cleft lip and palate: A system of management* (pp. 91–103). Baltimore, MA: Williams & Wilkins.

Trost-Cardamone, J. E. (1997). Diagnosis of specific cleft palate speech error patterns for planning therapy of physical management needs. In K. R. Bzoch (Ed.), *Communicative disorders related to cleft lip and palate* (vol. 4, pp. 313–330). Austin, TX: Pro-Ed.

Vallino, L. D. (1990). Speech, velopharyngeal function, and hearing before and after orthognathic surgery. *Journal of Oral & Maxillofacial Surgery, 48*(12), 1274–1281.

Vijayalakshmi, P., & Reddy, M. R. (2006). Assessment of dysarthric speech and an analysis on velopharyngeal incompetence. Conference Proceedings. *IEEE English Medical and Biological Society, 1,* 3759–3762.

Ward, E. C., McAuliffe, M., Holmes, S. K., Lynham, A., & Monsour, F. (2002). Impact of malocclusion and orthognathic reconstruction surgery on resonance and articulatory function: An examination of variability in five cases. *British Journal of Oral Maxillofacial Surgery, 40*(5), 410–417.

Warren, D. W., Dalston, R. M., & Mayo, R. (1993). Hypernasality in the presence of "adequate" velopharyngeal closure. *The Cleft Palate–Craniofacial Journal, 30*(2), 150–154.

Warren, D. W., Dalston, R. M., Trier, W. C., & Holder, M. B. (1985). A pressure-flow technique for quantifying temporal patterns of palatopharyngeal closure. *Cleft Palate Journal, 22*(1), 11–19.

Witt, P. D. (2009). Velopharyngeal dysfunction. In J. E. Lossee & R. E. Kirschner (Eds.), *Comprehensive Cleft Care* (pp. 627–640). New York, NY: McGraw-Hill.

Witt, P. D., O'Daniel, T. G., Marsh, J. L., Grames, L. M., Muntz, H. R., & Pilgram, T. K. (1997). Surgical management of velopharyngeal dysfunction: Outcome analysis of autogenous posterior pharyngeal wall augmentation. *Plastic and Reconstructive Surgery, 99*(5), 1287–1296; discussion 1297–1300.

Witzel, M. A., Rich, R. H., Margar-Bacal, F., & Cox, C. (1986). Velopharyngeal insufficiency after adenoidectomy: An 8-year review. *International Journal of Pediatric Otorhinolaryngology, 11*(1), 15–20.

Yanagisawa, E., Estill, J., Mambrino, L., & Talkin, D. (1991). Supraglottic contributions to pitch raising. Videoendoscopic study with spectroanalysis. *Annals of Otolology, Rhinolology, and Laryngology, 100*(1), 19–30.

Yanagisawa, E., Kmucha, S. T., & Estill, J. (1990). Role of the soft palate in laryngeal functions and selected voice qualities. Simultaneous velolaryngeal videoendoscopy. *Annals of Otology, Rhinology, and Laryngology, 99*(1), 18–28. (Erratum published 1990, *Annals of Otology, Rhinology, and Laryngology, 99*(6, Pt. 1), p. 431)

Yorkston, K. M., Beukelman, D. R., & Traynor, C. D. (1988). Articulatory adequacy in dysarthric speakers: A comparison of judging formats. *Journal of Communication Disorders, 21*(4), 351–361.

Yoshida, H., Michi, K., Yamashita, Y., & Ohno, K. (1993). A comparison of surgical and prosthetic treatment for speech disorders attributable to surgically acquired soft palate defects. *Journal of Oral and Maxillofacial Surgery, 51*(4), 361–365.

Ysunza, A., & Vazquez, M. C. (1993). Velopharyngeal sphincter physiology in deaf individuals. *The Cleft Palate–Craniofacial Journal, 30*(2), 141–143.

CREDITS

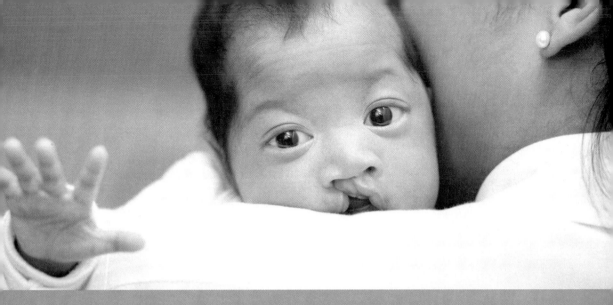

PART 3

Assessment Procedures: Speech, Resonance, and Velopharyngeal Function

CHAPTER 11

Speech and Resonance Assessment

CHAPTER OUTLINE

INTRODUCTION

Children with a cleft lip/palate or other craniofacial conditions are at risk for different types of communication disorders. If the child has a cleft of the primary palate, there is a risk of dental or occlusal abnormalities that can interfere with speech. If the child has a cleft of the secondary palate, there is a risk of velopharyngeal insufficiency that can affect speech and resonance. If the child has a craniofacial syndrome, there is a risk for neurological dysfunction that can affect language and cognition. Overall, the structural anomalies that are typical of cleft and craniofacial conditions can cause problems in the areas of speech sound production, resonance, phonation, and even language at different times in development.

The evaluation of speech, resonance, phonation, and velopharyngeal function begins with a perceptual evaluation. The purpose of the perceptual evaluation is to determine whether there is an abnormality that affects the quality and/or intelligibility of speech. It is also important to determine whether there are any characteristics of velopharyngeal dysfunction, such as hypernasality, nasal air emission, or compensatory articulation productions. When evaluating resonance and velopharyngeal function in particular, the knowledge and experience of the speech-language pathologist can make a difference between a correct and incorrect diagnosis (Smith & Kuehn, 2007).

The goal of the perceptual evaluation is to determine whether there is a disorder and, subsequently, the type, severity, and possible cause (Kummer, 2016; Kummer, 2018). Based on the results of the evaluation, further assessment may be indicated using instrumental procedures. The ultimate goal of the evaluation is to obtain enough information regarding the disorder to be able to make appropriate recommendations for treatment.

The purpose of this chapter is to review the perceptual evaluation process for individuals who have a history of cleft lip/palate, other craniofacial anomalies, suspected velopharyngeal dysfunction, or a resonance disorder from other causes. This chapter provides practical suggestions for an efficient and effective assessment of speech sound production and resonance. The focus of this chapter is on the perceptual assessment of velopharyngeal function, which is done by a speech-language pathologist. It should be noted that the evaluation and management of velopharyngeal insufficiency/incompetence (VPI) should be done in the context of a multidisciplinary team (Glade & Deal, 2016; Naran, Ford, & Losee, 2017).

Timetable for Assessment

Because children with clefts and other craniofacial conditions are at high risk for various communication disorders, speech-language evaluations should occur often enough so that issues are identified promptly and treatment can be initiated in a timely manner (American Cleft Palate–Craniofacial Association [ACPA], 2009). Information from the speech-language evaluation is also needed by the cleft/craniofacial team because it can affect surgical and dental management.

First Year

The first year of a child's life is usually a time of great joy for the parents. When the infant has a congenital anomaly, however, there is also significant anxiety over what will happen in the future and the ultimate results of treatment. Most people cope best with information rather than with uncertainty. Therefore, the parents should be counseled by various professionals, preferably by members of a cleft palate team, soon after the child's birth and again early in the first year. These professionals should explain the implication of the diagnosis or condition, the potential effect of the anomalies on function, what might happen in the future, the tentative treatment plan, and the ultimate prognosis.

During the child's first year, the primary speech-language pathology concerns are feeding, the development of the prerequisites for speech (i.e., cooing and babbling), and language development. The family should be assisted with feeding modifications as necessary. They should also be given written instructions on speech and language stimulation for before and after the palate repair. It should be emphasized that under the age of 3, language development should be the primary focus. In other words, the quantity of speech is more important than the quality of speech during those early years. The infant's development should be monitored through parent report, direct observation, or the use of infant scales. If problems in development are noted, further assessment and intervention should be initiated immediately.

Annual Screenings and Periodic Evaluations

From the age of 3 to the early school years, children are typically seen by the cleft/craniofacial team annually. At that time, a speech screening is usually done. If issues are noted, additional testing may be recommended.

In addition to the regular screenings, a comprehensive evaluation of speech, resonance, and informal assessment of language development should be done between age 3 and 4. At this age, the child is usually communicating with connected speech and at least attempting to produce a variety of speech sounds. This is important to obtain an accurate evaluation of velopharyngeal function. In addition, if the evaluation shows evidence of velopharyngeal insufficiency, the child should be big enough at this age to have corrective surgery without serious concerns for the airway. If the child's speech development and expressive language skills are delayed or if there are upper airway concerns, the assessment of resonance and velopharyngeal function should be done at a later time.

A perceptual assessment, along with instrumental measures, should always be done before recommending VPI surgery (e.g., pharyngeal flap or sphincter pharyngoplasty). A 3-month postoperative evaluation should also be done to determine the outcome of the VPI surgery and develop a follow-up treatment plan. Finally, an evaluation is sometimes needed after an adenoidectomy or maxillary advancement if there has been a noticeable change in speech (Pannbacker & Middleton, 1990; Smith & Guyette, 2004).

The Diagnostic Interview

Whether doing a comprehensive evaluation or merely a screening evaluation in a cleft palate clinic, the examiner can obtain valuable information from the family regarding the child's overall communication abilities (Hirschberg & Van Demark, 1997). Therefore, the speech pathology evaluation is usually preceded by an interview with the parent or other family members.

Many clinics send the family a pre-evaluation questionnaire to obtain medical and development history and to determine the current concerns about speech. This information helps the examiner to prepare for the evaluation and can shorten the interview process. However, even if background information was received through a questionnaire or medical record, at least a brief interview should be done before the formal assessment. Examples of interview questions for pediatric patients can be found in **TABLE 11-1**.

Parents are usually very good observers of their children and can often effectively compare their child's communication skills with those of siblings or peers. Therefore, a simple rule of thumb is as follows: If the parents are worried about their child's speech, there probably is a good reason (Glascoe, 1991).

Language Screening

Because children with cleft palate or craniofacial syndromes are at risk for language delay, it is important that their language development be closely monitored throughout the preschool years. This can be done through screenings at the time of the yearly visits to the cleft palate/craniofacial team. If language problems are suspected from the screening or the parents express concerns about their child's language development, a comprehensive language evaluation is warranted. A comprehensive language evaluation should routinely be done for children who have additional risk factors for language disorders (i.e., hearing loss, developmental delay, or neurological problems). If a language disorder is identified, intervention should be initiated as soon as possible to ensure the best outcome.

The methods for language evaluation are beyond the scope of this chapter. Instead, the

TABLE 11-1 **Sample Questions for Parents**

Following are a few questions that can be used to obtain diagnostic information. Questions should be selected based on the child's age and developmental level.

Current Concern

- What concerns you about your child's speech?
- When did you first become concerned?
- Who referred your child for the evaluation, and what was that person's concern?

Speech Production

- What types of sounds does your child use during vocal play—vowels only or some consonants?
- If the child uses consonants, what are some of the consonants that you hear?
- Are the consonants produced individually or in repetitive syllables?
- Does your child "jabber" or use jargon?
- Does your child leave out sounds in words?
- Do you understand your child's speech all of the time, most of the time, some of the time, or hardly at all?
- How well do strangers understand your child's speech?
- Are there any particular speech sounds that are difficult for your child to produce?

Resonance

- Does your child sound nasal? If so, does it sound like your child is talking through her nose, or does it sound like she is stopped up or has a cold?
- Do you ever hear air coming through her nose during speech?
- Do you ever hear a bubbling sound or snorting during speech?
- When did you first notice the problem with nasality?
- If the onset was sudden, what event preceded it?
- Has your child had an adenoidectomy? If so, did it change her speech?
- Does your child's speech vary with the weather, allergies, fatigue, or any other factors?

Language

- Does your child communicate with gestures, single words, short phrases, incomplete sentences, or complete sentences?
- How many words does your child usually put together in an utterance?
- Does your child leave out the little words (e.g., "of," "to," "the," or "is") in sentences?
- Is your child communicating as well as other children her age?
- Have you ever had a concern about how well your child understands the speech of others or follows directions?

Medical History

- Was your child born with any congenital problems? If so, what were they? How and when were they treated?
- Does your child have any medical problems, medical diagnoses, or conditions?
- What surgeries has your child undergone?
- Does your child take any medications on a regular basis?
- Does your child hear normally? When was the last hearing test?
- Has your child had many ear infections? If so, how were they treated?
- Does your child have any problems with vision?
- Where is your child on the growth chart?

Developmental History

- Was your child quiet, about average, or very vocal as an infant?
- Did you have any concerns about initial speech development?
- Did your child begin to use words before or after her first birthday?
- When your child was learning to sit up, stand, and walk, did she seem normal or behind other children?
- Did your child walk before or after her first birthday?

- Does your child have any difficulty learning in preschool or school?
- Does your child have any problems with fine motor or gross motor skills?

Feeding and Oral-Motor Skills
- Does your child have any difficulty chewing, sucking, or swallowing?
- Did your child have any feeding problems as an infant?
- Does your child ever have liquid come out of her nose or food in her nose?
- Does your child drool or keep her mouth open during the day?

Airway
- Does your child snore at night?
- Does your child ever gasp for breath at night or sleep restlessly?
- Is your child hard to wake up in the morning?
- Does your child seem rested or tired during the day?
- Does your child like to breathe through her nose or through her mouth during the day?
- Is your child's breathing ever noisy during the day?
- Does your child have allergies, asthma, or chronic congestion?

Treatment History
- Has your child ever had a speech-language evaluation or therapy?
- Is your child currently receiving therapy? If yes, what are the goals?
- Has your child's speech improved in the past 6 months? If so, in what way?
- Has your child ever had occupational or physical therapy?

interested reader should consult one of the many books available on this subject. However, a discussion regarding screening methods may be helpful, particularly as they apply to a clinic setting.

There are several formal screening tests that allow the examiner to sample the child's communication abilities using a more structured format. Screening tests for children under the age of 3 include the *Receptive-Expressive Emergent Language Test* (REEL-3), 3rd edition (Bzoch, League, & Brown, 2003); the *Early Language Milestone* (ELM) Scale-2, 2nd edition (Coplan, 1993); and *The Rossetti Infant-Toddler Language Scale* (Rossetti, 2006). These tests are scored through direct observation and parent report. For children between the ages of 2 and 6, the *Fluharty-2 Preschool Speech and Language Screening Test*, 2nd edition (Fluharty, 2000), can be used to screen both articulation and language development. Other preschool language tests include the *Clinical Evaluation of Language Fundamentals® Preschool*, 5th edition (CELF-P®-5) (Semel, Wiig, & Secord, 2013), and the *Preschool Language Scales*, 5th edition (PLS™-5) (Zimmerman, Steiner, & Pond, 2011).

Although formal screening tests provide structure and a set format, they are not always necessary for language screening. In fact, most experienced examiners can determine whether a child's language is close to age level through a combination of the parent interview and/or questionnaire, observations of the child, and informal testing (Scherer & D'Antonio, 1997). The use of parent questionnaires alone has been found to be a valid means of screening language development compared with other methods (Scherer & D'Antonio, 1995). The questions must be understandable enough for the parents to answer with confidence and detailed enough to be of value to the examiner.

An informal language screening assessment can be done by these means:

- Observe play behaviors and the type and complexity of gestures and spontaneous utterances.
- Have interesting toys available and observe spontaneous vocalizations and utterances.
- Listen to the child's spontaneous speech while he is talking to the parent.

TABLE 11-2 Sample Questions to Elicit Language and Speech	
Either/Or Questions	**Open-Ended Questions**
What do you like best? • Puppy dogs or kitty cats? • Baby dolls or teddy bears? • Singing or dancing? • Cupcakes or cookies? • Vanilla ice cream or chocolate ice cream? • Baseball or basketball? • Playing inside or outside? What do you do in a chair? Sit or stand? What do you wear on your foot? A shirt or a shoe? What do you like to eat? Cheese or a chair?	What do you want to be when you grow up? Why? What does a fireman do? What does a policeman do? What does a teacher do? How do you make a peanut butter and jelly sandwich? What do you like to do when you are playing outside? What are your favorite animals?

- Ask the child to point to certain objects or follow certain commands.
- Ask simple either/or questions to get the child talking.
- Once the child is talking, ask questions that do not require a yes/no answer. In particular, ask for descriptions or explanations (see TABLE 11-2).
- Have the child repeat sentences, such as those listed in the articulation screening test (see Table 11-3). Have the child repeat sentences of increasing complexity. Even in repeating, the child will usually revert to his own form of syntax and morphology, which gives an indication of expressive language abilities.

Through these simple methods, the examiner should be able to determine the primary method of communication (e.g., gestures, signs, single words, short utterances, short sentences, or complete sentences). If the child is communicating with sentences, the examiner should also be able to determine whether the sentences are complete or merely telegraphic, the approximate mean length of utterance (MLU), and whether there are errors of syntax and morphology. Overall, the behaviors of the child, as noted through observation and parent report, can be compared to norms to estimate the child's developmental level and determine whether formal language testing is necessary.

Speech Assessment

The most important tool that we have to assess speech, resonance, and voice is the "examiner's ear" (Smith & Kuehn, 2007). In fact, in a survey of speech-language pathologists and cleft palate surgeons in the United States, 99.2% of the 126 respondents who were associated with a cleft palate team reported that they always include a perceptual assessment in the assessment of VPI (Kummer, Clark, Redle, Thomsen, & Billmire, 2011).

As part of the perceptual evaluation, the examiner should determine whether speech sound production is affected by abnormal structure (e.g., velopharyngeal insufficiency or dental malocclusion) versus abnormal function. This determination is particularly important because it affects the treatment plan (Kummer, 2011; Kummer, 2016; Kummer, 2018).

In addition to assessing speech sound production, the ear is used to analyze the acoustic product of velopharyngeal function to make inferences about the function of the velopharyngeal valve. With thorough analysis of what is perceived, a determination can be made regarding the status of velopharyngeal function and its potential for change. If there is no abnormality, as judged by a perceptual evaluation, then it does not matter what the instrumental procedures show. It is only when the perceptual evaluation shows an abnormality that treatment is ever initiated (Trindade, Genaro, Yamashita, Miguel, & Fukushiro, 2005).

Finally, the perceptual evaluation should include a judgment of phonation. This is important because dysphonia is often found in children with cleft palate or craniofacial syndromes from congenital abnormalities and acquired conditions, such as vocal nodules.

Some children are naturally loquacious, and little or no effort is needed to elicit spontaneous connected speech. These children will cooperate for the speech assessment by repeating whatever is asked. Other children need some prodding. In fact, anyone who works with young children knows that if a child does not want to talk, you can't make that child talk. Instead, you have to find ways to make the child want to talk.

If the child refuses to talk or repeat what you ask, a great technique to get the child talking is to ask either/or questions (see Table 11-2). Children are much more likely to respond to an either/or question than an open-ended one or a request to repeat. If the child doesn't answer the question at first, say what you like better, and then move on to the next question. Once the child is responding to the either/or questions, then gradually begin asking the child to repeat the test speech samples. If the child still refuses to repeat, do an informal assessment of all speech sounds through either/or questions only. If the child will not answer the questions, ask the parent to try to elicit words or conversation from the child while you pretend to do something else.

Speech Samples

During the assessment, it is important to select an appropriate speech sample to obtain the information that is needed for a definitive diagnosis. When testing a child, the speech sample must be developmentally appropriate in the areas of speech sound production and syntax.

Formal Articulation Tests

There are several formal articulation tests that can be used for assessment of speech production. Although a formal articulation test with single words is a popular method to assess speech sound accuracy, there are many disadvantages to the use of a single word test. The disadvantages include the following:

- Some children are able to produce a sound at the single-word level but not in connected speech, where there is an increase in utterance length and phonemic complexity. Therefore, single words are not a good representation of the child's actual speech abilities.
- Single-word tests are designed to assess each phoneme in one word position rather than many words in connected speech.
- The test phoneme may be affected by the phonemic context of the word. For example, the word "window" is not appropriate for testing medial /d/ because the /n/ sound (a continuant with the same placement) is just before it.
- The tests and test forms are expensive, which increases the ultimate cost of care.
- Single-word articulation tests that involve naming pictures are time consuming to administer, increase costs, negatively affect net revenue, and decrease access to care. This is a particular issue considering the changes in healthcare financing, waiting lists for services, and large caseload sizes.

In comparison to single-word articulation tests, tests that involve repetition, particularly repetition of sentences, provide better diagnostic information and are actually more valid in representing normal speech production (Hirschberg & Van Demark, 1997). In addition, they take less time to complete and there is nothing to purchase.

The following sections describe how repetition can be used in the assessment of speech sound production and even nasal emission, resonance, and phonation.

Single Sounds

If the child has limited connected speech or the examiner wants to isolate specific phonemes for assessment, the child should be asked to repeat single sounds or single syllables. Vowels, voiced continuants (for example, /v/ and /z/), and voiceless consonants can be produced in isolation. Voiced plosives and the voiced affricate (e.g., /bɑ, bi, dɑ, di, gɑ, gi, dʒɑ, dʒi/) can be produced only with a vowel. By having the child attempt to imitate all speech sounds in isolation or in syllables, the examiner can determine the child's ability to achieve appropriate speech sound placement at this basic level.

Imitation of isolated phonemes can also be used to test resonance and determine whether there is nasal emission. To test for hypernasality, prolongation of a vowel should be used, because vowels are purely resonance sounds. Comparing resonance between a low vowel (e.g., /ɑ/) and a high vowel (e.g., /i/) can help determine there is consistent hypernasality on all vowels, or whether it occurs only on the high vowel. To test for nasal emission, a pressure-sensitive consonant should be used. The best consonant for this purpose is /s/ because it is voiceless and also a continuant, so it requires sustained airflow. If hyponasality or cul-de-sac resonance is suspected, prolongation of the /m/ sound is a good test. With the lips totally closed, the sound has to travel through the pharynx and nasal cavity. If there is obstruction in either cavity, prolongation of the /m/ will be noticeably difficult.

Syllable Repetition

Instead of using a formal test of articulation, an informal test using syllable repetition can be done. This test is faster and cheaper and provides more diagnostic information than a standard articulation test.

In the syllable repetition test, the child is asked to produce syllables repetitively to assess each speech sound individually (i.e., /pɑ, pɑ, pɑ, pɑ, pɑ, pɑ, pɑ/). The initial position of the sound is always tested with these syllables. With repetition, the sound is also placed in a medial position. Although not always necessary, the final position can also

be tested through syllable repetition by having the child repeat syllables where the vowel precedes the consonant (i.e., /ɑp, ɑp, ɑp, ɑp, ɑp, ɑp, ɑp/).

One diagnostic advantage of the syllable repetition test is that it allows the examiner to assess one consonant and one vowel at a time and eliminates the effects of other contiguous consonant sounds. This makes it easier for the examiner to identify specific speech sound errors. In addition, certain syllables can be selected to test for nasal emission on consonants or hypernasality on vowels. Rapid repetition of syllables has an additional advantage in that it may uncover evidence of oral-motor dysfunction (e.g., childhood apraxia of speech).

To test for nasal emission, the child is asked to repeat syllables with high-pressure consonants (plosives, fricatives, and affricates) where the consonant is voiceless (e.g., /pɑ, pɑ, pɑ/, /pi, pi, pi/, /tɑ, tɑ, tɑ/, /ti, ti, ti/). The voiceless phoneme is used rather than its voiced cognate because nasal emission is easier to hear when there is no phonation. In addition, voiceless consonants have a higher amount of airflow than their voiced cognates (where the vocal folds attenuate the flow), and therefore, audible nasal emission is more likely to occur on these sounds.

Each of the pressure-sensitive phonemes should be tested with a low vowel (such as /ɑ/) and then again with a high vowel (such as /i/). This type of test allows the examiner to assess not only articulation placement and the presence of nasal emission on each individual consonant, but it also allows the examiner to determine whether hypernasality occurs on all vowels or is specific to high vowels only (Kummer, 2009; Kummer, 2011; Kummer, 2016; Lee, Wang, & Fu, 2009).

Sentence Repetition

To test speech and resonance in connected speech (and to also obtain some clues regarding expressive language), the examiner should have a battery of sentences for the child to repeat. A sample list of sentences for evaluation of articulation placement in addition to characteristics of velopharyngeal function can be found in **TABLE 11-3**.

TABLE 11-3	**Sample Sentences for Assessment of Speech Sound Production and Velopharyngeal Function**
Have the child repeat the following sentences:	
p	Popeye plays in the pool.
b	Buy baby a bib.
m	My mommy made lemonade.
w	Wade in the water.
j	You have a yellow yo-yo.
h	He has a big horse.
t	Take Teddy to town.
d	Do it for Daddy.
n	Nancy is not here.
k	I eat cake and cookies.
g	Go get the wagon.
ŋ	Put the ring on her finger.
f	Fred has five fish.
v	Drive a van.
1	I like yellow lollipops.
s	I see the sun in the sky.
z	Zip up your zipper.
ʃ	She went shopping.
tʃ	I ride a choo-choo train.
ʤ	John told a joke to Jim.
r	Randy has a red fire truck.
ɚ	The teacher and doctor are here.
θ	Thank you for the toothbrush.
blends	splash, sprinkle, street

Each sentence should contain phonemes that are similar in articulatory placement (e.g., "Take Teddy to town"). When evaluating for nasal emission, the sample should contain many pressure-sensitive consonants, particularly those that are voiceless (e.g., "I see the sun in the sky"). When testing for hypernasality, the sample should contain voiced oral sounds (e.g., "Buy baby a bib"). To make it even easier to test for hypernasality, the examiner can separate out the effects of nasal air emission or compensatory errors by using a sample of sentences with a large number of low-pressure consonants (e.g., "How are you?"). Sample sentences can be found in TABLE 11-4. Finally, to test for hyponasality, the examiner should use sentences with a high frequency of nasal phonemes (e.g., "My mama made lemonade for me"). Sample nasal sentences can also be found in TABLE 11-5.

By asking the child to repeat these sentences, the examiner can quickly and easily test for articulation errors, abnormal resonance, and nasal emission in a connected speech environment. The examiner can also determine whether there is consistent or inconsistent nasal emission in connected speech.

TABLE 11-4	**Sample Sentences for Evaluation of Hypernasality**
Have the child repeat the following sentences:	
How are you?	
Who are you?	
Where are you?	
Why are you here?	
You are here.	
They are here.	
Where are they?	
They are where you are.	

TABLE 11-5 Sample Sentences for Evaluation of Hyponasality
Have the child repeat the following sentences:
My mom made lemonade.
My name is Amy Minor.
My mom makes money at the market.
Many men are at the mine.
Ned made nine points in the game.
My nanny is not mean.
Nan needs a dime to call home.
My mom's home is many miles away.
Many men are moving the piano.

Counting

Connected speech can often be elicited from a young child by having him count or recite the alphabet. Counting from 60 to 70 or simply repeating "60, 60, 60, 60" can be particularly informative because these numbers contain a combination of a high vowel (/i/), the sibilant /s/, plosives, and even a triple blend (/kst/). This combination of sounds requires a continuation of intraoral airflow for /s/ and a buildup of air pressure for the plosives. This can particularly tax the velopharyngeal mechanism and may overwhelm a tenuous velopharyngeal valve. Counting from 70 to 79 can be diagnostic because this series contains a nasal phoneme (/n/) followed by an alveolar plosive. (The /t/ in 70 is usually pronounced as /d/ in American English). This speech sample can uncover timing issues (usually associated with apraxia) with opening and closing the velopharyngeal valve. If there are concerns regarding hyponasality, counting from 90 to 99 allows the examiner to assess the production of the nasal /n/ in connected speech.

Connected Speech

Although a single-word test helps the examiner isolate the production of individual phonemes, it is important to assess articulation and particularly resonance in connected speech. Connected speech increases the demands on the velopharyngeal valving system to achieve and maintain closure. As a result, hypernasality and nasal emission are more apparent in connected speech than in single words. An increase in articulation errors is also common during the production of continuous utterances. Connected speech can be spontaneous, or the examiner can ask the child to repeat syllables or sentences over and over to simulate connected speech.

What to Evaluate

Children with clefts or craniofacial conditions often have disorders of speech sound production, resonance, and voice. Thus, these areas should be the focus of an evaluation. For children under the age of 6, a screening of language should also be done, with further in-depth assessment as needed.

Speech Sound Production

When assessing articulation, the examiner analyzes the placement of each speech sound to determine whether there are speech sound substitutions, omissions, or distortions. The examiner also decides whether there are any phonological patterns to the errors and whether any of the errors are purely developmental in nature considering the child's age. When there are structural anomalies that have the potential to affect speech, the examiner must determine whether there are any obligatory distortions or compensatory errors as a result. If the child is at risk for VPI, the examiner must also observe whether there is nasal emission during the production of pressure-sensitive phonemes or nasalization of voiced oral consonants. All of this information is used as a basis for determining appropriate treatment.

As noted previously, an obligatory distortion occurs when the articulation placement (the function) is normal, but the structural abnormality causes distortion of speech sound. For example, when there is a large velopharyngeal opening, the placement of articulation may be normal, but the manner of production is altered from oral to nasal because of the lack of velopharyngeal closure. As a result, voiced plosives may sound closer to their nasal cognates (m/b, n/d, and ŋ/g). These nasal sounds for oral sounds are not actual substitutions, but are obligatory distortions because articulation placement is normal. Whenever nasal phonemes are primarily heard with connected speech, the examiner should suspect VPI as the cause. Nasal emission on consonants, despite normal articulation placement, is another type of obligatory distortion.

Compensatory articulation errors are common in individuals with a VPI, particularly when the velopharyngeal opening is large enough to cause significant nasal emission of the airstream. When compensatory errors occur as a result of VPI, the manner of production is usually maintained (e.g., a plosive is substituted with another plosive, and a fricative is substituted with another fricative). However, the placement of production is moved posteriorly to the pharynx, where there is airflow. In other cases, the placement is similar, but the manner is changed to a voiced nasal sound. For example, if the child cannot build up pressure for an /s/ sound or other sibilants, a compensation may be to produce an /n/ (which has a similar placement) instead. A description of various compensatory errors is found in the chapter *Speech/ Resonance Disorders and Velopharyngeal Dysfunction* and therefore will not be repeated here.

Some compensatory productions can be co-articulated with the normal oral sound. For example, plosives can be produced with normal placement in the oral cavity but co-articulated with a glottal stop (/ʔ/) for the "plosion." Fricatives and affricates (particularly sibilants) can be co-articulated with a pharyngeal or posterior nasal fricative for the "friction."

To determine the true placement of the sound, the examiner should listen carefully and if necessary try to imitate the sound. By imitating the production, the examiner can usually determine the place of production and thus identify the cause of the error. The examiner should also watch the production of each phoneme. Glottal stops, for example, result in exaggerated laryngeal movements that can be seen and felt on the patient's neck during articulation.

If the patient is using glottal stops for consonants, without co-articulating the oral placement, this may be confused with a simple consonant omission. To make a distinction between a glottal stop and a true omission, it should be remembered that glottal stops are produced with a rapid voice onset (like a grunt). If the phoneme is completely omitted, the voice onset is smooth with the initiation of the vowel, and the vowel is longer in duration than if the consonant is substituted by a glottal stop. A final clue to the production of glottal stops is the observation of increased laryngeal activity that can be seen and felt in the throat area.

A pharyngeal fricative can sound similar to a lateral lisp to an inexperienced listener. To make this distinction, the examiner should determine whether the airstream is in the oral or pharyngeal area. This is easily done by closing the child's nose during production. If the sound stops, then it is being produced in the pharynx.

The scoring of an articulation test is traditionally done by using phonetic diacritics from the International Phonetic Alphabet (IPA) (Bronsted et al., 1994). However, this system does not include symbols for compensatory productions that are typical of individuals with velopharyngeal dysfunction. Therefore, a set of diacritic symbols for compensatory productions has been proposed by Trost-Cardamone (Trost, 1981; Trost-Cardamone, 1997). The examiner may choose to use these diacritics or just the words (e.g., glottal stop, pharyngeal fricative) to describe the errors (which would actually enhance communication with those who are unfamiliar with these symbols).

Childhood apraxia of speech (CAS) is often found in children with craniofacial syndromes that affect neurodevelopment, such as velocardiofacial/22q11.2 deletion syndrome (VCFS/22q deletion syndrome) (Kummer, Lee, Stutz, Maroney, & Brandt, 2007). Apraxia can cause a severe speech sound disorder. It can also cause inconsistent hypernasality or mixed resonance caused by the difficulty in coordinating the movements of the velopharyngeal valve during speech. With apraxia, placement errors and errors of velopharyngeal closure tend to increase with an increase in utterance length or phonemic complexity.

There are several formal tests of apraxia that go from a nonspeech oral level to the sentence level of speech production (Hickman, 1997; Kaufman, 1995). Apraxia can also be tested informally by using the diadochokinetic exercises, which involve having the child rapidly repeat various two-syllable and three-syllable combinations, using the /p/, /t/, and /k/ sounds (e.g., /pʌtʌ, pʌtʌ, pʌtʌ/ and /pʌtʌkʌ, pʌtʌkʌ, pʌtʌkʌ, pʌtʌkʌ/). Additionally, the child can be asked to produce difficult multisyllabic words repetitively (e.g., baseball bat, kitty cat, puppy dog, teddy bear, patty cake, basketball, ice cream cone). To determine whether there is apraxia in the presence of VPI, the examiner should use words with nasal sounds (e.g., "money," "mommy," "many more"). If the examiner finds that the child can produce individual sounds accurately but struggles to produce sounds in various combinations, CAS should be strongly suspected.

Stimulability is the ability to correct an abnormal speech sound production when given minimal cues. Stimulability is a good prognostic indicator for whether a speech sound can be corrected with speech therapy and how quickly. An assessment of stimulability is an important component of the perceptual evaluation of resonance and velopharyngeal function. This is because some compensatory placement errors actually *cause* nasal emission and even hypernasality. For example, the production of a glottal stop, pharyngeal fricative, or nasal fricative is done with the velopharyngeal valve open (Henningsson & Isberg, 1991; Moller, 1991). Therefore, the examiner should determine whether the child is stimulable for elimination of nasal emission or hypernasality with a correction of articulatory placement. If the child is able to produce the sound without nasal air emission or hypernasality merely by changing placement, then the problem is functional, and hence, there is a good prognosis for correction with speech therapy.

Nasal Emission

As part of the articulation assessment, the speech-language pathologist should assess for the presence of audible nasal emission of the airstream. If present, it is important to determine whether the nasal emission is low in intensity, which is usually the result of a larger velopharyngeal opening, or is the "bubbly" nasal rustle (also known as turbulence), which is the result of a small opening (Kummer, Briggs, & Lee, 2003; Kummer, Curtis, Wiggs, Lee, & Strife, 1992). The examiner should also note the occurrence of a nasal snort, which is produced most often with /s/ blends. A nasal grimace commonly accompanies nasal air emission, and this should be reported if it is observed.

The consistency of the nasal air emission should be noted during the articulation test. If nasal emission typically occurs during the production of all pressure-sensitive phonemes, including plosives, then it is considered consistent. If it occurs occasionally on most pressure-sensitive phonemes, then it is inconsistent. If it occurs consistently but only on specific phonemes, such as sibilants, then it may be phoneme-specific nasal emission (PSNE), which is related to faulty articulation rather than VPI. In particular, the production of pharyngeal fricatives or posterior nasal fricatives results in PSNE because the airflow is in the pharynx and therefore can be released only through the nose.

It is always important to assess for nasal air emission in connected speech. Many patients are able to achieve velopharyngeal closure for short segments, and therefore nasal emission may not be noted, even at the sentence level. Because connected speech increases the demands on the velopharyngeal mechanism, nasal air emission is more likely to be noted at this level. At times, it is necessary to ask the patient to produce difficult or multisyllabic words (e.g., "60," "basketball") quickly and repetitively to try to tax the velopharyngeal mechanism to determine whether there is tenuous closure.

Nasal emission reduces the volume of airflow available in the oral cavity for speech, thus causing the consonants to be weak in intensity and pressure. The adequacy of intraoral airflow for the production of plosives, fricatives, and affricates should be noted by having the child repeat sentences loaded with these pressure-sensitive phonemes. If these consonants seem to be weak,

CASE REPORT

Velocardiofacial/22q11.2 Deletion Syndrome and Apraxia of Speech

Maddie, age 3 years 10 months, had a diagnosis of velocardiofacial/22q11.2 deletion syndrome (VCFS/22q deletion syndrome). Medical history included a submucous cleft, a ventricular septal defect (VSD), and an interrupted aortic valve. Maddie was very small for her age, staying consistently under the 10th percentile for both weight and height. She had airway problems as an infant. Early feeding problems were also reported, and Maddie continued to have difficulty with certain textures. According to the parents, Maddie's development of gross motor milestones was essentially within normal limits, and her understanding of language seemed normal. However, fine motor skills were abnormal, and speech development was delayed.

An assessment revealed that Maddie could put words together and even sing nursery rhymes. However, her speech was mostly unintelligible. She communicated primarily with gestures and signs. She had a limited phonemic repertoire consisting of only nasal consonants (/m/, /n/), glottal sounds (/h/, glottal stops), and vowels. Occasionally, she was able to produce a /d/ approximation. Vowels were on target most of the time.

Although Maddie was able to produce nasal sounds in isolation, she was unable to produce them in certain word positions or with certain vowels. She was also unable to combine them for words such as "mommy," "money," "naming," or "many." When attempting to imitate oral pressure sounds or blow, there was only nasal air emission.

Given all this information gathered in the evaluation, it was determined that Maddie had significant VPI complicated by significant oral-motor dysfunction (childhood apraxia of speech).

Recommendations include surgical intervention for correction of the VPI. However, given her age, size, and history of airway obstruction, it was decided to delay the surgery for a few months until she was a little bigger. In the meantime, speech therapy, with active involvement of the parents, was recommended to improve articulation placement and the ability to combine different articulation positions, starting with the nasal sounds. This was done with the help of a nose clip both during therapy and at home.

it might be assumed that intraoral airflow is compromised because of nasal emission (which is probably inaudible). Inaudible nasal emission and weak consonants occur with hypernasality and are caused by a large velopharyngeal opening.

The leak of airflow through the nose also causes the speaker to take more frequent breaths to replenish the airflow. This shortens utterance length. To test utterance length, the examiner should observe the phrasing of utterances in connected speech. Utterance length can also be tested by asking the child to count to 20 and noting when he takes another breath. Most normal speakers will count at least to 15 on one breath.

Resonance

When evaluating resonance, the examiner should first determine whether it is normal or abnormal by listening to connected speech. If resonance is found to be abnormal, the examiner should determine the type of abnormal resonance (e.g., hypernasal, hyponasal, cul-de-sac, or mixed). The type of resonance is important to determine because it will give clues as to the causation, which has implications for treatment (Kummer, 2009; Kummer, 2011; Kummer, 2016). As a general rule, if nasal sounds are heard more frequently than normal or are substituted for oral sounds, the resonance is hypernasal. On the other hand, if oral sounds are heard as a substitution for nasal sounds, the resonance is hyponasal. If necessary, the examiner can have the individual repeat sentences loaded with oral sounds and then repeat sentences loaded with nasal sounds if the type of resonance is hard to determine in spontaneous speech. Cul-de-sac resonance sounds as if the voice is muffled and remains in the head. Mouth breathing or a history of upper airway obstruction may suggest either hyponasality or cul-de-sac resonance. Finally, mixed resonance occurs when there is hypernasality on oral sounds and hyponasality on nasal sounds. This is usually very inconsistent when it occurs.

Determining the type of resonance is very important, but determining the severity is usually irrelevant. This is because severity of the resonance doesn't affect the treatment (Bzoch, 1979). Even if there is mild hypernasality from VPI, physical management will be required for treatment. Despite this, several authors have suggested the use of an equal-appearing interval scale to rate the severity of deviant resonance with up to seven levels (McWilliams, Morris, & Shelton, 1990; Subtelny, Van Hattum, & Myers, 1972). Although these rating scales have a high degree of face validity, the reliability of these scales continues to be questioned. In fact, the more levels on the scale, the less reliable the scale will be. In addition, the severity of hypernasality in a patient who has VPI is usually inconsistent because it depends on many factors, including utterance length, the speed of production, and effort versus fatigue. If the examiner wants to rate severity, however, it may be best to use a simple four-point scale that includes normal, mild, moderate, and severe as descriptors.

Hypernasality can be phoneme-specific, occurring only on the high vowel /i/. This occurs if the patient holds the back of the tongue up too high during production of this vowel. This can be determined by asking the child to produce syllables with the /i/ vowel and then syllables with the /ɑ/ vowel.

Phonation

Dysphonia is common in individuals with VPI or craniofacial syndromes. Dysphonia may be caused by congenital anomalies of the larynx or vocal folds or acquired conditions, such as vocal nodules (McWilliams, Lavorato, & Bluestone, 1973; McWilliams et al., 1990). As part of the evaluation, therefore, the examiner should listen for characteristics of dysphonia, including hoarseness, breathiness, roughness, strain, glottal fry, hard glottal attack, inappropriate pitch level, restricted pitch range, diplophonia, and inappropriate loudness (Kummer & Marsh, 1998). These auditory perceptual aspects of vocal quality can be rated using the Consensus Auditory-Perceptual Evaluation of Voice (CAPE-V), which is a standardized protocol developed in 2002 as a result of a consensus meeting of voice specialists (Kempster, Gerratt, Verdolini Abbott, Barkmeier-Kraemer, & Hillman, 2009; Stemple, Glaze, & Gerdeman, 1995; Wilson, 1987).

In addition to ratings of various vocal characteristics, the ability to sustain phonation for 10 seconds or longer should be observed. Dysphonic characteristics may not be noted until the end of the prolonged vowel as the child begins to run out of air. Finally, the quality of breath support and the type of breathing pattern should be noted. If the patient has obvious dysphonia, a more comprehensive evaluation of voice should be considered and may include aerodynamic measures, endoscopy, or stroboscopy.

Supplemental Evaluation Procedures

Experienced clinicians may be able to evaluate all of the above characteristics by merely listening to spontaneous speech or repetition of sounds and sentences. The assessment of experienced evaluators tends to be very reliable (Paal, Reulbach, Strobel-Schwarthoff, Nkenke, & Schuster, 2005). However, less experienced clinicians may find it helpful to employ some supplemental tests to more clearly define the speech characteristics and their potential cause. Therefore, the following is a list of simple low-tech and "no-tech" evaluation procedures that may be useful in evaluating resonance and nasal emission (Kummer, 2009; Kummer, 2011).

Visual Detection

There are ways to visualize the effects of nasal emission during speech by using a mirror, an "air paddle," and the See-Scape™. It should be noted that these tools do not give any indication of hypernasality, however.

- **Mirror test:** Some clinicians use the mirror test to determine the presence of nasal emission. For this test, a small mirror (preferably a dental mirror with a narrow rim) is placed under the nares while the patient produces pressure-sensitive sounds (**FIGURE 11-1**). If the mirror clouds up with condensation, it indicates nasal emission. This technique can give false positives if not done correctly, however. The mirror must be placed under the naris after the patient has already begun talking, or it will pick up condensation from normal nasal breathing. In addition, it has to be removed before the patient stops talking because at the end of an utterance, the velum lowers and a puff of air is expelled through the nares. Even when done correctly, this technique does not give information on whether the nasal emission is consistent or just occurred on one phoneme.

- **Air paddle:** The examiner can see the effects of nasal emission by using an air paddle, as first described by Bzoch (1979). An air paddle can be cut (or even torn) from a piece of paper and placed underneath the nares during the production of repetitive syllables with pressure-sensitive consonants (**FIGURE 11-2**). It is best to use voiceless

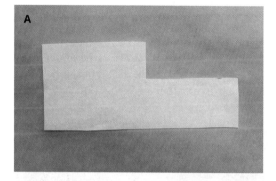

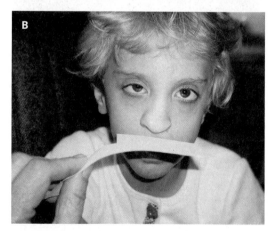

FIGURE 11-2 (A) An air paddle to be used in testing for nasal air emission. The paddle can be cut (or even torn) from a piece of paper. **(B)** The paddle is placed underneath the nares during the production of repetitive syllables that have pressure-sensitive consonants. If the paddle moves during speech, this confirms that there is nasal emission during speech. This works only when there is a significant amount of nasal emission.

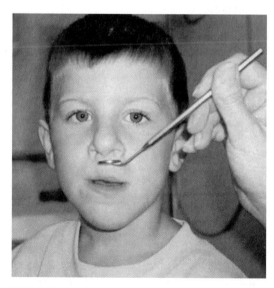

FIGURE 11-1 A dental mirror for testing nasal air emission. A dental mirror can be held under the nares during speech to evaluate nasal air emission. The evaluation is based on the appearance of condensation and should be done carefully to be sure the condensation is not from breathing. Also, this test does not indicate the sound during which the nasal emission occurred.

consonants because they have more airflow than their voiced cognates, and therefore, if there is nasal emission, it will be more apparent on this test. If the paddle moves during the production of these sounds, this confirms that there is nasal emission. This test is not very sensitive and actually works only when there is a lot of nasal emission.

- **See-Scape™:** The See-Scape is a pneumatic device that is sold by several distributors (Pro-Ed, Mayer Johnson, Slosson Educational Publications, AliMed). A "nasal olive" is placed in the child's nostril. The nasal olive is attached to a flexible tube that is connected to a rigid plastic vertical tube. As the child repeats pressure-sensitive phonemes, a Styrofoam° float will rise in the vertical tube when there is nasal air emission (**FIGURE 11-3**).

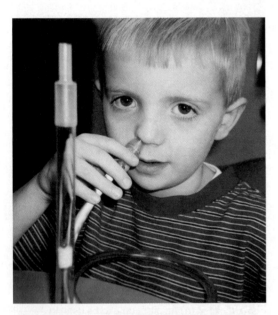

FIGURE 11-3 The use of a See-Scape (Super Duper, Greenville, SC) for testing nasal emission. The patient places the nasal olive at the entrance to the nostril. If there is nasal emission during speech production, the Styrofoam float will rise in the tube. Because the Styrofoam cannot be disinfected, this device is not recommended.

Although this device shows nasal emission when it occurs, it has several disadvantages. First, the retail cost of over $100 is not insignificant. Perhaps the biggest concern, however, relates to infection control. Although this device should be thoroughly cleaned and disinfected between uses, cleaning cannot be done with the Styrofoam float. In addition, the Styrofoam will shrink over time, which makes the device useless.

Tactile Detection

- **Feeling the sides of the nose:** Vibration from hypernasality can sometimes be felt by placing the fingers lightly on the side of the patient's nose (**FIGURE 11-4**). This feeling can be simulated by prolonging an /m/ and feeling the vibration on the nasal cartilage. This is not a very sensitive test, however. Nasal emission from a large velopharyngeal opening cannot be felt on the side of the nose. On the other hand, if there is a nasal rustle from a small opening, this can easily be felt on the cartilage of the nose.

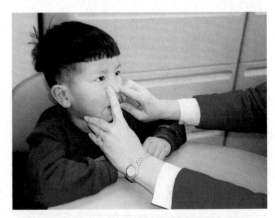

FIGURE 11-4 A tactile test of nasal air emission and hypernasality. Nasal emission, particularly a nasal rustle, can sometimes be felt by placing the index fingers lightly on the cartilage of the nose. Hypernasality can sometimes be felt on the bones and cartilage of the nose.

Auditory Detection

Although visual and tactile detection can be helpful, by far the best evaluation procedures are those that use auditory detection because what is being evaluated is an auditory event (Kummer, 2009; Kummer, 2011; Kummer, 2014; Kummer 2016). In addition, the auditory tests are more reliable when using an appropriate speech sample.

- **Nasal cul-de-sac test:** The nasal cul-de-sac test is done by having the patient produce an oral speech segment with the nose unoccluded and then repeat the same speech segment with the nostrils pinched closed (Bzoch, 1979; Haapanen, 1991) (**FIGURE 11-5**). To test for hypernasality, the child is asked to prolong a vowel or repeat a sentence that is devoid of nasal consonants (Kuehn & Henne,

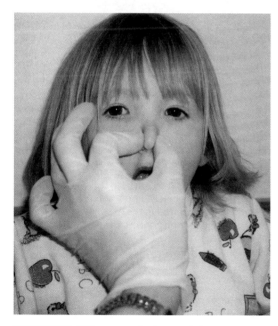

FIGURE 11-5 The nose pinch, or cul-de-sac, test. The examiner asks the patient to produce a speech segment with only oral sounds and then repeat the segment with the nostrils occluded to determine whether there is a difference. A difference in resonance indicates hypernasality.

2003). If the velopharyngeal valve is functioning normally and there is no hypernasality, there should be no change in resonance with the closed nose. On the other hand, if there is hypernasality, the resonance will noticeably change. This is because sound in the nasal cavity will be blocked from exiting, causing nasal cul-de-sac resonance. Therefore, a difference in quality with closure of the nares during oral sound production always indicates hypernasality. To assess for nasal air emission, the child is asked to repeat syllables or sentences loaded with pressure-sensitive consonants. If there is an increase in volume and oral pressure on consonants with closure of the nose, this suggests significant nasal emission. Finally, to assess hyponasality, the child is asked to produce a nasal sound repetitively (such as /mɑ, mɑ, mɑ/) or prolong an /m/. If there is little or no difference in the quality of the speech with the nose closed, then this confirms a diagnosis of hyponasality.

- **Stethoscope:** A stethoscope is a great tool for evaluating resonance and nasal emission. The drum of the stethoscope can be placed on either side of the nose or under the nose during speech. The stethoscope is even more effective, however, if the drum is removed and the tube is placed directly within a nostril (**FIGURE 11-6**). The only disadvantage of this method is that the tubing has to be appropriately disinfected between patients.

- **Listening tube:** A plastic tube works just like the stethoscope in helping to detect hypernasality and nasal emission. Suction tubing is readily available in a hospital and can be used for this purpose. It should be cut into smaller, perhaps 2-foot-long, pieces. When using a tube as part of the evaluation, one end of the tube is placed just within the child's nostril, and the other end is placed near the examiner's ear (**FIGURE 11-7A**). Even a toy whistle can be used for this purpose (**FIGURE 11-7B**).

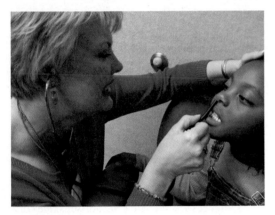

FIGURE 11-6 The use of a stethoscope. The drum is taken off the end, and the tube is placed in the opening of the nostril. This requires disinfection after each use.

The advantage of the tube is that you can make it any length for comfort. The disadvantage is that the examiner needs to be careful not to forget which end went in the child's nose and which end went in her ear. In addition, the tube needs to be either disinfected or discarded after use.

- **Straw:** A simple straw (preferably a bending straw) can actually be just as effective as a stethoscope or a listening tube in evaluating resonance or nasal emission (**FIGURE 11-8**). The short end of a bending straw is placed just inside the child's nostril, and the other end is placed near the examiner's ear.

With one end of the tube (e.g., stethoscope, listening tube, or straw) in the child's nostril and the other end near the examiner's ear, the child should be asked to repeat oral sounds in isolation (i.e., /s/), in repetition, and/or in sentences. If there is either hypernasality or nasal emission, it will be heard loudly through the tube. In fact, the sound is actually amplified as it travels up the narrow tubing, which is what happens with a stethoscope. Therefore, the examiner can hear hypernasality or nasal emission that is not easily detected in connected speech without amplification.

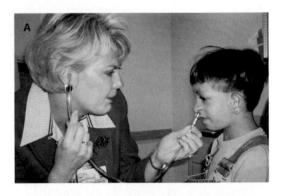

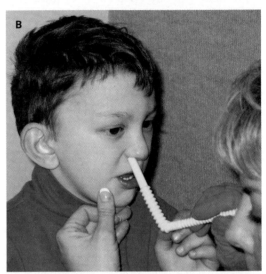

FIGURE 11-7 Tubing. **(A)** A listening tube for a test of nasal air emission and hypernasality. One end of a plastic tube is placed in the child's nostril, and the other end is placed in the examiner's ear. As the child produces sounds or sentences, the examiner can hear occurrences of nasal air emission or hypernasality. **(B)** A toy whistle can also be used as a listening tube. It can then be given to the child to take home as a prize.

The tube can also be used to determine whether there is hyponasality from a blockage in the vocal tract. In this case, the child is asked to repeat nasal sounds in isolation (i.e., /m/), in repetition, and/or in sentences. If there is no sound or very little sound heard through the straw during the production of nasal sounds,

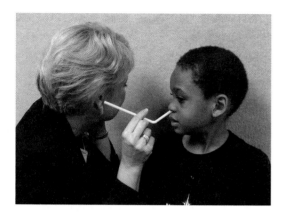

FIGURE 11-8 A straw for amplification of nasal emission and/or hypernasality. A straw is placed in the child's nostril as he produces a speech segment with only oral sounds. If there is nasal air emission or hypernasality, it can be heard loudly through the straw.

then hyponasality and nasal airway blockage are suggested.

Of all these supplemental tests, the straw is the ultimate low-cost, "no-tech" instrument—yet it may be the best way to evaluate hypernasality and nasal emission for several reasons. First, the straw amplifies the sound, just like a stethoscope. Therefore, the examiner is able to easily determine whether there is hypernasality merely by noting whether there is sound through the tube. In addition, the examiner can hear nasal emission clearly even if it is inaudible in regular speech. If the velopharyngeal valve is only slightly inefficient in closing, a click can be heard when amplifying the sound with a straw. The examiner can hear hypernasality and nasal emission even in a noisy clinic environment because the straw acts almost as a low-tech hearing aid. This "equipment" is cheap (less than a penny each) and readily available wherever there is food and drink. The straw is disposable, so it requires no cleaning. In addition, infection control is not an issue. Finally, this method has better validity than visual or tactile detection in that it involves an auditory assessment of an auditory event. For these reasons, the straw is recommended as the best tool for evaluation of resonance and nasal emission.

Differential Diagnosis of Cause

The primary purpose of an evaluation is to gather relevant information to make a differential diagnosis regarding the type of speech/resonance disorder and probable cause. This information is important because it has a direct effect on the treatment recommendations (Garrett, Deal, & Prathanee, 2002; Kummer, 2009; Kummer, 2011; Kummer, 2014; Kummer, 2016; Marsh, 2004; Shprintzen & Golding-Kushner, 1989).

Abnormalities of structure, such as dental malocclusion or velopharyngeal insufficiency, can cause obligatory distortions of speech or compensatory productions. Differential diagnosis is important because obligatory distortions require physical correction only, whereas compensatory errors require correction of structure and speech therapy. **TABLE 11-6** is designed to help the examiner with this differential diagnosis.

Lateral distortion of sibilant sounds and even lingual-alveolar sounds is very common as an obligatory distortion when the teeth interfere with tongue movement. Lateral distortion can be confirmed by placing a straw at the front of the patient's dental arch during production of a /t/ and then an /s/ sound. If the production is normal, the airstream will be heard through the straw. If the airstream is not heard, the straw should be placed at different positions on the side of the dental arch during the production of the /s/ sound. If the airstream is lateralized, it will be heard through the straw at some point on the side of the dental arch rather than in the front.

If there is nasal emission with the production of pressure-sensitive consonants, it is important to determine the type. This can give a clue as to the size of the velopharyngeal opening and the cause. For example, loud nasal emission with an inconsistent nasal rustle indicates a small opening. In contrast,

TABLE 11-6 Obligatory Distortions versus Compensatory Errors

Causes and Treatment	Obligatory Distortions	Compensatory Errors
Definition	• Articulation placement is normal • Distortion is caused by structure only	• Articulation placement is abnormal • Substitution increases intelligibility
Class II malocclusion (severe)	• Distortion on lingual-alveolars, sibilants	• Labiodentals for bilabials • Backing of lingual-alveolars
Class III malocclusion or severe anterior crossbite	• Frontal distortion	• Reverse labiodentals for labiodentals and bilabials • Palatal–dorsal productions of sibilants, causing lateral distortion
VPI	• Nasalized phonemes (e.g., /m/ and /b/) • Hypernasality • Nasal emission on plosives, fricatives, and affricates	• /n/ and /s/ substitution • Glottal stop • Pharyngeal plosive • Pharyngeal and/or post-nasal fricative

inaudible nasal emission that causes weak consonants and short utterance length indicates a large opening. The consistency of nasal emission is also important to note. If nasal emission occurs on all pressure-sensitive sounds, including plosives, it is caused by VPI. If it occurs only on certain sounds so that it is phoneme-specific, then it is caused by misarticulation. TABLE 11-7 can assist the examiner in determining the type of nasal emission and the probable cause.

Differential diagnosis of the cause of nasal emission can be particularly challenging if the child has an oronasal fistula. If the fistula is small, it is unlikely to cause nasal emission during speech because the airflow in the oral cavity primarily flows horizontally across the opening. If the fistula is 5 mm or more in diameter, nasal emission may be noted with the production of sibilants, which are anterior sounds. If the fistula is very large, there may be hypernasality as well as nasal emission.

There are two ways to determine whether nasal emission is from a fistula, from VPI, or from both. One way is to occlude the fistula with chewing gum or Fruit Roll-ups (which are dry and

sticky) and compare the amount of nasal emission with occlusion and without occlusion. This is time consuming and messy, however. A better way is to compare the amount of nasal emission on /k/ with the amount of nasal emission on /t/ and /s/. Because most fistulas occur in the hard palate, which is anterior to the placement of a /k/, the airstream from /k/ flows horizontally to the opening and not up into the fistula. In contrast, the tongue tip movement on /t/ and /s/ can direct the airstream into the fistula. Considering these facts, if there is no nasal emission on /k/ but nasal emission on anterior sounds, then the source of the nasal emission is the fistula. If there is nasal emission on the /k/, then there is VPI. If there is more nasal emission on anterior sounds than /k/, then it is caused by both VPI and the fistula. This is shown on TABLE 11-8.

If there is a nasal rustle, determining the cause is important because it can be caused by either abnormal structure or abnormal function. For example, a nasal rustle commonly occurs with a small velopharyngeal opening from a structural defect. However, it also occurs during production of a posterior velar fricative. The differential

TABLE 11-7　Types of Nasal Emission

Type of Nasal Emission	Characteristics
Inaudible nasal emission	• Cause: large velopharyngeal opening • Characterized by: no resistance to the flow • Usually accompanied by: 　- Severe hypernasality 　- Weak or omitted consonants 　- Short utterance length 　- Nasal grimace 　- Compensatory articulatory productions • Treatment: surgery
Audible nasal emission	• Cause: medium-sized velopharyngeal opening • Characterized by: resistance to airflow so nasal emission is audible • Often accompanied by: 　- Moderate hypernasality 　- Weak consonants 　- Nasal grimace 　- Compensatory articulatory productions • Treatment: surgery
Nasal rustle (nasal turbulence)	• Cause: small velopharyngeal opening • Characterized by: very audible distortion from friction and bubbling of secretions at the velopharyngeal port • Often accompanied by: 　- Mild hypernasality 　- Audible nasal emission • Treatment: surgery
Phoneme-specific nasal emission (PSNE)	• Cause: pharyngeal articulation on certain sounds, resulting in an open velopharyngeal valve • Characterized by: nasal emission or nasal rustle that consistently occurs on certain sounds only, typically one or more of the sibilants • Treatment: speech therapy

TABLE 11-8　Fistula versus VPI as a Cause of Nasal Emission

Nasal Emission Occurs On:	Cause
All sounds (/k/, /t/, /s/)	VPI, maybe also the fistula
All sounds, but more on anterior sounds (/t/, /s/)	VPI and the fistula
Anterior sounds (/t/, /s/) only, but not on the /k/	Fistula only, no VPI

diagnosis is important because structural defects require surgical intervention, whereas articulation placement errors require speech therapy. TABLE 11-9 will help the examiner make a differential diagnosis of the cause of a nasal rustle. Stimulability testing can also be helpful in making the correct diagnosis. Eliminating a nasal rustle with a correction of articulation placement

TABLE 11-9 Structure versus Function as a Cause of Nasal Rustle	
Abnormal Structure (Small Gap)	**Abnormal Function (Misarticulation)**
Inconsistent: occurs inconsistently on all pressure-sensitive sounds, including plosives (/p/, /t/, /k/)	Consistent: occurs consistently on certain phonemes, particularly /s/ and other sibilants
Occurrence increases with utterance length and complexity	Occurs on single words as well as connected speech
Articulation placement is normal	Articulation placement is in the pharynx
Treatment: surgery	Treatment: speech therapy

TABLE 11-10 Differential Diagnosis of Resonance Disorders		
Hypernasality	**Hyponasality**	**Cul-de-Sac Resonance**
Noted on vowels and voiced oral consonants	Noted on vowels and voiced nasal consonants	Noted primarily on vowels
Oral plosives sound like their nasal cognates (/m/ and /b/, /n/ and /d/, /ŋ/ and /g/)	Nasals sound like their oral cognates (/b/ and /m/, /d/ and /n/, /g/ and /ŋ/)	Can affect the volume of either oral or nasal sounds, depending on the location of the obstruction
Resonance changes when you plug the nose on oral sounds	Resonance does not change when you plug the nose on oral sounds	Resonance does not change or changes only slightly when you plug the nose on oral sounds
There is low volume	Speech sounds "stopped up"	There is low volume and speech seems muffled
Usually caused by VPI	Usually caused by obstruction	Usually caused by obstruction
Refer to a craniofacial team	Refer to an ear, nose, and throat doctor (ENT)	Refer to an ENT

confirms that the cause is faulty articulation and not VPI. (For specific suggestions on changing articulatory placement for stimulability testing and therapy, see the chapter *Speech Therapy*.)

In evaluating resonance, it is important to first determine whether resonance is normal or abnormal. If abnormal, a differential diagnosis needs to be made regarding the type of resonance. TABLE 11-10 can be used as a tool toward making a differential diagnosis of the type of resonance and probable cause.

If the child has evidence of VPI, the speech characteristics can be considered together to predict the size of the opening. In general, hypernasality with weak consonants is a predictor of a large velopharyngeal opening, whereas normal resonance with very audible nasal emission suggests a small velopharyngeal opening. TABLE 11-11 will help the examiner to consider the speech characteristics and predict the size of the velopharyngeal opening in connected speech.

TABLE 11-11 Estimation of the Size of the Velopharyngeal Gap

Small Gap	Medium-Sized Gap	Large Gap
Very audible because of friction and bubbling of secretions Often called a nasal rustle	Somewhat audible	Not audible
Is inconsistent (unless phoneme-specific), but increases with utterance length, rate, and fatigue	Usually consistent on pressure-sensitive sounds	Occurs on all pressure-sensitive sounds
Consonants are normal in pressure and intensity	Consonants are somewhat weak in pressure and intensity	Consonants are very weak in intensity and pressure or seem to be omitted
Utterance length is not affected	Utterance length is slightly affected	Utterance length is short because of the frequent need to take a breath to replenish the loss of airflow through the nasal cavity
Can be phoneme-specific because of abnormal articulation placement in the pharynx, and if so, can be corrected with speech therapy	Is never phoneme-specific, so always requires physical management (surgery or prosthesis)	Is never phoneme-specific, so always requires physical management (surgery or prosthesis)
Associated with normal resonance	Associated with mild to moderate hypernasality	Associated with severe hypernasality

CASE REPORT

Phoneme-Specific Nasal Emission

Jeff was a 36-year-old man with a history of nasality, although he was not born with a cleft palate. When Jeff was a child, his parents were told that he would need surgery to correct the problem. They opted not to have the surgery done. In his early 20s, Jeff sought another opinion and was again told that he would require surgery for correction. Because of his hesitancy to go through with the procedure, the surgery was never done. When he came to our clinic at the age of 36, Jeff reported that his speech had been a barrier in his work and social life and therefore he was finally ready for the surgery.

Upon examination, the velum appeared to be normal. An assessment of speech revealed the substitution of a pharyngeal fricative for all sibilant sounds (s, z, ʃ, ʒ, ʧ, ʤ). Because the pharyngeal fricative is produced in the pharynx, the air is released through an open velopharyngeal valve and then through the nasal cavity. There was no nasal emission on other consonants, and resonance was normal.

Given these findings, it was apparent that Jeff had been misdiagnosed with VPI. Instead, he demonstrated phoneme-specific nasal emission, which is a speech sound disorder.

(continues)

CASE REPORT

Phoneme-Specific Nasal Emission *(continued)*

Jeff proved to be stimulable for correct production of all misarticulated sounds when given appropriate cues. (See the chapter *Speech Therapy* for techniques to change articulation placement.) With the change in placement from pharyngeal to oral, there was a total elimination of nasal emission. Therefore, rather than recommending a surgical procedure, as had been recommended in the past, speech therapy was recommended. Within a few months, he was producing sibilants normally with no nasal air emission and was therefore discharged from therapy.

This case illustrates the importance of a differential diagnosis. In Jeff's case, the nasal emission was from misarticulation rather than VPI. It is fortunate that he did not have unnecessary surgery but unfortunate that he had not received speech therapy for correction when he was a child.

Follow-Up

The purpose of an evaluation is to determine appropriate treatment recommendations for the patient. In some cases, recommendations may have to be deferred if there is a need for additional testing or consultation from other professionals. The speech-language pathologist should continue to be actively involved with the patient and family until final treatment recommendations are made.

Recommendations

Depending on the evaluation results, additional diagnostic procedures may be recommended (e.g., a nasopharyngoscopy evaluation, a videofluoroscopic speech study, a videofluoroscopic swallow study, an ear, nose, and throat [ENT] evaluation, or a sleep study). Before making referrals for additional evaluations, the speech-language pathologist should always discuss the recommendations with the primary care physician and the referring physician. This is not only common courtesy but is consistent with the "medical model," where the primary care physician manages the child's overall plan of care.

Based on the child's speech characteristics, the examiner is able to determine whether there is velopharyngeal dysfunction and if so whether it has a structural versus functional cause. The speech characteristics even allow the examiner to estimate the size of the velopharyngeal gap (see Table 10-3). With this information, the examiner can make appropriate recommendations for physical management (surgery or prosthetic device), speech therapy, or both. **TABLE 11-12**

TABLE 11-12 Recommendations Based on Causality
Velopharyngeal Insufficiency (Structural Abnormality)
• Surgery (postoperative speech therapy as needed)
• Prosthesis—speech bulb or palatal lift if the velum is long enough past the velar eminence
• Speech therapy for articulation errors and compensatory productions
Velopharyngeal Incompetence (Neurophysiological Abnormality)
• Surgery (postoperative speech therapy as needed)
• Prosthesis—palatal lift
• Speech therapy for articulation errors and compensatory productions
Velopharyngeal Mislearning
• Speech therapy only
Symptomatic Oronasal (Palatal) Fistula
• Surgery
• Prosthesis—obturator
• Speech therapy for articulation errors and compensatory productions

has a list of recommendations that can be considered for each cause (Glade & Deal, 2016).

Recommendations should not only be based on the cause of the speech disorder but should also be made considering the potential for improvement, the associated risks (particularly airway obstruction and obstructive sleep apnea), the patient's quality of life, and the desires of the patient and family. The examiner must be careful not to impose her own value system and personal preferences on the patient and the family. They are the ones who have to live with the consequences of the decision; therefore, they should be the ones to make informed decisions about the recommended interventions.

Family Counseling

Family counseling is important to help the family make informed decisions about treatment and to train them to work with the child at home. Handouts with labeled drawings are particularly useful in helping the family to understand the anatomy, the problem with speech, and any surgical procedures that are being proposed. Many centers give out their own handouts and brochures that contain specific information regarding their program and facility. Informational brochures are also available through the ACPA Family Services website (ACPA, n.d.).

Evaluation Report

There is a great need for standardization of assessment protocols and methods of recording and reporting evaluation results (Golding-Kushner et al., 1990; Hirschberg & Van Demark, 1997; Sell, Harding, & Grunwell, 1999). Despite general agreement that standardization is needed, there is still great variability among centers and providers in the way evaluation results are reported.

The purpose of the evaluation report is to effectively communicate results and recommendations to other professionals and, in some cases, to the family. Therefore, a good evaluation report is one that is clear and concise. Many professionals fail to consider their "customers" when writing the report. Long reports are usually not read and not appreciated by busy professionals. (Some speech-language pathologists forget that the quality of the evaluation is not judged by the quantity of pages in the report.) The report should contain appropriate language and medical terminology but should also be understandable to the readers. (Phonetic symbols are not understood by other professionals and families.) The report should focus on the examiner's impressions (based on the evaluation results) and the recommendations. It is important to be correct and confident in the stated conclusions and recommendations because they will often result in surgical management.

SUMMARY

A perceptual assessment of speech and resonance gives the examiner information regarding the presence of VPI and its effect on speech production. It is important to assess articulation to determine whether there are any obligatory distortions or compensatory errors resulting from VPI. The examiner should determine whether there is nasal emission and whether this is causing weak consonants or short utterance length. If resonance is abnormal, the examiner should determine the type of resonance but not be particularly concerned about rating the severity. Phonation should also be assessed because dysphonia is common in individuals with clefts, VPI, and craniofacial syndromes.

Although there are instrumental procedures to evaluate velopharyngeal function, a perceptual assessment remains the best method for judging abnormal speech and resonance. To augment the perceptual assessment, the use of a straw (or other type of tube) is the most appropriate and effective method of assessing the speech correlates of velopharyngeal dysfunction. Finally, differential diagnosis of the cause of speech/resonance disorders is very important for determination of the appropriate method of treatment.

FOR REVIEW AND DISCUSSION

1. What should be the focus of concern for the speech-language pathologist when the child is a newborn? What should be the focus of concern when the child is a toddler? At what age can velopharyngeal function usually be evaluated? Why can't it be evaluated earlier?

2. What type of information is important to obtain in the diagnostic interview with the parent or guardian?

3. Discuss different types of speech stimuli that can be used in an assessment and the advantages of each type.

4. List the types of errors and distortions that should be identified in a test of speech sound production. Why is it important to identify the type of error?

5. Why is it important to test stimulability? If the child responds well to stimulation, what might that suggest?

6. What sounds would you use to test for hypernasality? What sounds would you use to test for nasal emission? What sounds would you use to test for hyponasality? Explain the reason for each.

7. Describe methods for informally detecting hypernasality. What is the advantage of auditory detection over visual or tactile detection? What is the advantage of using a straw or listening tube over using a mirror for detection of nasal emission?

8. Your patient has normal resonance but inconsistent nasal emission. He has a small fistula in the middle of the palate. What would you do to determine whether the nasal emission is caused by the fistula or VPI?

9. Why is a differential diagnosis of the cause of abnormal resonance or nasal emission so important? Discuss possible repercussions of making the wrong diagnosis.

10. How can you differentiate an obligatory distortion from a compensatory error? How can you determine whether a nasal rustle is caused by abnormal structure or abnormal function? How can you determine whether a fistula is a cause of nasal emission?

REFERENCES

American Cleft Palate–Craniofacial Association (ACPA). (n.d.). ACPA Family Services: Resources for your cleft journey. Retrieved from http://www.cleftline.org/parents-individuals/.

American Cleft Palate–Craniofacial Association (ACPA). (2009). Parameters for evaluation and treatment of patients with cleft lip/palate or other craniofacial anomalies. *The Cleft Palate–Craniofacial Journal, 30* (Suppl.), 1–16.

Bronsted, K., Grunwell, P., Henningsson, G., Jansonius, K. J. K., Meijer, M., Ording, U., . . . Wyatt, R. (1994). A phonetic framework for the cross-linguistic analysis of cleft palate speech. *Clinical Linguistics and Phonetics, 8,* 109–125.

Bzoch, K. R. (1979). Clinical assessment, evaluation and management of 11 categorical aspects of cleft palate speech. In K. R. Bzoch (Ed.), *Communicative disorders related to cleft lip and palate* (vol. 4, pp. 261–311). Austin, TX: Pro-Ed.

Bzoch, K. R., League, R., & Brown, V. L. (2003). *Receptive-Expressive Emergent Language Test: A method for assessing the language skills of infants* (3rd ed.). Austin, TX: Pro-Ed.

Coplan, J. (1993). *Early Language Milestone (ELM) Scale-2* (2nd ed.). Austin, TX: Pro-Ed.

Fluharty, N. B. (2000). *Fluharty-2: Preschool Speech and Language Test* (2nd ed.). Austin, TX: Pro-Ed.

Garrett, J. D., Deal, R. E., & Prathanee, B. (2002). Velopharyngeal assessment procedures for the Thai cleft palate population. *Journal of the Medical Association of Thailand, 85*(6), 682–692.

Glade, R. S., & Deal, R. (2016). Diagnosis and management of velopharyngeal dysfunction. *Oral and Maxillofacial Surgery Clinics of North America, 28*(2), 181–188.

Glascoe, F. P. (1991). Can clinical judgment detect children with speech-language problems? *Pediatrics, 87*(3), 317–322.

Golding-Kushner, K. J., Argamaso, R. V., Cotton, R. T., Grames, L. M., Henningsson, G., Jones, D. L., . . . Marsh, J. L. (1990). Standardization for the reporting of nasopharyngoscopy and multiview videofluoroscopy: A report from an international working group. *Cleft Palate Journal, 27*(4), 337–347; discussion 347–348.

Haapanen, M. L. (1991). A simple clinical method of evaluating perceived hypernasality. *Folia Phoniatrica, 43*(3), 122–132. (Erratum published 1991, *Folia Phoniatrica, 43*(4), p. 2003)

Henningsson, G., & Isberg, A. (1991). A cineradiographic study of velopharyngeal movements for deviant versus nondeviant articulation. *The Cleft Palate–Craniofacial Journal, 28*(1), 115–117; discussion 117–118.

Hickman, L. A. (1997). *Apraxia profile: A descriptive assessment tool for children.* San Antonio, TX: Communication Skill Builders.

Hirschberg, J., & Van Demark, D. R. (1997). A proposal for standardization of speech and hearing evaluations to assess velopharyngeal function. *Folia Phoniatrica et Logopedica, 49*(3/4), 158–167.

Kaufman, N. R. (1995). *Kaufman Speech Praxis Test for Children (KSPT).* Detroit, MI: Wayne State University Press.

Kempster, B., Gerratt, B., Verdolini Abbott, K., Barkmeier-Kraemer, J., & Hillman, R. E. (2009). Consensus auditory-perceptual evaluation of voice: Development of a standardized clinical protocol, *American Journal of Speech-Language Pathology, 18,* 124–132.

Kuehn, D. P., & Henne, L. J. (2003). Speech evaluation and treatment of patients with cleft palate. *American Journal of Speech-Language Pathology, 12,* 103–109.

Kummer, A. W. (2009). Assessment of velopharyngeal function. In J. E. Losee & R. E. Kirschner (Eds.), *Comprehensive cleft care* (pp. 589–605). New York, NY: McGraw-Hill.

Kummer, A. W. (2011). Perceptual assessment of resonance and velopharyngeal function. *Seminars in Speech and Language, 32*(2), 159–167.

Kummer, A. W. (2014). Speech evaluation for patients with cleft palate. *Clinics in Plastic Surgery, 41*(2), 241–251.

Kummer, A. W. (2016). Evaluation of speech and resonance for children with craniofacial anomalies. *Facial Plastic Surgery Clinics of North America, 24*(4), 445–451.

Kummer A. W. (2018). A pediatrician's guide to communication disorders secondary to cleft lip/palate (CLP). *Pediatric Clinics of North America, 65*(1), 31–46.

Kummer, A. W., Briggs, M., & Lee, L. (2003). The relationship between the characteristics of speech and velopharyngeal gap size. *The Cleft Palate–Craniofacial Journal, 40*(6), 590–596.

Kummer, A. W., Clark, S. L., Redle, E. E., Thomsen, L. L., & Billmire, D. A. (2011). Current practice in assessing and reporting speech outcomes of cleft palate and velopharyngeal surgery: A survey of cleft palate/craniofacial professionals. *The Cleft Palate–Craniofacial Journal, 49*(2), 146–152.

Kummer, A. W., Curtis, C., Wiggs, M., Lee, L., & Strife, J. L. (1992). Comparison of velopharyngeal gap size in patients with hypernasality, hypernasality and nasal emission, or nasal turbulence (rustle) as the primary speech characteristic. *The Cleft Palate–Craniofacial Journal, 29*(2), 152–156.

Kummer, A. W., Lee, L., Stutz, L., Maroney, A., & Brandt, J. W. (2007). The prevalence of apraxic characteristics in patients with velocardiofacial syndrome as compared to other populations. *The Cleft Palate–Craniofacial Journal, 44*(2), 175–181.

Kummer, A. W., & Marsh, J. H. (1998). Pediatric voice and resonance disorders. In A. F. Johnson & B. H. Jacobson (Eds.), *Medical speech-language pathology: A practitioner's guide.* New York, NY: Thieme.

Lee, G. S., Wang, C. P., & Fu, S. (2009). Evaluation of hypernasality in vowels using voice low tone to high tone ratio. *The Cleft Palate–Craniofacial Journal, 46*(1), 47–52.

Marsh, J. L. (2004). The evaluation and management of velopharyngeal dysfunction. *Clinics in Plastic Surgery, 31*(2), 261–269.

McWilliams, B. J., Lavorato, A. S., & Bluestone, C. D. (1973). Vocal cord abnormalities in children with velopharyngeal valving problems. *Laryngoscope, 83*(11), 1745–1753.

McWilliams, B. J., Morris, H. L., & Shelton, R. L. (1990). Diagnosis of phonation and resonance. In B. J. Williams, H. L. Morris, & R. L. Shelton (Eds.), *Cleft palate speech* (pp. 311–319). Philadelphia, PA: B. C. Decker.

Moller, K. T. (1991). An approach to the evaluation of velopharyngeal adequacy for speech. *Clinics in Communication Disorders, 1*(1), 61–65.

Naran, S., Ford, M., & Losee, J. E. (2017). What's new in cleft palate and velopharyngeal dysfunction management? *Plastic and Reconstructive Surgery, 139*(6), 1343e–1355e.

Paal, S., Reulbach, U., Strobel-Schwarthoff, K., Nkenke, E., & Schuster, M. (2005). Evaluation of speech disorders in children with cleft lip and palate. *Journal of Orofacial Orthopedics, 66*(4), 270–278.

Pannbacker, M., & Middleton, G. (1990). Integrating perceptual and instrumental procedures in assessment of velopharyngeal insufficiency. *Ear, Nose & Throat Journal, 69*(3), 161–175.

Rossetti, L. (2006). *The Rossetti Infant-Toddler Language Scale*. East Moline, IL: Lingui-Systems.

Scherer, N. J., & D'Antonio, L. L. (1995). Parent questionnaire for screening early language development in children with cleft palate. *The Cleft Palate–Craniofacial Journal, 32*(1), 7–13.

Scherer, N. J., & D'Antonio, L. L. (1997). Language and play development in toddlers with cleft lip and/or palate. *American Journal of Speech-Language Pathology, 6*(4), 48–54.

Sell, D., Harding, A., & Grunwell, P. (1999). GOS. SP.ASS/98: An assessment for speech disorders associated with cleft palate and/or velopharyngeal dysfunction (Revised). *International Journal of Language and Communication Disorders, 34*(1), 17–33.

Semel, E., Wiig, E. H., & Secord, W. A. (2013). *Clinical Evaluation of Language Fundamentals®—Preschool* (5th ed.). New York, NY: Pearson.

Shprintzen, R. J., & Golding-Kushner, K. J. (1989). Evaluation of velopharyngeal insufficiency. *Otolaryngologic Clinics of North America, 22*(3), 519–536.

Smith, B., & Guyette, T. W. (2004). Evaluation of cleft palate speech. *Clinics in Plastic Surgery, 31*(2), 251–260.

Smith, B. E., & Kuehn, D. P. (2007). Speech evaluation of velopharyngeal dysfunction. *The Journal of Craniofacial Surgery, 18*(2), 251–260.

Stemple, J. C., Glaze, L. E., & Gerdeman, B. K. (1995). *Clinical voice pathology: Theory and management.* San Diego, CA: Singular Publishing Group.

Subtelny, J. D., Van Hattum, R. J., & Myers, B. B. (1972). Ratings and measures of cleft palate speech. *Cleft Palate Journal, 9*(1), 18–27.

Trindade, I. E., Genaro, K. F., Yamashita, R. P., Miguel, H. C., & Fukushiro, A. P. (2005). Proposal for velopharyngeal function rating in a speech perceptual assessment. *Pro Fono, 17*(2), 259–262.

Trost, J. E. (1981). Articulatory additions to the classical description of the speech of persons with cleft palate. *Cleft Palate Journal, 18*(3), 193–203.

Trost-Cardamone, J. E. (1997). Diagnosis of specific cleft palate speech error patterns for planning therapy of physical management needs. In K. R. Bzoch (Ed.), *Communicative disorders related to cleft lip and palate* (vol. 4, pp. 313–330). Austin, TX: Pro-Ed.

Wilson, D. K. (1987). *Voice problems of children* (vol. 3). Baltimore, MD: Williams & Wilkins.

Zimmerman, I. L., Steiner, V. G., & Pond, R. E. (2011). *Preschool language scales* (5th ed.). New York, NY: Pearson.

CREDITS

Part/Chapter opener photo: © PeopleImages/Getty Images

All photos courtesy of the Cleft and Craniofacial Center at Cincinnati Children's Hospital Medical Center.

CHAPTER 12

Orofacial Examination

CHAPTER OUTLINE

INTRODUCTION

In speech pathology, an orofacial examination (sometimes called an oral-peripheral examination or perioral examination) involves assessment of oral structures and other facial structures that may be relevant for speech. An intraoral examination (sometimes called an oral mechanism examination) is part of a complete orofacial examination.

An orofacial examination should always be done as part of a speech or resonance evaluation, especially if the individual has a history of cleft or craniofacial anomalies. Unfortunately, many speech-language pathologists have not been taught how to perform a thorough intraoral examination. In fact, research shows that even medical students are not given sufficient instruction or experience in performing oral examinations (Shanks, Walker, McCann, & Kerin, 2011). By performing regular orofacial examinations, speech-language pathologists can increase their familiarity with normal oral structures and will be able to recognize abnormalities more easily (Thomas & Bender, 1993).

Knowledge of the oral structures and their potential effect on speech production and resonance is extremely important to make appropriate recommendations for treatment. If there are structural factors that cause or contribute to the deviant speech or resonance, these structural problems should be corrected as soon as possible. When there are obligatory distortions, correcting the structure alone will correct these distortions. In contrast, compensatory productions need to be corrected with speech therapy after the structure is normalized.

The examiner should be aware that an assessment of velopharyngeal function cannot be made based on an intraoral examination (Smith & Guyette, 2004; Smith & Kuehn, 2007). Velopharyngeal closure occurs behind the velum, usually on the plane of the hard palate. Therefore, it is well above the level that is viewed through the oral cavity. In addition, the examiner cannot see the point of maximum lateral pharyngeal wall movement from an intraoral perspective. In fact, at the oral level, the lateral pharyngeal walls may actually appear to bow outward during phonation. Finally, velopharyngeal function cannot be judged during a sustained vowel only.

Despite these limitations, the examiner can evaluate all of the oral structures that can affect speech and resonance, including the status of labial competence, dental occlusion, the hard palate, the oral surface of the velum, the uvula, the tonsils, and the tongue (Smith & Kuehn, 2007). As such, an intraoral assessment can provide valuable information that can affect the examiner's overall impressions and recommendations.

This chapter describes the methodology for a comprehensive examination of relevant structures and function for the production of normal speech and resonance. In addition, appropriate procedures for infection control are discussed.

General Methodology

An evaluation of the oral cavity is an important part of a speech and resonance evaluation. It is important to determine whether there are structural anomalies that are affecting speech. If there are such anomalies, the treatment requires physical correction of the structure before considering the need for speech therapy (unless there are speech errors that are unrelated to the abnormal structures). The following sections describe methods for conducting a thorough evaluation of the oral cavity so that appropriate treatment recommendations can be made.

Tools for an Intraoral Examination

An intraoral examination can often be done without special equipment or materials. There are some things that are helpful to have on hand, however, including the following:

- Gloves: Used for protection of the patient and the examiner.
- Flashlight: Used for illumination of the oral cavity.
- Tongue blades: Used to press the back of the tongue down (when necessary) to observe the velum and uvula. Also used to inspect the dentition and occlusion by pulling the lips and cheeks away from the teeth. (Flavored tongue blades should be considered for children.)
- Dental mirror: Used like a tongue blade to press the back of the tongue down (when necessary) to observe the velum and uvula. Also used to assess the palate for a fistula or for looking up into the pharynx.

- Alcohol swabs or towelettes: Used to clean contaminated instruments or surfaces.
- Sanitizing gel: Used to sanitize hands, particularly if soap and water are not available.

Examination of the Oral Cavity

If done correctly, a physical examination of the morphology and function of the oral cavity can reveal important information that relates to speech sound production. Instead of a quick look in the mouth, however, the examiner should carefully inspect all the structures and also view some of these structures during function.

When conducting an intraoral examination, most healthcare professionals ask the patient to open the mouth and say /ɑ/ (as in "father"). Because production of this vowel results in a drop of the mandible and thus the anterior part of the tongue, this vowel works well for evaluation of the anterior oral structures, including the hard palate. However, during production of this vowel, the back of the tongue is high and retracted, thus obstructing the view of the posterior section of the oral cavity and pharynx. In fact, production of this vowel makes it impossible for the examiner to view the posterior portion of the oral cavity, including the velum, tip of the uvula, tonsils, and pharynx. It is because of high posterior tongue position that a tongue blade is used to depress the back of the tongue so that the examiner can view the posterior structures.

Children are usually very resistant to the use of a tongue blade, which can limit their cooperation. Fortunately, a good intraoral examination can be obtained with many children without a tongue blade by having the child say /æ/ (as in "hat") rather than /ɑ/. At the same time, the child is instructed to stick her tongue out and down as far as it will go (**FIGURE 12-1**). A young child can be instructed to point her tongue to her shoes or to try to touch her chin with her tongue. This technique brings the back of the tongue down and forward, which opens the view to the back of the oral cavity. This provides the examiner with

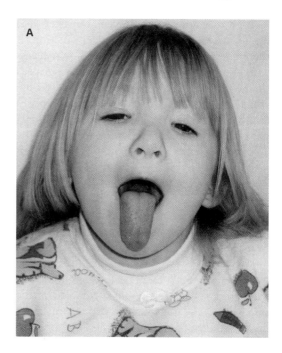

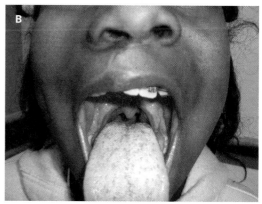

FIGURE 12-1 Having the child produce the vowel /æ/ rather than /ɑ/ will provide a better view of the back of the oral cavity because the back of the tongue goes down for this vowel. In most cases, this eliminates the need for a tongue blade. At the same time, the patient can be instructed to stick her tongue out and down to try to touch her chin.

a much better view of the velum, uvula, tonsils, and pharynx. In some young children, the tip of the epiglottis can even be seen (Shinohara & Takahashi, 2005).

If a tongue blade is needed, however, it is important to place it in the proper position. If the blade is placed too far forward, which is a common mistake, pushing downward causes the posterior part of the tongue to mound up, which further obscures rather than exposes the back of the oral cavity and the pharynx. If the tongue blade is placed behind the circumvallate papilla (a line of prominent taste buds that form an inverted "V" on the posterior tongue), it often elicits the gag reflex. The gag can give the examiner a good view, but it is a quick view and may be the last one that the patient will allow. The correct technique is to place the tongue blade approximately three-quarters of the way back on the tongue. The examiner should then press the tongue downward firmly, while scooping it forward at the same time. The tongue is a strong, muscular organ, so firm pressure is often required to push against resistance.

As the individual phonates, there may be vigorous upward movement of the velum or very little movement, even in normal speakers. To stimulate movement to see the pharynx and the tip of the uvula, the child can be asked to produce the vowel repetitively or to pant ("like a puppy dog"). If this does not stimulate movement, then the examiner can ask the child to do a big yawn with the tongue protruded. This helps to elevate the velum to its fullest extent.

Positioning of the patient is another consideration when performing an intraoral examination. The patient's head should be tilted slightly backward so that the examiner can look directly to the back of the pharynx. The examiner's eye level should be at the level of the patient's oral cavity.

For an infant or toddler, it is helpful to place the child on the parent's lap, facing the parent. The child is then laid back so her head is slightly lower than the rest of her body. The examiner should sit opposite the caregiver so that there is a good view of the child's oral cavity from above (albeit upside down). Although this position usually promotes an open-mouth posture, the tongue may fall back into the pharynx, requiring the use of a tongue blade. If the child doesn't open wide enough, the examiner can place a tongue blade between the teeth and apply steady downward pressure on the tongue and mandible. The jaw muscles closing the mouth are powerful but fatigue rapidly, so constant, firm pressure will allow insertion of the tongue blade within a few seconds. When the blade reaches the posterior tongue, the gag reflex causes the mouth to open fully. Alternatively, closing the nose forces the mouth to open for breathing. Finally, crying is not always a bad thing because it does allow the examiner a better intraoral view, especially in this position.

If a submucous cleft is suspected, palatal palpation of the hard palate can be done to determine whether there is a notch in the posterior border. If the examiner is inexperienced or not well trained in this area, palatal palpation can be difficult—not only for the examiner but especially for the patient. The key to successful palpation is to be gentle and slow in feeling the palate. Surprises in the area of the gag reflex are not well received by the child! However, careful palpation of the roof of the mouth with a gloved finger does not cause discomfort. If there is an open cleft or a fistula, it should be remembered that this is a variation in structure—not an open wound.

In preschool and school-aged children, it is best to use the fifth (or little) finger for palpation. This finger is long enough to reach the back of the palate of children in this age group. In addition, this finger is narrow enough to feel a small notch in the palatal bone. For teenagers and adults, the fifth finger is usually not long enough to reach to the back of the hard palate. Therefore, the index finger must be used.

To begin the examination, it is important that the examiner wash his or her hands thoroughly and then don gloves. For a young child, the examiner should begin by merely rubbing or stimulating the outside gums above the maxillary teeth. This helps the patient to become more comfortable and accepting of the examiner's finger in the mouth. The examiner should then stimulate the alveolar ridge behind the teeth by moving the finger from the front of the ridge to the back in the area of the molars. Once the patient is comfortable with that amount of stimulation, the examiner should glide the finger directly behind the last molar and then slowly move the finger horizontally along the back edge

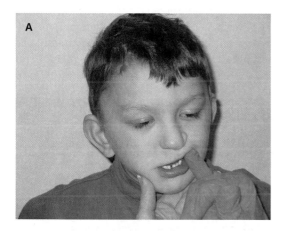

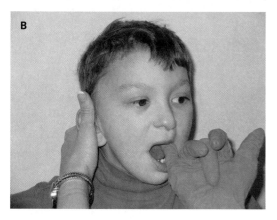

FIGURE 12-2 Method for palpating the hard palate. **(A)** Using the little finger for children, the examiner should start by putting the finger under the lips and palpating the gum ridge. **(B)** The finger is then moved between the cheek and gum, around the molars, and then along the back end of the hard palate until it is in midline.

of the hard palate until it reaches the midline (**FIGURE 12-2**). This is the point where the notch should be felt if it exists. To feel for the notch, the examiner should try to gently probe the midpoint of the posterior border of the hard palate. With the little finger, the examiner is more likely to feel a small or narrow defect than if the larger index finger is used.

To visualize the surface of the hard palate or velum, a dental mirror can be especially helpful (**FIGURE 12-3**). The mirror should be placed under the palate, and the light of a flashlight should be directed to the mirror. The light will be reflected off the mirror and will therefore illuminate the surface of the palate above it. This is particularly useful when examining the hard palate for a fistula. If the velum is very short, the dental mirror can also be used to look up into the nasopharynx.

Finally, the examiner should assess the skeletal relationship between the maxillary and the mandibular arches during occlusion. The child should be asked to bite on her back teeth so that her normal bite can be viewed. Once the child has obtained her normal bite, the examiner should insert a tongue blade between the lateral teeth and the cheeks and then pull the cheeks away from the teeth to view the occlusal relationship (**FIGURE 12-4**).

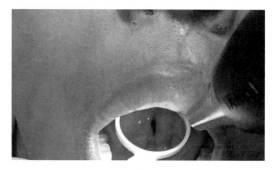

FIGURE 12-3 A dental mirror can be especially helpful in visualizing the palate to see a palatal fistula. The light should be directed onto the mirror rather than the palate so that it bounces upward to illuminate the fistula.

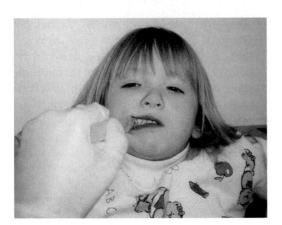

FIGURE 12-4 By inserting a tongue blade between the lateral teeth and the cheeks, the examiner can pull the cheeks away from the teeth to view the occlusal relationship.

Important Observations

When conducting an orofacial examination, it is important to keep in mind that there are normal variations in structure, which may result in characteristics that are unusual but not necessarily abnormal or significant. In addition, there may be minor anomalies that have no effect on function, including speech.

It is very important, however, that speech-language pathologists and other healthcare providers are attentive observers of dysmorphology in patients that they serve. This is because whenever there are anomalies on the outside of the head (face and/or skull), there are usually corresponding anomalies on the inside of the head. In addition, whenever there are anomalies on the inside of the head, there are often corresponding functional abnormalities. For example, the observation of external ear malformations would suggest the possibility of internal ear anomalies of the ossicles and perhaps even of the cochlea. The internal anomalies would lead to the functional problem of hearing loss. In another example, the observation of hypertelorism (wide-spaced eyes) and abnormal skull shape may suggest internal brain anomalies that could result in functional problems with cognition and language. Outside anomalies typically

affect appearance and aesthetics. Inside anomalies typically affect function (i.e., cognition, language, speech, resonance, hearing, feeding, and swallowing). These functional disorders are typically treated by speech-language pathologists. TABLE 12-1 lists how anomalies of craniofacial structures could potentially affect function.

An orofacial examination begins with observation of the external anatomy of the head and face. The examiner should inspect the eyes, ears, nose, mouth, and facial profile for evidence of abnormality or dysmorphology. The examiner should also watch facial gestures, the tongue, and the jaw movement during speech. Most importantly, the examiner should conduct a thorough intraoral

TABLE 12-1 Effects of External Anomalies on Internal Structures and Function		
External Structures	**Internal Structures**	**Possible Functional Problems**
Skull	Brain	Language, learning/cognition, motor skills
Eyes	Eyes	Vision
Ears	Auditory canal, ossicles, cochlea	Hearing (conductive and/or sensorineural hearing loss)
Nose	Nasal cavity	Breathing and resonance (hyponasality or cul-de-sac resonance)
Jaws	Teeth	Dentition, dental occlusion, articulation, and resonance

examination. The following sections describe what should be observed with specific structures.

Eyes

Normally, the eyes should be about one eye's width apart. In certain craniofacial syndromes, however, the spacing between the eyes and the appearance of the eyes is often abnormal. There may be excessive spacing between the eyes, called hypertelorism (**FIGURE 12-5A**), or too little spacing between the eyes, called hypotelorism. The opening between the eyelids, called palpebral fissures, should also be observed. Narrow palpebral fissures are a phenotypic feature in congenital conditions, such as velocardiofacial/22q11.2 deletion syndrome (VCFS/22q deletion syndrome; see **FIGURE 12-5B**). Finally, the presence of epicanthal folds might be noted. These are excess folds of tissue that extend from the upper eyelid to the lower part of the orbit at the inner canthus or corner of the eye. This is often seen in Down syndrome and other syndromes, although epicanthal folds are normal in the Asian population.

Ears

The shape and location of the ears should be observed. Many craniofacial syndromes include malformed ears, such as a simplified helix, or microtia (**FIGURE 12-6**), which is hypoplasia, or absence of the pinna or auricle of the ear. This is often accompanied by aural atresia, which is the congenital absence of the external auditory canal. Aural atresia usually results in a conductive hearing loss, and of course, this can have an effect on the quality of speech, and possibly resonance, when it is bilateral. Ears that are low set (below the level of the eyes), malformed, or bent may also be suggestive of a syndrome.

Lips

The lips should be assessed for bilabial incompetence (the inability to achieve and maintain bilabial closure at rest) because it has the potential to affect production of bilabial and labiodental phonemes. Bilabial incompetence

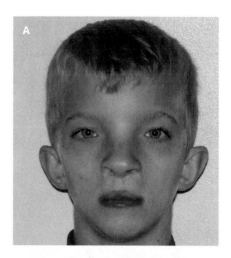

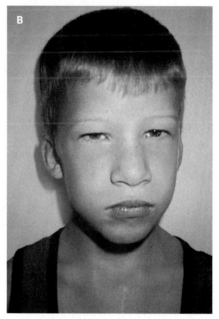

FIGURE 12-5 Eye anomalies. **(A)** Hypertelorism (wide-spaced eyes), which is common with several syndromes. **(B)** Narrow palpebral fissures (eye openings) in a child with velocardiofacial/22q11.2 deletion syndrome.

may occur if there is contraction of the scar from the lip repair, a protruding premaxilla, or a Class II malocclusion (**FIGURE 12-7**).

The examiner should note whether there is an open-mouth posture at rest. A chronic open-mouth posture can be from malocclusion, but it

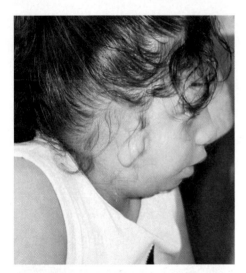

FIGURE 12-6 Microtia in a child with hemifacial microsomia.

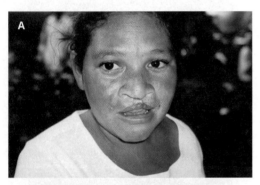

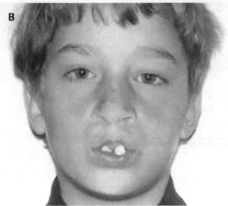

FIGURE 12-7 (A) A short upper lip from the lip repair. **(B)** A protruding premaxilla and short upper lip. Both affect bilabial competence at rest and during speech.

can also be indicative of low facial tone or upper airway obstruction. An open-mouth posture can cause or exacerbate sialorrhea (drooling). This can be subtle, with just a little moisture on the chin, or it can be copious so that the child wears a bib or carries a cloth. If the child has feeding difficulties by history or by observation, copious drooling could also be an indication of oral-motor dysfunction.

In patients with cleft lip and/or cleft palate, the examiner should look for lip pits, which are small bilateral depressions in the bottom lip (**FIGURE 12-8**). If there is scarring on the bottom lip, the examiner should ask whether there were lip pits that were surgically removed. The finding of lip pits is indicative of Van der Woude syndrome, which is autosomal dominant, so it has a 50% recurrence risk for all future pregnancies.

Uncommonly, there is reduced mobility of the upper lip from scarring. To assess this, the patient should be asked to sustain exaggerated /i/ (as in "heat") and /u/ (as in "who") sounds. The symmetry and range of lip movement should be noted. Observing the patient produce quick repetitions of the /p/ or /b/ sounds will allow the examiner to assess the ability to make rapid movements with the lips.

Nose and Airway

Anomalies of the nose can cause upper airway obstruction and hyponasality or nasal cul-de-sac resonance. Therefore, the examiner should note whether there is a flat nasal bridge or evidence of stenosis of one or more of the nares. Additional characteristics of upper airway obstruction include suborbital coloring (darkness under the eyes), pinched nostrils, and a face that appears elongated and narrow caused by the downward position of the mandible. These characteristics have been referred to as the adenoid facies because they are commonly seen in individuals with upper airway obstruction from adenoid enlargement (Elluru, 2005). Other signs of upper airway obstruction include strident breathing; snoring at night; sleep apnea; and, of course, hyponasality.

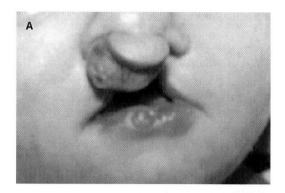

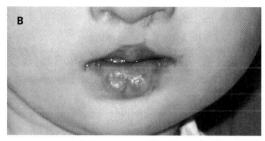

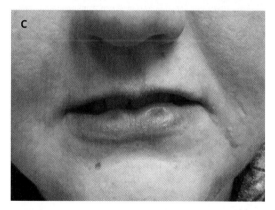

FIGURE 12-8 Bilateral lip pits, which indicate Van der Woude syndrome. This is an important finding because this syndrome is autosomal dominant.

To test the nasal airway, the examiner should ask the patient to close the lips and breathe nasally for several minutes. Before opening the mouth, the child should be asked to inspire deeply through the nose and then exhale through the nose. The examiner should observe whether there is any difficulty with nasal breathing or pinching of the nostrils during inspiration. The patency of each nostril can be assessed

by having the child close one nostril and then forcibly inspire through the other. If there is obstruction, this will be difficult to do and will result in a high-pitched sound, with the highest sound in the most obstructed nostril. Another test is to ask the patient to prolong an /m/ (which requires the lips to be closed). If there is significant blockage, the patient will be unable to do this easily.

Facial Bones and Profile

The examiner should note the bony structures of the face as they relate to each other. The facial profile, which can give an indication of the dysmorphology of the other facial bones, can be evaluated by having the patient turn so that the examiner is viewing the side of the person's face. For a normal profile, imaginary points on the forehead, bridge of the nose, base of the nose, and chin button should all line up in a vertical plane. The examiner should note whether there is maxillary retrusion with midface deficiency and whether the mandible is either micrognathic or prognathic.

Dentition and Occlusion

Dental anomalies (i.e., rotated or supernumerary teeth, crossbite, overbite, overjet, and underjet) are common contributors to speech problems in children with clefts or other craniofacial conditions. A crossbite with a narrow maxillary arch can be particularly problematic for speech (**FIGURE 12-9**). To determine whether dental anomalies are interfering with tongue placement or movement for speech, the child should be asked to prolong an /s/. The examiner should then determine whether the tongue is anterior to the alveolar ridge and maxillary teeth because of a crossbite (which would cause a frontal distortion) or touching a tooth or teeth because of their abnormal position or oral cavity crowding (which would cause a lateral distortion).

Malocclusion, where there is a discrepancy in the relationship between the maxilla

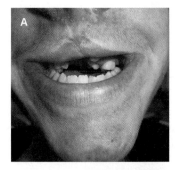

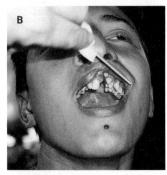

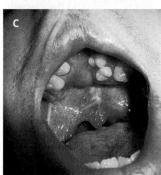

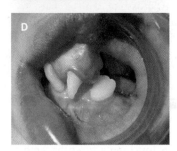

and mandible, can be particularly problematic for speech. Because the tongue always resides within the mandible, the position of the mandible in relationship to the maxilla can affect tongue tip articulation against the alveolar ridge and bilabial competence. With Class II malocclusion from micrognathia, the tongue tip may be under the palate rather than the alveolar ridge (**FIGURE 12-10**). With Class III malocclusion, the tongue tip may be anterior to the alveolar ridge (**FIGURE 12-11**). Therefore, when malocclusion is noted, the examiner should assess the position of the tongue tip relative to the position of the alveolar ridge and also assess bilabial competence.

Finally, the status of oral hygiene should be assessed. Poor oral hygiene is common in patients with misaligned teeth because thorough cleaning is much more difficult and they often

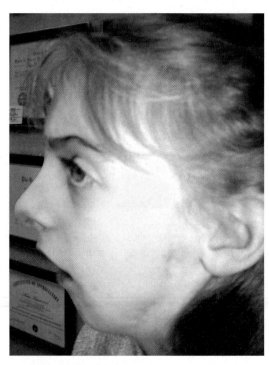

FIGURE 12-9 Crossbites. **(A)–(B)** Crossbites with missing and misplaced teeth. **(C)** Note the anterior fistula just under the lip. **(D)** Lateral crossbite and missing teeth.

FIGURE 12-10 Class II malocclusion with micrognathia. This causes the tongue tip to rest under the hard palate rather than under the alveolar ridge.

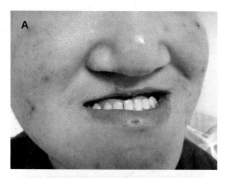

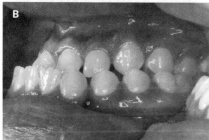

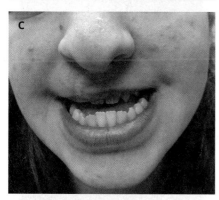

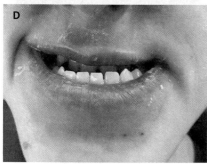

FIGURE 12-11 Class III malocclusion. This results in an anterior tongue position relative to the position of the alveolar ridge.

have an aversion to looking at their teeth. If the examiner notices poor oral hygiene or obvious caries, a referral for dental care should be included in the overall recommendations following the assessment.

Tongue

As noted previously, the position of the tongue tip relative to the alveolar ridge is particularly important to note. In addition, the size of the tongue relative to the mandibular arch, the palatal arch, and the overall oral cavity space should be assessed. If the tongue does not fit within the oral cavity during attempts to close the teeth, this may suggest macroglossia, which can affect both dentition and speech (**FIGURE 12-12A**). Multiple lobulations of the tongue may be noted in a child with oral–facial–digital syndrome (**FIGURE 12-12B**). If the patient has had a tongue flap for closure of an oronasal fistula, the scarring and effect on function should be noted. Even with extensive scarring after a tongue flap, there is usually no effect on lingual function with articulation.

The possibility of a tongue thrust should be considered if there is an anterior open bite. This can be determined by gently scratching the tip of the tongue with a tongue blade to provide a tingling sensation and then having the child take a drink of water. After the swallow, the examiner asks the child to report whether the tongue tip went up (against the alveolar ridge), forward (against or between the incisors), or down (against the mandibular incisors). If the child consistently reports that the tongue goes forward or down with the swallow, a tongue thrust should be suspected (Dahan, Lelong, Celant, & Leysen, 2000; Eslamian & Leilazpour, 2006; Fraser, 2006; Peng, Jost-Brinkmann, Yoshida, Chou, & Lin, 2004; Piyapattamin, Soma, & Hisano, 2002). If the child is unable to report the direction of the tongue movement, the movement can be observed by asking the child to swallow while the lips are held open with a tongue blade. If there is an anterior open bite, observing the tongue movement during swallowing is usually easy.

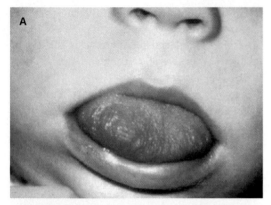

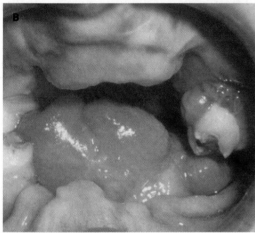

FIGURE 12-12 Tongue anomalies. **(A)** Macroglossia in a patient with Beckwith–Wiedemann syndrome. **(B)** Lobulated tongue in a patient with oral–facial–digital syndrome. This typically does not affect speech.

Ankyloglossia, commonly called tongue-tie, is a condition where the person cannot elevate the tongue tip sufficiently to touch the roof of the mouth—*with mouth open*—and cannot protrude the tongue tip past the mandibular gingival ridge or mandibular incisors (**FIGURE 12-13**). During protrusion, the tongue tip often resembles the top of a heart because the restricted lingual frenulum causes an indentation in the midline.

Ankyloglossia is not likely to cause abnormal speech—particularly for English speakers (Kummer, 2005). To determine whether the ankyloglossia is affecting articulation, the examiner

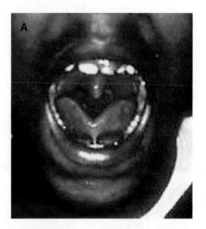

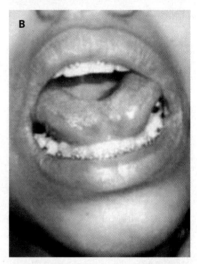

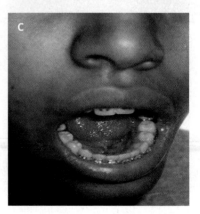

FIGURE 12-13 Ankyloglossia (tongue-tie). Note the heart shape at the tip of the tongue in **(A)**.

should evaluate production of /l/ (where there is usually lingual elevation) and /θ/ (where there is lingual protrusion). It should be noted that /l/ can be produced with the tongue tip down and the dorsum up. In addition, the /θ/ sound can be produced with the tongue tip against the back of the incisors or even just under the alveolar ridge, so very little protrusion is actually required. If the child is able to produce these sounds with slight modifications, frenulectomy should not be recommended. On the other hand, the trilled /r/ sound used in Spanish and some other languages may be difficult to produce with ankyloglossia. Of note, ankyloglossia can be a hindrance for patients with concomitant oral-motor difficulties and has the potential to affect early feeding and moving a bolus around the mouth.

Tonsils

The presence of tonsils and their relative size should be evaluated. Otolaryngologists rate the size of tonsils on the following scale, based on their position within the tonsillar fossa (space within the faucial pillars):

Grade 0 Tonsils are within the tonsillar fossa

Grade 1+ Tonsils extend just outside the faucial pillars and occupy ≤ 25% of the oropharyngeal width

Grade 2+ Tonsils occupy 26–50% of the oropharyngeal width

Grade 3+ Tonsils occupy 51–75% of the oropharyngeal width

Grade 4+ Tonsils occupy > 75% of the oropharyngeal width

In addition to extending medially, tonsils can extend forward in the oral cavity or backward into the pharynx. If one tonsil is larger than the other and intrudes into the pharynx, it will push against the posterior faucial pillar, which will make the uvula bend to the side of the large tonsil (**FIGURE 12-14**). If the tonsils are markedly asymmetric in size, this may be a sign of malignancy in the larger tonsil, so a referral to an otolaryngologist would be appropriate. Enlarged tonsils are always important to identify because they can interfere with velopharyngeal function, causing nasal emission or

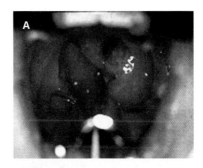

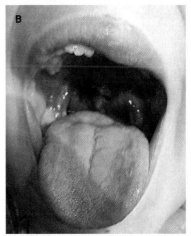

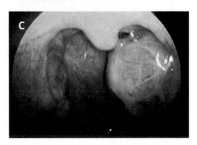

FIGURE 12-14 Large tonsil unilaterally. Note the deviation of the uvula in all cases. This suggests that the tonsil is intruding into the oropharynx.

a blockage of sound and airflow from entering the oral cavity and resulting in weak consonants and pharyngeal cul-de-sac resonance. They can even interfere with posterior tongue placement for velar sounds (/k/, /g/, /ŋ/). Finally, enlarged tonsils can affect the airway, causing obstructive sleep apnea (OSA).

Alveolar Ridge and Hard Palate

As noted previously, the position of the alveolar ridge as it relates to the position of the tongue tip is important to observe. Significant jaw discrepancy can affect this relationship, causing difficulty with normal speech production.

For a child with cleft lip and/or palate, the examiner should rule out a fistula. One indication of a nasolabial fistula is a report of food coloring (e.g., chocolate or red sauce) in the child's nostril after meals. To inspect for a nasolabial fistula, the examiner should use a tongue blade or dental mirror to gently raise the upper lip. Using a gloved finger, the fistula usually can be palpated by feeling the top of the gum area, just under the buccal sulcus. This type of fistula causes nasal regurgitation but does not affect speech because it is out of the way of articulation and airflow. In addition, it will eventually be closed with the bone graft, so it is not a concern.

An oronasal fistula in the hard palate that is dime sized or larger can affect speech and cause nasal regurgitation (**FIGURE 12-15**). Therefore, the hard palate should be inspected with the help of a dental mirror and flashlight. Despite the use of the mirror, the size of a fistula is often difficult to estimate. It may appear small on the oral surface yet open considerably on the nasal surface. In addition, there may be a furrow or a small depression in the palate that appears to be a fistula but is actually just a blind pouch that does not go all the way through. If a fistula is identified, its approximate size and location should be noted because these factors are the determinants as to whether the fistula may be symptomatic.

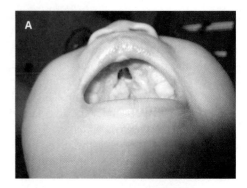
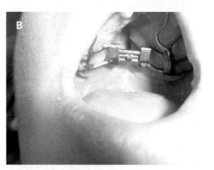
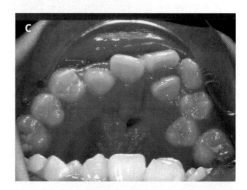
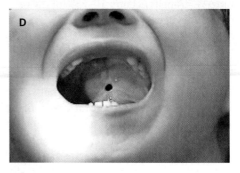

FIGURE 12-15 Examples of oronasal fistulas.

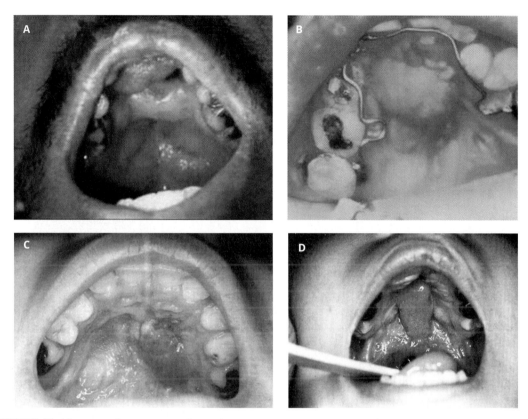

FIGURE 12-16 Tongue flap. A tongue flap is done to correct a large oronasal fistula. In **(A)**, there is still a remaining opening on the right side (patient's left).

An examination of the hard palate will reveal the overlying mucosa, which is normally uniform in color (Jones, 1989; Schacher et al., 2010). At times, the examiner will notice tissue on the palate that is a different color or texture than the other palatal mucosa. This may be caused by a tongue flap or buccal flap that was used to surgically close an oronasal fistula (**FIGURE 12-16**). The examiner should be sure that the flap is not so bulky that it interferes with normal articulation.

The palatal vault should be evaluated in relationship to the size of the tongue. A low palatal vault or narrow maxillary arch can reduce the space available for lingual articulation and also affect oral resonance. To compensate for intraoral crowding, the mandible will often lower, and the tongue may be forced down and forward during speech.

Finally, if present, a V shape in the hard palate should be noted because it indicates a submucous cleft that extends through the hard palate. A submucous cleft can extend as far as the position of the incisive foramen (just behind the alveolar ridge).

Occasionally, an examination of the hard palate reveals a palatal torus. A **torus** is a slow-growing nodular protuberance of bone that can occur in either the hard palate or mandible. There is evidence that both types of tori (plural form of torus) are hereditary. They occur almost twice as often in females than in males (Buddula, 2009; Nortje, 2006; Papadopoulos & Lawhorn, 2008; Schwartz, 2005). A **torus palatinus**, also called a

CASE REPORT

Oronasal Fistula

Gerald presented as a new patient at the age of 11. He had a bilateral complete cleft lip and palate, which were repaired in another state. He also had had a pharyngeal flap for correction of velopharyngeal insufficiency at the age of 4. Gerald received speech therapy for several years in school. The mother reported that her primary concern was Gerald's nasality.

Upon examination, Gerald's speech was found to be minimally intelligible. His articulation pattern consisted of backing of anterior phonemes. Many compensatory productions were used. Resonance was hyponasal, and mouth breathing was noted, suggesting upper airway obstruction. An obstructing pharyngeal flap was suspected.

The surprise came with the intraoral inspection, however. When examining the hard palate, a very large oronasal fistula was observed. However, it was packed with food. Gerald was taken to the otolaryngologist, who cleaned out the fistula and the nasal cavity.

Once the fistula was cleaned out and opened, the speech was reevaluated and found to be hypernasal with nasal air emission. The pattern of backing of phonemes was obviously developed as a means to compensate for the position of the open fistula.

Nasopharyngoscopy showed both lateral ports around the flap to be stenosed, which was the cause of the hyponasality and upper airway obstruction when the fistula was impacted. With this information in mind, a fistula repair and lateral port revisions were recommended.

This case study illustrates the importance of an intraoral examination. Although it is not possible to observe velopharyngeal function with an intraoral examination, some observations made in the intraoral examination relate directly to the cause of the speech or resonance disorder.

palatal torus, is a bony protuberance in the midline of the hard palate (**FIGURE 12-17**). It can have a flat, spindled, nodular, or lobular configuration. It is usually asymmetric and is rarely a source of

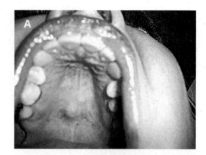
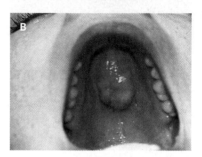
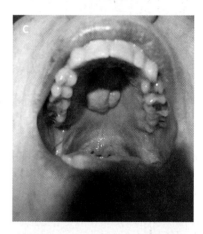
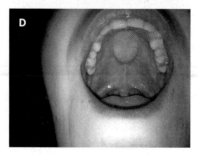

FIGURE 12-17 Examples of a torus palatinus. Note that in **(C)** there is also a bifid uvula and subtle evidence of a submucous cleft in the velum.

discomfort unless the mucosal surface becomes ulcerated. Therefore, it is of little clinical significance. A torus palatinus does not interfere with speech or any other function unless it is very large.

Velum and Uvula

The examiner should always examine velar morphology and movement. A normal velum should be consistent in color and may have a white line down the middle, called the median palatine raphe.

In children with cleft palate, it is important to inspect the velum for a fistula, just as is done with the hard palate. If the fistula is anterior to the velar dimple (the point where the velum bends during phonation from the contraction of the levator muscles), it may be symptomatic during speech because this location is near the area of maximum airflow as it enters the oral cavity. On the other hand, a fistula that is posterior to the area of the velar dimple will not affect resonance because it is below the area of velopharyngeal closure and in the area of velar redundancy (the vertical area of velum that is under the point of contact against the posterior pharyngeal wall).

Although not common, a portion or all of the velum can dehisce (pull apart) days or weeks after the palate repair. This may look like an unrepaired, incomplete cleft palate (**FIGURE 12-18**). In addition, a large velar defect can be noted as a result of a previous tumor removal (**FIGURE 12-19**).

During phonation, the velum may appear to be short relative to the position of the posterior pharyngeal wall. This can be deceiving, however, because the oral view is well below the level of actual velopharyngeal contact. The effective length of the velum can be estimated, however, by the position of the velar dimple during contraction, which is where the levator veli palatini muscles interdigitate in the velum to pull it up and back during phonation (Veerapandiyan et al., 2011). The section of the velum that is anterior to the dimple is the effective length because it spans the length of the pharynx that is needed to obturate the nasopharyngeal port during speech. During sustained phonation, the velar dimple should appear to be back approximately 80% of the length of the velum (Mason

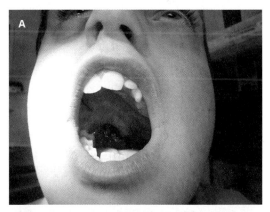

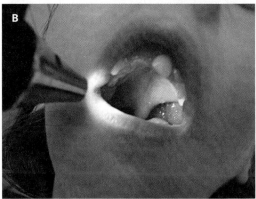

FIGURE 12-19 Velar defect after tumor resection. **(A)** Defect is on the patient's right side. **(B)** Defect is on the patient's left side.

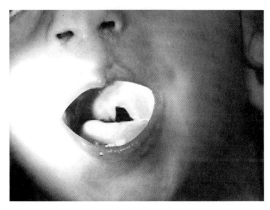

FIGURE 12-18 Dehisced velum following cleft palate repair.

& Simon, 1977). If the velar dimple is closer to the hard palate than to the uvula, the effective length may be too short, which can cause velopharyngeal insufficiency. On the other hand, a velar dimple that is very close to the uvula suggests a short velum with too little vertical surface to close firmly against the pharyngeal wall. When this is the case, the uvula can often be observed to flip backward during phonation.

If there is no history of cleft palate, the examiner should look for characteristics of a submucous cleft. Signs of a submucous cleft include a zona pellucida, which is a bluish-appearing area in the middle of the velum (Reiter, Brosch, Wefel, Schlomer, & Haase, 2011). This appearance occurs when the velum is thin and hence transparent as a result of the lack of muscle in this area. A thin velum is important to note because, in the absence of velopharyngeal insufficiency/incompetence (VPI) it can be the cause of nasal resonance, resulting from transmission of sound energy through it.

If there is a submucous cleft that extends through the velum, the velum may appear to "tent up" in an upside down V shape during phonation (**FIGURE 12-20**). When this occurs, it is because the levator veli palatini muscles are inserted on the edge of the posterior hard palate rather than in the midline of the velum. The contraction of these muscles results in the V shape in the velum. The V-shaped defect may be noted even without phonation, particularly if the submucous cleft extends through velum and the bony hard palate. Even when there is no apparent evidence of a submucous cleft through an intraoral examination, it cannot be ruled out. There may be an occult submucous cleft in the muscles or mucosa on the nasal side of the velum that can be detected only through nasopharyngoscopy (Finkelstein, Hauben, Talmi, Nachmani, & Zohar, 1992; Rourke, Weinberg, Marazita, & Jabbour, 2017). In addition, it should be remembered that even with clear evidence of a submucous cleft, there may be normal resonance and velopharyngeal function.

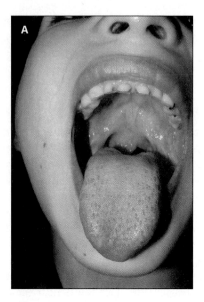

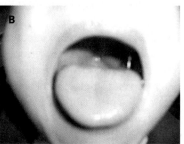

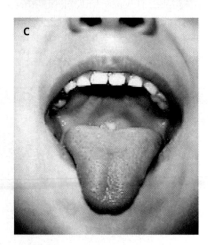

FIGURE 12-20 Submucous cleft. During phonation, the velum appears to tent up in an inverted V shape from the abnormal orientation of the levator muscles.

After examining the basic morphology of the velum, velar function should be observed during phonation of a vowel, preferably during phonation of the /æ/ vowel. The observation of poor velar movement during phonation is common with phonation of a single vowel. Eliciting the gag reflex can confirm the presence of neuromotor function and also show the maximum excursion of the velum. However, this does not correlate well with movement potential for speech. As noted previously, the best way to elicit velar movement is by having the child produce the vowel repetitively.

With normal velopharyngeal movement, the velum should raise symmetrically, and the velar dimple and uvula should be in midline. Two lateral velar dimples observed during phonation suggests diastasis of the levator veli palatini muscles, which is consistent with a submucous cleft (Boorman & Sommerland, 1985). Asymmetrical velar movement suggests velopharyngeal incompetence from unilateral paralysis or paresis (weakness) of the velum. In this case, the velar dimple may not be in midline but instead may be skewed to the better side. In addition, the uvula may point to the better side during phonation. Asymmetric velar movement usually causes a lateral, rather than central, velopharyngeal gap, which is important to note when making surgical recommendations. The examiner should particularly look for unilateral velar paralysis or paresis in individuals with hemifacial microsomia.

Velopharyngeal incompetence (generalized poor movement of the velum) should be considered in children with neuromotor dysfunction related to dysarthria, apraxia, or velar paralysis or paresis. Poor velar movement can also be caused by enlarged adenoids that interfere with the upward movement of the velum or an anterior inclination of the pharyngeal wall in the nasopharynx, making extensive velar movement unnecessary for speech. Finally, the individual may have a sagittal pattern of closure, making velar movement less important.

Inspection of the uvula is important because its appearance may give a clue to a submucous cleft (Finkelstein et al., 1992). Either a bifid uvula (with two separate tags) or a hypoplastic uvula that is short and stubby can suggest a submucous cleft (**FIGURE 12-21**). In some cases, the uvula may appear to be intact because the saliva helps to "glue" the tags of a bifid uvula together. If the examiner suspects that the uvula is bifid but is unsure, this can often be determined by placing the tip of a tongue blade just behind the uvula and then flipping it forward (Rivron, 1989; Vilacosta & Canadas Godoy, 2008). If there are two tags, they will separate with this maneuver. (This is not recommended for a young child, however.) It should be remembered that a bifid uvula is a relatively common finding in the general population and does not always indicate a submucous cleft (Bagatin, 1985; Wharton & Mowrer, 1992). In many cases, the defect includes only the uvula and does not involve the velum. To be safe, however, it is important to counsel individuals with a bifid uvula that they may be at risk for developing or exacerbating hypernasality following an adenoidectomy.

Posterior and Lateral Pharyngeal Walls

The depth of the posterior pharyngeal wall should be viewed relative to the length of the velum during phonation. When the posterior pharyngeal wall is very deep (and/or the velum is very short), the examiner may be able to look up into the nasopharynx with a dental mirror and flashlight. In most cases, however, the examiner cannot determine whether the pharyngeal wall is too deep or the velum is too short for closure because there is no way to know how the pharynx curves as it courses superiorly and then anteriorly to form the nasal cavity. The pharynx may appear to be very deep at the oral level but may curve sufficiently during the incline so that velopharyngeal closure can be obtained. In addition, the velum may be closing against a large

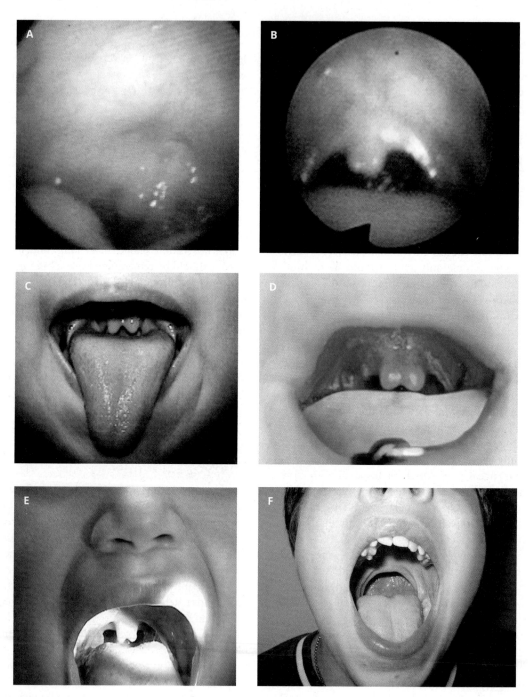

FIGURE 12-21 Abnormal uvulae that can suggest a submucous cleft. **(A)** and **(B)**. The uvula is hypoplastic with a faint line in the middle. **(C–E)** The uvula is clearly bifid. **(F)** The uvula is absent, which is often the case after a cleft palate repair. This does not affect speech.

adenoid pad rather than the posterior pharyngeal wall, which cannot be noted with an intraoral examination.

Lateral and posterior pharyngeal wall movement on the oral level can be observed during phonation. There may be very vigorous movement of the pharyngeal walls, which can substantiate that the nervous supply to the pharynx is intact. However, it doesn't necessarily indicate good pharyngeal wall movement in the area of velopharyngeal closure. In addition, poor movement of the lateral pharyngeal walls is not necessarily an indication of a problem. In fact, at the oral level, the lateral pharyngeal walls may actually bow outward during phonation while bowing inward at a higher plane to assist with closure. Bowing outward at the oral level during phonation is actually a good thing because that opens the oropharynx to facilitate the transmission of airflow and sound into the oral cavity.

If the adenoids are enlarged, the inferior border of the adenoid pad can occasionally be observed on the posterior pharyngeal wall. It appears as lobulated tissue just behind and under the velum during phonation.

The examiner may notice a Passavant's ridge when the child phonates for the oral examination (**FIGURE 12-22**). It appears as a shelf-like ridge that bulges forward from the posterior pharyngeal wall at the oropharyngeal level during phonation and the gag reflex (Yamawaki, 2003). If a Passavant's ridge is observed from an intraoral view, it is positioned too low to assist with velopharyngeal closure. Therefore, it is no more than an interesting observation.

If the patient has had previous surgery for VPI, there may be visible evidence on the posterior pharyngeal wall. For example, a vertical white line on the posterior pharyngeal wall can be a scar from the donor site of a pharyngeal flap. In some cases, the actual flap from the surgery (pharyngeal flap or sphincter pharyngoplasty) can be viewed from an intraoral perspective. This usually indicates that the flap is too low to be effective for speech. In addition, a low flap is more likely to cause sleep apnea (and even swallowing problems)

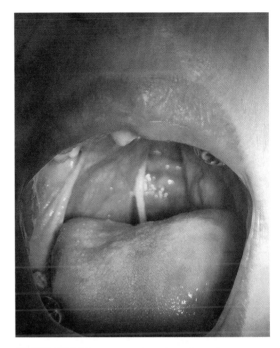

FIGURE 12-22 Passavant's ridge. This ridge can sometimes be seen on the posterior pharyngeal wall through an intraoral examination during phonation. It is caused by contraction of the superior constrictor muscles.

because it is near the level of the base of the tongue (see the chapter *Surgical Management* for more information).

Epiglottis

The epiglottis is located just below the base of the tongue and is relatively high in the hypopharynx in young children. As such, it can sometimes be viewed during an intraoral assessment of a young child, particularly if the child protrudes the tongue to say /æ/ (Shinohara & Takahashi, 2005) (**FIGURE 12-23**). This is not a reason for concern. As the tongue goes forward, the epiglottis is pulled upward toward the oropharyngeal isthmus. The epiglottis is not usually seen in adults because the larynx descends in the neck with age, minimizing its ability to be viewed during oral examinations.

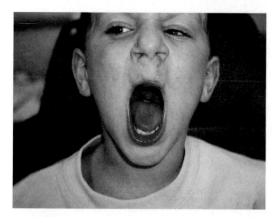

FIGURE 12-23 Epiglottis. Because the epiglottis is closer to the base of the tongue in children than in adults, it can sometimes be seen popping up when the child opens his mouth and sticks out his tongue.

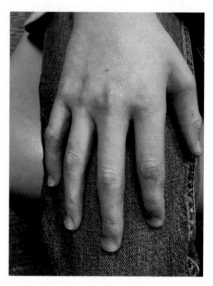

FIGURE 12-24 Long and tapered fingers, which are often found with velocardiofacial/22q11.2 deletion syndrome.

Putting It All Together

During the orofacial examination, the examiner should determine the physical factors that appear to be interfering with articulation and/or resonance. Although the examiner should focus on assessing anomalies that can contribute to a speech or resonance disorder, other anomalies should also be noted. This is because they may require additional referral or follow-up (e.g., dental caries), or they could provide evidence of an unidentified syndrome (e.g., hypertelorism). Even non-orofacial features, such as short stature or long and slender digits (**FIGURE 12-24**), can provide clues to a syndrome. (These particular features are suggestive of VCFS/22q deletion syndrome.) Some relevant anomalies or medical conditions that are not readily seen, such as heart or kidney anomalies, may be recorded in the medical record or reported by the parents. When anomalies are noted that require additional evaluation or follow-up, the speech-language pathologist should discuss the findings with the primary care physician and referring physician and suggest referrals to other specialists as appropriate.

Infection Control during the Examination

A discussion of the intraoral examination would not be complete without a section on infection control. Knowledge of infection control is important to protect the healthcare provider and prevent the spread of infection to those individuals who are being served. Speech-language pathologists should practice good infection control procedures because they are in close physical contact with the individuals in their care and are often working around and even in the mouth. Unfortunately, most speech-language pathologists have had little training on appropriate infection control procedures unless they have obtained it from on-the-job experience (Bankaitis, Kemp, Krival, & Bandaranayake, 2006; Mosheim, 2005).

The most common causes of communicable diseases in healthcare environments are the human immunodeficiency virus (HIV), hepatitis B virus (HBV), cytomegalovirus I (CMV), methicillin-resistant staphylococcus aureus (MRSA) bacteria, clostridium difficile (C-diff) bacteria, and the tuberculosis bacteria. Professionals must also be concerned about the transmission of minor diseases, such as the common cold and influenza. Pediatric settings are a particular concern because children generally have poor personal hygiene habits yet are very susceptible to infection (Krewedl, 1999).

In 1988, the Centers for Disease Control and Prevention (CDC) in Atlanta published guidelines for infection control called Universal Blood and Body Fluid Precautions (UBBFP). They have since been revised and are now called Standard Precautions (CDC, 2005). Standard precautions contain recommended procedures that are designed to protect the patient, the professional, and all others in a healthcare environment from the spread of infection. These procedures are based on the assumption that every patient and healthcare provider is a potential carrier of an infectious disease and that any body fluid may contain contagious microorganisms. The American Speech-Language-Hearing Association (ASHA) adopted these guidelines and recommended them to its membership in 1990. There are now documents and links on the ASHA website related to standard precautions and infection control (ASHA, 2012). Despite the fact that standard precautions have been recommended for more than two decades, there is evidence to suggest that they are not consistently or appropriately used by many healthcare professionals (Aultman & Borges, 2011).

Handwashing

The role of the human hands in the transmission of infection was recognized even before the establishment of microbiology as a science (Kerr, 1998). For many years, handwashing has been considered the single most important means of preventing the spread of infection in a healthcare setting (Akyol, Ulusoy, & Ozen, 2006; CDC, 2005; CDC, 2013; Gallagher, 1999; Ginsberg & Clarke, 1972; Horton, 1995; Kiernan, 1999; World Health Organization [WHO], 2009). Handwashing reduces the number of potential pathogens on the hands and interrupts the opportunity of transferring organisms to patients and others.

Unfortunately, healthcare workers are not always compliant in washing their hands as often as they should (Aultman & Borges, 2011). As a result, nosocomial infections (hospital acquired) continue to be a principal cause of morbidity and even mortality in healthcare settings (Brunetti et al., 2006; Kennedy, Elward, & Fraser, 2004; Picheansathian, Pearson, & Suchaxaya, 2008). It is widely believed that if all healthcare providers used the proper technique for handwashing and this became a habit, infection rates in healthcare facilities would drop dramatically (Brown & Persivale, 1995). Certainly, greater awareness of this problem may help to generate improvement.

Hands should be washed before and after every patient contact and especially before and after an intraoral examination. It is best if hands are washed in front of the parents and child because this models appropriate hygienic behavior (Bellet, 1996). The use of examination gloves does not eliminate the need for handwashing (Bowman & Nicholas, 1990; Hopkins, 1989; Ripper, 1988; Shogren, 1988). It is important that the examiner wash his or her hands before putting the gloves on because there can be a perforation in the glove that is not readily visible. Handwashing is also necessary after glove removal because the warm, moist environment in the glove is conducive to rapid bacterial multiplication (Mayone-Ziomek, 1998). Finally, hands should be washed after contact with potentially contaminated surfaces.

Both the CDC and the WHO have published guidelines on appropriate handwashing in a hospital environment (CDC, 2005; CDC, 2013; WHO, 2009). The WHO recommendations for proper handwashing with soap and water are stated as follows:

- Wet hands with water.
- Apply enough soap to cover all hand surfaces.
- Rub hands palm to palm, right palm over left dorsum with interlaced fingers and vice versa.

- Rub hands palm to palm with fingers interlaced.
- Rub backs of fingers to opposing palms with fingers interlocked.
- Rub rotationally, left thumb clasped in right palm and vice versa.
- Rub rotationally backward and forward, with clasped fingers of right hand in left palm and vice versa.
- Rinse hands with water.
- Dry hands thoroughly with a single use towel.
- Use towel to turn off faucet.

For more information or to see illustrations, go to the WHO website at http://whqlibdoc.who .int/publications/2009/9789241597906_eng.pdf.

If soap and water are not immediately available or hands are not visibly dirty or contaminated, antimicrobial handwipes or gels can be used for antisepsis. Antimicrobial handwashing products (e.g., 2% chlorhexidine gluconate, triclosan) should be used before contact with newborns, immunocompromised patients and patients on high-risk units, and before an invasive procedure.

Gloves

With the standard precautions approach to infection control, the examiner should assume that all human secretions, including saliva, could be infectious or contain bloodborne pathogens. Therefore, the examiner must wear personal protective equipment (PPE) when performing any task that has the risk of contact with the patient's secretions or requires physical contact with the patient's mouth or nose. Therefore, gloves should always be worn during an intraoral examination, during a feeding evaluation or therapy, and while performing a nasopharyngoscopy exam.

Until recently, latex gloves were used in most healthcare settings. However, latex allergies have become very common. To minimize sensitization of healthcare workers and exposure to latex-sensitive patients, most institutions have now eliminated the use of latex gloves. Hospital gloves are now made of vinyl, nitrile, or another synthetic material.

Gloves should fit tightly because loosely fitted gloves interfere with the manipulation of objects. Gloves should be changed immediately if holes, rips, or tears are visible and as needed during the patient's care. When removing gloves, they should be pulled off so that they are inside out and then immediately discarded (**FIGURE 12-25**). This prevents physical contact with the contaminated

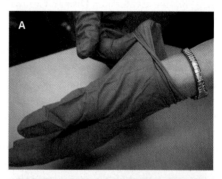

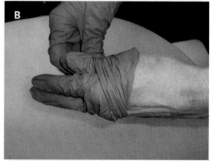

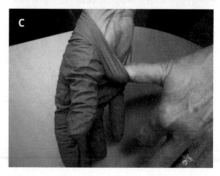

FIGURE 12-25 Proper way to remove gloves.
(A) Grab the glove at the wrist. **(B)** Pull the glove off so that it is inside out. **(C)** Put thumb under the wrist of the second glove and pull it off inside out.

surface of the gloves. Because all gloves are designed for single-patient use, they are discarded in the waste can after each patient.

Patient Equipment and Supplies

Tongue blades, dental mirrors, and other tools for an intraoral assessment should not be placed directly on a desk or table after use. Instead, these tools should be placed on a clean paper towel or tissue until they can be cleaned or discarded.

Disposable items should be used for intraoral examinations or manipulation whenever possible. It is easier to dispose of an item and use a new one for the next person than to have to wash and disinfect the item between uses. Items that are manufactured to be disposable usually cannot be adequately washed or disinfected and therefore they should be discarded immediately after use.

Items that are not disposable, such as a dental mirror, should be cleaned and sanitized in a dishwasher if possible. Alternatively, the item can be thoroughly cleansed with hot, soapy water and then wiped down with alcohol. Both ethyl alcohol and isopropyl alcohol have a broad spectrum of antimicrobial activity that counteracts vegetative bacteria, fungi, and viruses (including HIV) (Widmer & Frei, 1999). In addition, alcohol has many qualities that make it suitable for low-level and intermediate-level disinfection, including the fact that it is fast acting (15–30 seconds) and readily evaporates. Sterilization, as opposed to disinfection, is required to destroy bacterial spores, however. Items contaminated with saliva only and intact mucous membranes are resistant to bacterial spores. Therefore, sterilization is usually not necessary unless the instruments have the potential for exposure to blood. On the other hand, C-diff bacteria are not killed with alcohol, so if this disease is a concern, chlorine bleach wipes should be used.

All patient equipment and supplies should be stored in a clean and safe manner that protects the items from exposure or contamination to body fluids, known soiled items, dust, particulate matter, and moisture. Supplies should always be stored a minimum of 4–6 inches off the floor to enable floor cleaning and to protect from accidental damage or contamination with floor cleaning solutions.

Surface Disinfection

Flat surfaces, such as tables and armchairs, can be contaminated with saliva or mucous during a session. Therefore, all therapy or patient care rooms should be equipped with spray disinfectant products and disinfectant towelettes (Bankaitis et al., 2006). Surfaces should be cleaned and disinfected between patients.

SUMMARY

Speech-language pathologists and other healthcare providers should be keen observers of dysmorphic craniofacial features in their patients or students. This can be helpful in the prediction and timely treatment of related functional problems, including problems with speech and resonance. A thorough orofacial examination is important for children with clefts and known craniofacial syndromes. It is also important for children who demonstrate disorders of speech and/or resonance. Observations from the orofacial examination can help the speech-language pathologist determine which speech errors are from abnormal structure and therefore require physical management instead of speech therapy or before initiating speech therapy.

FOR REVIEW AND DISCUSSION

1. Describe the best method for viewing the intraoral structures with the least amount of stress or discomfort for the patient.

2. What are the particular anomalies that can be observed of the eyes, ears, nose, lips, and facial bones? Why are these observations an important part of a speech pathology examination?

3. What is the purpose of palatal palpation? Describe how this is done and what should be felt.

4. What observations of the velopharyngeal mechanism can be made through an intraoral examination? Why can't velopharyngeal function be viewed by looking in the mouth?

5. Describe a method for evaluating dental occlusion. Why is it important to assess occlusion? What are the implications for treatment recommendations?

6. Discuss the evaluation of the structure and function of the tongue and what should be considered. Why is ankyloglossia an unlikely cause of speech disorders?

7. Describe methods of infection control when performing an intraoral examination.

REFERENCES

Akyol, A., Ulusoy, H., & Ozen, I. (2006). Handwashing: A simple, economical and effective method for preventing nosocomial infections in intensive care units. *Journal of Hospital Infection, 62*(4), 395–405.

American Speech-Language-Hearing Association (ASHA). (2012). Infection control in speech-language pathology. Retrieved from http://www.asha.org/slp/infectioncontrol.htm.

Aultman, J. M., & Borges, N. J. (2011). The ethical and pedagogical effects of modeling "not-so-universal" precautions. *Medical Teacher, 33*(1), e43–e49.

Bagatin, M. (1985). Submucous cleft palate. *Journal of Maxillofacial Surgery, 13*(1), 37–38.

Bankaitis, A. U., Kemp, R. J., Krival, K., & Bandaranayake, D. (2006). *Infection control for speech-language pathology.* St. Louis, MO: Auban.

Bellet, P. S. (1996). Physical examination. In R. C. Baker (Ed.), *Pediatric primary care.* Philadelphia, PA: Lippincott Williams & Wilkins.

Boorman, J. G., & Sommerland, B. C. (1985). Levator veli palati and palatal dimples: Their anatomy, relationship, and clinical significance. *British Journal of Plastic Surgery, 38,* 326–332.

Bowman, A. M., & Nicholas, T. J. (1990). Improving compliance with universal blood and body fluid precautions in a rural medical center. *Journal of Nursing Quality Assurance, 5*(1), 73–81.

Brown, J. W., & Persivale, E. J. (1995). Managing the front line of infection control: Handwashing. *Director, 3*(1), 36–37.

Brunetti, L., Santoro, E., De Caro, F., Cavallo, P., Boccia, G., Capunzo, M., & Motta, O. (2006). Surveillance of nosocomial infections: A preliminary study on hand hygiene compliance of healthcare workers. *Journal of Preventive Medicine and Hygiene, 47*(2), 64–68.

Buddula, A. (2009). Staining of palatal torus secondary to long-term minocycline therapy. *Journal of Indian Society of Periodontology, 13*(1), 48–49.

Centers for Disease Control and Prevention (CDC). (2005). Appendix 11: Recommendations for application of standard precautions for the care of all patients in all healthcare settings. Retrieved from http://www.cdc.gov/sars/guidance/I-infection/app1.html.

Centers for Disease Control and Prevention (CDC). (2013). Handwashing: Clean hands save lives. Retrieved from http://www.cdc.gov/handwashing/.

Dahan, J. S., Lelong, O., Celant, S., & Leysen, V. (2000). Oral perception in tongue thrust and other oral habits. *American Journal of Orthodontics and Dentofacial Orthopedics, 118*(4), 385–391.

Elluru, R. G. (2005). Adenoid facies and nasal airway obstruction: Cause and effect? *Archives of Otolaryngology-Head & Neck Surgery, 131*(10), 919–920.

Eslamian, L., & Leilazpour, A. P. (2006). Tongue to palate contact during speech in subjects with and without a tongue thrust. *European Journal of Orthodontics, 28*(5), 475–479.

Finkelstein, Y., Hauben, D. J., Talmi, Y. P., Nachmani, A., & Zohar, Y. (1992). Occult and overt submucous cleft palate: From perioral examination to nasendoscopy and back again. *International Journal of Pediatric Otorhinolaryngology, 23*(1), 25–34.

Fraser, C. (2006). Tongue thrust and its influence in orthodontics. *International Journal of Orthodontics Milwaukee, 17*(1), 9–18.

Gallagher, R. (1999). This is the way we wash our hands. *Nursing Times, 95*(10), 62–65.

Ginsberg, F., & Clarke, B. (1972). Handwashing is simple, effective infection control, so why won't people wash their hands? *Modern Hospital, 119*(4), 132.

Hopkins, C. C. (1989). AIDS: Implementation of universal blood and body fluid precautions. *Infectious Disease Clinics of North America, 3*(4), 747–762.

Horton, R. (1995). Handwashing: The fundamental infection control principle. *British Journal of Nursing, 4*(16), 926, 928, 930–933.

Jones, J. A. (1989, October 30). Integrating the oral examination into clinical practice. *Hospital Practice, 24*(10A), 23–27, 30, 39.

Kennedy, A. M., Elward, A. M., & Fraser, V. J. (2004). Survey of knowledge, beliefs, and practices of neonatal intensive care unit healthcare workers regarding nosocomial infections, central venous catheter care, and hand hygiene. *Infection Control and Hospital Epidemiology, 25*(9), 747–752.

Kerr, J. (1998). Handwashing. *Nursing Standards, 12*(51), 35–39; quiz 41–42.

Kiernan, M. (1999). Handwashing in infection control. *Community Nurse, 5*(7), 19–20.

Krewedl, A. (1999, August 23). Infection control in pediatric settings. *Advance*, pp. 26–27.

Kummer, A. W. (2005, December 27). To clip or not to clip? That's the question. *The ASHA Leader, 10*(17), 6–7, 30.

Mason, R. M., & Simon, C. (1977). An orofacial examination checklist. *Language, Speech, and Hearing Services in the Schools, 8*(3), 155–163.

Mayone-Ziomek, J. M. (1998). Handwashing in healthcare. *Dermatological Nursing, 10*(3), 183–188.

Mosheim, J. (2005, October 24). Infection control: Protocols protect the clinician and patient. *Advance*

for Speech-Language Pathologists & Audiologists, pp. 7–9.

Nortje, C. J. (2006). General practitioners radiology. Case 39. Diagnosis. Palatal torus. *Journal of the South African Dental Association, 61*(2), 81.

Papadopoulos, H., & Lawhorn, T. (2008). Use of a palatal flap for torus reduction. *Journal of Oral and Maxillofacial Surgery, 66*(9), 1969–1970.

Peng, C. L., Jost-Brinkmann, P. G., Yoshida, N., Chou, H. H., & Lin, C. T. (2004). Comparison of tongue functions between mature and tongue-thrust swallowing: An ultrasound investigation. *American Journal of Orthodontics and Dentofacial Orthopedics, 125*(5), 562–570.

Picheansathian, W., Pearson, A., & Suchaxaya, P. (2008). The effectiveness of a promotion programme on hand hygiene compliance and nosocomial infections in a neonatal intensive care unit. *International Journal of Nursing Practice, 14*(4), 315–321.

Piyapattamin, T., Soma, K., & Hisano, M. (2002). Temporary tongue thrust: Failure during orthodontic treatment. *Australian Orthodontic Journal, 18*(1), 39–46.

Reiter, R., Brosch, S., Wefel, H., Schlomer, G., & Haase, S. (2011). The submucous cleft palate: Diagnosis and therapy. *International Journal of Pediatric Otorhinolaryngology, 75*(1), 85–88.

Ripper, M. (1988). Universal blood and body fluid precautions. *Journal of Advances in Medical Surgical Nursing, 1*(1), 21–25.

Rivron, R. P. (1989). Bifid uvula: Prevalence and association in otitis media with effusion in children admitted for routine otolaryngological operations. *Journal of Laryngology & Otology, 103*(3), 249–252.

Rourke, R., Weinberg, S. M., Marazita, M. L., & Jabbour, N. (2017). Diagnosing subtle palatal anomalies: Validation of video-analysis and assessment protocol for diagnosing occult submucous cleft palate. *International Journal of Pediatric Otorhinolaryngology, 100*, 242–246.

Schacher, B., Burklin, T., Horodko, M., Raetzke, P., Ratka-Kruger, P., & Eickholz, P. (2010). Direct thickness measurements of the hard palate mucosa. *Quintessence International, 41*(8), e149–e156.

Schwartz, A. J. (2005). Insertion of a folded laryngeal mask airway around a palatal torus. *American Association of Nurse Anesthetics Journal, 73*(3), 211–216.

Shanks, L. A., Walker, T. W., McCann, P. J., & Kerin, M. J. (2011). Oral cavity examination: Beyond the core curriculum? *British Journal of Oral and Maxillofacial Surgery, 49*(8), 640–642.

Shinohara, E. H., & Takahashi, A. (2005). View of the epiglottis during examination of the oral cavity. *British Journal of Oral and Maxillofacial Surgery, 43*(3), 264.

Shogren, E. (1988). An ounce of prevention is worth a pound of cure: Using universal blood and body fluid precautions in your work setting. *MNA Accent, 60*(2), 35–36.

Smith, B., & Guyette, T. W. (2004). Evaluation of cleft palate speech. *Clinics in Plastic Surgery, 31*(2), 251–260.

Smith, B. E., & Kuehn, D. P. (2007). Speech evaluation of velopharyngeal dysfunction. *The Journal of Craniofacial Surgery, 18*(2), 251–260.

Thomas, J. E., & Bender, B. S. (1993). What to look for after you say "Open wide." *Postgraduate Medicine, 93*(7), 109–110.

Veerapandiyan, A., Blalock, D., Ghosh, S., Ip, E., Barnes, C., & Shashi, V. (2011). The role of cephalometry in assessing velopharyngeal dysfunction in velocardiofacial syndrome. *Laryngoscope, 121*(4), 732–737.

Vilacosta, I., & Canadas Godoy, V. (2008). Images in clinical medicine: Bifid uvula and aortic aneurysm. *New England Journal of Medicine, 359*(2), e2.

Wharton, P., & Mowrer, D. E. (1992). Prevalence of cleft uvula among school children in kindergarten through grade five. *The Cleft Palate–Craniofacial Journal, 29*(1), 10–12; discussion 13–14.

Widmer, A. F., & Frei, R. (1999). Decontamination, disinfection, and sterilization. In P. R. Murray, E. J. Baron, M. A. Pfaller, F. C. Tenover, & R. H. Yolken (Eds.), *Manual of clinical microbiology* (pp. 138–164). Washington, DC: ASM Press.

World Health Organization (WHO). (2009). *WHO guidelines on hand hygiene in health care.* Geneva, Switzerland: WHO Press. Retrieved from http://www.who.int/gpsc/5may/tools/9789241597906/en/.

Yamawaki, Y. (2003). Forward movement of posterior pharyngeal wall on phonation. *American Journal of Otolaryngology, 24*(6), 400–404.

CREDITS

Chapter opener photo: © PeopleImages/Getty Images

All photos courtesy of the Cleft and Craniofacial Center at Cincinnati Children's Hospital Medical Center.

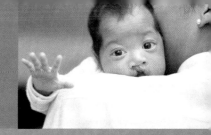

CHAPTER 13

Overview of Instrumental Procedures

CHAPTER OUTLINE

INTRODUCTION

A knowledgeable speech-language pathologist can diagnose velopharyngeal insufficiency/incompetence (VPI) versus velopharyngeal mislearning based solely on the results of a perceptual speech evaluation (Hinton, 2009). However, instrumental assessment of velopharyngeal function provides important additional information that can be used to determine the best surgical procedure for the patient and to assess the outcomes of the surgical and/or therapeutic intervention (Karnell, 2011).

The purpose of this chapter is to provide an overview of the two basic categories of instrumental procedures for evaluation of velopharyngeal function—those that give indirect yet objective information and those that give direct yet subjective information. The uses and relative advantages and disadvantages of each procedure are discussed.

Indirect Procedures

Indirect instrumental procedures for evaluation of velopharyngeal function (e.g., nasometry and speech aerodynamics) are those that give objective data regarding the physical correlates of the function of the velopharyngeal valve, such as acoustic output or measures of airflow and air pressure. The advantage of objective data is that a comparison can be made between the patient's measures versus standardized norms. In addition, data from these instruments can be used to determine the outcomes of surgery or therapy, or they can be used to compare treatment outcomes between professionals and centers. The disadvantage of indirect procedures is that they do not allow visualization of the structures or the velopharyngeal opening.

Nasometry

Nasometry is a method of measuring the acoustic correlates of resonance, audible nasal emission, and velopharyngeal function through a computer-based instrument. It provides an easy, noninvasive method for obtaining objective data by analyzing the acoustic energy from both the oral and nasal cavities during speech.

The Nasometer™ II (PENTAX Medical, Montvale, NJ) includes a Nasometer Headset (**FIGURE 13-1A**) or a Hand-Held Separator (**FIGURE 13-1B**), each of which has microphones on either side of a sound separator plate—one for the oral cavity and one for the nasal cavity.

The sound separator plate is placed between the child's upper lip and nose during data capture (**FIGURE 13-2**).

The speech sample for nasometry usually consists of standardized passages with normative data. The first passages to have normative data were the Zoo Passage (Fletcher, 1972), the Rainbow Passage (Fairbanks, 1960), and Nasal Sentences (Fletcher, 1978). Later, the MacKay-Kummer Simplified Nasometric Assessment Procedures-Revised (SNAP-R) (Kummer, 2005) was developed to provide more diagnostic value and to also make it easier for evaluation of children. When an individual's score is compared to normative data for that passage, a judgment can be made regarding the normalcy of resonance. High scores in comparison to normative data suggest hypernasality, whereas low scores in comparison to normative data suggest hyponasality.

During production of the speech passage, the Nasometer II captures data regarding acoustic energy from both the nasal (N) cavity and the oral (O) cavity during speech in real time. The Nasometer II then calculates the average ratio of nasal over total (nasal plus oral) acoustic energy and converts this to a percentage value called the nasalance score (also known as mean nasalance score. The nasalance score can be depicted as follows: Nasalance = N ÷ (N + O) × 100. This score gives the examiner information about the percentage of nasality in speech.

Nasometry is useful in that it supplements what is heard through the perceptual evaluation

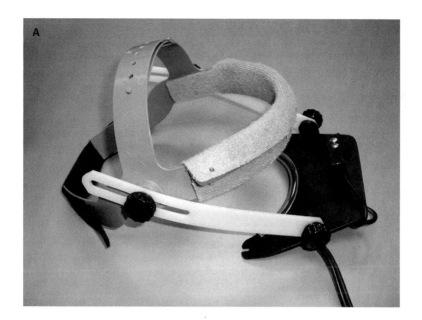

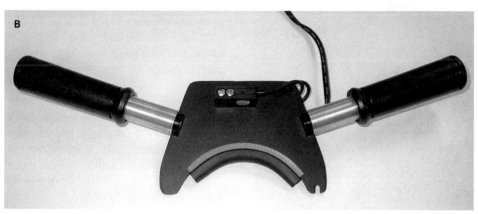

FIGURE 13-1 (A) The Nasometer II Headset. **(B)** The Nasometer II Hand-Held Separator.

and what is seen through direct instrumental measures (Karnell, 2011; Kummer, 2016; Perry & Schenck, 2013; Sweeney & Sell, 2008). In addition to evaluating characteristics of velopharyngeal dysfunction, nasometry can be used to assess hyponasality from upper airway obstruction. It has even been used to evaluate and treat resonance of children with hearing impairment. Nasometry can be used effectively for pre- and post-surgical comparisons. Finally,

it can provide visual feedback for the patient during therapy.

Speech Aerodynamics

Speech aerodynamics (sometimes called the pressure-flow technique) is a procedure to measure the aerodynamic properties of airflow and air pressure during speech production (**FIGURE 13-3**). The aerodynamic procedure is

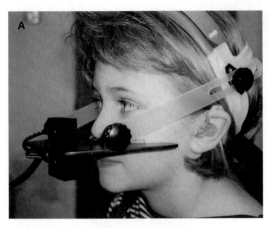
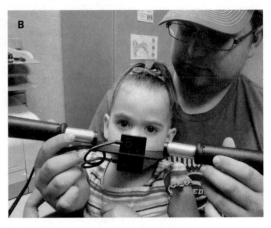

FIGURE 13-2 (A) Placement of the Nasometer II Headset on a patient. The sound separator plate should be perpendicular to the face or in a horizontal position. The microphones should be directly in front of the mouth and the nose. **(B)** Placement of the Hand-Held Separator. The separator plate should be placed in the same position as the Headset.

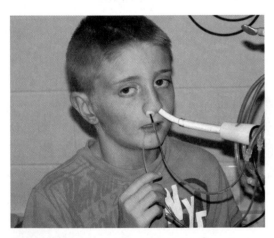

FIGURE 13-3 The pressure-flow technique to estimate velopharyngeal orifice areas during speech production. A flow tube is placed in the nose, and pressure catheters are placed in the mouth and nostril.

based on using a known relationship between air pressure and airflow to determine the size of the velopharyngeal opening. This technique involves simultaneous measurements of nasal airflow and the pressure in the oral and nasal cavities. Based on a formula developed by Warren and DuBois (1964), the size of the velopharyngeal (VP)

opening is estimated from the ratio of airflow to a pressure difference in the oral and nasal cavities.

The flow measurement is taken using a tube connected to a **pneumotachograph** (an instrument capable of measuring flow rates), and pressure measurements are taken using pressure **transducers**, which convert the detected air pressure or flow into electrical signals. Both instruments are based on a principle of converting a property of the flow to a measurable electrical signal. More information on how these instruments work can be found in the textbook of Baken and Orlikoff (2000).

Aerodynamic instrumentation has been used in the evaluation of VPI because it can provide a good approximation of intraoral air pressure levels and the amount of nasal air emission during speech. The data collected allow the examiner to calculate an estimate of velopharyngeal orifice size during consonant production and determine the patency of the nasal airway during breathing (Smith & Kuehn, 2007; Zajac & Mayo, 1996).

Although aerodynamic instrumentation is used in a few clinics, it is not widely used at this time. In fact, only 4.3% of respondents to the 2009 survey reported using it clinically (Kummer, Clark, Redle, Thomsen, & Billmire, 2012). Perhaps

TABLE 13-1 Advantages of Aerodynamics and Nasometry

Advantages of Aerodynamics
- Gives a rough estimate of velopharyngeal gap size based on nasal airflow (e.g., emission)

Advantages of Nasometry
- Measures both nasal airflow (emission) and hypernasality (resonance)
- Uses connected speech rather than a single consonant
- Provides differential diagnosis of phoneme-specific nasal emission or phoneme-specific hypernasality versus VPI
- Provides differential diagnosis of a symptomatic fistula versus VPI
- Can be used for speech biofeedback in therapy

this is because the system is costly and clinicians find the procedures hard to follow. In addition, the speech sample used is very limited because of practical constraints of the placement of the oral pressure-sensing tube. Finally, there are many flaws with the accuracy of the flow-pressure instruments (Liran Oren, PhD, research assistant professor and expert in flow dynamics, Department of Otolaryngology-Head and Neck Surgery, University of Cincinnati College of Medicine, personal communication). For example, the model used by Warren and DuBois (1964) to develop the relationship between pressure-flow and the size of the opening was not based on an anatomically realistic model, and the model considered changes in only the diameter of the VP opening, not the height (i.e., length). In addition, the pressure-flow measurement technique requires sealing one nostril (for pressure measurements) and occluding the other (for flow measurement). These modifications of how the airflow is allowed to exit from the nasal cavity cause the static pressure to artificially increase, thus likely making the VP opening larger than it actually is (from the pressure buildup).

Because of the limitations of this procedure and the fact that it is not commonly used clinically, there is no full chapter in this book on aerodynamic procedures.

Comparison of Indirect Methods

In late 2009, a survey was sent to plastic surgeons, otolaryngologists, and speech-language pathologists who are members of the American Cleft Palate–Craniofacial Association (ACPA) and work with patients with VPI. Of the 126 respondents, more participants reported using nasometry (28.9%) than aerodynamic measures (4.3%) (Kummer et al., 2012). Still, less than a third of respondents reported using instrumentation as part of their evaluation to obtain objective measures. For a comparison of advantages of each direct procedure, see TABLE 13-1.

Direct Procedures

Direct instrumental procedures for evaluation of velopharyngeal function, such as videofluoroscopy and nasopharyngoscopy, allow the examiner to visualize the structures and function of the velopharyngeal valve during speech (de Stadler & Hersh, 2015).

The advantage of direct visualization through these procedures is that the examiner can view both the anatomy of the velopharyngeal structures and the physiology during speech. In addition, the examiner can determine the location of a velopharyngeal gap and the potential anatomic and physiologic causes of VPI. This information is important for surgical planning. Finally, direct procedures can be helpful in assessing the placement of a prosthetic device or evaluating the results of surgical procedures for correction of VPI. The disadvantage of direct procedures is that they do not provide objective data and are dependent on clinical interpretation.

Videofluoroscopy

Videofluoroscopy is a radiological procedure used to obtain real-time moving images of internal structures. This is done through the use of a fluoroscope, which consists of an X-ray source, a fluorescent screen, and a video capture system. A videofluoroscopic speech study provides visualization of the velopharyngeal valve during speech, along with a simultaneous audio recording. Note that videofluoroscopy is also used to assess swallowing function in a procedure that is called either a modified barium swallow (MBS) or videofluoroscopic swallowing study (VSS).

Because videofluoroscopy involves two-dimensional imaging, a videofluoroscopic speech study requires several views in order to see all aspects of the velopharyngeal port (Dudas, Deleyiannis, Ford, Jiang, & Losee, 2006; Lam et al., 2006; Perry & Schenck, 2013; Smith & Kuehn, 2007; Ysunza, Carmen Pamplona, & Santiago Morales, 2011; Ysunza, Pamplona, Ortega, & Prado, 2008). On the lateral (sagittal) view, where the beam goes through the side of the head from

ear to ear, the examiner can see the occlusion of the jaws, the hard palate, tongue, velum, posterior pharyngeal wall, adenoids, and larynx. During speech, the movement of the velum and the tongue can be observed (**FIGURE 13-4**). On the frontal view, also called the anterior–posterior (AP) view because the beam goes from the front of the face to the back, the examiner can see the nasal septum and lateral pharyngeal walls (**FIGURE 13-5**). Finally, on the base view, where the beam goes from under the chin up through the port, the examiner can see the outline of the lateral and posterior pharyngeal walls and, to some extent, the velum (**FIGURE 13-6**). There are other supplementary views that can be used as needed. Regardless, to obtain an impression of the function of the entire velopharyngeal valve, several views must be considered together.

One disadvantage with videofluoroscopy is that the pharyngeal walls cannot be easily viewed without a coating of barium. Therefore, barium is needed for the frontal and base views. Barium is usually squirted into the pharynx through a rubber catheter that goes through the nose and back to the pharynx. Barium in the nose and pharynx causes a mild burning sensation (similar to water in the nose). Unfortunately, if the child cries, the

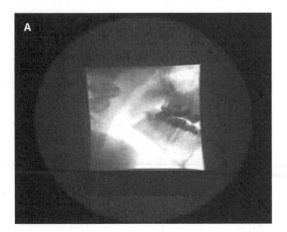
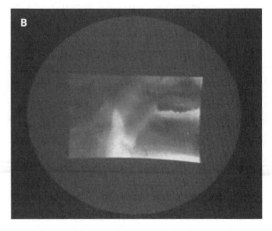

FIGURE 13-4 (A) Lateral view showing a short velum relative to the posterior pharyngeal wall, which results in velopharyngeal insufficiency. **(B)** Lateral view showing a velum of normal length but poor movement during speech, which results in velopharyngeal incompetence.

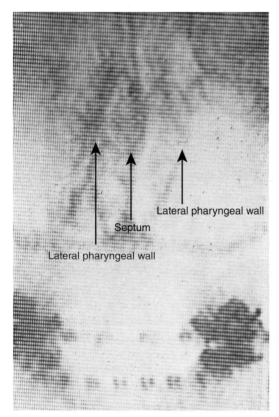

FIGURE 13-5 Frontal (anterior–posterior) view showing the nasal septum in midline. The lateral pharyngeal walls are well coated with barium and bow outward during nasal breathing, as noted in this frame.

secretions wash out the barium so that it needs to be squirted in again.

Videofluoroscopy for speech is done in a radiology department by a radiologist and/or a radiology technician. However, the speech pathologist should determine an appropriate speech sample for the patient. In addition, these studies should always be interpreted by both a radiologist and a speech-language pathologist.

Nasopharyngoscopy

Nasopharyngoscopy (also called nasendoscopy or video nasendoscopy) is a minimally invasive nasopharyngeal endoscopic procedure that

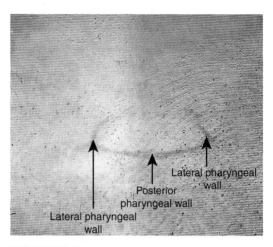

FIGURE 13-6 Base view with the posterior pharyngeal wall at the bottom of the screen. The open port can clearly be seen.

allows direct visual observation and analysis of the velopharyngeal mechanism during speech (Karnell, 2011; Kummer, 2016; Perry & Schenck, 2013; Ramamurthy, Wyatt, Whitby, Martin, & Davenport, 1997; Shetty, Frampton, & Patel, 2009; Smith & Kuehn, 2007; Strauss, 2007). The required equipment includes at least a flexible fiberoptic nasopharyngoscope and a cold light source. In addition, it is preferable to have a video monitor and a video recording system.

With this procedure, the nasal cavity is numbed with a nose spray. Then, the nasopharyngoscope is inserted into the nose while the examiner views the nasal cavity through a monitor (or eyepiece if a monitor is not available) (**FIGURE 13-7A**). The scope is passed through the middle meatus and then directed back to the pharynx (**FIGURE 13-7B**). Once in the pharynx, the examiner turns the tip of the scope with a lever so that the scope turns down to provide a view of the nasopharyngeal structures from above. Nasopharyngoscopy allows the examiner to view the nasal surface of the velum and the entire velopharyngeal valve during speech (**FIGURE 13-8**). In addition, other nasopharyngeal structures can be viewed, including the nasal cavity and turbinates, the eustachian tube orifices,

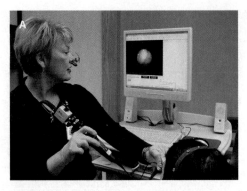 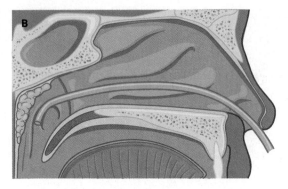

FIGURE 13-7 (A) The nasopharyngoscopy procedure with the patient positioned to see the monitor. **(B)** Position of the nasopharyngoscope as it goes through the middle meatus and then is turned downward to view the velopharyngeal valve from above.

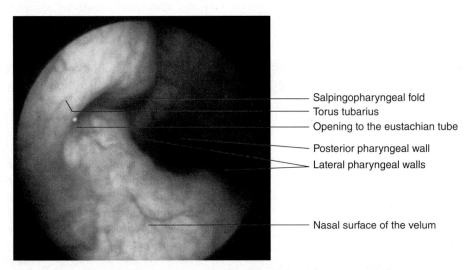

FIGURE 13-8 A nasopharyngoscopy view of normal velopharyngeal structures. The nasal surface of the velum is always at the bottom of the screen, and the posterior pharyngeal wall is always at the top of the screen. The opening to the eustachian tube can be seen on the left side of the view.

the posterior pharyngeal wall, the adenoids, and the vocal folds. This procedure allows the examiner to clearly view a velopharyngeal opening if it occurs during speech (**FIGURE 13-9**).

In addition to its use in assessing VPI, nasopharyngoscopy is also used for postoperative evaluations after surgery for VPI because the examiner is able to directly view the results of the surgical procedure and determine whether it has been effective. In addition to its use in the evaluation of velopharyngeal function, nasopharyngoscopy is also commonly used in the evaluation of swallowing, upper airway obstruction, and voice disorders.

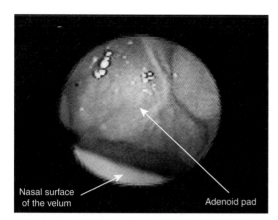

Nasal surface
of the velum

Adenoid pad

FIGURE 13-9 Nasopharyngoscopy view of a coronal velopharyngeal opening during speech.

Nasopharyngoscopy is often done by otolaryngologists, but it is also within the scope of practice for specially trained speech-language pathologists. Regardless of who passes the scope, the speech-language pathologist should be present for the evaluation and provide the speech sample. In addition, the recorded study should be reviewed by both the surgeon and speech pathologist to determine the appropriate course of treatment based on the findings.

Speech Samples

The composition of the speech sample used during a videofluoroscopy or nasopharyngoscopy examination is very important. This is because if the speech sample does not adequately tax the velopharyngeal mechanism, the study may not identify mild or inconsistent VPI or a phoneme-specific opening. In general, the speech sample may include a combination of repetition of syllables, counting, and repetition of sentences loaded with pressure-sensitive phonemes. In addition, it is often helpful to have the patient prolong vowel sounds, which are continuants and therefore require sustained velopharyngeal

closure. (See the chapter *Speech and Resonance Assessment* for specific speech samples.)

Reporting the Results

Some centers report results of nasopharyngoscopy and videofluoroscopy with a purely narrative report. Others use a numeric scale or a checklist format to rate various parameters of structure and function. In 1990, a multidisciplinary group proposed a system for reporting direct observations of the movement of the velopharyngeal structures from their resting position to the opposing structure using a ratio scale (Golding-Kushner et al., 1990). It is not known how often this scale is used today. Regardless of the method used, what is more important is that there is consistency in the observations that are made in each study and in the way that the studies are reported. Fortunately, precise measurements are not necessary for determination of treatment. Instead, the information that is most important in determining appropriate intervention is the following:

- The relative size of the opening (e.g., pinhole sized, small, medium, large, very large)
- The closure pattern (e.g., coronal, sagittal, circular, and "bowtie," where there is closure in midline but bilateral openings)
- The location of the opening (e.g., midline, right of midline, left of midline)
- The probable cause of the opening (e.g., cleft palate, submucous cleft, adenoidectomy, irregular adenoids, neurological dysfunction)

Although the results are used primarily to determine treatment recommendations, they should be shared with the family. After the initial explanation, it may also be helpful to play the videotape of the procedure and point out the structures and their function. All medical terms should

TABLE 13-2 **Advantages of Videofluoroscopy and Nasopharyngoscopy**

Advantages of Videofluoroscopy
- Can see tongue movement during speech
- Can see the entire posterior pharyngeal wall during speech
- Can see the point on the posterior pharyngeal wall of velar contact[a]

Advantages of Nasopharyngoscopy
- Can see all structures of the velopharyngeal mechanism in great detail and almost at the same time
- Can determine the location, size, shape, and cause of the opening, even if it is very small
- Has the best resolution and is in natural color
- Can see morphology of the nasal surface of the velum and identify an occult submucous cleft
- Can see the entire adenoid, including irregularities in the surface that can affect the velopharyngeal seal
- Can see pulsations of medially displaced carotid arteries in patients with velocardiofacial/22q11.2 deletion syndrome
- Can see tonsils intruding into the pharynx, which can affect resonance and velopharyngeal (VP) function
- Can view the vocal folds and determine the presence of vocal nodules
- Can determine the effectiveness of VPI surgery because the ports after a pharyngeal flap or sphincter pharyngoplasty can be viewed directly
- Is done without radiation or injection of barium in the nasopharynx
- Can allow the parent to hold the child in his lap during the procedure
- Can give the parents the results and recommendations immediately after the procedure
- Can be used for speech biofeedback

[a]Some surgeons want this information to know where to position a flap or sphincter in the pharynx. Others argue that you should just place it as high in the pharynx as possible and therefore this view is not needed.

be clearly defined. When discussing the function of the velopharyngeal mechanism, supplementary pictures and diagrams are very helpful.

Comparison of Direct Methods

Videofluoroscopy was the gold standard for evaluation of velopharyngeal function in the 1970s. In the 1980s, flexible nasopharyngoscopy became an option. In the same survey, more respondents reported using nasopharyngoscopy routinely (59.3%) than videofluoroscopy (19.2%) (Kummer et al., 2012). For a comparison of advantages of each direct procedure, see TABLE 13-2.

Imaging for Research

Clinicians and researchers are always looking for new methods to evaluate the structure and function of the velopharyngeal valve. Some technologies are particularly useful for clinical care,

while others are more suited for expanding our knowledge through research. One relatively new method for studying the velopharyngeal valve is the use of magnetic resonance imaging.

Magnetic Resonance Imaging

Magnetic resonance imaging (MRI) is a noninvasive method of producing a very clear and detailed view of internal body structures using a magnetic field and radio waves. MRI can provide high-resolution images of the structures of the velopharyngeal sphincter in all planes. Therefore, it has proved to be an effective method of imaging and examining the morphology of the velum and in particular the levator veli palatini muscles (Atik et al., 2008; Drissi et al., 2011; Perry, Kuehn, Sutton, & Fang, 2017). It has also been effective in viewing the dysmorphology of a submucous cleft palate (Kuehn, Ettema, Goldwasser, & Barkmeier, 2004).

A primary disadvantage of MRI as a clinical tool is the static nature of the imaging. In addition, MRI typically shows a two-dimensional view, although the use of serial images and computer modeling to obtain three-dimensional images can be done (Perry et al., 2017; Serrurier & Badin, 2008). Other disadvantages to clinical use of this technology include noise in the scanner, the potential for claustrophobia during the exam, and current expense. Because of these disadvantages, MRI is not currently a standard procedure for clinical evaluation of velopharyngeal function. However, it is a valuable research tool and has provided important information to enhance our understanding of normal and abnormal velopharyngeal morphology.

SUMMARY

The best way to evaluate resonance disorders and velopharyngeal dysfunction is through a perceptual examination. Despite that, instrumental procedures can provide very valuable additional information to augment the perceptual evaluation results. Indirect procedures (e.g., aerodynamic instrumentation and nasometry) provide objective data relative to the function of the velopharyngeal valve. Objective data can be used for measuring patient outcomes and for comparison of treatment results between professionals and centers. Direct procedures (e.g., videofluoroscopy and nasopharyngoscopy) provide visual information about the structures and function of the velopharyngeal valve. This information is important because it helps the examimer determine the cause of the velopharyngeal dysfunction and the location of the gap which is particularly useful for surgical planning. MRI is useful for in-depth imaging of the structures of the velopharyngeal valve. It is currently used for research but may be used as a clinical tool in the future.

Because instrumentation is expensive and requires specialty training for use, these procedures are usually done in a medical center, particularly one that has a craniofacial program. There are low-tech instruments, however, that can be used effectively in other clinical settings.

FOR REVIEW AND DISCUSSION

1. If the perceptual assessment is sufficient in diagnosing VPI, what are the reasons for using instrumentation?

2. What is the difference between direct procedures and indirect procedures? What are the advantages and disadvantages of each type of procedure?

3. What are the primary advantages and disadvantages of nasometry versus aerodynamic procedures?

4. What are the primary advantages and disadvantages of nasopharyngoscopy versus videofluoroscopy?

5. What type of speech sample would be most appropriate with each type of instrumentation?

6. Why is MRI technology particularly useful for research? Why is it not used clinically at this point?

7. Why is instrumentation typically available only in certain specialty centers?

REFERENCES

Atik, B., Bekerecioglu, M., Tan, O., Etlik, O., Davran, R., & Arslan, H. (2008). Evaluation of dynamic magnetic resonance imaging in assessing velopharyngeal insufficiency during phonation. *Journal of Craniofacial Surgery, 19*(3), 566–572.

Baken, R. J., & Orlikoff, R. F. (2000). *Clinical measurement of speech and voice* (2nd ed.). San Diego, CA: Singular.

de Stadler, M., & Hersh, C. (2015). Nasometry, videofluoroscopy, and the speech pathologist's evaluation and treatment. *Advances in Oto-Rhino-Laryngology, 76,* 7–17.

Drissi, C., Mitrofanoff, M., Talandier, C., Falip, C., Le Couls, V., & Adamsbaum, C. (2011). Feasibility of dynamic MRI for evaluating velopharyngeal insufficiency in children. *European Radiology, 21*(7), 1462–1469.

Dudas, J. R., Deleyiannis, F. W., Ford, M. D., Jiang, S., & Losee, J. E. (2006). Diagnosis and treatment of velopharyngeal insufficiency: Clinical utility of speech evaluation and videofluoroscopy. *Annuals of Plastic Surgery, 56*(5), 511–517; discussion 517.

Fairbanks, D. (1960). *Voice and articulation drill book.* New York, NY: Harper and Row.

Fletcher, S. G. (1972). Contingencies for bio-electronic modification of nasality. *Journal of Speech and Hearing Disorders, 37,* 329–346.

Fletcher, S. G. (1978). *Diagnosing speech disorders from cleft palate.* New York, NY: Grune & Statton.

Golding-Kushner, K. J., Argamaso, R. V., Cotton, R. T., Grames, L. M., Henningsson, G., Jones, D. L., . . . Marsh, J. L. (1990). Standardization for the reporting of nasopharyngoscopy and multiview videofluoroscopy: A report from an international working group. *Cleft Palate Journal, 27*(4), 337–347; discussion 347–348.

Hinton, V. A. (2009). Instrumental measures of velopharyngeal function. In J. E. Lossee & R. E. Kirschner (Eds.), *Comprehensive cleft care* (pp. 607–617). New York, NY: McGraw-Hill.

Karnell, M. P. (2011). Instrumental assessment of velopharyngeal closure for speech. *Seminars in Speech and Language, 32*(2), 168–178.

Kuehn, D. P., Ettema, S. L., Goldwasser, M. S., & Barkmeier, J. C. (2004). Magnetic resonance imaging of the levator veli palatini muscle before and after primary palatoplasty. *The Cleft Palate–Craniofacial Journal, 41*(6), 584–592.

Kummer, A. W. (2005). The MacKay-Kummer Simplified Nasometric Assessment Procedures-Revised (SNAP-R). Retrieved from https://www.researchgate .net/publication/273060845_The_MacKay -Kummer_SNAP_Test-R_Simplified_Nasometric _Assessment_Procedures_Revised_2005.

Kummer, A. W. (2016). Evaluation of speech and resonance for children with craniofacial anomalies. *Facial Plastic Surgery Clinics of North America, 24*(4), 445–451.

Kummer, A. W., Clark, S. L., Redle, E. E., Thomsen, L. L., & Billmire, D. A. (2012). Current practice in assessing and reporting speech outcomes of cleft palate and velopharyngeal surgery: A survey of cleft palate/craniofacial professionals. *The Cleft Palate–Craniofacial Journal, 49*(2), 146–152.

Lam, D. J., Starr, J. R., Perkins, J. A., Lewis, C. W., Eblen, L. E., Dunlap, J., & Sie, K. C. (2006). A comparison of nasendoscopy and multiview videofluoroscopy in assessing velopharyngeal insufficiency. *Otolaryngology-Head and Neck Surgery, 134*(3), 394–402.

Perry, J., & Schenck, G. (2013). Instrumental assessment in cleft palate care. *Perspectives on Speech Science and Orofacial Disorders, 23*(2), 49–61.

Perry, J. L., Kuehn, D. P., Sutton, B. P., & Fang, X. (2017). Velopharyngeal structural and functional assessments of speech in young children using dynamic magnetic resonance imaging. *The Cleft Palate–Craniofacial Journal, 54*(4), 408–422.

Ramamurthy, L., Wyatt, R. A., Whitby, D., Martin, D., & Davenport, P. (1997). The evaluation of velopharyngeal function using flexible nasendoscopy. *Journal of Laryngology & Otology, 111*(8), 739–745.

Serrurier, A., & Badin, P. (2008). A three-dimensional articulatory model of the velum and nasopharyngeal wall based on MRI and CT data. *Journal of the Acoustic Society of America, 123*(4), 2335–2355.

Shetty, S., Frampton, S., & Patel, N. (2009). Flexible nasendoscopy. *Clinical Otolaryngology, 34*(2), 169–171.

Smith, B. E., & Kuehn, D. P. (2007). Speech evaluation of velopharyngeal dysfunction. *Journal of Craniofacial Surgery, 18*(2), 251–261; quiz 266–267.

Strauss, R. A. (2007). Flexible endoscopic nasopharyngoscopy. *Atlas of the Oral and Maxillofacial Surgery Clinics of North America, 15*(2), 111–128.

Sweeney, T., & Sell, D. (2008). Relationship between perceptual ratings of nasality and nasometry in

children/adolescents with cleft palate and/or velopharyngeal dysfunction. *International Journal
of Language & Communication Disorders, 43*(3),
265–282.

Warren, D. W., & DuBois, A. (1964). A pressure-flow
technique for measuring velopharyngeal orifice area
during continuous speech. *Cleft Palate Journal, 1,*
52–71.

Ysunza, A., Carmen Pamplona, M., & Santiago
Morales, M. A. (2011). Velopharyngeal valving
during speech, in patients with velocardiofacial
syndrome and patients with non-syndromic palatal

clefts after surgical and speech pathology management. *International Journal of Pediatric Otorhinolaryngology, 75*(10), 1255–1259.

Ysunza, A., Pamplona, M. C., Ortega, J. M., & Prado,
H. (2008). Video fluoroscopy for evaluating adenoid
hypertrophy in children. *International Journal of
Pediatric Otorhinolaryngology, 72*(8), 1159–1165.

Zajac, D. J., & Mayo, R. (1996). Aerodynamic and temporal aspects of velopharyngeal function in normal
speakers. *Journal of Speech, Language and Hearing
Research, 39*(6), 1199–1207.

CREDITS

Chapter opener photo: © PeopleImages/Getty Images
Figure 13-3: Courtesy of David J. Zajac, PhD, University of North Carolina at Chapel Hill

All other photos courtesy of the Cleft and Craniofacial
Center at Cincinnati Children's Hospital Medical
Center.

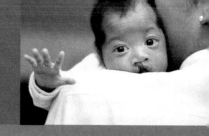

CHAPTER 14

Nasometry

CHAPTER OUTLINE

INTRODUCTION

Nasometry is a method of measuring the acoustic correlates of resonance and velopharyngeal function through a computer-based instrument. Nasometry testing gives the examiner a nasalance score, which is the percentage of nasal acoustic energy of the total (nasal plus oral) acoustic energy. Because nasometry does not include visualization of the velopharyngeal structures, it is considered an **indirect instrumental procedure**. The advantage of nasometry is that it provides objective data that can be compared to standardized norms for interpretation.

Nasometry is useful in the evaluation of resonance because it supplements what is heard through the perceptual evaluation and what is seen through direct instrumental measures (Sweeney & Sell, 2008). It can also be used effectively for pre- and post-treatment comparisons. Finally, nasometry can be a valuable treatment tool because it provides visual feedback for the patient.

The purpose of this chapter is to describe nasometry and its use in the evaluation and treatment of individuals with resonance disorders. In addition, this chapter describes the procedures used with nasometry for the clinician.

Nasometry and Its Clinical Uses

Nasometry was developed as a means to quantify the acoustic correlates of velopharyngeal function during speech. Nasometry supplements the perceptual assessment of resonance which, by its nature, is subjective.

Development of Nasometry

The first instrument to measure nasal and oral acoustic energy was developed by Samuel Fletcher in 1970. This instrument was called TONAR, which is an acronym for The Oral-Nasal Acoustic Ratio (Fletcher & Bishop, 1970). TONAR was later updated, revised, and then renamed TONAR II (Fletcher, 1976a; Fletcher, 1976b). Although the TONAR instruments provided objective data regarding the acoustic product of speech, the data acquisition was somewhat unreliable (Dalston, 1997). Therefore, Samuel Fletcher, along with colleagues Larry Adams and Martin McCutcheon at the University of Alabama, developed the Nasometer™ based on Fletcher's early work. It was first introduced by Kay Elemetrics Corporation in 1986 (Fletcher, 1970; Fletcher, Adams, & McCutcheon, 1989).

In 2002, a second version of the Nasometer was released as Nasometer II, Model 6400. Although the Nasometer II is fundamentally the same as the original version, it captures data through both analog and digital circuitry rather than just analog circuitry. Additionally, Nasometer II records the speech signal, which can be played back.

The latest hardware/software version is the Nasometer II, Model 6450 (PENTAX Medical). This version contains a built-in sound chip in the hardware. The hardware connects to the host computer via a USB interface. This design allows the Nasometer II to be used with laptop as well as desktop computers.

Two other instruments have been developed to measure nasalance: the NasalView (Tiger Electronics, Seattle, WA) and the OroNasal System (Glottal Enterprises, Syracuse, NY). These instruments are not as widely used perhaps because there are no published normative studies for their use. In addition, it has been shown that there are significant differences in the nasalance scores of these instruments, so norms established for the Nasometer cannot be used with them (Bressmann, 2005; Lewis & Watterson, 2003). Because of these findings and the fact that the Nasometer is widely used internationally, the remainder of this chapter focuses on nasometry using the Nasometer II, Model 6450.

What Is a Nasometer?

A **Nasometer** is a computer-based instrument used to measure the acoustic correlates of resonance, audible nasal emission, and velopharyngeal function (Karnell, 2011; Kummer, 2016; Perry & Schenck, 2013). It provides an easy, non-invasive method for obtaining objective data by analyzing the acoustic energy from both the oral and nasal cavities during speech. As such, it can be a valuable tool in both the evaluation of resonance disorders and in the treatment of functional resonance problems.

The Nasometer provides data of the relative amount of nasal resonance in speech for a passage. This is done by capturing data regarding acoustic energy in both the nasal (N) cavity and oral (O) cavity during speech in real time. The Nasometer software then calculates the average ratio of nasal over total (nasal plus oral) acoustic energy for the passage. This ratio is converted to a percentage value called the nasalance score. The nasalance score can be depicted, therefore, as follows: Nasalance = N ÷ (N + O) × 100.

When an individual's score is compared to normative data, a judgment can be made regarding the normalcy of resonance. High scores in comparison to normative data suggest hypernasality, whereas low scores in comparison to normative data suggest hyponasality.

Clinical Uses

Since its introduction, the Nasometer has been a useful tool in the evaluation of resonance and velopharyngeal function of patients with a history of cleft palate (Dalston, 1997; Dalston, Warren, & Dalston, 1991b; Dalston, Warren, & Dalston, 1991c; Hardin, Van Demark, Morris, & Payne, 1992; Karnell, 1995; Karnell, 2011; van der Heijden, Hobbel, van der Laan, Korsten-Meijer, & Goorhuis-Brouwer, 2011). It has even been used to evaluate and treat resonance of children with hearing impairment (Hassan et al., 2011; Tatchell, Stewart, & Lapine, 1991). Nasometry has been used to assess upper airway obstruction and hyponasality based on the acoustic correlates of airway obstruction during speech (Dalston,

Warren, & Dalston, 1991a; Dalston et al., 1991b; Hardin et al., 1992; Hong, Kwon, & Jung, 1997; Nieminen, Lopponen, Vayrynen, Tervonen, & Tolonen, 2000; Parker, Clarke, Dawes, & Maw, 1990). It has even been suggested as a means of selecting at-risk individuals for adenoidectomy (Kummer, Myer, Smith, & Shott, 1993; Parker, Maw, & Szallasi, 1989; Williams, Eccles, & Hutchings, 1990; Williams, Preece, Rhys, & Eccles, 1992).

Very often, nasometry is used to measure changes in resonance following surgical procedures (Dejonckere & van Wijngaarden, 2001; Eckardt, Teltzrow, Schulze, Hoppe, & Kuettner, 2007; Mueller, Neuber, Schelhorn-Niese, & Schumann, 2007; Soneghet et al., 2002; Van Lierde, De Bodt, Baetens, Schrauwen, & Van Cauwenberge, 2003; Van Lierde, Monstrey, Bonte, Van Cauwenberge, & Vinck, 2004). It is also used to show the effects of various forms of treatment, including continuous positive airway pressure, or CPAP (Sweeney, Sell, & O'Regan, 2004), prosthetic management (Rieger, Wolfaardt, Seikaly, & Jha, 2002), and speech therapy.

Equipment

The Nasometer requires a host computer, specialized software, an external module, a headset, and a means for calibration. These components are described here.

Hardware and Software

The Nasometer II requires the use of a host computer and specialized software. The system components include a Nasometer II external module box (**FIGURE 14-1**) and either a Nasometer headset with a sound separator plate (**FIGURE 14-2A**) or a Nasometer handheld sound separator plate (**FIGURE 14-2B**). The sound separator plate has two directional microphones on either side—one to pick up sound from the nasal cavity and the other to pick up sound from the oral cavity. The equipment

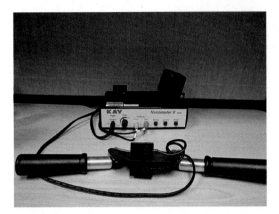

FIGURE 14-1 Basic Nasometer equipment. The Nasometer requires the use of a host computer, a Nasometer box, and a sound separator plate for data collection.

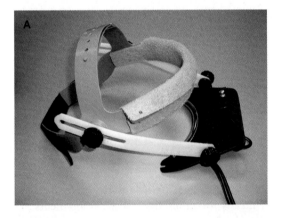

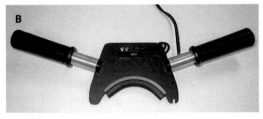

FIGURE 14-2 (A) The Nasometer II headset. **(B)** The Nasometer II handheld separator.

connection and software installation instructions can be found in the Nasometer II, Model 6450 Installation, Operations, and Maintenance Manual (PENTAX Medical, n.d.)

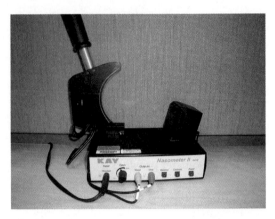

FIGURE 14-3 Calibration. During calibration, the separator plate should be placed so that both microphones are equidistant from the Nasometer box and about 12 inches in front of the calibration speaker.

Calibration

Before its first use and at regular intervals, the Nasometer should be calibrated according to the manufacturer's instructions. This is necessary to be sure that data collection and analyses are accurate. The sound separator plate is placed in the calibration stand located on the top of the Nasometer II external hardware module. The provided calibration slot ensures that both microphones are equidistant from the calibration speaker (approximately 6 inches [15 cm]) (**FIGURE 14-3**). When a tone from the external module is presented to the microphones, both the nasal and oral microphones register the tone equally. If the two microphones are not balanced so that the tone registers above or below the 50% mark, calibration adjustments are automatically made in the Nasometer II software to balance any detected sensitivity differences between the two microphones.

Nasometric Procedures

For comprehensive information about nasometric procedures, the reader should consult the Nasometer II manual that comes with the equipment. Although extensive instruction regarding nasometry procedures is beyond the scope of this text, some basic information is important to cover.

Placing the Sound Separator Plate

Either the Nasometer II headset or the handheld sound separator plate can be used for data collection. Before use (and also after use), the examiner should wipe the sound separator plate and plastic guard with a chlorine wipe to disinfect and sanitize it. The device is then plugged into the external module.

If the headset is used, it should be placed on the individual's head and then secured using the top adjustment band and the Velcro® strip in the back. When in place, the sound separator plate should fit snugly between the child's upper lip and nose. The microphones should be directly in front of the mouth and the nose, and the plate should be perpendicular to the face (or in a horizontal position). An angle in excess of 15 degrees in either direction can affect the integrity of the data (PENTAX Medical, n.d.). Once the plate is in proper position, the top and then the bottom adjustment knobs should be tightened to keep the plate in place and add further stability. The plastic tubing along the plate promotes a tight seal and softens the force against the face. The proper placement of the Nasometer II headset is seen in **FIGURE 14-4A** and **B**.

Positioning the headset on young children can be a challenge. Despite the examiner's best efforts, there are times when the child simply refuses to put it on. In addition, young children are often not tolerant of keeping it on during the time that the examiner is recording the data in between passages. The headset has another disadvantage in that the headgear must be sanitized between uses.

Because of the challenges in using the headset and the problem with disinfection, the use of the newer handheld separator plate is preferred (**FIGURE 14-4C** and **D**). This device has two handles to hold the separator plate in place so there is no need for the headgear. In some cases, the handheld separator plate can be held in place by the child. For young children, however, it is preferable to have the child sit in the parent's lap and then have the parent hold the device in place from behind. The device can be set down in between passages, and it is easier to clean than the original headset.

Preparing the Child for the Exam

Most young children cooperate very well for nasometry (van der Heijden et al., 2011). To ensure best cooperation, the child should be told what to expect before the day of the appointment. This can be done by sending parents information describing the exam and a picture or drawing of the Nasometer. The speech samples that will be used in the exam should be included so that the child can practice repeating them at home. At Cincinnati Children's, a coloring book that explains the nasometry procedure is sent to the family before the appointment (**FIGURE 14-5**).

To ease the child's fears and promote cooperation for the evaluation, the examiner should make the procedure as nonthreatening as possible. For example, at Cincinnati Children's, we may tell the child that he will be playing a computer game and wearing a "superhero" mask. He will talk to the computer through the microphones because "computers don't have ears." When the computer can hear him talk, it will make lots of blue "mountains." It helps to have the child feel the plate and the plastic tubing that will come in contact with his face. The examiner can explain that the separator plate will "hug" his face during the exam. Even if the child is not fully cooperative, a few syllables or short utterances usually result in useful collection of data.

Data Collection

Once the separator plate is in place, the child is asked to read or repeat standardized speech

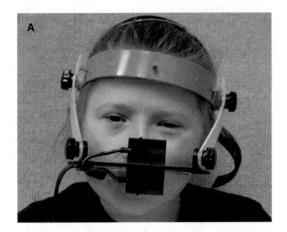
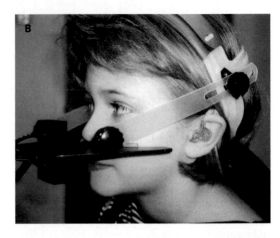
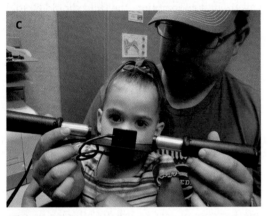
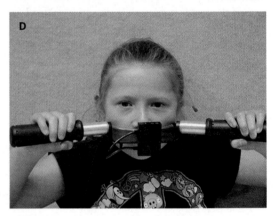

FIGURE 14-4 (A) and **(B)** Placement of the Nasometer II headset on a patient. The sound separator plate should be perpendicular to the face or in a horizontal position. The microphones should be directly in front of the mouth and the nose. **(C)** and **(D)** Placement of the handheld separator. The separator plate should be placed in the same position as the headset.

passages (**FIGURE 14-6**). To start data collection, the examiner presses the F12 key. To stop data collection, the examiner presses the space bar. The microphones pick up acoustic energy from the oral cavity and nasal cavity simultaneously.

To compare the individual's performance with normative data, a standardized speech segment must be used. There are several standardized passages in English that are incorporated in the Nasometer II software, so they can be displayed on the screen.

Normed Passages in English

There are three types of standardized passages with normative data for nasometry. They include passages that contain only oral consonants, passages that contain primarily nasal consonants, and passages that have a mixture of both oral and nasal consonants.

To evaluate velopharyngeal function or hypernasality, the oral passages are used. An abnormally high score on these passages suggests velopharyngeal insufficiency/incompetence (VPI) with hypernasality and/or nasal emission.

Do you like computer games? We hope so because the speech pathologist has one for you to play. With this game, you get to wear a super hero mask that fits around your face.

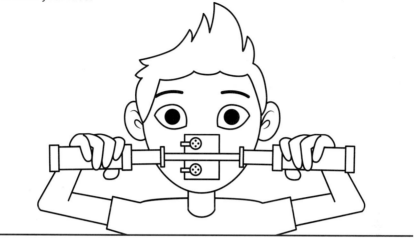

When you talk into microphones on the mask, you will see funny blue lines on the computer screen.

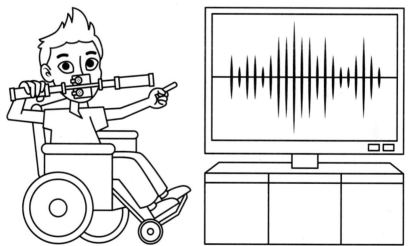

FIGURE 14-5 Page from a coloring book used to prepare the patient for the examination.

To evaluate for hyponasality or even cul-de-sac resonance, the nasal passages are used. An abnormally low score on these passages suggests hyponasality and probable nasopharyngeal blockage. A nasal passage should always be used following surgery to correct VPI because these procedures have the potential to cause upper airway obstruction with obstructive sleep apnea (OSA). In evaluating the effect of timing of velopharyngeal opening and closing, a passage containing a mixture of nasal and oral consonants should be used (Sweeney & Sell, 2008). Overall, however, a passage with a mixture of oral and nasal consonants is generally less valuable from a diagnostic standpoint.

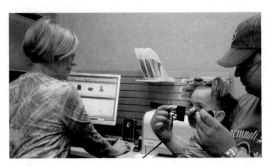

FIGURE 14-6 Nasometer procedure for data collection. The individual is asked to read or repeat certain speech passages for data collection.

Original Passages

The first nasometric norms were established for the following three passages: the Zoo Passage (Fletcher, 1972), the Rainbow Passage (Fairbanks, 1960), and Nasal Sentences (Fletcher, 1978). These passages for Nasometer II and their norms (mean scores and standard deviations) can be found in **APPENDIX 14A**.

The Zoo Passage consists of sentences with oral consonants only (no nasal sounds). The Rainbow Passage has a mixture of oral and nasal consonants. In fact, 11.5% of the consonants in this passage are nasals, which is representative of the percentage of nasal consonants in Standard American English. The Nasal Sentences passage is loaded with nasal consonants. It has more than three times as many nasal sounds, about 35% of the passage, as would normally occur in Standard American English.

Although the original passages are still commonly used, particularly with adults, they have certain disadvantages. They are hard to use with children who have a limited attention span or have limited compliance. The Zoo and Rainbow passages are long and awkward, and some of the sentences are semantically and syntactically complex. Some of the words are difficult to pronounce, especially for children who have incomplete phonological acquisition. When the passage is produced with articulation substitutions or deletions, the nasalance score associated with it

loses some validity. A pause with the use of "um" is particularly problematic.

The biggest problem with these passages, however, is the phonetic heterogeneity of the oral passages, which limits their diagnostic use. For example, it makes it impossible to isolate the effects of phoneme-specific nasal emission, phoneme-specific hypernasality, or a fistula versus the effects of VPI.

SNAP Test

In an effort to determine the most efficient way to collect nasometric data while avoiding the pitfalls of the original passages, some investigators have found that reliable measures of nasalance can be obtained using much shorter passages (Kummer, 2005; Watterson, Lewis, & Foley-Homan, 1999; Wozny, Kuehn, Oishi, & Arthur, 1994). In addition, it has been reported that the clinically relevant information provided in the Rainbow Passage can be obtained using the other speech samples (Dalston & Seaver, 1992).

Given the limitations of the original passages, the *MacKay-Kummer Simplified Nasometric Assessment Procedures* (*SNAP Test*) was developed for the purpose of providing more appropriate standardized passages for children while enhancing the diagnostic value of nasometry (MacKay & Kummer, 1994). Normative data was obtained for this test using the Nasometer I, Model 6200. With the introduction of Nasometer II, the *Simplified Nasometric Assessment Procedures-Revised* (*SNAP Test-R*) was developed, and another normative study was conducted using this newer equipment (Kummer, 2005). This test, along with its normative data, can be found in **APPENDIX 14B**.

The SNAP Test-R consists of a battery of passages divided into three subtests. Any or all of these subtests can be used by the examiner, but they are usually selected based on the age of the child; the anticipated level of cooperation; the child's ability to read; and most importantly, the specific characteristics or etiologies that need to be evaluated.

Subtest I, the *Syllable Repetition/Prolonged Sounds Subtest*, includes 14 consonant–vowel

(CV) syllables of pressure-sensitive consonants (plosives and fricatives) and nasal sounds (/m/ and /n/) combined with either the low vowel /ɑ/ (as in "father") or the high vowel /i/ (as in "tea"). Subtest I also includes two prolonged vowels, /ɑ/ and /i/, and two prolonged consonants, /s/ and /m/. The child is asked to produce the syllables repetitively until the screen is full of relatively even peaks. The prolonged sounds are produced until the screen is full.

There are several advantages of Subtest I. First, it can be used with younger children who have a short attention span, poor cooperation, or a limited phonemic repertoire. In addition, it has better diagnostic value than longer passages that contain a mixture of consonants and vowel types. With a single consonant and single vowel per passage, it is easier for the examiner to isolate the phonemes that are affected by VPI, a fistula, or phoneme-specific nasality. For example, the examiner can identify phoneme-specific nasal emission by comparing the relative nasalance on sibilant phonemes (particularly /s/) versus plosive sounds. The examiner may determine that there is abnormally high nasalance on high vowels as compared to low vowels, suggesting either a high tongue position or thin velum as possible causes. Finally, higher nasalance scores on anterior sounds (/tɑ/ or /sɑ/) versus posterior sounds (/kɑ/) suggest that there is a fistula that is symptomatic for speech.

Subtest II, the *Picture-Cued Subtest*, contains passages that elicit connective speech yet are phonetically homogeneous, thus enhancing the diagnostic value of the test. For each passage, one carrier phrase (e.g., "Pick up the . . .") is used with three pictures to complete three sentences (e.g., "Pick up the book," "Pick up the pie," or "Pick up the baby"). In this subtest, there is a passage that focuses on each of the following: bilabial plosives, lingual-alveolar plosives, velar plosives, sibilant fricatives, and nasals. There are pictures on the computer screen to cue the child, or the child can read the sentences (**FIGURE 14-7**). The child can also repeat the sentences after the examiner. Ideally, the child should say the set of three sentences twice so that there is a total of six sentences produced for each passage.

Subtest III, the *Paragraph Subtest*, consists of two short, easy-to-read passages (**FIGURE 14-8A and B**). The first passage contains primarily plosive phonemes, whereas the second passage is loaded with the /s/ consonant. The examiner can select either or both passages depending on the articulation ability of the individual and the diagnostic goals of the examiner. These passages are more phonetically heterogeneous than the other two subtests and include some nasals but are still more homogeneous than the Zoo and Rainbow passages. As with the other subtests, these passages can either be read or repeated after the examiner.

Normative Studies for Other Languages

Some authors suggest that nasalance scores can vary with language (Anderson, 1996; Leeper, Rochet, & MacKay, 1992; Santos-Terron, Gonzalez-Landa, & Sanchez-Ruiz, 1990; van Doorn & Purcell, 1998). This may be true, depending on the balance of high vowels versus low vowels in the language. However, the nasalance score for a particular passage is greatly dependent on its vowel content regardless of the language.

Passages with more voiced consonants and/or high vowels have higher average nasalance scores in comparison to passages with more voiceless consonants and/or low vowels, regardless of language (Awan, Omlor, & Watts, 2011; Kummer, 2005; Mandulak & Zajac, 2009). High vowels, with the high tongue position, have about 17% nasalance, whereas low vowels have only about 7% nasalance (Kummer, 2005). Therefore, different passages in the same language will have different normative nasalance scores. The relative nasalance between languages cannot be directly compared unless the passages have the same high-vowel/low-vowel composition.

Several normative studies have found that nasalance scores vary with dialect when the same

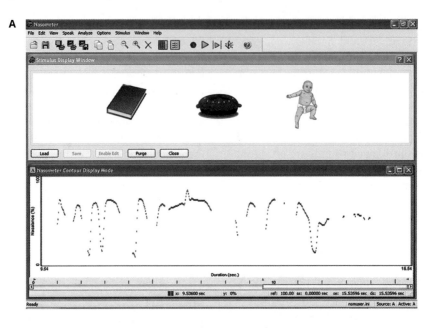

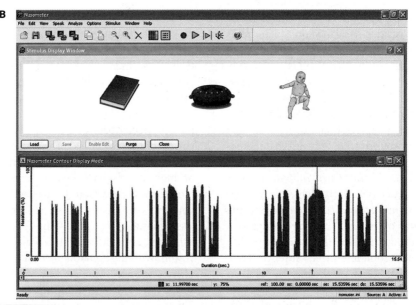

FIGURE 14-7 Nasometer displays after data collection. The nasalance percentage points are displayed on the computer screen in real time as the individual is speaking. For normal speech and the production of only oral sounds, the data points are usually between 10 and 20 percentage points above the baseline. **(A)** A contour display of data from the Bilabials Passage of the SNAP Test of a patient with VPI. Pictures from the test are displayed on the screen. **(B)** A filled contour display of the same data.

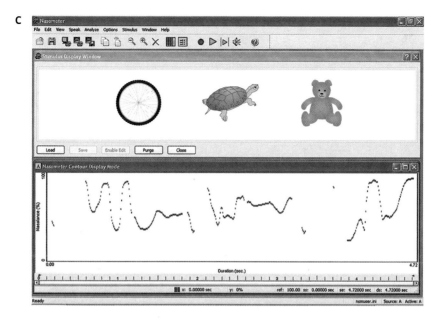

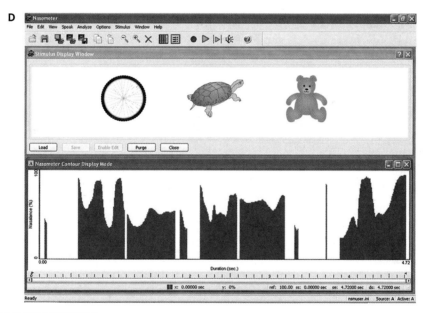

FIGURE 14-7 (CONTINUED) (C) A contour display of data from the Lingual-Alveolars Passage of the SNAP Test of another patient with VPI. The pictures are displayed on the screen. **(D)** A filled contour display of the same data.

A

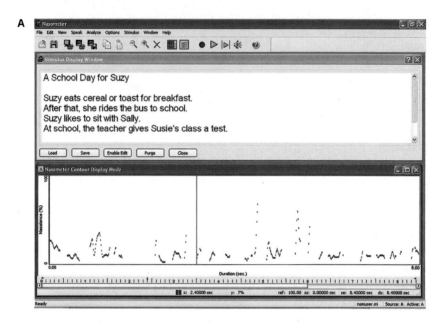

B

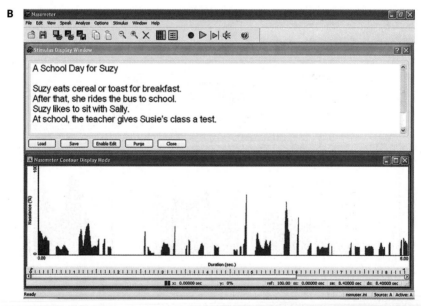

FIGURE 14-8 (A) A contour display of data from the Paragraph Subtest of the SNAP Test. **(B)** A filled contour display of the same data.

passage is used (Awan et al., 2015; Leeper et al., 1992; Seaver, Dalston, Leeper, & Adams, 1991) and even with racial group or culture (Mayo, Floyd, Warren, Dalston, & Mayo, 1996). Because consonants are produced essentially the same, regardless

of dialect, and many are voiceless, these differences are likely to be in the production of the vowels. Nasalized vowels are presumably the cause of a nasal twang, which is exaggerated nasality, as noted in some dialects (perhaps the Southern dialect in

American English because this dialect seems to use more high vowels than other English dialects). It might be assumed that dialects, accents, or even languages that use a higher posterior tongue position on some vowels might be expected to have slightly higher nasalance scores as compared to those with a lower posterior tongue position on vowels (Lewis & Watterson, 2003). There may also be a difference in dialects between the timing of closure when transitions are made between nasal consonants and vowels (Mayo et al., 1996).

Nasometric Results

As data is collected during the speech segment, a visual depiction of the relative amount of nasal acoustic energy in the speech is displayed on the monitor. Once the speech segment is completed, descriptive statistic summaries can be obtained and saved.

Display of the Speech Signal

As the individual is speaking, the speech signal enters the microphones, and the software computes the nasalance score, which as noted previously, is the percentage of nasal acoustic energy of the total energy. This nasalance value is displayed during speech in real time on the bottom of the screen as a nasogram.

A **nasogram** is a contour display of the individual data points in sequence as they are collected in real time during the production of a passage. The nasogram is recorded and can be saved for later review along with the auditory playback feature. The contour display can be changed to a bar graph, which is helpful in therapy. For young children, there are also games and animated graphics to help keep the child engaged.

The default nasogram is the Contour Display mode (Figures 14-7A and C and 14-8A), where the percentage nasalance is displayed on the vertical (x) axis and the time is displayed on the horizontal (y) axis. The contour can be filled in as an option (Figures 14-7B and D and 14-8B). The Bar Display mode also shows nasalance on the horizontal axis in real time, but only one frame of data shows at a time (**FIGURE 14-9**).

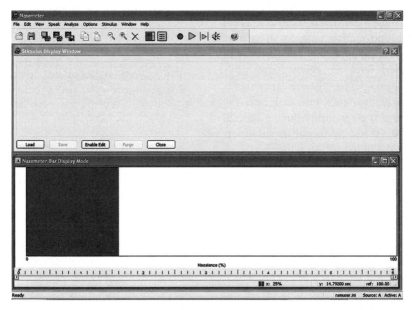

FIGURE 14-9 Horizontal bar graph shows nasalance results in real time. It can be used to provide feedback in therapy.

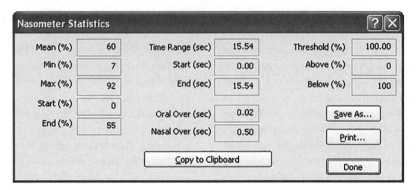

FIGURE 14-10 Summary statistics of the results. The "Mean (%)" is the mean of all the percentage points for the entire passage.

Result Statistics

Once the passage has been read or repeated, the examiner can obtain descriptive statistics for that segment of speech. This is done by clicking Analyze and then Compute Result Statistics from the menu, which brings up a statistics box (**FIGURE 14-10**). **TABLE 14-1** shows the definitions of each value.

For evaluation, the most important statistic is the mean nasalance score, which is the mean of all nasalance score data points during production of the passage. The mean nasalance score is compared to normative data to determine whether there is an abnormality and, if there is, the approximate degree of severity. The minimum and maximum percentage nasalance scores give the range of nasalance and can help the examiner to judge the variability during speech. For treatment, the threshold can be useful in setting a target for the individual to achieve.

Because there is variability in the scores of normal speakers and the scores do not always match perceptual impressions, Bressmann and colleagues (Bressmann et al., 2000) suggested adding two new measures to the nasometric evaluations: the nasalance distance, which they define as the range between maximum and minimum nasalance, and the nasalance ratio, which is the minimum nasalance divided by maximum nasalance. These numbers give an indication of the variability of nasalance within a passage.

TABLE 14-1 Important Nasometry Statistics

- Mean (%)—the mean nasalance percentage points for the entire passage
- Min (%)—the lowest nasalance value in the data, excluding zero values (important when assessing hyponasality)
- Max (%)—the highest nasalance value in the data (important when assessing hypernasality)
- Threshold (%)—an assigned target nasalance value that is indicated by the placement of the reference cursor
- Above (%)—the percentage of the nasalance trace that is greater than the ratio value set by the location of the reference cursor
- Below (%)—the percentage of the nasalance trace that is less than the ratio value set by the location of the reference cursor

Sensitivity and Specificity of the Nasalance Score

Several studies have been conducted to evaluate the sensitivity and specificity of the nasalance score as it is correlated to another measure of velopharyngeal function (Dalston, Neiman, & Gonzalez-Landa, 1993; Dalston et al., 1991b; Dalston et al., 1991c). The sensitivity refers to the extent to which the score is able to correctly identify individuals with abnormal resonance. The specificity refers to the extent to which the score correctly excludes individuals with normal speech from the abnormal group.

Dalston and colleagues (Dalston et al., 1991c) conducted a study to determine the extent to which nasometric results using Nasometer I corresponded with aerodynamic estimates of velopharyngeal orifice area. Using an oral speech passage and a cutoff nasalance score of 32, the sensitivity of the Nasometer scores in correctly identifying the presence or absence of velopharyngeal areas in excess of 0.10 cm was 0.78 and 0.79, respectively. As a second part of the study, the nasalance results were compared to clinical judgments of hypernasality. Again, using the score of 32 as the threshold of abnormality, the sensitivity and specificity of nasometry in correctly identifying subjects with more than mild hypernasality in their speech was 0.89, whereas the specificity was 0.95. Hardin and colleagues conducted a similar study but used a cutoff score of 26 (Hardin et al., 1992). In this study, a sensitivity coefficient of 0.87 and a specificity coefficient of 0.93 were obtained. Of the nasometry-based classifications, 91% accurately reflected listener judgments of hypernasality. Watterson, McFarlane, and Wright (1993) also found a significant correlation between nasalance and judgments of hypernasality on an oral speech passage. These results suggest that the Nasometer is an appropriate instrument that can be of value in assessing individuals suspected of having VPI.

Dalston and associates (Dalston et al., 1991b) conducted a complementary study to determine the extent to which nasometric scores corresponded with clinical judgments of hyponasality and aerodynamic measurements of nasal cross-sectional area. The sensitivity of the nasalance scores in correctly identifying individuals with hyponasality was 0.38, whereas the specificity was 0.92. The sensitivity and specificity of nasometry in correctly identifying the presence or absence of hyponasality as determined by perceptual assessment was 0.48 and 0.79, respectively. However, when individuals with audible nasal emission were eliminated from analysis, the sensitivity rose to 1.0, and the specificity rose to 0.85. This study

suggests that the sensitivity of nasometry in the identification of hyponasality with nasal air emission is not as strong as the sensitivity for identification of hypernasality or hyponasality alone.

Karnell (1995) suggested that one reason for a lack of agreement between perceptual measures and the nasalance results is that nasometry does not permit discrimination between nasal acoustic energy caused by hypernasality and nasal acoustic energy caused by audible nasal emission. Hypernasal resonance occurs on vowels, and audible nasal air emission occurs during the production of consonants. However, the presence of either can give the impression of "hypernasality" as judged by the listener.

To test resonance, without the effect of nasal air emission, Karnell used a "low-pressure" speech sample that contained only consonants that do not require intraoral air pressure. The nasalance results from this sample were compared to the results of the "high-pressure" sentences from the Zoo Passage. He found that the scores for some individuals were significantly different in the two passages. From this study, he suggested that those individuals with hypernasal resonance obtain elevated nasalance scores on the low-pressure and high-pressure speech samples because the resonance occurs primarily on the vowels. In contrast, those individuals with normal resonance but with nasal air emission, especially the nasal rustle, will have low or normal scores on the low-pressure sample but will have higher nasalance scores on the speech sample with high-pressure consonants. This observation seems true in clinical experience and is another reason to consider the nasalance score based on what is heard perceptually.

Interpretation of Nasometric Results

Many factors can affect the nasalance score. As noted previously, the expected nasalance score for a given passage is dependent on the vowel composition of that passage. This is why the normative score is not exactly the same for all oral passages in the same language. In addition, the score must be interpreted with knowledge of the patient's speech sound production during the passage. This is because the use of glottal stops or pharyngeal sounds elevates the score, even in the presence of a normally functioning velopharyngeal valve.

Expected Nasalance Results

The degree of nasalance in normal speech is partly dependent on whether the consonants are voiced or voiceless. Voiceless oral consonants in normal speech actually have no nasalance. This is because there is no phonated sound (and therefore no nasal resonance), and there is no audible nasal emission of the airstream. Therefore, when producing a sustained /s/, for example, the nasalance score is 0, and there is no tracing on the screen. In contrast, all voiced consonants have some nasal resonance. This can be demonstrated by producing a sustained /z/ and contrasting it with the voiceless cognate /s/. Although the nasalance score varies according to voicing, it does not seem to vary between the low-pressure and high-pressure consonants (Watterson, Lewis, & Deutsch, 1998).

Because all vowels are voiced, they all have some degree of nasalance. This can be seen on the screen when prolonging a vowel. The degree of nasalance varies depending on the type of vowel produced (Lewis & Watterson, 2003). There is more nasalance on high vowels than on low vowels, as can be noted on the SNAP Test-R (Kummer, 2005). In fact, the nasalance for /i/ is usually at least 10 percentage points higher than that for the low vowel /ɑ/.

One might question how it is possible to have nasal resonance, as represented by nasalance, on voiced oral sounds when the velopharyngeal valve is completely closed. There are actually two possible reasons for this. One is that the sound separator plate cannot totally block reception of the signal from one side of the plate to the other side. Therefore, there may be some spillover

between the microphones during the production of voiced phonemes, particularly vowels (PENTAX Medical, n.d.). The other reason is that there seems to be transpalatal transmission of sound during production of voiced phonemes, particularly vowels (Awan et al., 2011; Blanton, Watterson & Lewis, 2015; Gildersleeve-Neumann & Dalston, 2001). It can be assumed that the hard palate is like a brick wall and allows little sound to go through it. On the other hand, the soft palate is more like a heavy curtain—allowing some sound to pass through into the nasal cavity.

High vowels have more nasal resonance than low vowels because the high tongue position results in a smaller oral passage and hence, increased impedance to the sound going through the oral cavity. At the same time, there is increased sound pressure against the soft tissues of the velum (S. G. Fletcher, personal communication, May 12, 1999). In contrast, low vowels result in a larger oral opening and less impedance. Therefore, there is less nasalance on low vowels. Overall, a normal nasalance score for a passage with all voiced oral sounds is typically under 20%.

In evaluating nasal resonance, a prolonged nasal sound often results in scores that are in the 90s. However, when nasal consonants are combined with oral consonants in connected speech, the resulting nasalance score is between 50% and 70%.

Interpretation of the Nasalance Score

Because nasalance and resonance are on a continuum, there is a borderline area between clearly normal and clearly abnormal. Therefore, there is no single score that serves as an absolute or definitive cutoff point between normal and abnormal resonance. Suggested thresholds (based on about two standard deviations from the mean) are given for the various passages of the SNAP Test-R. In looking at all the norms for a passage devoid of nasal phonemes, it can be said that in general, a score under about 20% suggests no hypernasality, scores between 30% and 40% are in the mild range, and scores over 40% can be considered clearly hypernasal (Smith & Kuehn, 2007).

Given the large borderline range and the variability of scores based on phonemic content of the passage, the results of nasometric testing must always be interpreted by the speech pathologist in the context of the perceptual assessment. This is important because many factors can affect the nasalance score. For example, an individual's nasalance score can be in the normal range, even in the presence of audible nasal air emission. On the other hand, the nasalance score may be as much as two standard deviations above the normative mean, yet the person may still have very acceptable speech.

If there is obstruction in the vocal tract causing cul-de-sac resonance, the obstruction may impede the transmission of resonance in both the oral and nasal cavities, resulting in an essentially normal nasalance score because the nasalance score is a ratio of the two. In the same way, if there is a combination of hyponasality and hypernasality, both aspects are combined for the average nasalance score (Dalston et al., 1991a). If there is a nasal rustle, this may result in a high nasalance score because of the degree of nasal distortion, even though it may be caused by a small velopharyngeal opening. On the other hand, a large

velopharyngeal opening with blockage caused by enlarged adenoids may give a moderate nasalance score because of the lack of intensity of both oral and nasal acoustic energy. A breathy vocal quality or low volume can even influence the nasalance score to some degree as well.

Articulation errors can also affect the nasalance score. If pharyngeal fricatives or posterior nasal fricatives are substituted for sibilant phonemes, the nasal emission associated with these articulation productions will produce an elevated nasalance score, particularly on passages that contain a large number of sibilants. The same is true if nasal sounds are substituted for oral sounds (for example, the substitution of /ŋ/ for /l/). Although these errors are because of faulty articulation placement rather than VPI, this cannot be distinguished by the Nasometer if heterogeneous passages are used. Because there are so many factors that can affect the nasalance score, nasometry should always serve as a supplement to clinical judgment but not as a substitute for it.

With prior information from the perceptual examination, the examiner can interpret the nasalance scores with more confidence. In addition, certain patterns of scores can be diagnostic, as can be seen through the case reports in **TABLE 14-2**.

TABLE 14-2 Case Reports of Nasometry Scores and Analysis of Causality

CASE 1	
Oral Passages	*Nasalance Score (Mean %)*
Bilabial plosives	11
Lingual-alveolar plosives	11
Velar plosives	13
Sibilant fricatives	46

Analysis: All passages are within the normal range except the sibilants. This suggests phoneme-specific nasal emission on sibilants caused by the use of pharyngeal fricatives as a substitution. This can be corrected with speech therapy.

(continues)

TABLE 14-2 Case Reports of Nasometry Scores and Analysis of Causality	*(continued)*

CASE 2	
Oral Passages	*Nasalance Score (Mean %)*
Bilabial plosives	30
Lingual-alveolar plosives	48
Velar plosives	13
Sibilant fricatives	43

Analysis: Velar phonemes are normal, but anterior phonemes show high nasalance scores. This indicates normal velopharyngeal function but a symptomatic fistula that is just above the tongue tip.

CASE 3	
Oral + /ɑ/ Syllables	*Nasalance Score (Mean %)*
pɑ, pɑ, pɑ . . .	5
tɑ, tɑ, tɑ . . .	8
kɑ, kɑ, kɑ . . .	8
sɑ, sɑ, sɑ . . .	7
ɑ, ɑ, ɑ . . .	7
Oral + /i/ (as in "tea") Syllables	*Nasalance Score (Mean %)*
pi, pi, pi . . .	38
ti, ti, ti . . .	37
ki, ki, ki . . .	37
si, si, si . . .	39
i, i, i . . .	37

Analysis: Low-vowel syllables are normal, but high-vowel syllables are abnormally high. This suggests phoneme-specific hypernasality on high vowels caused by an abnormally high tongue position. Another possibility is a thin velum.

Interpretation of the Nasogram

In addition to the nasalance scores, the configuration of the nasogram on the screen can be useful in the diagnostic process (**FIGURE 14-11**). Some general guidelines in interpretation are as follows:

During production of an oral passage with no nasals:

- Normal oral resonance is typically between 10 and 15 percentage points.

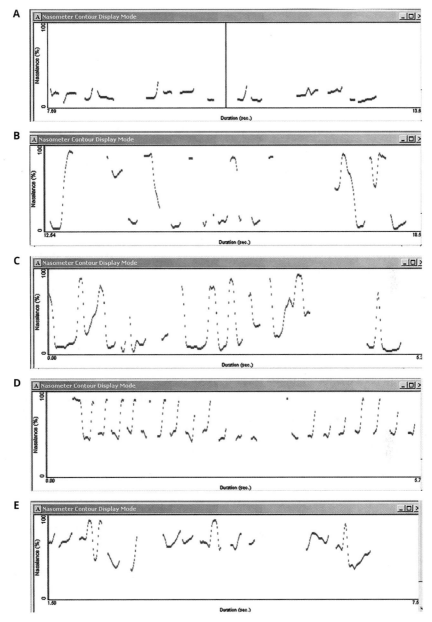

FIGURE 14-11 Nasograms. **(A)** A normal nasogram for an oral passage. **(B)** and **(C)** Normal resonance as noted by the solid lines at the bottom but audible nasal emission as noted by the high dotted lines. **(D)** and **(E)** Hypernasality and nasal emission as noted by the high solid lines and dotted lines.

- The expected difference between vowels /ɑ/ and /i/ is about 10 percentage points when combined with oral consonants and about 20 percentage points when combined with nasal consonants.

- The higher the contour is on the screen, the more hypernasality there will be in speech.

- If most of the data points appear normal (and the nasalance score is normal) but there are occasional high peaks, this indicates normal resonance but inconsistent nasal emission.

- A gradual rise in the curve throughout the passage suggests muscle fatigue, which could indicate neuromotor problems.
- There should be no data points during production of a prolonged /s/ or /ʃ/. If there is a break in velopharyngeal closure during prolongation of the sound, it will be seen on the screen.
- If one or more of the sibilant sounds is high in isolation or in syllables yet all other phonemes are normal, consider phoneme-specific nasal emission caused by the substitution of a pharyngeal fricative or posterior nasal fricative for these sounds.
- If lingual-alveolars and bilabials are significantly higher than velars, this indicates a symptomatic fistula.
- If vowels are high but prolonged /s/ is zero, a thin velum, high tongue position, or vowel-specific hypernasality could be the cause.

During production of a nasal passage:

- If the data points are low and remain toward the bottom of the screen, this indicates hyponasality and also upper airway obstruction.

The nasogram can be particularly helpful in counseling individuals and their families. With the visual display, it is easier for the examiner to explain what is happening during speech as well as the relative severity of the problem.

Use in Treatment

In addition to its utility as a diagnostic tool, nasometry can be useful in the therapy process by providing the individual with real-time visual feedback regarding nasality. In this way, it is useful in eliminating nasal emission or hypernasality that is phoneme specific. It can also be useful in helping the patient learn to use the velopharyngeal mechanism after VPI surgery. As a form of biofeedback, it may be used to modify resonance in selected cases of VPI caused by a neuromotor condition (Heppt, Westrich, Strate, & Mohring, 1991).

Although the Nasometer is a great tool for providing biofeedback in therapy, it should be noted that *biofeedback is effective only if the individual's velopharyngeal mechanism is anatomically and physiologically capable of achieving and maintaining normal velopharyngeal closure during connected speech.* If there is VPI, physical management (a prosthetic device or surgery) is needed for improvement or correction of speech.

To motivate young patients who are receiving therapy, games are provided as part of the software (**FIGURE 14-12**). The options on the Nasometer games can be changed to access different display formats, including the filled contour display, bar display, or inverted contour display, depending on the therapy task (**FIGURE 14-13**). The green reference cursor line can be placed on the nasogram according to the patient's therapy goals. The patient is asked to try to keep the nasalance trace below the reference-line level during speech.

To address specific errors, such as a phoneme-specific nasal emission on /s/, the child is instructed to eliminate the high spikes on the nasogram that occur when she produces the /s/ phoneme. It may be helpful to contrast minimal paired words with and without the /s/ phoneme. For example, because the /s/ phoneme should not be visible on the nasogram, words such as "mile" and "smile" should look similar, as noted in **FIGURE 14-14A**. When there is a phoneme-specific nasal rustle, an obvious difference can be noted in the tracings, as can be seen in **FIGURE 14-14B**.

A

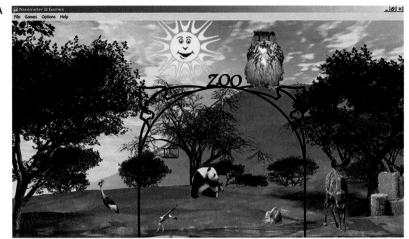

Look at this book with us. It's a story about a zoo. That is where bears go. Today it's very cold out of doors, but we see a cloud overhead that's a pretty white fluffy shape. We hear that straw covers the floor of cages to keep the chill away; yet a deer walks through the trees with her head high. They feed seeds to birds so they're able to fly.

| PLAY | Click PLAY or press Space Bar to start game. | 48.93 % | 11 sec. |

B

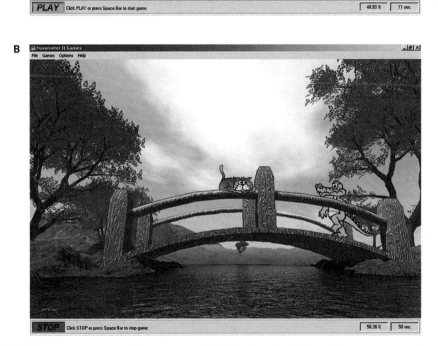

| STOP | Click STOP or press Space Bar to stop game. | 58.38 % | 50 sec. |

FIGURE 14-12 Nasometer games. All games provide biofeedback with the ability to set a nasalance threshold. When achieving the desired threshold, the child is rewarded with an emerging picture. This should be used only with nasality caused by abnormal placement.

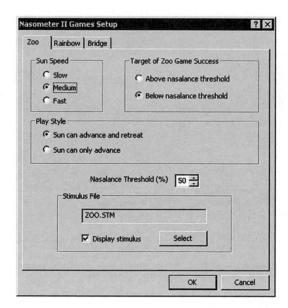

FIGURE 14-13 The options on the Nasometer games can be changed to meet the needs of each therapy session.

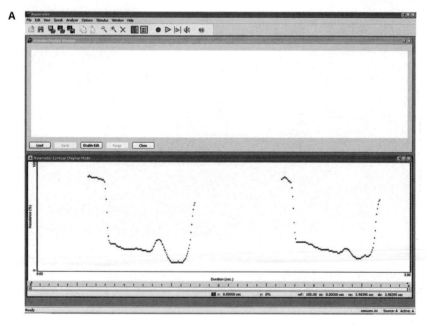

FIGURE 14-14 The words "mile" and "smile." **(A)** Normal speech production of the word "mile" and then "smile." Note that the two tracings are normal in appearance because there is no nasalance on the /s/ sound.

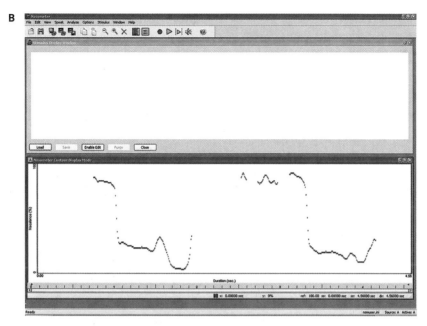

FIGURE 14-14 (CONTINUED) (B) Production of the word "mile" and then "smile" with a nasal rustle on /s/. Note that in this case, there is a high squiggly line at the beginning of the word "smile" because of the nasal rustle on /s/.

One big advantage of the Nasometer is that the nasogram with the audio can be replayed for the child again and again. This allows the child to see and hear the nasal emission. In addition, after the speech task has been completed, the clinician can open the statistics box to obtain the percentage above and below the threshold. This can serve as a basis for charting progress.

SUMMARY

Nasometric testing is an easy, noninvasive procedure used to obtain objective data regarding the acoustic correlates of velopharyngeal function (Hirschberg et al., 2006). The nasalance score can be compared to normative data to gauge the type and degree of nasality. Nasometry is an excellent means of substantiating the subjective findings of the speech pathologist. In addition, the Nasometer provides a visual display that is helpful in counseling individuals and families. Finally, nasometry is an excellent means for providing visual biofeedback during therapy when working on functional causes of hypernasality and/or nasal emission.

Although nasometry can be a very valuable part of an evaluation of resonance and velopharyngeal function, it should not be viewed as an independent diagnostic measure. Because the nasalance score can be affected by articulation errors, production errors, mixed nasality, and other factors, the objective measurements provided by nasometry should be interpreted based on an accompanying perceptual evaluation by a speech pathologist. In addition, just like with aerodynamic instrumentation, nasometry can give objective scores but cannot show the cause of velopharyngeal dysfunction or the location and size of the opening as direct measures can do. Therefore, the results of the nasometry must be integrated into a test battery for a complete evaluation of velopharyngeal function.

FOR REVIEW AND DISCUSSION

1. What is the Nasometer, and what are the equipment components?

2. What does the nasalance score measure? How is it calculated?

3. What are the standardized tests for use with nasometry? What type of passage should be used for testing hyponasality? What type of passage would be appropriate for testing hypernasality?

4. If the child has only plosives in his phonemic repertoire, what passages could be used?

5. Why is the nasalance score 0 during prolongation of the /s/ sound?

6. Why is the nasalance score not 0 with normal connected speech?

7. If the child has a high nasalance score on the sibilants passage but other scores are normal, what might you conclude? What would you recommend?

8. If a child with a history of cleft palate has a high nasalance score on plosives and lingual-alveolars but a normal score on velars, what might you suspect to be the cause? What would you do next? What would you recommend?

9. Which passage would have the higher nasalance score in normal speech: repetitive /pi/ or repetitive /pɑ/? Why?

REFERENCES

Anderson, R. T. (1996). Nasometric values for normal Spanish-speaking females: A preliminary report. *The Cleft Palate–Craniofacial Journal, 33*(4), 333–336.

Awan, S. N., Bressmann, T., Poburka, B., Roy, N., Sharp, H., & Watts, C. (2015). Dialectical effects on nasalance: A multicenter, cross-continental study. *Journal of Speech, Language, and Hearing Research, 58*(1), 69–77.

Awan, S. N., Omlor, K., & Watts, C. R. (2011). Effects of computer system and vowel loading on measures of nasalance. *Journal of Speech, Language, and Hearing Research, 54*(5), 1284–1294.

Blanton, A., Watterson, T., Lewis, K. (2015). The differential influence of vowels and palatal covering on nasalance scores. *The Cleft Palate–Craniofacial Journal, 52*(1), 82–87.

Bressmann, T. (2005). Comparison of nasalance scores obtained with the Nasometer, the Nasal View, and the OroNasal System. *The Cleft Palate–Craniofacial Journal, 42*(4), 423–433.

Bressmann, T., Sader, R., Whitehill, T. L., Awan, S. N., Zeilhofer, H. F., & Horch, H. H. (2000). Nasalance distance and ratio: Two new measures. *The Cleft Palate–Craniofacial Journal, 37*(3), 248–256.

Dalston, R. M. (1997). The use of nasometry in the assessment and remediation of velopharyngeal inadequacy. In K. R. Bzoch (Ed.), *Communicative disorders related to cleft lip and palate* (vol. 4, pp. 331–346). Austin, TX: Pro-Ed.

Dalston, R. M., Neiman, G. S., & Gonzalez-Landa, G. (1993). Nasometric sensitivity and specificity: A cross-dialect and cross-culture study. *The Cleft Palate–Craniofacial Journal, 30*(3), 285–291.

Dalston, R. M., & Seaver, E. J. (1992). Relative values of various standardized passages in the nasometric assessment of patients with velopharyngeal impairment. *The Cleft Palate–Craniofacial Journal, 29*(1), 17–21.

Dalston, R. M., Warren, D. W., & Dalston, E. T. (1991a). The identification of nasal obstruction through clinical judgments of hyponasality and nasometric assessment of speech acoustics. *American Journal of Orthodontics and Dentofacial Orthopedics, 100*(1), 59–65.

Dalston, R. M., Warren, D. W., & Dalston, E. T. (1991b). A preliminary investigation concerning the use of nasometry in identifying patients with hyponasality and/or nasal airway impairment. *Journal of Speech and Hearing Research, 34*(1), 11–18.

Dalston, R. M., Warren, D. W., & Dalston, E. T. (1991c). Use of nasometry as a diagnostic tool for identifying patients with velopharyngeal impairment. *The Cleft Palate–Craniofacial Journal, 28*(2), 184–188; discussion 188–189. (Erratum published 1991, *The Cleft Palate–Craniofacial Journal,* 1991, *28*(4), p. 446)

Dejonckere, P. H., & van Wijngaarden, H. A. (2001). Retropharyngeal autologous fat transplantation for congenital short palate: A nasometric assessment of functional results. *Annals of Otology, Rhinology, & Laryngology, 110*(2), 168–172.

Eckardt, A., Teltzrow, T., Schulze, A., Hoppe, M., & Kuettner, C. (2007). Nasalance in patients with maxillary defects: Reconstruction versus obturation. *Journal of Craniomaxillofacial Surgery, 35*(4–5), 241–245.

Fairbanks, D. (1960). *Voice and articulation drill book.* New York, NY: Harper and Row.

Fletcher, S. G. (1970). Theory and instrumentation for quantitative measurement of nasality. *Cleft Palate Journal, 7,* 601–609.

Fletcher, S. G. (1972). Contingencies for bio-electronic modification of nasality. *Journal of Speech and Hearing Disorders, 37,* 329–346.

Fletcher, S. G. (1976a). "Nasalance" vs. listener judgments of nasality. *Cleft Palate Journal, 13,* 31–44.

Fletcher, S. G. (1976b). Theory and use of Tonar II: A status report. *Biocommunications Research Reports, 1,* 1–38.

Fletcher, S. G. (1978). *Diagnosing speech disorders from cleft palate.* New York, NY: Grune & Statton.

Fletcher, S. G., Adams, L., & McCutcheon, M. J. (1989). Cleft palate speech assessment through oral-nasal acoustic measures. In K. R. Bzoch (Ed.), *Communicative disorders related to cleft lip and palate* (pp. 246–257). Boston, MA: College Hill Press.

Fletcher, S. G., & Bishop, M. E. (1970). Measurement of nasality with Tonar. *Cleft Palate Journal, 7,* 610–621.

Gildersleeve-Neumann, C. E., & Dalston, R. M. (2001). Nasalance scores in noncleft individuals: Why not zero? *The Cleft Palate–Craniofacial Journal, 38*(2), 106–111.

Hardin, M. A., Van Demark, D. R., Morris, H. L., & Payne, M. M. (1992). Correspondence between nasalance scores and listener judgments of hypernasality and hyponasality. *The Cleft Palate–Craniofacial Journal, 29*(4), 346–351.

Hassan, S. M., Malki, K. H., Mesallam, T. A., Farahat, M., Bukhari, M., & Murry, T. (2011). The effect of cochlear implantation on nasalance of speech in postlingually hearing-impaired adults. *Journal of Voice, 26*(5), pp. 669.e17–669.e22.

Heppt, W., Westrich, M., Strate, B., & Mohring, L. (1991). Nasalance: A new concept for objective analysis of nasality. *Laryngorhinootologic, 70*(4), 208–213.

Hirschberg, J., Bok, S., Juhasz, M., Trenovszki, Z., Votisky, P., & Hirschberg, A. (2006). Adaptation of nasometry to Hungarian language and experiences with its clinical application. *International Journal of Pediatric Otorhinolaryngology, 70*(5), 785–798.

Hong, K. H., Kwon, S. H., & Jung, S. S. (1997). The assessment of nasality with a Nasometer and sound spectrography in patients with nasal polyposis. *Otolaryngology-Head & Neck Surgery, 117*(4), 343–348.

Karnell, M. P. (1995). Nasometric discrimination of hypernasality and turbulent nasal airflow. *The Cleft Palate–Craniofacial Journal, 32*(2), 145–148.

Karnell, M. P. (2011). Instrumental assessment of velopharyngeal closure for speech. *Seminars in Speech and Language, 32*(2), 168–178.

Kummer, A. W. (2005). The MacKay-Kummer Simplified Nasometric Assessment Procedures-Revised (SNAP-R). In PENTAX Medical *Instruction manual for Nasometer II: Model 6450.* PENTAX Medical, Retrieved from www.researchgate.net /publication/273060845_The_MacKay-Kummer _SNAP_Test-R_Simplified_Nasometric_Assessment _Procedures_Revised_2005

Kummer, A. W. (2016). Evaluation of speech and resonance for children with craniofacial anomalies.

Facial Plastic Surgery Clinics of North America, 24(4), 445–451.

Kummer, A. W., Myer, C. M. L., Smith, M. E., & Shott, S. R. (1993). Changes in nasal resonance secondary to adenotonsillectomy. *American Journal of Otolaryngology, 14*(4), 285–290.

Leeper, H. A., Rochet, A. P., & MacKay, I. R. A. (1992). Characteristics of nasalance in Canadian speakers of English and French. *Proceedings of the International Conference on Spoken and Language Processes, 5,* 49–52.

Lewis, K. E., & Watterson, T. (2003). Comparison of nasalance scores obtained from the Nasometer and the NasalView. *The Cleft Palate–Craniofacial Journal, 40*(1), 40–45.

MacKay, I. R. A., & Kummer, A. W. (1994). Simplified nasometric assessment procedures. In Kay Elemetrics Corp. (Ed.), *Instruction manual: Nasometer model 6200-3* (pp. 123–142). Lincoln Park, NJ: Kay Elemetrics Corp.

Mandulak, K. C., & Zajac, D. J. (2009). Effects of altered fundamental frequency on nasalance during vowel production by adult speakers at targeted sound pressure levels. *The Cleft Palate–Craniofacial Journal, 46*(1), 39–46.

Mayo, R., Floyd, L. A., Warren, D. W., Dalston, R. M., & Mayo, C. M. (1996). Nasalance and nasal area values: Cross-racial study. *The Cleft Palate–Craniofacial Journal, 33*(2), 143–149.

Mueller, K., Neuber, B., Schelhorn-Niese, P., & Schumann, D. (2007). Diagnostic value of nasometry: Representative study of patients with cleft palate and normal subjects. *Folia Phoniatrica et Logopaedica, 59*(5), 219–226.

Nieminen, P., Lopponen, H., Vayrynen, M., Tervonen, A., & Tolonen, U. (2000). Nasalance scores in snoring children with obstructive symptoms. *International Journal of Pediatric Otorhinolaryngology, 52*(1), 53–60.

Parker, A. J., Clarke, P. M., Dawes, P. J., & Maw, A. R. (1990). A comparison of active anterior rhinomanometry and nasometry in the objective assessment of nasal obstruction. *Rhinology, 28*(1), 47–53.

Parker, A. J., Maw, A. R., & Szallasi, F. (1989). An objective method of assessing nasality: A possible aid in the selection of patients for adenoidectomy. *Clinical Otolaryngology, 14*(2), 161–166.

PENTAX Medical. (n.d.). Installation, operations, and maintenance manual: Nasometer II, Model 6450. Lincoln Park, NJ: PENTAX Medical.

Perry, J., & Schenck, G. (2013). Instrumental assessment in cleft palate care. *SIG 5 Perspectives on Speech Science and Orofacial Disorders, 23*(2), 49–61.

Rieger, J., Wolfaardt, J., Seikaly, H., & Jha, N. (2002). Speech outcomes in patients rehabilitated with maxillary obturator prostheses after maxillectomy: A prospective study. *International Journal of Prosthodontics, 15*(2), 139–144.

Santos-Terron, M. J., Gonzalez-Landa, G., & Sanchez-Ruiz, I. (1990). Nasometric patterns in the speech of normal child speakers of Castilian Spanish. *Revista Espanola de Foniatrica, 4,* 71–75.

Seaver, E. J., Dalston, R. M., Leeper, H. A., & Adams, L. E. (1991). A study of nasometric values for normal nasal resonance. *Journal of Speech and Hearing Research, 34*(4), 715–721.

Smith, B. E., & Kuehn, D. P. (2007). Speech evaluation of velopharyngeal dysfunction. *The Journal of Craniofacial Surgery, 18*(2), 251–261.

Soneghet, R., Santos, R. P., Behlau, M., Habermann, W., Friedrich, G., & Stammberger, H. (2002). Nasalance changes after functional endoscopic sinus surgery. *Journal of Voice, 16*(3), 392–397.

Sweeney, T., & Sell, D. (2008). Relationship between perceptual ratings of nasality and nasometry in children/adolescents with cleft palate and/or velopharyngeal dysfunction. *International Journal of Language and Communication Disorders, 43*(3), 265–282.

Sweeney, T., Sell, D., & O'Regan, M. (2004). Nasalance scores for normal-speaking Irish children. *The Cleft Palate–Craniofacial Journal, 41*(2), 168–174.

Tatchell, J. A., Stewart, M., & Lapine, P. R. (1991). Nasalance measurements in hearing-impaired children. *Journal of Communication Disorders, 24*(4), 275–285.

van der Heijden, P., Hobbel, H. H., van der Laan, B. F., Korsten-Meijer, A. G., & Goorhuis-Brouwer, S. M. (2011). Nasometry cooperation in children 4–6 years. *International Journal of Pediatric Otorhinolaryngology, 75*(3), 420–424.

van Doorn, J., & Purcell, A. (1998). Nasalance levels in the speech of normal Australian children. *The Cleft Palate–Craniofacial Journal, 35*(4), 287–292.

Van Lierde, K. M., De Bodt, M., Baetens, L., Schrauwen, V., & Van Cauwenberge, P. (2003). Outcome of treatment regarding articulation, resonance, and voice in Flemish adults with unilateral and bilateral cleft palate. *Folia Phoniatrica et Logopedica, 55*(2), 80–90.

Van Lierde, K. M., Monstrey, S., Bonte, K., Van Cauwenberge, P., & Vinck, B. (2004). The long-term speech outcome in Flemish young adults after two different types of palatoplasty. *International Journal of Pediatric Otorhinolaryngology, 68*(7), 865–875.

Watterson, T., Lewis, K. E., & Deutsch, C. (1998). Nasalance and nasality in low-pressure and high-pressure speech. *The Cleft Palate–Craniofacial Journal, 35*(4), 293–298.

Watterson, T., Lewis, K. E., & Foley-Homan, N. (1999). Effect of stimulus length on nasalance scores. *The Cleft Palate–Craniofacial Journal, 36*(3), 243–247.

Watterson, T., McFarlane, S. C., & Wright, D. S. (1993). The relationship between nasalance and nasality in children with cleft palate. *Journal of Communication Disorders, 26*(1), 13–28.

Williams, R. G., Eccles, R., & Hutchings, H. (1990). The relationship between nasalance and nasal resistance to airflow. *Acta Otolaryngology (Stockholm), 110*(5/6), 443–449.

Williams, R. G., Preece, M., Rhys, R., & Eccles, R. (1992). The effect of adenoid and tonsil surgery on nasalance. *Clinical Otolaryngology & Allied Sciences, 17*(2), 136–140.

Wozny, C. G., Kuehn, D. P., Oishi, J. T., & Arthur, J. L. (1994, November). *Effect of passage length on nasalance values in normal adults.* Paper presented at the American Speech-Language-Hearing Association, New Orleans, LA.

CREDITS

Standard Nasometric Passages Supplied by Kaypentax

Zoo Passage[a]

Look at the book with us. It's a story about a zoo. That is where bears go. Today it's very cold out of doors, but we see a cloud overhead that's a pretty, white, fluffy shape. We hear that straw covers the floor of cages to keep the chill away, yet a deer walks through the trees with her head high. They feed seeds to birds so they're able to fly.

Rainbow Passage[b]

When the sunlight strikes raindrops in the air, they act like a prism and form a rainbow. The rainbow is a division of white light into many beautiful colors. These take the shape of a long round arch, with its path high above and its two ends apparently beyond the horizon.

There is, according to legend, a boiling pot of gold at one end. People look, but no one ever finds it. When a man looks for something beyond his reach, his friends say he is looking for the pot of gold at the end of the rainbow.

Nasal Sentences[c3]

Mama made some lemon jam.
Ten men came in when Jane rang.
Dan's gang changed my mind.
Ben can't plan on a lengthy rain.
Amanda came from Bounding, Maine.

Normative data for standardized passages collected on 40 adult subjects using Nasometer II (PENTAX Medical, n.d.):

Test Passage	Mean Nasalance	SD of Mean
Zoo Passage	11.25	5.63
Rainbow Passage	31.47	6.65
Nasal Sentences	59.55	7.96

a The Zoo Passage excludes nasal consonants.
b In the Rainbow Passage, 11.5% of the consonants are nasal consonants.
c The Nasal Sentences Passage is loaded with nasal phonemes so that 35% of the total phonemes in these sentences are nasal consonants. This is more than three times as many as would be expected in Standard American English sentences.

CREDITS

Appendix opener photo: PeopleImages/Getty Images

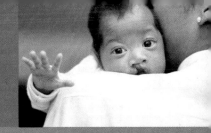

APPENDIX 14B

Score Sheet for the SNAP Test-Revised

The MacKay-Kummer SNAP Test-R
Simplified Nasometric Assessment Procedures Revised 2005

Name: _____   Date: _____

Age: _____   Examiner: _____

Subtest I: Syllable Repetition/Prolonged Sounds Subtest

Instructions: Repeat or prolong until the screen is full.

Oral + /ɑ/ Syllables	Norms	SD	Score (Threshold: ≥ 15)
pɑ, pɑ, pɑ . . .	6	3	
tɑ, tɑ, tɑ . . .	7	4	
kɑ, kɑ, kɑ . . .	7	4	
sɑ, sɑ, sɑ . . .	7	5	
ʃɑ, ʃɑ, ʃɑ . . .	7	4	

Oral + /i/ Syllables	Norms	SD	Score (Threshold: ≥ 35)
pi, pi, pi . . .	17	7	
ti, ti, ti . . .	17	7	
ki, ki, ki . . .	18	8	
si, si, si . . .	17	8	
ʃi, ʃi, ʃi . . .	16	8	

Nasal + /a/ Syllables	Norms	SD	Score (Threshold: ≤ 40)
mɑ, mɑ, mɑ . . .	53	13	
nɑ, nɑ, nɑ . . .	53	11	

Nasal + /i/ Syllables	Norms	SD	Score (Threshold: ≤ 60)
mi, mi, mi . . .	72	13	
ni, ni, ni . . .	74	11	

Prolonged Sounds	Norms	SD	Score (Threshold: +/−2 SDs)
Prolonged /ɑ/	6	3	
Prolonged /i/	19	9	
Prolonged /s/	0	0	
Prolonged /m/	93	3	

Subtest II: Picture Cued Subtest

Instructions: Produce a sentence with the carrier phrase and picture. Do each twice.

Oral Passages	Norms	SD	Score (Threshold: ≥ 22)
Bilabial plosives	11	5	
Lingual-alveolar plosives	11	5	
Velar plosives	13	6	
Sibilant fricatives	12	5	

Nasal Passage	Norms	SD	Score (Threshold: ≤ 45)
Nasals	54	9	

Subtest III: Paragraph Subtest

Instructions: Read or repeat each passage.

Passages (Reading)	Norms	SD	Score (Threshold: > 25)
Bilabial plosives (w/nasals)	16	5	

Passages (Reading)	Norms	SD	Score (Threshold: > 20)
Sibilant fricatives (w/o nasals)	10	4	

Notes:

_____

_____

_____

_____

Important: The threshold value for each test is an approximation of the beginning of a borderline range of abnormal resonance. These values were estimated based on standard deviations (about 2 higher for orals, about 1 lower for nasals) and clinical experience. It should be noted that a small number of normal speakers will score outside 2 standard deviations of the mean for both orals and nasals. Therefore, the suggested threshold values should be used as general guidelines and not as absolute markers between normal and abnormal resonance. The scores on nasometry should always be used as a means to support clinical judgment but never to replace it.

Picture Cued Subtest

Pick up the . . .

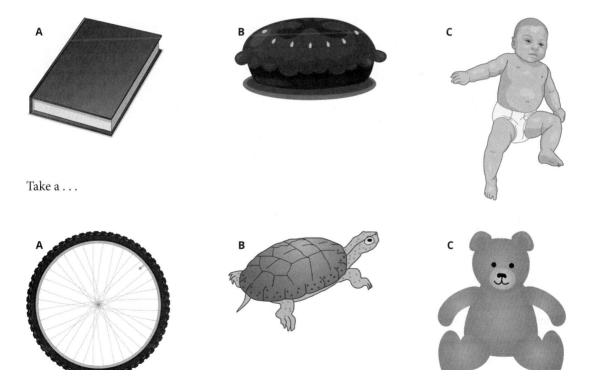

A

B

C

Take a . . .

A

B

C

Go get a . . .

A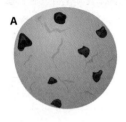

B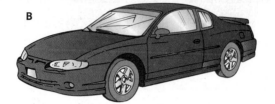

C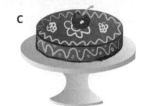

Suzy sees the . . .

A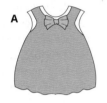

B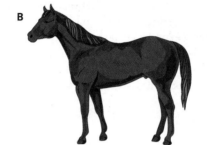

C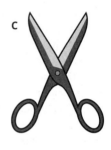

Mama made some . . .

A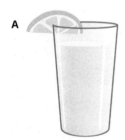

B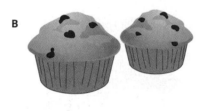

C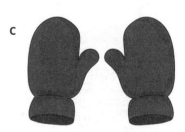

Paragraph Subtest

Instructions: Read the title with the passage.

Bobby and Billy Play Ball

Bobby and Billy go to play ball.
They get a bat, a ball, and a glove.
They go to the ball park.
Billy took a turn at bat.
Bobby tried to throw the ball.
Billy hit the ball up high.
Bobby and Billy like to play ball.

A School Day for Suzy

Suzy eats cereal or toast for breakfast.
After that, she rides the bus to school.
Suzy likes to sit with Sally.
At school, the teacher gives Suzy's
class a test.
Suzy likes her school.
She also likes her teacher.

CREDITS

Appendix opener photo: PeopleImages/Getty Images

CHAPTER 15

Videofluoroscopy

CHAPTER OUTLINE

INTRODUCTION

Velopharyngeal insufficiency/incompetence (VPI) can be diagnosed based on the characteristics of the speech as determined through a perceptual speech evaluation alone. However, instrumental assessment of the velopharyngeal valve, as can be done through videofluoroscopy, is usually indicated to determine the cause, the approximate size, and particularly the location of the velopharyngeal opening. This information is important to obtain so that the best form of surgical intervention can be determined.

Videofluoroscopy is an imaging technique used to obtain real-time moving images of internal structures. This is done through the use of a fluoroscope, which consists of an X-ray source and fluorescent screen. A **videofluoroscopic speech study** is the use of videofluoroscopy to evaluate velopharyngeal function during speech (Dudas, Deleyiannis, Ford, Jiang, & Losee, 2006; Lam et al., 2006; Rowe & D'Antonio, 2005; Shprintzen, 1995; Smith & Kuehn, 2007; Ysunza, Pamplona, Ortega, & Prado, 2008; Ysunza, Pamplona, Ortega, & Prado 2011). Videofluoroscopy can help the examiner assess both the anatomical and physiological abnormalities that cause VPI. This information is important so that the optimal surgical or prosthetic treatment for the patient can be determined. Videofluoroscopy is also used to assess swallowing and is called either a **modified barium swallow (MBS)** or **videofluoroscopic swallowing study (VFSS)**.

Videofluoroscopy was first used for direct visualization of velopharyngeal function in the late 1960s and early 1970s, and it has been used ever since. With the advent of nasopharyngoscopy, it is not used as extensively as it once was, but it is still used occasionally by many centers. Therefore, the professionals who treat patients with velopharyngeal dysfunction should be knowledgeable of its uses, advantages, and disadvantages. In addition, videofluoroscopy continues to be a powerful tool in the evaluation of swallowing disorders.

The purpose of this chapter is to explain how videofluoroscopy is used in evaluating velopharyngeal function. The specific procedures for a videofluoroscopic speech study are reviewed, and the interpretation of images is discussed as it relates to the diagnosis of VPI and recommendations for treatment.

History of Radiography for VPI

Radiography refers to the use of the roentgen ray (X-ray) to image internal body parts. As the ray goes through the body, it creates an image on the other side. The image then shows structures as light images and airspace as dark images. Because the beam goes entirely through a structure, it projects the summation of all parts of that structure through which the beam passes. In other words, it shows matter, whether the matter is consistent throughout or occurring only in a small portion of the line of the beam.

Conventional radiography depends on the natural attenuation of the different tissues. **Attenuation** is the combined absorption and scattering of radiation proton particles by the tissues. When there is greater attenuation, as in bone, fewer radiation particles reach the image. This results in less exposure and hence, an image that is near the white end of the spectrum. When there is less attenuation (as in air), more radiation particles reach the film. This results in more exposure, so the image is near the black end of the spectrum.

Traditionally, radiographic images were recorded on film and then on videotape. Systems now use high-resolution digital imaging. The advantages of digital radiographs include the fact that they can be viewed on a computer, are of greater resolution, and can be stored electronically.

Most radiographic images are planar, or two dimensional, in nature. To image a three-dimensional volume structure adequately, it must be examined in three mutually perpendicular planes to fully appreciate that structure (Pelo, Tassiello, Boniello, Gasparini, & Longobardi, 2006; Skolnick & Cohn, 1989; Skolnick, McCall, & Barnes, 1973). Of course, the velopharyngeal port is a three-dimensional volume structure. Therefore, multiple views for a complete assessment are required.

Lateral Cephalometric X-Rays

Lateral cephalometric X-rays are still radiographic images of the midsagittal plane of the head. They are typically taken in a dental professional's office, using a standard head holder. Through a process called laminography, which involves careful measurement of the distances and angles between particular landmarks on the image, orthodontists and oral surgeons use lateral cephalometric images to study and measure the craniofacial bones and parameters of growth.

The lateral "ceph" is a still picture that can be taken during phonation of a vowel or production of a prolonged /s/. It shows the hard palate, the velum at rest, velar length and height during phonation, and the posterior pharyngeal wall. The lateral ceph illustrates the cervical spine, angle of the cranial base, and the morphologic features of the facial skeleton. Cervical spine and cranial base anomalies that affect the position of the pharyngeal wall for velopharyngeal closure can be identified through this procedure. In the 1950s, lateral cephalometric X-rays were used extensively in cleft palate research. In fact, the role of adenoid tissue in velopharyngeal closure was better understood with the use of this procedure (Smith & Kuehn, 2007).

Despite its value in certain circumstances, cephalometric images are no longer used for routine assessment of velopharyngeal function for several reasons. First, the lateral ceph shows only the midsagittal section of the velopharyngeal portal. Therefore, lateral pharyngeal walls cannot be viewed. As a result, the examiner is likely to misdiagnose the presence or absence of velopharyngeal insufficiency about 30% of the time as compared to the use of a multiview technique (Major, Flores-Mir, & Major, 2006). Another problem is that the lateral ceph is a still image that can show structure but not velar movement during speech (Kuehn & Henne, 2003). Finally, the image is a summation of all of the parts through which the beam travels. If the velum is touching on just one part of the posterior pharyngeal wall, it looks like there is complete closure on the lateral view because of this summation effect. Therefore, small openings may not be detected.

Cineradiography

The use of cineradiography as a method for evaluating velopharyngeal function was first introduced in the early 1950s. Often referred to as a cine study, this technique involved taking a series of 16 to 24 frames of radiographs per second, which were recorded on motion picture film. Multiple views were taken for appreciation of all aspects of the velopharyngeal valve. Although this procedure was far better than a single lateral ceph, which showed only one view and no movement, there was no way to simultaneously record sound, so correlating movement patterns with speech phonemes was not possible (Shprintzen, 1995). Another major disadvantage of this procedure was the relatively high dosage of radiation per study.

Videofluoroscopy

A significant methodological advancement was made with the introduction of a radiographic procedure using videofluoroscopy (Skolnick, 1969; Skolnick 1970; Skolnick & McCall, 1971). Through the use of multiple views, videofluoroscopy allows the examiner to visualize both the structures and function of the velopharyngeal mechanism (Skolnick & Cohn, 1989). Unlike cineradiography, it allows simultaneous audio recording of the speech.

Multiview videofluoroscopy has many important uses. It can be used to confirm the presence of a velopharyngeal opening and estimate the size of that opening (Lam et al., 2006). The cause of VPI can be differentiated between a short velum and poor velar movement. In comparison with nasopharyngoscopy, videofluoroscopy is superior in showing the vertical movement of the velum during speech. It also provides a view of the entire length of the posterior pharyngeal wall during closure, which cannot be seen with nasopharyngoscopy. Videofluoroscopy can help the examiner determine surgical and prosthetic options for the treatment of VPI. It can be helpful in assessing the placement of a prosthetic device, particularly a palatal lift. Finally, it can be used to evaluate the effects of some surgical procedures, such as adenoidectomy, maxillary advancement, and a retropharyngeal implant (Havstam et al., 2005; Kendall, Leonard, & McKenzie, 2004). In comparison to nasopharyngoscopy, videofluoroscopy is not a good method for evaluating small, localized openings; seeing the entire port at once; or examining the effectiveness of VPI surgery.

Before using videofluoroscopy for evaluation of velopharyngeal function, the speech-language pathologist should refer to the practice document regarding videofluoroscopy, published by the American Speech-Language-Hearing Association (ASHA, 2004).

Preparation of the Patient

Most patients who require an evaluation of velopharyngeal function are children. For best results, it helps to prepare the patient and the family for the procedure before the day of the exam. Many centers send information to the family regarding the videofluoroscopy procedure at the time that the appointment is scheduled. Information about what to expect should also be sent to the child, preferably in the form of a storybook or coloring book. The child can even be given a list of the standard phrases and sentences to practice at home. When the patient and family receive information before the examination, the child is more likely to be cooperative during the procedure.

Regardless of prior preparation, the child may be nervous during the examination. Therefore, it is important that the speech-language pathologist and/or X-ray technologist speak calmly and softly to the child. It is best to tell the child exactly what will be done before it is done. The parents can help by encouraging the child and offering the child a reward for completing the study.

Videofluoroscopy Procedure

The velopharyngeal port is a three-dimensional structure that operates as a sphincter, with movement from all sides of the port. With fluoroscopic imaging, however, only two-dimensional views can be obtained (Shprintzen, 1995; Shprintzen, Rakof, Skolnick, & Lavorato, 1977; Skolnick, 1975; Skolnick et al., 1973). Therefore, to evaluate the motion of the entire velopharyngeal valve, it is necessary to obtain multiple views (Skolnick & Cohn, 1989; Skolnick & McCall, 1971).

The views most commonly used with videofluoroscopy for speech include the lateral view, the frontal view, and the base view. The name of the view (e.g., lateral view) denotes the direction in which the radiation beam passes through the body. In addition to the standard views, there are some supplemental views (Towne's view and oblique view) that can also be used for certain diagnostic circumstances. These views are further described as follows.

Lateral View

For the lateral view, the beam goes through the side of the head to reveal a midsagittal section. As such, this view shows the velum and posterior pharyngeal wall. Through this view, the examiner is able to view the effective length of the velum, velar movement and height during speech, the entire posterior pharyngeal wall, tongue movement during speech, and the patency of an oronasal fistula when barium is injected in the nasal cavity.

For the lateral view, the patient is ideally placed in an upright position. The fluoroscopic table is positioned vertically, and the patient stands or sits between the table and the fluoroscopic screen (**FIGURE 15-1**). The head remains in a neutral position with the patient looking straight ahead. For a young child who has difficulty holding still, the child can be placed on his side with a special pillow to support and stabilize the head (**FIGURE 15-2**). An initial concern in using this position was that gravity may affect velar movement. However, if there is an effect of gravity, it is likely to be negligible (Perry, 2011).

Regardless of the position used, the X-ray technician must position the head so that the rami on both sides of the mandible are superimposed

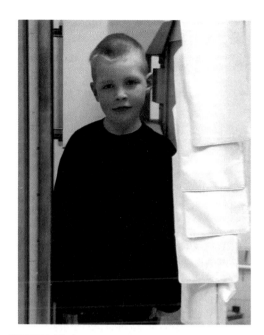

FIGURE 15-1 Patient position for the lateral view. The fluoroscopic table is vertically positioned, and the patient stands or sits between the table and the fluoroscopic screen. The head remains in a neutral position with the patient looking straight ahead.

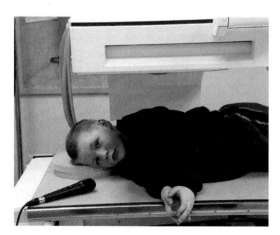

FIGURE 15-2 Alternate patient position for the lateral view. This is used if the patient needs more head support. For a young child who has difficulty holding still, the child can lie on the table on his side. A special pillow is used to support and stabilize the head. The disadvantage of this position is the potential effect of gravity on velar movement, although this effect is probably negligible.

on the view. This helps to ensure that the head is not rotated or tilted during the study. If the head is not lined up correctly to obtain a true lateral view, the beam will go through tissue (rather than the opening), which makes it appear that there is closure when there is not.

Frontal View

For the frontal view, also called the anterior–posterior (AP) view, the X-ray beam is directed through the nose so that it is tangential to the plane of the velar eminence (top of the velum) during oral speech. As a result, the velar eminence appears as an arc between the lateral pharyngeal walls. The frontal view is done to visualize the lateral pharyngeal walls at rest and during speech.

For the frontal view, the patient is positioned to face forward so that the beam is directed straight through the front of the nose. The patient can be upright or placed in a supine position (**FIGURE 15-3**).

As with the lateral view, it is very important that the head be centered and not rotated for the frontal view. The X-ray technician does this by making sure that the nasal septum appears in

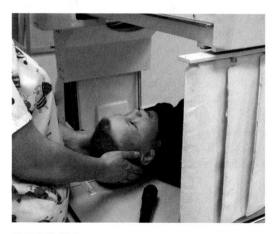

FIGURE 15-3 Patient position for the frontal, or AP (anterior–posterior), view. The patient is placed in a supine position and the head is centered. This can be determined by observing the nasal septum through the fluoroscope and making sure that it appears to be in midline.

midline. The septum should be equidistant from the lateral margins of the maxillary cavity, and the incisor teeth should appear to be on either side of the nasal septum (allowing for deviations in structures, of course). During nasal breathing, the lateral pharyngeal walls can be seen to bow outward on either side of the nasal septum. With speech, the lateral pharyngeal walls bow inward to close against the velum. However, because this is a two-dimensional view, the lateral walls appear to close against the septum when there is normal velopharyngeal closure.

Base View

For the base view, also called the en face view, the beam enters through the base of the chin and then up through the velopharyngeal port. This allows the examiner to see the entire velopharyngeal sphincter from the bottom up (Kuehn & Henne, 2003). With this orientation, the relative contributions of the velum, the lateral pharyngeal walls, and posterior pharyngeal wall closure can be determined. The border of the velum is not as easy to appreciate as the pharyngeal walls with this view. Also, the presence of large adenoids can affect the interpretation of this view (Witt, Marsh, McFarland, & Riski, 2000).

For the base view, the patient is placed on the X-ray table in a prone position. The patient is then asked to assume a "sphinx position" by pulling the head up and placing the upper body weight on the arms and elbows (**FIGURE 15-4**). The head and the back are then hyperextended so that the X-ray beam can be directed vertically through the base of the chin. The correct positioning of the base view is actually very difficult because the beam must be directly at right angles to the plane of closure. Otherwise, the port will not be visualized or the dimensions of the port will be severely distorted.

Towne's View

For the Towne's view, the beam goes down into the port from above. It has been described as an

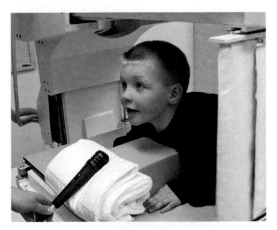

FIGURE 15-4 Patient position for the base view. The patient is placed on the X-ray table in a prone position and then asked to assume a "sphinx position" by pulling the head up and placing the upper body weight on the arms and elbows. The head and the back are then hyperextended so that the X-ray beam can be directed vertically through the base of the chin and then up through the velopharyngeal port. The correct positioning is important because the beam must be directly at right angles to the plane of closure.

alternative to the base view because it also provides an en face orientation, although from above rather than below (Stringer & Witzel, 1986; Stringer & Witzel, 1989). As such, the Towne's view shows the perimeter of the velopharyngeal valve.

For the Towne's view, the patient is seated upright with the chin tucked and the head hyperflexed (Kuehn & Henne, 2003). The beam goes through the top of the head and intersects the plane of the velopharyngeal port in a perpendicular manner. When the adenoids are large, the Towne's view may provide a better view of the velopharyngeal port than the base view (La Rossa, Brown, Cohen, & Spackman, 1980; Stringer & Witzel, 1986; Stringer & Witzel, 1989).

Oblique View

For the oblique view, the beam is projected at 45 degrees from midline or between where the frontal and lateral beams would go. Therefore, the oblique view shows the relationship between movements of the velum (as seen on the lateral view) and each lateral pharyngeal wall on each side (as seen on the frontal view). The oblique view can be helpful in visualizing asymmetrical movement of the lateral pharyngeal walls, which is actually quite common (Argamaso, Levandowski, Golding-Kushner, & Shprintzen, 1994; D'Antonio, Muntz, Marsh, Marty-Grames, & Backensto-Marsh, 1988). This view might also be chosen if a satisfactory base view cannot be obtained because of large adenoids or the inability to hyperextend the neck (Skolnick & Cohn, 1989).

The oblique view is performed by having the patient sit facing forward. With the fluoroscopy on, the patient slowly rotates the head and body as a single unit so that it moves 45 degrees to one side, back to the midline, and then 45 degrees to the other side. This allows the examiner to view each lateral wall and its relationship to the velum separately and then compare the movements on each side.

Use of Contrast Material

On the lateral view, the velum and posterior pharyngeal wall can be easily visualized without the need for a contrast substance. However, on the other views, a radiopaque contrast substance is necessary to visualize the lateral pharyngeal walls.

The most commonly used substance for contrast is a suspension of barium sulfate. This can be purchased as a premixed liquid or as a powder that is mixed with water until it is the consistency of heavy cream (Skolnick & Cohn, 1989). Flavoring can be added to the mixture as well.

When the barium is added for the other views, it is sometimes helpful to repeat the lateral view. Barium can make a Passavant's ridge more obvious on the lateral view (Cohn, Rood, McWilliams, Skolnick, & Abdelmalek, 1984). It can also be helpful in determining the patency of an oronasal fistula. If the fistula is patent, the barium can often be seen dripping from the nasal cavity through the fistula to the oral cavity (Clark, D'Antonio, Liu, & Welch, 1992; Skolnick, Glaser, & McWilliams,

1980). In addition, as the patient swallows, barium may be seen going up into the fistula. Finally, barium on the lateral view can sometimes outline a defect in the nasal surface of the velum as a result of a submucous cleft. Because barium can produce artifacts or occasionally obscure structures on the lateral view, it is recommended that lateral videofluoroscopy always be performed without barium first and then again with barium only if specific information is needed.

With all views, barium may be helpful in the identification of small gaps that cannot otherwise be seen because of the resolution of the views. This is because with small gaps, the high pressure of the airflow that is released through the opening can cause bubbling of the barium at the top of the valve. The observation of bubbling, therefore, always indicates a small velopharyngeal gap. However, the absence of bubbling is not similarly diagnostic. When there is a larger velopharyngeal gap, there is less concentrated air pressure going through the opening, and therefore bubbling is less likely to occur.

There are different methods for instilling barium into the nasopharynx. One method is to use a soft rubber catheter and syringe. The catheter is inserted into a nostril and pushed through the nose to the nasopharynx. The barium is then delivered to the pharynx through the syringe (**FIGURE 15-5**). Some centers administer a mixture of topical anesthesia (e.g., tetracaine or pontocaine) and a decongestant (e.g., xylometazoline or oxymetazoline) into the nose a few minutes prior to inserting the catheter. This numbs the nasal cavity and opens up the nasal passages for more comfortable insertion. In addition, a small amount of viscous lidocaine can be applied to the tip of the catheter to help ease it through the nasal meatus. These steps are not required, however, because there is very little discomfort with the catheter insertion.

Another method for instilling the barium is to simply drip it through the nares using a large nose dropper or pipette. The patient is placed in a supine position, and the head is hyperextended so that gravity helps to move the barium back to the

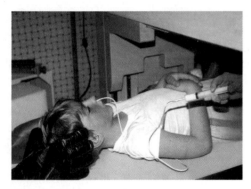

FIGURE 15-5 A method for instilling barium into the nasopharynx is through the use of a large syringe and catheter. The barium is squeezed through the catheter to the nasopharynx.

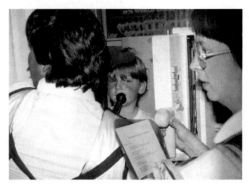

FIGURE 15-6 The X-ray technician asks the patient to repeat syllables and standard sentences. A microphone is placed near the patient's head so that it can record the speech simultaneously with the visual images.

nasopharynx. The patient is asked to sniff the barium, and the head of the patient is rotated to be sure that the soft palate and pharyngeal walls become adequately coated with the contrast material.

Regardless of the method used, approximately 1 to 3 mL of barium are needed in each nostril for adequate coverage. Complete coverage is important because without an adequate and even coating of barium over all the structures, these views may be useless to the examiner.

One big issue with the use of barium is that it causes the eyes to water and gives the sensation of having water in the nose. A mild burning sensation in the nasopharynx also occurs, and this can last for an hour or more following its introduction. Although the barium can cause some discomfort and minor irritation, most children tolerate the procedure fairly well, especially if they are prepared for what to expect. However, if the child cries during this procedure, the secretions can wash the barium down. When that occurs, more barium has to be passed into the nasopharynx for the study.

Speech Sample

During the projection for each view, the patient should first be asked to swallow. With the act of swallowing, the velopharyngeal structures come together forcefully and are easy to identify. This helps the X-ray technologist ensure that the

orientation is correct. It can also be useful when the study is interpreted because it orients the evaluators to the location of the structures. The technologist then asks the patient to repeat syllables or standard sentences. A microphone is placed near the patient's head to record the speech simultaneously with the visual images (**FIGURE 15-6**).

The patient should be asked to repeat a combination of sentences loaded with pressure-sensitive phonemes (see Table 11-3 in the chapter *Speech and Resonance Assessment*), produce a repetition of pressure-sensitive syllables, and count from 60 to 70. Because there is an inherent risk with radiation exposure, the speech sample needs to be long enough to obtain needed information but as short as possible to avoid unnecessary radiation exposure (Isberg, Julin, Kraepelien, & Henrikson, 1989). If the speech sample is carefully chosen, no more than 30 seconds is needed to obtain an adequate speech sample for each view.

Interpretation
Team Interpretation of the Results

A videofluoroscopic speech study can be performed by the X-ray technologist or radiologist. However, the biggest challenge is the analysis and interpretation of the findings. In all cases, the radiologist and the speech-language pathologist must work together to review and interpret the study. The radiologist has a thorough understanding of the anatomy, physiology, and imaging of the velopharyngeal structures. The speech-language pathologist also understands the anatomy and physiology but particularly understands the physiology of speech and the correlation between velopharyngeal function and the acoustic product of speech. With both perspectives, the interpretation of the study is more complete and accurate.

Interpretation of the Lateral View

On the lateral view, the examiner should observe the length, thickness, and contour of the velum both at rest and during phonation. During phonation, the velum should elevate to the approximate level of the hard palate. There should be a bend in the velum at a point that is about two-thirds of the distance from the hard palate to the tip of the uvula. This bend, where there is "knee action," is at the point of insertion of the levator veli palatini muscles and occurs as the levator sling contracts to pull the velum up and back. When the velum makes contact with the posterior pharyngeal wall, the extent of contact between the velar eminence (the high point on the top of the "knee") and the vertical part of the velum should be noted (Kuehn & Henne, 2003). The extent of the contact area gives an indication of the firmness of closure. If the contact area is small, it might be assumed that the closure is tenuous.

On the posterior pharyngeal wall, the presence and approximate size of an adenoid pad should be noted. The adenoid pad usually appears as a smooth, convex structure that is either on the same plane as the hard palate or slightly higher. If there is no adenoid mass, the depth and contour of the pharyngeal wall should be assessed. The examiner should note the relative depth of the pharynx during nasal breathing and any anterior motion of the posterior pharyngeal wall, if this occurs, with speech. When a Passavant's ridge is

present, it can be viewed as a shelf-like projection on the posterior pharyngeal wall, but only during speech. Tonsillar tissue can be seen somewhat on this view. It appears as an oval mass that is superimposed over the area of the posterior tongue. Finally, tongue movement during articulation can be assessed with this view.

Evidence of abnormality may include a short velum relative to the posterior pharyngeal wall, a thin velum, or poor knee action of the velum during speech. **FIGURE 15-7A** and **B** shows a lateral view of patients with a short velum relative to the posterior pharyngeal wall, resulting in velopharyngeal insufficiency. **FIGURE 15-7C** shows a velum with poor movement and little knee action, resulting in velopharyngeal incompetence. An estimate of the size of the velopharyngeal opening as a result of these abnormalities should be made.

On the lateral view, the examiner may also see evidence of a patent oronasal fistula if barium is used. Other abnormalities may include a localized indentation on the posterior pharyngeal wall following the removal of the adenoids. The appearance of hypertrophic tonsils or adenoids that intrude into the airway should be noted.

The movement of the tongue tip, dorsum, the posterior tongue, and even the larynx should be observed to determine whether there are compensatory productions, such as generalized backing of phonemes, glottal stops, pharyngeal plosives, pharyngeal fricatives, or palatal–dorsal productions. In some cases, the patient will use the posterior portion of the tongue to assist in elevating the velum during speech as a compensatory strategy. If this is occurring, then the apparent movement of the velum and the resultant closure is actually very deceptive.

Interpretation of the Frontal View

The purpose of the frontal view is to assess the extent of lateral pharyngeal wall motion and the symmetry of movement between the two sides. When there is normal velopharyngeal function, the point of maximum lateral pharyngeal

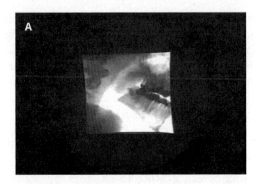

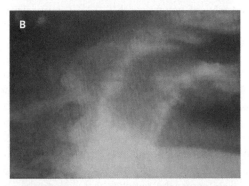

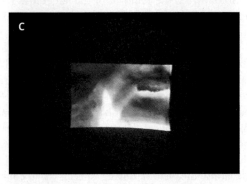

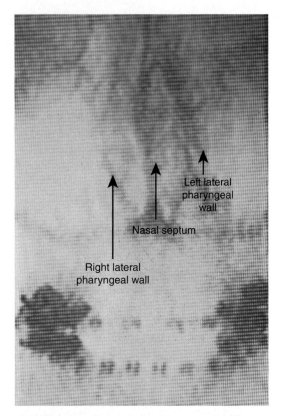

FIGURE 15-8 Frontal view. This view shows the nasal septum in midline. The lateral pharyngeal walls are well coated with barium and bow outward during nasal breathing as noted in the frame.

FIGURE 15-7 Lateral view. **(A)** and **(B)** Short effective length of the velum relative to the posterior pharyngeal wall, which results in velopharyngeal insufficiency. **(C)** Normal velar length, but poor movement during speech, which results in velopharyngeal incompetence.

wall movement is just below the plane of the velar eminence (Skolnick & Cohn, 1989). Interpreting this view is a challenge because of the superimposition of the vomer and facial structures. The examiner should also remember that, because this view goes from the front to the back, the lateral wall on the right side of the screen is on the patient's left side and vice versa. The side of deficiency should be reported based on the patient's right or left rather than on the examiner's orientation. Standard markers can be used on the image to reduce reporting errors concerning the side of the body.

The observation of poor lateral wall movement may suggest a problem with velopharyngeal closure. On the other hand, the patient may merely have a coronal pattern of closure, which requires only minimal lateral wall movement. **FIGURE 15-8** shows the frontal view of a patient. The barium-coated lateral pharyngeal walls can be seen on either side of the septum. When there is a small velopharyngeal opening, bubbling of

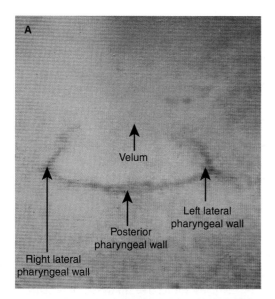

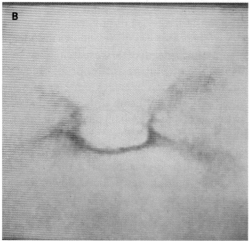

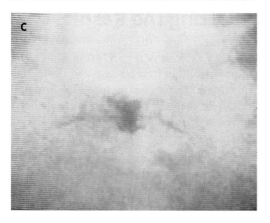

barium is often noted on this view. The examiner should note whether the bubbling is in the midline or seems to be skewed to one side.

In some cases, the lateral pharyngeal walls appear asymmetrical in their position at rest and during speech. Asymmetry with lateral wall movement can suggest a velopharyngeal opening on the side with the lesser amount of movement. Before making this judgment, however, it is important to be sure that the orientation of the view is appropriate and that the head was not turned slightly to give a false impression. If there is true asymmetry, this is important to document because it can affect the surgical management.

Interpretation of the Base View

If the head is positioned properly for the base view so that the beam goes directly through the velopharyngeal port, the margins of the port appear as an oval or round structure during nasal breathing. The lateral and posterior pharyngeal walls can be seen easily with this view if there is an adequate coating of barium and the position is correct. The velum, which appears at the top of the oval, is harder to visualize because it does not pick up as much barium.

During speech, the structures can be observed to narrow and then close the lumen as a sphincter. Depending on the basic pattern of closure, a black horizontal line (with a coronal pattern), a vertical line (with a sagittal pattern), or a circle (with a circular pattern) remain in the middle of the closure area. **FIGURE 15-9A** shows an open nasopharyngeal port through the base view. The port begins to close in **FIGURE 15-9B** and is entirely closed in **FIGURE 15-9C**, leaving a small circle. On

FIGURE 15-9 Base view. The posterior pharyngeal wall is at the bottom of the screen. The velum is at the top but not well visualized because it does not pick up the barium well. **(A)** The entire port is open for nasal breathing. **(B)** The port is partially closed. **(C)** The port is totally closed. This represents a circular pattern of closure.

this view, the examiner should be careful not to confuse movement of the tongue and vocal folds with velopharyngeal movement. In addition, the large foramen magnum can be seen on this view and should not be mistaken for the velopharyngeal port.

When there is velopharyngeal dysfunction, the pharyngeal lumen does not appear to totally close. In fact, an opening during speech is a clear indication of VPI. The examiner should also observe the symmetry of both sides of the port and note asymmetrical movement during speech. As with the frontal view, the left lateral wall is on the right side of the screen and vice versa. With a small velopharyngeal gap, bubbling of barium can often be seen on this view as well.

Interpretation of the Towne's View

Because the Towne's view is similar to the base view (only looking from above), the same observations and cautions apply. Again, the examiner should note that the patient's left lateral wall is seen on the right side of the screen and vice versa.

Interpretation of the Oblique View

The oblique view can be difficult to interpret because of the superimposition of multiple structures over the area of interest. A coating of barium can make interpretation easier, and a swallow prior to the speech sample can help to orient the examiner to the structures of concern. As in the frontal, base, and Towne's views, the patient's right side is seen on the left side of the screen and vice versa.

On the oblique view, the examiner can observe each lateral wall individually. The lateral wall should be viewed at rest and then during speech to determine whether it closes against the velum. A notation should be made if there is an apparent gap between the lateral wall and velum on that side. As with the other views, bubbling of the barium should be noted because it indicates a small velopharyngeal opening (Sell, Mars, & Worrell, 2006).

Overall Results

Based on the information obtained from all views, the examiner must assimilate the information to make a determination of the extent of closure, the approximate gap size, the gap location, and the basic pattern of closure. This information is especially important because it allows the surgeon to design the surgical correction based on the child's specific defect.

Interpretation of the various views typically involves subjective analyses only. Direct measurement is difficult to do because the image on the screen is not life size and depends on a variety of factors. However, measurements are sometimes needed for research purposes. This is done by putting a ruler or an object of a known dimension in each view. For the view that is of interest, the examiner compares a still image of the velopharyngeal valve at rest with an image of the valve during the patient's best attempt at closure. Quantifiable measurements can then be made, using the ruler (or other object) in the view with a known dimension as reference (Williams, Henningsson, & Pegoraro-Krook, 1997).

Reporting the Results

Some centers report the results of videofluoroscopy with a narrative report, using a few short paragraphs. Other centers use a scale to rate various parameters of structure and function as noted on each view. The first published rating scale was developed by McWilliams-Neely and Bradley (1964). Since that time, others have made additions and modifications to this basic scale.

In 1990, the American Cleft Palate–Craniofacial Association assembled a group of clinicians to develop a standardized method for interpreting and reporting the results from videofluoroscopy and nasopharyngoscopy (Golding-Kushner et al., 1990). They developed a procedure that attempts to quantify the movement of the velopharyngeal structures relative to each structure's resting position and the resting position of the opposing structure. This is done as a ratio rather than as an absolute measurement. For example, the resting position of the velum is at the 0.0 point, and the point of closure against the pharyngeal wall is 1.0. If the velum raises and closes 50% of the opening, then velar displacement is at a rating of 0.5 along the trajectory toward the posterior pharyngeal wall. This estimation is done for each lateral wall and for the posterior pharyngeal wall as well. Although some may use this system, it is complicated and inter- and even intra-judge reliability has been an issue. Most importantly, the size of the opening does not usually affect treatment recommendations. Instead, it is the location of the opening and the cause that are most important to determine. Therefore, this rating scale is not widely used.

Regardless of the specific rating scale used or whether a narrative report is done, it is important to be consistent in the observations that are made and in the way they are reported. This is particularly important if preoperative and postoperative studies are done for comparison.

Advantages and Limitations of Videofluoroscopy

The most commonly used methods for direct visualization of the velopharyngeal mechanism are videofluoroscopy and nasopharyngoscopy (Rowe & D'Antonio, 2005). There are differences in opinion as to the best method of assessment in all cases. The examiner should consider what is more important to visualize in each patient's case and the relative benefits and risks of each procedure before determining which type of assessment to use.

Although videofluoroscopy is most commonly used for evaluation of swallowing dysfunction, it is also used for evaluation of velopharyngeal function. For this use, it has the particular advantage of providing a view of the entire length of the posterior pharyngeal wall. It also shows the point at which the velum contacts the pharyngeal wall during speech. With this view, it is easy to determine whether there is velopharyngeal insufficiency caused by a short velum or velopharyngeal incompetence because of poor velar movement. In comparison with nasopharyngoscopy, videofluoroscopy is superior in showing the length of the velum and its upward movement during speech. It also provides a view of the entire length of the posterior pharyngeal wall during closure. As such, it is better than nasopharyngoscopy for looking at the pharynx below the velum during speech (Witt et al., 2000). Videofluoroscopy also allows the examiner to view the movement of the tongue tip and back of the tongue during speech. The fact that the study is recorded (on video or digital images) allows the study to be viewed by multiple team members after completion of the study.

A primary disadvantage of videofluoroscopy is the radiation exposure, even with the new systems that require lower doses. As with any X-ray procedure, there is always a concern about the amount of radiation exposure associated with the test and its potential to cause somatic or genetic damage. Therefore, the aim of pediatric radiology is to keep the radiation dose to the minimum needed to obtain the required diagnostic information. In 1989, it was estimated that for 1 minute of videofluoroscopy in the lateral view, the radiation exposure is between 0.025 rad and 0.5 rad and for the frontal and base views, which require a higher radiation level for adequate resolution, the exposure is from 0.125 rad to 1.00 rad (Skolnick & Cohn, 1989). By way of comparison, a single lateral cephalometric X-ray is about 0.25 rad, and a single CT slice is between 1 and 4 rads. Since that time, digital radiographic techniques have significantly reduced the radiation dose, although very little work has been published on the estimated radiation dose used in such examinations (Zammit-Maempel, Chapple, & Leslie, 2007). This may be partly because the radiation dose varies depending on the patient's size and the thickness of the bones. In general, the radiation dosage for videofluoroscopy is low in comparison with many other types of X-ray procedures (Chan, Chan, & Lam, 2002; Chau & Kung, 2009). However, no amount of radiation is innocuous, and therefore the benefits gained from this procedure must always be weighed against the potential risks.

Another disadvantage of videofluoroscopy is that the overall resolution of a radiographic procedure is not as good as a direct view as with nasopharyngoscopy. In fact, the ability to visualize structures such as the velum and posterior pharyngeal wall depends on these structures being surrounded by air. However, as the velopharyngeal port narrows for closure, the amount of air between the velum and pharyngeal wall is markedly reduced and finally disappears during contact. Therefore, the ability to distinguish the margins of each structure becomes more difficult, if not impossible. As a result, a small gap is usually not seen. The only clue to its presence may be occasional bubbling of the barium. Gaps as a result of irregular adenoids cannot be seen. In addition, as noted previously, the X-ray beam goes through all of the structures in the plane, so the image represents a sum of all the parts. Therefore, if the velum touches the posterior pharyngeal wall at any point in the coronal plane, it will look as if there is complete closure even if the velum does not contact the pharyngeal wall at all points. Also, if the beam is not perfectly perpendicular to the opening, the gap may not be visualized. Finally, because each individual view is only two dimensional, the examiner must essentially extrapolate information from each view to imagine the three-dimensional structure and its function.

Videofluoroscopy is not a good procedure for evaluating the placement and the results of surgical procedures for VPI. It is very difficult to see a pharyngeal flap or sphincter pharyngoplasty with this procedure unless there is a very good coating of barium. In fact, the presence of either could actually be missed altogether. **FIGURE 15-10** is an example of a pharyngeal flap as viewed through videofluoroscopy with a good coating of barium.

Although some professionals consider videofluoroscopy to be less invasive than nasopharyngoscopy, the introduction of barium into the nasopharynx, especially with a catheter, is really no different than inserting a small scope into the nasopharynx. The barium can cause watering of the eyes and also a burning sensation in the nose and pharynx that can persist for an hour or more. With this procedure, the parents have to be separated from the child. Also, the large equipment can also be frightening to young children. Therefore, this procedure is actually not less traumatic for a child than nasopharyngoscopy.

Because of the limitations of videofluoroscopy and the relative advantages of nasopharyngoscopy, this X-ray procedure seems to be used less frequently as a primary means of evaluating velopharyngeal function. Most centers now use nasopharyngoscopy as their primary means of evaluating velopharyngeal function (D'Antonio, Achauer, & Vander Kam, 1993; Kuehn & Henne, 2003; Kummer, Clark, Redle, Thomsen, & Billmire, 2011; Lertsburapa, Schroeder, & Sullivan, 2010).

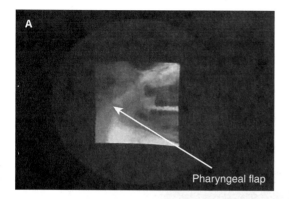
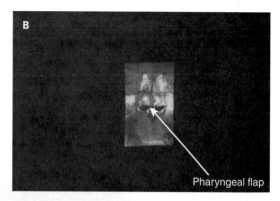

Pharyngeal flap

Pharyngeal flap

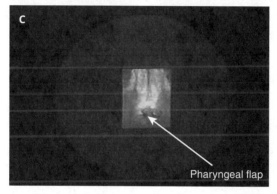

Pharyngeal flap

FIGURE 15-10 Videofluoroscopy of a pharyngeal flap. **(A)** Lateral view that shows the pharyngeal flap as a faint shadow that is low, near the base of the tongue. **(B)** Frontal, or AP (anterior–posterior), view that shows the flap in midline and the lateral ports coated with barium. **(C)** Base view that shows the flap in midline and the open lateral ports on each side.

SUMMARY

Instrumental assessment is not required for the diagnosis of velopharyngeal dysfunction because this can be determined through a perceptual assessment alone. However, videofluoroscopy is a useful procedure for visualizing the structures and function of the velopharyngeal valve. In particular, videofluoroscopy provides a view of the movement and knee action of the velum and its level of contact on the posterior pharyngeal wall. Information obtained from videofluoroscopy is used to determine the best surgical procedure for the patient to correct VPI. Videofluoroscopy can be used to determine the presence of obstruction in the vocal tract, particularly if it involves adenoid or tonsillar hypertrophy. Videofluoroscopy is also a very useful tool for evaluation of swallowing.

Videofluoroscopy is not ideal for evaluating small velopharyngeal openings or the results of surgery for VPI. It also has the disadvantage of exposing the child to radiation, although the dose is very small. In the past few decades, videofluoroscopy is used less as a standard evaluation procedure for individuals who exhibit resonance disorders or characteristics of velopharyngeal dysfunction. This is because most centers now rely more on nasopharyngoscopy.

FOR REVIEW AND DISCUSSION

1. In evaluating an X-ray, what color are the structures, and what color is the air? What causes this difference?

2. What are the current uses for lateral cephalometric X-rays? Why are lateral cephalometric X-rays no longer used for evaluation of velopharyngeal function?

3. Why are multiple videofluoroscopy views necessary for evaluation of velopharyngeal function?

4. What are the typical views used for evaluation of velopharyngeal function? For each

view, describe the structures that can be evaluated.

5. What contrast material is commonly used during a videofluoroscopic evaluation? Which views require this substance to view the structures adequately? How is this substance instilled into the nasopharynx?

6. Describe what the examiner should observe, and note when reviewing each of the views.

7. What are the advantages of videofluoroscopy? What are some of the limitations?

REFERENCES

American Speech-Language-Hearing Association (ASHA). (2004). Knowledge and skills needed by speech-language pathologists performing videofluoroscopic swallowing studies. Retrieved from www.asha.org/policy/KS2004-00076.htm

Argamaso, R. V., Levandowski, G. J., Golding-Kushner, K. J., & Shprintzen, R. J. (1994). Treatment of asymmetric velopharyngeal insufficiency with skewed pharyngeal flap. *The Cleft Palate–Craniofacial Journal, 31*(4), 287–294.

Chan, C. B., Chan, L. K., & Lam, H. S. (2002). Scattered radiation level during videofluoroscopy for swallowing study. *Clinical Radiology, 57*(7), 614–616.

Chau, K. H., & Kung, C. M. (2009). Patient dose during videofluoroscopy swallowing studies in a Hong Kong public hospital. *Dysphagia, 24*(4), 387–390.

Clark, D. E., D'Antonio, L. L., Liu, J. R., & Welch, T. B. (1992). Radiographic demonstration of oronasal fistulas in patients with cleft palate with the use of barium sulfate contrast. *Oral Surgery, Oral Medicine, Oral Pathology, Oral Radiology, and Endodontology, 74*(5), 661–670.

Cohn, E. R., Rood, S. R., McWilliams, B. J., Skolnick, M. L., & Abdelmalek, L. R. (1984). Barium sulphate coating of the nasopharynx in lateral view videofluoroscopy. *Cleft Palate Journal, 21*(1), 7–17.

D'Antonio, L. L., Achauer, B. M., & Vander Kam, V. M. (1993). Results of a survey of cleft palate teams concerning the use of nasendoscopy. *The Cleft Palate–Craniofacial Journal, 30*(1), 35–39.

D'Antonio, L. L., Muntz, H. R., Marsh, J. L., Marty-Grames, L., & Backensto-Marsh, R. (1988). Practical application of flexible fiberoptic nasopharyngoscopy for evaluating velopharyngeal function. *Plastic and Reconstructive Surgery, 82*(4), 611–618.

Dudas, J. R., Deleyiannis, F. W., Ford, M. D., Jiang, S., & Losee, J. E. (2006). Diagnosis and treatment of velopharyngeal insufficiency: Clinical utility of speech evaluation and videofluoroscopy. *Annals of Plastic Surgery, 56*(5), 511–517; discussion 517.

Golding-Kushner, K. J., Argamaso, R. V., Cotton, R. T., Grames, L. M., Henningsson, G., Jones, D. L., . . . Marsh, J. L. (1990). Standardization for the reporting of nasopharyngoscopy and multiview videofluoroscopy: A report from an International Working Group. *Cleft Palate Journal, 27*(4), 337–347; discussion 347–348.

Havstam, C., Lohmander, A., Persson, C., Dotevall, H., Lith, A., & Lilja, J. (2005). Evaluation of VPI-assessment with videofluoroscopy and nasoendoscopy. *British Journal of Plastic Surgery, 58*(7), 922–931.

Isberg, A., Julin, P., Kraepelien, T., & Henrikson, C. O. (1989). Absorbed doses and energy imparted from radiographic examination of velopharyngeal function during speech. *Cleft Palate Journal, 26*(2), 105–109.

Kendall, K. A., Leonard, R. J., & McKenzie, S. (2004). Airway protection: Evaluation with videofluoroscopy. *Dysphagia, 19*(2), 65–70.

Kuehn, D. P., & Henne, L. J. (2003). Speech evaluation and treatment of patients with cleft palate. *American Journal of Speech-Language Pathology, 12,* 103–109.

Kummer, A. W., Clark, S. L., Redle, E. E., Thomsen, L. L., & Billmire, D. A. (2011). Current practice in assessing and reporting speech outcomes of cleft palate and velopharyngeal surgery: A survey of cleft palate/craniofacial professionals. *The Cleft Palate–Craniofacial Journal, 49*(2), 146–152.

Lam, D. J., Starr, J. R., Perkins, J. A., Lewis, C. W., Eblen, L. E., Dunlap, J., & Sie, K. C. (2006). A comparison of nasendoscopy and multiview videofluoroscopy in assessing velopharyngeal insufficiency. *Otolaryngology-Head and Neck Surgery, 134*(3), 394–402.

La Rossa, D., Brown, A., Cohen, M., & Spackman, T. (1980). Videoradiography of the velopharyngeal portal using the Towne's view. *Journal of Maxillofacial Surgery, 8*(3), 203–205.

Lertsburapa, K., Schroeder, J. W., Jr., & Sullivan, C. (2010). Assessment of adenoid size: A comparison of lateral radiographic measurements, radiologist assessment, and nasal endoscopy. *International Journal of Pediatric Otorhinolaryngology, 74*(11), 1281–1285.

Major, M. P., Flores-Mir, C., & Major, P. W. (2006). Assessment of lateral cephalometric diagnosis of adenoid hypertrophy and posterior upper airway obstruction: A systematic review. *America Journal of Orthodontics and Dentofacial Orthopedics, 130*(6), 700–708.

McWilliams-Neely, B. J., & Bradley, D. P. (1964). A rating scale for evaluation of videotape recorded X-ray studies. *Cleft Palate Journal, 1,* 88–94.

Pelo, S., Tassiello, S., Boniello, R., Gasparini, G., & Longobardi, G. (2006). A new method for assessment of craniofacial malformations. *Journal of Craniofacial Surgery, 17*(6), 1035–1039.

Perry, J. L. (2011). Variations in velopharyngeal structures between upright and supine positions using upright magnetic resonance imaging. *The Cleft Palate–Craniofacial Journal, 48*(2), 123–133.

Rowe, M. R., & D'Antonio, L. L. (2005). Velopharyngeal dysfunction: Evolving developments in evaluation. *Current Opinion in Otolaryngology & Head & Neck Surgery, 13*(6), 366–370.

Sell, D., Mars, M., & Worrell, E. (2006). Process and outcome study of multidisciplinary prosthetic treatment for velopharyngeal dysfunction. *International Journal of Language Communication Disorders, 41*(5), 495–511.

Shprintzen, R. J. (1995). Instrumental assessment of velopharyngeal valving. In R. J. Shprintzen & J. Bardach (Eds.), *Cleft palate speech management: A multidisciplinary approach* (vol. 4, pp. 221–256). St. Louis, MO: Mosby.

Shprintzen, R. J., Rakof, S. J., Skolnick, M. L., & Lavorato, A. S. (1977). Incongruous movements of the velum and lateral pharyngeal walls. *Cleft Palate Journal, 14*(2), 148–157.

Skolnick, M. L. (1969). Video velopharyngography in patients with nasal speech, with emphasis on lateral pharyngeal motion in velopharyngeal closure. *Radiology, 93*(4), 747–755.

Skolnick, M. L. (1970). Videofluoroscopic examination of the velopharyngeal portal during phonation in lateral and base projections: A new technique for studying the mechanics of closure. *Cleft Palate Journal, 7,* 803–816.

Skolnick, M. L. (1975). Velopharyngeal function in cleft palate. *Clinics in Plastic Surgery, 2*(2), 285–297.

Skolnick, M. L., & Cohn, E. R. (1989). *Videofluoroscopic studies of speech in patients with cleft palate.* New York: Springer-Verlag.

Skolnick, M. L., Glaser, E. R., & McWilliams, B. J. (1980). The use and limitations of the barium pharyngogram in the detection of velopharyngeal insufficiency. *Radiology, 135*(2), 301–304.

Skolnick, M. L., & McCall, G. N. (1971). Radiological evaluation of velopharyngeal closure. *Journal of the American Medical Association, 218*(1), 96.

Skolnick, M. L., McCall, G. N., & Barnes, M. (1973). The sphincteric mechanism of velopharyngeal closure. *Cleft Palate Journal, 10,* 286–305.

Smith, B. E., & Kuehn, D. P. (2007). Speech evaluation of velopharyngeal dysfunction. *The Journal of Craniofacial Surgery, 18*(2), 251–260.

Stringer, D. A., & Witzel, M. A. (1986). Velopharyngeal insufficiency on videofluoroscopy: Comparison of projections. *American Journal of Roentgenology, 146*(1), 15–19.

Stringer, D. A., & Witzel, M. A. (1989). Comparison of multiview videofluoroscopy and nasopharyngoscopy in the assessment of velopharyngeal insufficiency. *Cleft Palate Journal, 26*(2), 88–92.

Williams, W. N., Henningsson, G., & Pegoraro-Krook, M. I. (1997). Radiographic assessment of velopharyngeal function for speech. In K. R. Bzoch (Ed.), *Communicative disorders related to cleft lip and palate* (vol. 4). Austin, TX: Pro-Ed.

Witt, P. D., Marsh, J. L., McFarland, E. G., & Riski, J. E. (2000). The evolution of velopharyngeal imaging. *Annals of Plastic Surgery, 45*(6), 665–673.

Ysunza, A., Pamplona, M. C., Ortega, J. M., & Prado, H. (2008). Video fluoroscopy for evaluating adenoid hypertrophy in children. *International Journal of Pediatric Otorhinolaryngology, 72*(8), 1159–1165.

Ysunza, A., Pamplona, M. C., Ortega, J. M., & Prado, H. (2011). Videofluoroscopic evaluation of adenoid hypertrophy and velopharyngeal closure during speech. *Gaceta Medica de Mexico, 147*(2), 104–110.

Zammit-Maempel, I., Chapple, C. L., & Leslie, P. (2007). Radiation dose in videofluoroscopic swallow studies. *Dysphagia, 22*(1), 13–15.

CREDITS

CHAPTER 16

Nasopharyngoscopy

CHAPTER OUTLINE

INTRODUCTION

Velopharyngeal insufficiency/incompetence (VPI) can be diagnosed based on the characteristics of speech as determined through a perceptual speech evaluation alone. However, instrumental assessment of the velopharyngeal valve, often done through nasopharyngoscopy, is usually indicated to determine the cause, the approximate size, and particularly the location of the velopharyngeal opening. This information is important to obtain so that the best form of surgical intervention can be determined for the patient.

Nasopharyngoscopy is a minimally invasive endoscopic procedure that allows visual observation and analysis of the velopharyngeal mechanism during speech (D'Antonio, Achauer, & Vander Kam, 1993; D'Antonio, Chait, Lotz, & Netsell, 1986; D'Antonio, Muntz, Marsh, Marty-Grames, & Backensto-Marsh, 1988; Ramamurthy, Wyatt, Whitby, Martin, & Davenport, 1997; Shetty, Frampton, & Patel, 2009; Smith & Kuehn, 2007; Strauss, 2007). Nasopharyngoscopy can help the examiner assess both the anatomic and physiologic abnormalities that are causing VPI so the optimal surgical or prosthetic treatment for the patient can be determined. Nasopharyngoscopy is not only a powerful tool in the evaluation of velopharyngeal function, but it is also commonly used in the evaluation of swallowing, upper airway obstruction, and the structure and function of the larynx and vocal folds.

The purpose of the chapter is to explain how nasopharyngoscopy is used in the evaluation of velopharyngeal function. The specific procedures for a nasopharyngoscopy assessment are reviewed, including methods for preparing a child for the examination and procedures for inserting the endoscope. The interpretation of the observations is discussed as it relates to the diagnosis of VPI and recommendations for treatment.

History of Endoscopy for VPI

By definition, endoscopy is a procedure that allows the visualization of the interior of a canal or hollow organ by means of a special instrument called an endoscope. Physicians have used endoscopy for many years to view anatomic structures and physiological function to make medical or surgical treatment decisions.

Early Endoscopic Procedures

In 1966, Taub described the use of a panendoscope for the assessment of velopharyngeal function. The panendoscope consisted of an optical tube that could be placed in the mouth and then turned upward for visualization of the velopharyngeal sphincter. This early scope had certain distinct disadvantages. Of course, placement of the tube in the mouth interfered with the normal production of speech. However, the optical tube was too big for insertion in the nose. Another problem was that the light bulb generated a dangerous amount of heat in addition to an electrical hazard for the individual. Therefore, use of this scope did not gain wide acceptance.

In 1969, Pigott, Bensen, and White described the use of a rigid endoscope that was slender enough to be inserted through the nose but large enough to allow observation of the velopharyngeal portal at rest and during speech. This endoscope provided a wide-angle view of about 70 degrees, which allowed visualization of most of the port (Pigott & Makepeace, 1982). Despite the large cone of view, this scope could not be maneuvered for additional assessment of the lateral edges of the port or to see farther down into the pharynx or vocal tract. In addition, because the scope was very straight and the diameter of the nasal cavity is not, the rigid scope was very difficult to insert, particularly if the patient had a septal deviation or stenosis of the naris. In addition, the pressure of the scope on the nasal septum and turbinates caused significant pain and was not well tolerated by most patients.

Flexible Fiberoptic Nasopharyngoscope

In the mid-1970s and the 1980s, the use of a flexible fiberoptic nasopharyngoscope began to appear in the literature. The flexible scope is smaller in circumference than the rigid scope.

Although it has a more restricted cone of view, its smaller size makes it much easier to pass transnasally and therefore, it is easier for patients to tolerate. This is particularly advantageous when evaluating young children.

In 1975, a side-viewing flexible endoscope was described by Miyazaki, Matsuya, and Yamaoka. With this design, the scope remained in a horizontal position, and the opening at the side of the scope gave the examiner the same view as with the rigid scope. However, because of the side opening, the scope could not be manipulated easily to provide a view of both the horizontal and vertical aspects of the port.

In the late 1970s and the 1980s, the end-viewing flexible endoscope was described by several authors (Croft, Shprintzen, & Rakoff, 1981; Shprintzen, 1979; Shprintzen et al., 1979). The tip of this scope was flexible, and with the use of a lever, the examiner could turn the tip down to view the velopharyngeal port from various angles. It could even be moved farther down the pharynx for a view of the larynx and the vocal folds. This type of endoscope is what is used today.

Nasopharyngoscopy Overview

Flexible fiberoptic nasopharyngoscopy is a minimally invasive endoscopic procedure that allows visual observation and analysis of the velopharyngeal mechanism or larynx during speech, phonation, or swallowing. Nasopharyngoscopy is now widely used for the clinical evaluation of velopharyngeal function (D'Antonio et al., 1993; Kuehn & Henne, 2003; Kummer, 2016; Perry & Schenck, 2013). Most clinicians feel that nasopharyngoscopy is superior to videofluoroscopy because of the excellent clarity of the view (in living color) and the maneuverability of the scope to see the entire port (Lam et al., 2006; Lertsburapa, Schroeder, & Sullivan, 2010). Most cleft/craniofacial centers in the United States use nasopharyngoscopy primarily or even exclusively over videofluoroscopy for the visual evaluation of

velopharyngeal function (Kummer, Clark, Redle, Thomsen, & Billmire, 2011).

Nasopharyngoscopy is a valuable tool for the evaluation of velopharyngeal function. The examiner can determine whether there is velopharyngeal closure during speech or an abnormal opening. In addition, the examiner can view the nasal surface of the velum and detect abnormalities. The posterior pharyngeal wall can be assessed for enlarged adenoids, a Passavant's ridge, or even a pulsating carotid artery. If the tonsils are enlarged, they can often be seen in the airway through the scope. Overall, nasopharyngoscopy is useful in determining the cause of resonance disorders and helping clinicians determine appropriate treatment.

When there is VPI, the information obtained through nasopharyngoscopy is very valuable for treatment planning. In fact, the observations provide a clear direction for the surgical procedure that is most likely to be successful for the patient (Osberg & Witzel, 1981; Shprintzen et al., 1979). If surgery is not an option, nasopharyngoscopy can help the prosthodontist design and modify an effective speech prosthetic device for the patient (D'Antonio et al., 1988; Hung & Cheng, 1989; Karnell, Rosenstein, & Fine, 1987) (see the chapter *Prosthetic Management* for information about prosthetic devices).

Nasopharyngoscopy is an excellent tool for evaluating the results of VPI surgery (Abdel-Aziz, 2007). If there is residual nasality or evidence of upper airway obstruction, nasopharyngoscopy can help the surgeon determine the cause and therefore the appropriate surgical revision procedure.

Although nasopharyngoscopy is primarily used for diagnostic purposes, it can also be used to provide biofeedback to the patient as part of the evaluation appointment (Brunner, Stellzig-Eisenhauer, Proschel, Verres, & Komposch, 2005; Witzel, Tobe, & Salyer, 1988; Ysunza, Pamplona, Femat, Mayer, & Garcia-Velasco, 1997). It should be noted that biofeedback is useful only when the problem with closure is functional (as in phoneme-specific nasal emission caused by misarticulation). It is not effective if the problem is caused by abnormal structure. (See the chapter *Speech Therapy* for more information about speech therapy).

It should be noted that nasopharyngoscopy for evaluation of velopharyngeal function is sometimes called nasendoscopy or video nasendoscopy. These terms are technically incorrect. The difference between the two procedures depends on the scope's journey and final destination. As such, if the scope is used to evaluate the nasal cavity, including where the sinuses drain, then it is correctly called nasendoscopy, also known as nasal endoscopy. However, if the scope is used to look at the nasopharynx, then it should be called nasopharyngoscopy.

This distinction in terminology may seem trivial, but it is very important from a billing standpoint (HCPro, 2008). The correct billing code for evaluation of the velopharyngeal valve through endoscopy is nasopharyngoscopy, Current Procedural Terminology (CPT) code 92511. When nasopharyngoscopy is done for evaluation of swallowing, it is referred to as the fiberoptic endoscopic evaluation of swallowing (FEES) procedure (Aviv et al., 1998; Bastian, 1991; Bastian, 1993; Bastian, 1998; Donzelli, Brady, Wesling, & Theisen, 2005; Langmore, Schatz, & Olsen, 1988; Leder, Acton, Lisitano, & Murray, 2005; Nacci et al., 2008). The correct code for evaluation of swallowing through nasopharyngoscopy is CPT code 92612.

Equipment

Nasopharyngoscopy equipment includes a flexible fiberoptic endoscope (**FIGURE 16-1**). Endoscopes can be purchased from several manufacturers (e.g., PENTAX Medical, Machida, Olympus, and Storz).

Scopes vary in the size of the distal tip (**FIGURE 16-2**). The smallest scope, often used in pediatrics, has a 2.2 mm diameter, and the largest scope is almost 5 mm in diameter. The 3.5 mm scope is commonly used because this

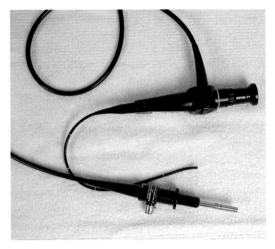

FIGURE 16-1 A flexible fiberoptic nasopharyngoscope. This instrument includes the long tubular endoscope. The body of the instrument, which is held in the examiner's hand, consists of an eyepiece and a control apparatus with a lever or wheel. The control apparatus allows the examiner to move the tip of the scope up and down like a periscope.

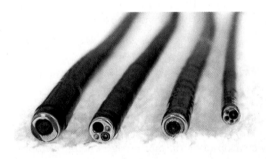

FIGURE 16-2 Nasopharyngoscopes of various sizes. The first scope on the left has a "chip in the tip" camera.

size provides a wide field of vision, yet it is easily tolerated by most individuals, including children. For very young children and infants (when the procedure is done to evaluate swallowing), a smaller scope is preferable.

The distal tip of each endoscope is slightly tapered for easy insertion. The tip is very flexible and can be bent or turned easily without distorting the image. When inspecting the lumen of the

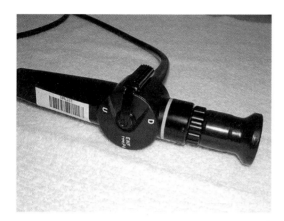

FIGURE 16-3 Eyepiece and control lever for moving the tip of the scope up and down.

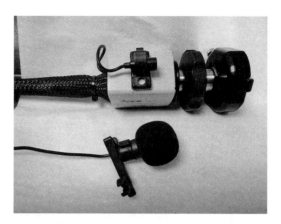

FIGURE 16-4 A very small, lightweight chip camera, which can be attached directly to the eyepiece of a nasopharyngoscope, and an external microphone.

scope, one can see the small lens in the middle for obtaining the image and the fiber bundles that encircle the lens for transmitting light.

The body of the scope, which is held in the examiner's hand, consists of an eyepiece and a control apparatus (**FIGURE 16-3**). The control apparatus contains a lever or wheel that allows the examiner to move the tip of the scope up and down. The scope has a cable that is plugged into a high-intensity light source (typically halogen or xenon) for illumination.

The flexible fiberoptic nasopharyngoscope and light source are the bare necessities for this examination. With this equipment alone, the examiner can perform a nasopharyngoscopy procedure at bedside or almost anywhere by viewing anatomic structures of interest through the endoscope's eyepiece. For standard evaluations in a clinic, however, a complete system, which includes a camera, microphone, video monitor, and recording system, is strongly recommended. In some cases, this may even be required for appropriate documentation and billing.

With the complete system, a specially designed camera is attached to the eyepiece, and an external microphone is used (**FIGURE 16-4**). There are newer "distal chip" endoscopes that come with the camera within the tip of the endoscope. These scopes offer significantly improved resolution compared to the traditional endoscopes so that even fine anatomical features, such as small capillaries, can be seen. However, the traditional fiberoptic scope with a camera mounted to the eyepiece is still far more typical and much less expensive than distal chip scopes.

In addition to the camera, a complete system includes a high-resolution monitor, which provides the examiner with a much better view than the single-person (and single-eye) eyepiece. In addition, the monitor allows others (including the parents and the patient) to see the exam as it is done.

A complete system also includes a high-quality digital video recorder and the use of an external microphone. With recording equipment, the videos can be reviewed frame by frame for in-depth analysis and reviewed later by the surgeon, who may not be present during the examination. The study can be shown to the patient and family to help them understand the problem and proposed treatment. The recordings allow for pre- and postoperative comparisons, which is important in improving outcomes. Videos and still images can be used in PowerPoint presentations for professional education. Finally, a high-quality color printer can also be useful for a hard copy of still pictures and a report of key examination findings. **FIGURE 16-5** shows

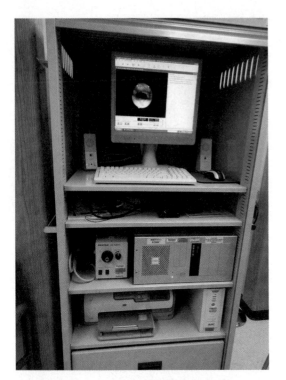

FIGURE 16-5 Complete nasopharyngoscopy system. In addition to the basic equipment, which includes the endoscope, camera, microphone, and cold-light source, a complete system for nasopharyngoscopy includes a computer, a monitor, a keyboard, speakers, video recording equipment, and a printer.

a system with a large high-definition monitor, a halogen cold-light source, and video recording equipment (PENTAX Medical, Montvale, NJ).

Preparation of the Patient

To obtain adequate information about the velopharyngeal valve with nasopharyngoscopy, the child should be able to repeat short sentences without crying. Therefore, the success of the nasopharyngoscopy procedure depends greatly on the child's developmental level and cooperation (Smith & Kuehn, 2007). With proper preparation, children as young as age 3 are generally able to cooperate sufficiently to obtain a useful nasopharyngoscopy examination.

Information Before the Exam Day

In a pediatric setting, preparing the child for what to expect can make the difference between a successful examination and one that is a waste of time, money, and everyone's patience. At Cincinnati Children's, the family receives a coloring book about the procedure a few weeks before the examination (see **APPENDIX 16A**). The coloring book even includes a list of sentences that will be used during the procedure. This helps the child and the parents understand what to expect and allows parents the opportunity to assist in preparing the child. Giving information in advance also reduces preparation time on the day of the examination.

Cooperation tends to improve with age, so obtaining a good examination with adults is usually not a problem. However, even adults can be nervous and apprehensive about the exam. Therefore, giving them information in advance of the examination is also helpful.

Perceptual Evaluation

Just before the nasopharyngoscopy evaluation, the speech-language pathologist should complete a perceptual evaluation. The information derived from the perceptual evaluation helps the examiner to determine what needs to be tested in the nasopharyngoscopy evaluation. For example, if the patient demonstrates nasal emission on sibilants only, the examiner should test these sounds in particular and determine whether, through instruction and biofeedback, closure can be obtained by altering the place of production. On the other hand, if hyponasality or cul-de-sac resonance is noted during the perceptual evaluation, the examiner would use nasal sounds and sentences to assess the source of obstruction.

When doing the perceptual assessment before the nasopharyngoscopy, the speech-language pathologist has an opportunity to develop a rapport with the child and help the child become comfortable within her surroundings (D'Antonio et al., 1986; Lotz, D'Antonio, Chait, & Netsell, 1993). It also provides a chance to practice the speech sample that will be used during the naso-pharyngoscopy procedure.

Infection Control

The examiner should always follow the Standard Precautions for the prevention of the spread of disease (American Speech-Language-Hearing Association [ASHA], n.d.; Centers for Disease Control and Prevention [CDC], 2005; CDC, 2013). This is not only for the protection of the patient but also for the protection of the examiner. Following these guidelines, thorough handwashing should be done as the first step, even before administration of the topical spray. The examiner should then wear gloves for the entire examination. The disinfected endoscope should always be hung or placed on a clean surface when not in use.

Nasal Anesthesia and Decongestion

Although nasopharyngoscopy can be done without topical anesthesia, especially with adults (Frosh, Jayaraj, Porter, & Almeyda, 1998), most clinicians use some form of numbing solution before the procedure. It is also helpful to open up the nasal passages before the examination with a topical decongestant. Before administering a topical anesthetic and/or decongestant, it is best to have the patient blow his nose. Excess secretions can interfere with the topical anesthetic and can also obscure the view of the velopharyngeal valve.

Topical anesthetics are medications that must be ordered by the physician but can be administered by the nurse or the speech-language pathologist. The speech-language pathologist should refer to the ASHA guidelines on the administration of topical anesthetics before beginning this practice (ASHA, 2005).

Several methods for numbing and decongesting the nasal cavity have been reported in the literature. Currently, most centers use a nasal spray to administer a mixture of topical anesthesia and a decongestant (**FIGURE 16-6**). However, the composition of the numbing medicine

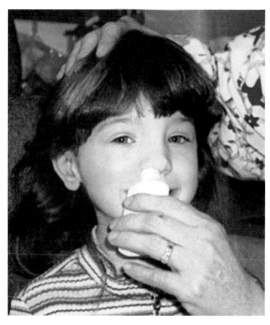

FIGURE 16-6 The use of a spray bottle to administer both the topical anesthesia and decongestant prior to the nasopharyngoscopy procedure.

and decongestant varies by center. Some centers use tetracaine or cophenylcaine (Douglas, Hawke, & Wormald, 2006; Smith & Rockley, 2002), whereas others dispute its benefits (Cain, Murray, & McClymont, 2002; Georgalas, Sandhu, Frosh, & Xenellis, 2005). Some centers use only a nasal decongestant, such as xylometazoline or oxymetazoline (Jonas et al., 2007; Sadek et al., 2001). Other centers recommend the use of water only as a lubricant and argue that a local anesthetic or other lubricant is not necessary (Nankivell & Pothier, 2008; Pothier, Raghava, Monteiro, & Awad, 2006).

At Cincinnati Children's, a one-to-one mixture of oxymetazoline (0.025%) is used to open the nasal passages and tetracaine (1%) for numbing, with a dosage of 0.3 mg/kg tetracaine per puff. Tetracaine is preferred because it also has a vasoconstrictor action, acts quickly, has infrequent side effects, and does not have a noxious odor. Although tetracaine affects the sensation, it does not affect velopharyngeal movement, so it has no negative effect on the study. Overall, this mixture is very effective in achieving the desired numbing while opening up the nasal passages for the scope.

The pharmacy dispenses this mixture in small individual spray bottles that are disposable. Each bottle contains about five or six puffs. Two or three puffs of spray are administered to each nostril so there is adequate coating of the turbinates and the nasal septum. After each nostril is sprayed, the child is asked to close the opposite nostril and then sniff hard to ensure that the solution is well distributed. A wait of only a few minutes is needed before the anesthetic takes effect.

The numbing spray should always be administered with the patient seated upright. If the medication is administered with the child in a reclined position, the spray may enter the hypopharynx and numb the airway, leading to aspiration and coughing episodes. This problem will spontaneously resolve after about 20 minutes, but this should be avoided by keeping the patient upright during administration of the spray (J. Paul Willging, M.D., personal communication, May 12, 2006).

For additional numbing, the sides of the scope are coated with viscous lidocaine (2%) gel or, as described for children, "special slime." (It is important to coat just the sides of the scope and not the viewing end.) This gel also acts as a lubricant for the scope to slide easily through the nose (Pothier, Awad, Whitehouse, & Porter, 2005). Using this technique, the examiner can ensure that the child has received adequate topical anesthesia to complete the procedure in relative comfort.

Explaining the Procedure

Before inserting the scope, the examiner should carefully explain what will be done and what to expect so that there are no surprises. If the patient is a child, it is important to talk on the child's level and to keep the atmosphere as light as possible. For example, the child can be asked whether he ever picks his nose and if he does, whether it hurts. The size of his "nose-picking finger" can then be compared to the size of the end of the scope, which of course is much smaller. You can even tell the child that you will be looking for the biggest boogers with your special "nose picker."

When explaining what to expect, it is important to be honest about what might be felt. For example, the explanation might be as follows:

> You will feel the scope (or my nose picker) in your nose, but because we put the medicine in there, it shouldn't hurt. Instead, you will feel a little pressure, and it may feel a little uncomfortable at first. When the scope is almost where it needs to be, there is a tight spot. As the scope goes through it, it might make you want to sneeze. [In fact, many children do sneeze repeatedly at this point, so it's good to stand clear!] It is very important to hold still, though, because if you move your head, it might make the scope bang around inside of your nose and that might hurt a little. Once the scope is in place, you need to repeat some silly sentences, and we will watch what happens on the monitor. When you finish saying all the sentences, we can take the scope out of your nose, and you are done.

Promising a reward at the end of the procedure can also provide some motivation for cooperation.

At times, children delay the procedure out of fear. If the child has further questions on what to expect, they should be answered. However, an extended delay is counterproductive and just increases the fear. The examiner should be mindful of this and be firm about doing the exam to complete it. If necessary, it is helpful to have someone else, perhaps a nurse, hold the child's head while the scope is inserted. Even the most apprehensive children who cry prior to the procedure are usually fine and very cooperative once the scope is in place.

When working with young children, nasopharyngoscopy often takes time and patience. If the child is prepared in advance and the examiner commits to spending whatever time is necessary, an adequate nasopharyngoscopy study can be obtained for children, even those as young as 3 years of age.

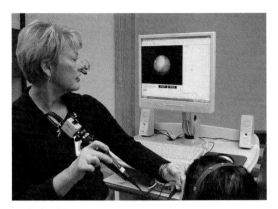

FIGURE 16-7 The nasopharyngoscopy procedure with the patient positioned to see the monitor.

Positioning the Patient

For best results in inserting the scope, the patient should be seated upright in a chair in front of the examiner. A young child should be seated on the parent's lap. The parent is then instructed to "hug" the child around the arms and hold the child's hands. This prevents the child from grabbing the scope during the procedure. It is also helpful to have another person gently hold the child's head to be sure that it does not move erratically during the exam. At times, it may be necessary for the parent to wrap her legs around the child's legs to keep the child from kicking. Older patients often want to be positioned so they can watch the procedure on the monitor (**FIGURE 16-7**).

Nasopharyngoscopy Procedure

With knowledge of the anatomy of the nose and a period of practice, the nasopharyngoscopy procedure is not difficult to perform. Tips on achieving a successful nasopharyngoscopy examination are described in the following sections.

Passing the Scope

Passing the scope for a nasopharyngoscopy procedure can be done by a physician (e.g., an otolaryngologist or plastic surgeon) or by a speech-language pathologist who has been trained in this procedure. Adequate training and experience are important so the procedure can be performed with good results and without causing undue discomfort for the patient.

Training for this procedure is usually not available (or even practical to provide) in a typical university setting. Instead, speech-language pathologists who are interested in passing the scope for nasopharyngoscopy evaluations (whether to evaluate velopharyngeal function, swallowing, or voice) should first review relevant documents on the ASHA website (2004a; 2004b). Clinical skills can then be obtained by attending specific focused courses, mentoring with an experienced professional, or reviewing videotapes of previous exams or by direct supervised experience. Although published in 1994, the book by Karnell titled *Videoendoscopy: From Velopharynx to Larynx* still provides useful information about this procedure.

Before inserting the scope, the examiner should check the camera to be sure the image is in focus. This can be done by placing the scope just above something in print and making adjustments to the focus as needed. The camera may also have to be turned slightly to be sure the image is upright. Some cameras require light balancing.

The examiner should try to determine the more patent side of the patient's nose for passage of the scope. This can be done by asking the child which side is better for breathing or by putting the scope at the entrance of each nostril to view each passageway. Another way is to have the patient close one nostril at a time and then inspire deeply through the other. The nostril with the higher pitch during inspiration is usually the one with the smaller passageway (Shprintzen, 1996). If one side is tried and there is resistance, the examiner should try the other side. When there is a unilateral cleft, usually the affected side is the more patent.

The best way to hold the scope is to place the camera end in one hand (usually the dominant hand) with the control lever on top for manipulation with the index finger. The thumb and fingers of the other hand should grasp the insertion end of the scope and gently pass it into the mid-section of the nostril (**FIGURE 16-8**). The examiner can rest her hand against the patient's nose or forehead for maximum control during insertion.

It is important to guide the scope into the correct nasal meatus for the comfort of the child and for the best view for the exam. The superior nasal meatus is too narrow for comfortable passage of the scope. The inferior nasal meatus (which is on the floor of the nose) is the largest opening and therefore the easiest for passage of the scope. The inferior meatus is often used to view an oronasal fistula from the nasal surface of the hard palate. It is also used when evaluating swallowing because the examiner is primarily interested in viewing residue after the swallow when the velum is back down. However, passing the scope through the inferior meatus does not provide an adequate view of velopharyngeal function. In fact, when the scope reaches the port, it will be directly on top of the velum and therefore the velopharyngeal valve cannot be viewed from above. In addition, the scope will bounce up and down with velar movement during speech, thus obscuring the examiner's view. Because of these issues, the middle meatus is used for evaluation of velopharyngeal function. The middle meatus is large enough for the scope to fit through easily,

and because of its position, it allows an unobstructed view of the port from above. To pass the scope through the middle meatus, it is guided up and over the inferior turbinate (**FIGURE 16-9**).

While passing the scope, the patient will feel pressure but should not feel pain. However, a deviated septum, narrow or stenotic nasal passage, choanal atresia, or even bone spurs can make passage of the scope uncomfortable for the patient and difficult for the examiner. If contact of the scope occurs, it will be felt by the examiner as resistance and by the patient as pressure or mild pain. The examiner can avoid contact with the scope by carefully observing its passage through the meatus and adjusting the position of the scope accordingly. It is always a good idea to tell the patient to let you know whether it hurts or is especially uncomfortable so that appropriate adjustments can be made in the position of the scope. The area that is the narrowest part of the canal and therefore the most sensitive is the back of the nose, just in front of the choana. As the scope passes through this area, it may cause the child's eyes to water and may even elicit a few sneezes. Once the scope goes through the choana, however, the area opens up, and there is less discomfort for the patient.

Once the scope is passed through the choana, the end of the scope should be turned down with the control apparatus (lever or wheel) on the scope. If the scope is not perpendicular to the port, there can be a significant error in

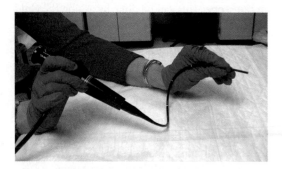

FIGURE 16-8 The best way to hold the scope is to place the viewing end in one hand (usually the dominant hand) with the tip control lever on top for manipulation with either the thumb or the index finger. The thumb and fingers of the other hand should grasp the insertion end of the scope and gently pass it into the nostril.

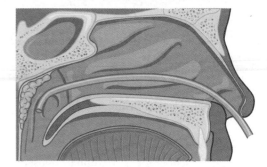

FIGURE 16-9 The scope is guided into the middle nasal meatus and then back to the nasopharynx, where it is tipped down to view the velum.

interpretation (Henningsson & Isberg, 1991). The examiner should also be careful not to place the scope too far down so that it is below the area of closure. This would give the false impression of a large velopharyngeal opening, when the true closure is occurring above the level of view.

To be sure that the scope is in good position, it is helpful to have the child swallow and then repeat some oral syllables. With both activities, the examiner should be able to view the velum moving at the bottom of the screen. If the velum is on one of the sides, the camera needs to be turned slightly until the velum is seen at the bottom of the screen.

Even when the scope is in good vertical position, the entire port is usually not seen at one time, particularly if the scope is a smaller diameter. To examine the entire area, the hand holding the scope should be rotated slightly from one side to the other. By moving the lever of the scope up and down and turning the scope from side to side, the examiner can view all areas of the velopharyngeal port, including the lateral pharyngeal walls, from just one side. It is important to remember that because the patient is facing the examiner, the left side of the screen will show the patient's right lateral pharyngeal wall and vice versa.

Sometimes, during insertion of the scope or during the examination, the field of view will become opaque or totally unclear. A totally white appearance indicates that the light is bouncing off a close object. To eliminate this whiteout effect, the examiner should withdraw the scope slightly and then reposition it before advancing farther. A foggy scope indicates that it is covered by secretions. When this occurs, the examiner should ask the child to sniff hard and then swallow several times. If that does not clear the scope, the examiner can push the scope to touch the pharyngeal wall, which usually clears the scope immediately. If the scope is still foggy, despite several attempts to clear it, it will be necessary to remove it, wipe the end with rubbing alcohol, and then try again. For copious secretions in the nasopharynx that interfere with the view of the velopharyngeal port, suctioning the nose (if available in the clinic) may be necessary to eliminate the secretions that obstruct the view. Suctioning can be done with

the scope in place by putting the suction catheter in the same or opposite naris but along the floor of the nose (inferior meatus).

Once the velopharyngeal valve has been adequately assessed, the scope can be passed down the pharynx to observe the vocal cords. The individual is asked to prolong an /i/ as long as possible so that vocal fold movement can be observed. Some children have difficulty with the concept of prolonging the sound. When this occurs, the speech-language pathologist can help by producing the sound simultaneously with the child in a contest to see who can hold it longer.

Management of Crying

Although there may be some minor discomfort with the nasopharyngoscopy procedure, particularly as the scope goes through the choana, it should not be painful. Once the scope is in place (which takes only a few seconds), there should be minor discomfort at most. Therefore, most children tolerate this procedure very well, especially if they are adequately prepared (**FIGURE 16-10**).

Despite preparation and nasal cavity numbing, it is not uncommon for a young child to still be fearful and therefore cry before and during the examination. Because crying affects the function of the velopharyngeal valve, it is important to get the child to repeat the speech sample without crying. There are several methods to stop the crying.

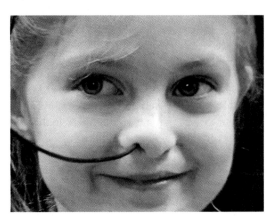

FIGURE 16-10 The scope in place in a patient who obviously has no discomfort.

One thing that exacerbates the crying is when all the adults in the room try to talk to the child at once to encourage the child to cooperate. When this occurs, everyone ends up yelling over each other, which has the opposite effect of the one intended. To prevent this, it is best to tell everyone in the room, including the parents, to be quiet during the examination so the speech-language pathologist is the only person talking to the child. Then, it is important to talk softly and calmly to the child. In a firm, yet gentle way, the child should be told that he must stop crying and say the words so that the scope can be taken out.

There are a few other techniques that can be used to stop the crying and increase cooperation. One technique is to get the child to open her eyes. Because children close their eyes when they are crying, getting the child to open her eyes to look at you usually stops or reduces the crying. Having a stuffed animal, a puppet, or a picture in front of the child can help to get the eyes open and distract the child. Finally, a bottle of bubbles can be useful in distracting the child. If the child agrees to blow some bubbles while the scope is in place, the act of blowing will stop the crying.

Speech Sample

The speech sample for a nasopharyngoscopy examination should include a combination of repeated syllables, sentences loaded with pressure-sensitive phonemes, and counting (see Table 11-3 in the *Speech and Resonance Assessment* chapter). As noted previously, the speech-language pathologist should determine the specific speech sounds for focus based on the results of the perceptual evaluation. When a small or inconsistent velopharyngeal opening is suspected, it is important to particularly tax the velopharyngeal valve by asking the child to speak rapidly so that the velopharyngeal opening can be found. Unlike videofluoroscopy, there is no inherent danger to the individual with this procedure; therefore, there is no need to restrict the length of time spent eliciting speech, unless the patient's cooperation is limited.

If hyponasality or upper airway obstruction is a concern, the examiner should assess the patency of the velopharyngeal port during nasal breathing,

forced nasal inspiration, and the production of nasal sounds. The child should be asked to repeat sentences with nasal phonemes, count from 90 to 100, repeat nasal syllables (e.g., /ma, ma, ma/; / mi, mi, mi/; /na, na, na/; /ni, ni, ni/) and then prolong an /m/ as long as possible. During all of these activities, the opening of the pharyngeal port should be assessed. If a pharyngeal flap or sphincter pharyngoplasty is in place, the patency of the port(s) should be carefully examined during nasal breathing and production of nasal sounds. This is done by placing the scope directly above the port.

Occasionally, a child will continue to cry or refuse to talk with the scope in the nose. In these cases, "desperate measures" are needed. For testing velopharyngeal function, sentences like "Stop sticking this scope in my nose!" or "Take this scope out of my nose" may be used. If nasal phonemes are needed, the child can repeat "No, no, no!" or "Not now, not now!"

Potential Complications

Complications with nasopharyngoscopy occur very rarely. However, it is possible for the patient to experience a vasovagal event, causing fainting. Fainting is usually the result of anxiety and can be avoided by watching the patient carefully and giving a great deal of reassurance as needed. The fainting response is not limited to the patient. The parent may actually be the one to faint!

If the patient (or parent) appears ashen, the procedure should be terminated immediately. The individual should be placed in a reclined position with the head lower than the legs or in a sitting position with the head below the knees.

Another rare complication is epistaxis, which is a nosebleed. Even when this occurs, the bleeding is usually slight and resolves quickly. A nasal decongestant can help stop the bleeding because it acts as a vasoconstrictor. However, with a little pressure, the bleeding stops on its own in most cases (J. Paul Willging, M.D., personal communication, May 12, 2006). Although the risk of medical complication is very slight, nasopharyngoscopy should be always performed in a setting where medical support is available.

Interpretation

The biggest challenge in nasopharyngoscopy is the analysis and interpretation of the findings and the formulation of appropriate recommendations. The recommendations are not always obvious or clear cut. Therefore, it is preferable to use a team approach when analyzing the results and determining the best treatment for the patient (D'Antonio et al., 1986; Willging, 2003).

Team Interpretation of the Results

The most appropriate team for nasopharyngoscopy evaluations is a speech-language pathologist and a VPI surgeon (e.g., pediatric otolaryngologist or plastic surgeon). Because speech and resonance (and of course phonation) are highly dependent on the structures of the vocal tract, it is always helpful to have an otolaryngologist as part of the team, particularly in cases of noncleft VPI. It makes no difference which professional passes the scope as long as both professionals take part in the interpretation of the results and formulation of the recommendations.

In the team assessment, each professional brings a different perspective to the evaluation. The speech-language pathologist evaluates the velopharyngeal structures and function as they relate to the acoustic characteristics of speech and resonance. The speech-language pathologist can also determine whether the velopharyngeal opening is caused by abnormal structure (requiring surgical correction) or abnormal function (requiring speech therapy). The surgeon assesses structural abnormalities of the nasal cavity, oral cavity, pharynx, and velopharyngeal valve. The surgeon can also determine the appropriate medical or surgical approaches to treatment for any abnormalities that are found.

The nasopharyngoscopy assessment is most valuable when it is viewed by both professionals simultaneously and when there is immediate discussion about findings and recommendations. This way, a separate referral and evaluation are often avoided, and recommendations for treatment can be made on the spot.

Clinical Observations

Nasopharyngoscopy provides a view of the entire velopharyngeal valve from above (**FIGURE 16-11**). As such, the examiner can evaluate the integrity of the velopharyngeal structures, their movement during speech production, and whether the velopharyngeal valve closes completely when appropriate. If there is VPI, the examiner can determine the relative size of the opening, the location, and the probable cause. Finally, the examiner can identify other abnormalities of the pharynx that may affect resonance and upper airway patency. Specific observations that the examiner should make during a nasopharyngoscopy examination are described as follows.

Velopharyngeal Closure

The adequacy of velopharyngeal closure should be assessed during connected speech. If there is a velopharyngeal opening, it is important to determine the relative size (e.g., pinhole, small, medium, large, very large), shape (e.g., circular, sagittal, coronal, bowtie), and location (e.g., midline, right corner, left corner) of the opening. When reporting location, it is important to keep in mind that the left side of the screen is the individual's right side and vice versa. Observations of the size, shape, and location of the opening are important in determining the surgical procedure that will have the best outcome in correcting VPI for the patient (Shprintzen et al., 1979). **FIGURE 16-12** shows velopharyngeal openings of different sizes, shapes, and locations. For a simple checklist of observations that should be made through nasopharyngoscopy, see **APPENDIX 16B**.

A very small opening may not be directly seen through nasopharyngoscopy. However, a small opening can be identified by bubbling of secretions (Figure 16-12A). Bubbling of secretions occurs when air is forced through a small velopharyngeal opening. The small size of the opening increases the pressure of the airflow. As the air is released on the top of the valve, the pressure causes the bubbling of secretions. This bubbling is often loud and is perceived as a nasal rustle (Kummer, Curtis, Wiggs, Lee, & Strife, 1992).

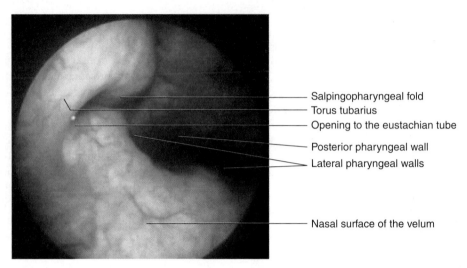

Salpingopharyngeal fold
Torus tubarius
Opening to the eustachian tube

Posterior pharyngeal wall
Lateral pharyngeal walls

Nasal surface of the velum

FIGURE 16-11 A nasopharyngoscopy view of normal velopharyngeal structures. The nasal surface of the velum is always at the bottom of the screen, and the posterior pharyngeal wall is always at the top of the screen. The opening to the eustachian tube can be seen on the left side of the photo.

Again, the location of the opening is important to document for surgical correction.

When there is velopharyngeal dysfunction for any reason, it is fairly common for the opening to occur inconsistently and/or for the size of the opening to vary. For example, with mild VPI, there may be complete closure or just a small opening with single sounds or short utterances or with effort. However, the opening may occur more consistently or be much larger with longer utterances, a faster rate, prolonged speaking, or fatigue. As such, the individual may be able to achieve better closure in certain circumstances but not be able to maintain it all day.

Inconsistent closure can also occur because of apraxia of speech or misarticulations. Children with apraxia of speech often have difficulty coordinating velopharyngeal movement with oral articulation movement. As a result, they may demonstrate complete velopharyngeal closure on single words or short utterances but inconsistent velopharyngeal closure with longer utterances. Finally, a velopharyngeal opening may occur only on certain speech sounds because of an articulation placement error. For example, if a sibilant sound is incorrectly substituted by a pharyngeal fricative, the velopharyngeal valve will open during

production of that sound, resulting in phoneme-specific nasal air emission (Peterson-Falzone, 1985; Peterson-Falzone & Graham, 1990).

Because of the inconsistency in closure, the examiner may not immediately see the velopharyngeal opening during the nasopharyngoscopy examination. If that occurs, the examiner should attempt to tax the velopharyngeal valve as much as possible with long utterances and a fast rate until the opening that is heard through the perceptual evaluation can be found. This can be done by asking the patient to count from 60 to 70 or repeat syllables and sentences rapidly.

Nasal Surface of the Velum

In addition to viewing the velopharyngeal port, the examiner should view the nasal surface of the velum. If the patient had a cleft palate repair, the examiner should be sure that the palate is intact. In some cases, there is an indentation in the posterior border of the velum, which can cause a gap during speech. If the patient has no history of cleft, the velum should be inspected for signs of a submucous cleft palate (**FIGURE 16-13**). This might include hypoplastic musculus uvulae muscles, which appear as flattening or concavity

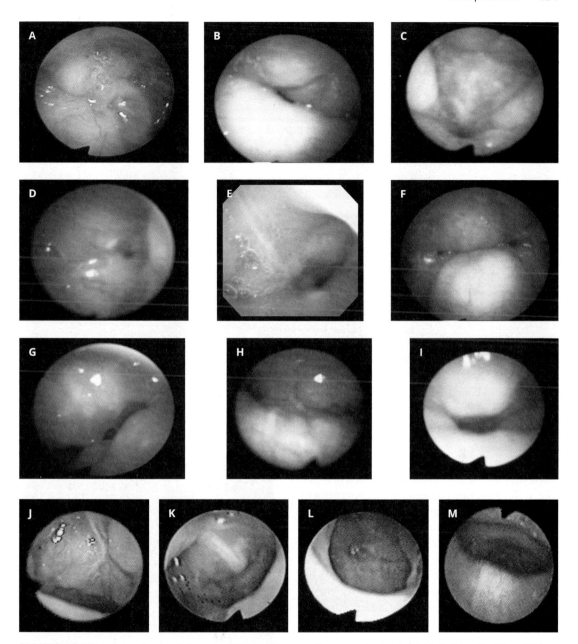

FIGURE 16-12 Various sizes and shapes of VPI. **(A)** Very small gap on the (patient's) left side of midline. (This is on the right side of the figure.) This is noted by the bubbling in that area during speech. **(B)** Small central gap with a coronal pattern of closure. **(C)** Small central gap with a circular pattern of closure. **(D)** Small opening to the (patient's) left of midline. **(E)** Larger opening to the (patient's) left of midline. **(F)** Bowtie closure with closure in the midline, but small openings on both sides. **(G)** Narrow coronal opening with touch closure in midline. **(H)** Bowtie closure with medium-sized openings on both sides. **(I)** Midsized opening with a circular pattern of closure. **(J)** Midsized coronal opening. **(K)** Large velopharyngeal opening caused by a short velum. **(L)** and **(M)** Very large velopharyngeal opening.

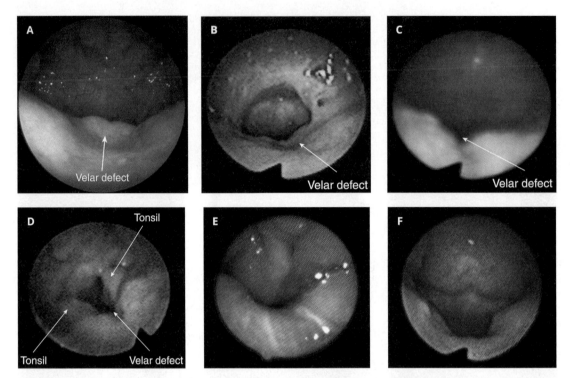

FIGURE 16-13 Examples of submucous clefts as seen on the nasal surface of the velum through nasopharyngoscopy. Note that in all cases, there is a notch in the midline and a depression on the end of the velum where there should be a bulge from the musculus uvulae muscles. Note in (D), large tonsils are intruding into the oropharynx.

in the area where there should be a convex shape. There may also be a depression or a notch in midline at the posterior border of the velum, which usually causes a velopharyngeal opening in midline (Gosain, Conley, Marks, & Larson, 1996; Lewin, Croft, & Shprintzen, 1980; Shprintzen, 1995; Shprintzen, 1996; Shprintzen & Golding-Kushner, 1989). If there is an oronasal fistula in the hard palate, it can be seen through the endoscope if it is passed through the inferior meatus (**FIGURE 16-14**).

Lateral Pharyngeal Walls

The degree of lateral pharyngeal wall movement should be observed. If there is asymmetry of lateral pharyngeal wall movement, it should be reported because it has implications for surgical correction. The relative contribution of all of these structures to

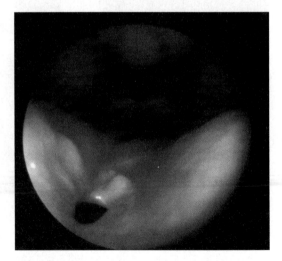

FIGURE 16-14 View of an oronasal fistula in the hard palate as seen through nasopharyngoscopy by going through the inferior meatus.

closure should be assessed. Based on these observations, the basic closure pattern (coronal, circular, or sagittal) can be determined (Croft et al., 1981; Finkelstein, Lerner, et al., 1993; Igawa, Nishizawa, Sugihara, & Inuyama, 1998; Shprintzen, Rakof, Skolnick, & Lavorato, 1977; Siegel-Sadewitz & Shprintzen, 1982; Skolnick, Shprintzen, McCall, & Rakoff, 1975; Witzel & Posnick, 1989).

Posterior Pharyngeal Wall and Adenoids

Although the posterior pharyngeal wall is relatively passive during velopharyngeal closure, it is still important to inspect during the nasopharyngoscopy examination. In particular, the examiner should view the adenoid pad and its effect on closure. The examiner may also note a Passavant's ridge or a medially displaced carotid artery.

The adenoid pad should be inspected for its size, surface, and location (Lertsburapa et al., 2010). The adenoid tissue may be large and

blocking the nasopharynx, the opening of the choana (see Figure 5-18 in the chapter *Facial, Oral, and Pharyngeal Anomalies*), or the opening to one or both eustachian tubes. It may also have an irregular surface with protrusions or fissures that prohibit the velum from achieving a tight veloadenoidal seal (Finkelstein, Berger, Nachmani, & Ophir, 1996; Gereau & Shprintzen, 1988; Siegel-Sadewitz & Shprintzen, 1986; Williams, Preece, Rhys, & Eccles, 1992) (**FIGURE 16-15**). In addition to the adenoids, the examiner should note other findings on the pharyngeal wall, such as the scar band as seen in **FIGURE 16-16**.

If the patient has a Passavant's ridge, it can sometimes be seen with nasopharyngoscopy but typically only if there is a large velopharyngeal opening (**FIGURE 16-17**). This is because a Passavant's ridge occurs only during phonation and it is usually located below the area of velopharyngeal closure (Finkelstein et al., 1991; Finkelstein, Lerner, et al., 1993; Witzel & Posnick, 1989).

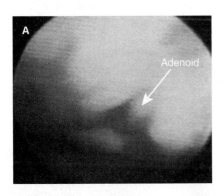
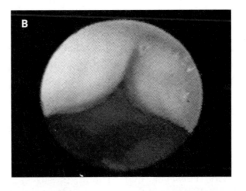
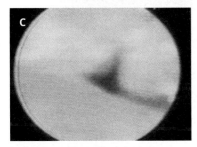
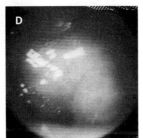
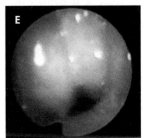

FIGURE 16-15 Irregular adenoids, as can be seen at the top of each view. **(A)** and **(B)** A notch in the adenoid pad, which will interfere with a tight velopharyngeal seal. **(C)–(E)** A small velopharyngeal opening during veloadenoidal closure as a result of the adenoid irregularity.

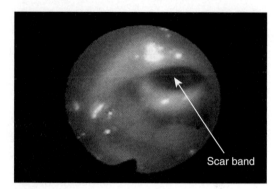

FIGURE 16-16 Scar band on the pharyngeal wall (at the top of the screen) that occurred following a tonsillectomy. The patient was prone to keloids.

Medial displacement of one or both of the carotid arteries is commonly seen in patients with velocardiofacial/22q11.2 deletion syndrome (VCFS/22q deletion syndrome) (D'Antonio & Marsh, 1987; Finkelstein, Zohar, et al., 1993; MacKenzie-Stepner, Witzel, Stringer, Lindsay, et al., 1987; Ross, Witzel, Armstrong, & Thomson, 1996; Witt, Miller, Marsh, Muntz, & Grames, 1998). This can be seen as pulsations on the posterior pharyngeal wall, especially during quiet breathing (**FIGURE 16-18**). It is important to look for pulsations on the pharyngeal wall with all patients diagnosed with VCFS/22q deletion syndrome but also in other patients with VPI of unknown etiology.

Tonsils

The tonsils sit between the faucial pillars in the oral cavity. However, hypertrophic tonsils can become so large that they push past the posterior faucial pillars and intrude into the pharynx. This can be seen through nasopharyngoscopy (**FIGURE 16-19A** and **B**). Large tonsils can cause both functional and mechanical interference with lateral pharyngeal wall movement (Finkelstein, Nachmani, & Ophir, 1994; Henningsson & Isberg, 1988; Kummer, Billmire, & Myer, 1993; MacKenzie-Stepner, Witzel, Stringer, & Laskin, 1987). In rare cases, the tonsils can become so large that they extend up to the area between the velum and posterior pharyngeal wall, thus

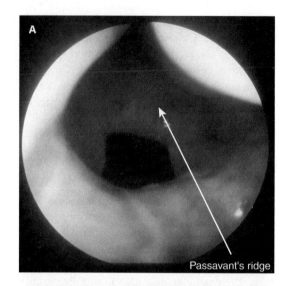

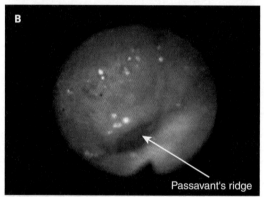

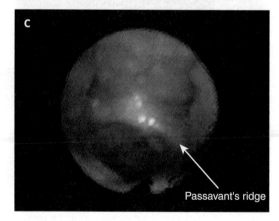

FIGURE 16-17 Passavant's ridge as seen from above through nasopharyngoscopy.

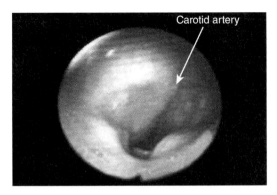

FIGURE 16-18 View of a medially displaced carotid artery on the left of the picture, which is commonly seen in patients with velocardiofacial/22q11.2 deletion syndrome.

interfering with velopharyngeal closure (see Figure 10-18B and C in the chapter *Speech/Resonance Disorders and Velopharyngeal Dysfunction*). Whenever hypertrophic tonsils are seen in the pharynx through nasopharyngoscopy, the examiner should consider their effect on velopharyngeal function and also on the airway. Nasopharyngoscopy can also identify hypertrophy of the lingual tonsils (**FIGURE 16-19C**). Tonsillectomy is usually indicated for tonsillar hypertrophy that causes interference of velopharyngeal function or airway obstruction.

Larynx and Vocal Folds

In addition to viewing the velopharyngeal structures, nasopharyngoscopy allows the examiner to view the larynx and vocal folds (Karnell, 1994; Karnell & Langmore, 1998). Because laryngeal abnormalities are often found in individuals with craniofacial anomalies and there is a high incidence of vocal nodules in individuals with velopharyngeal insufficiency, an examination of the vocal folds is often done as part of the nasopharyngoscopy exam (D'Antonio et al., 1988; Lewis, Andreassen, Leeper, Macrae, & Thomas, 1993; Zajac & Linville, 1989). By viewing the vocal folds, the examiner can determine whether there are vocal nodules (**FIGURE 16-20**), a

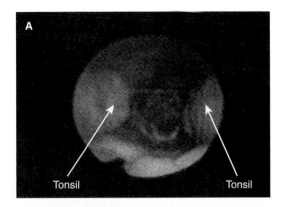

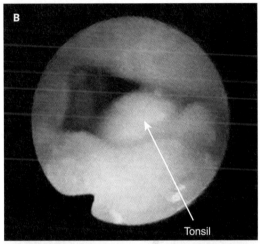

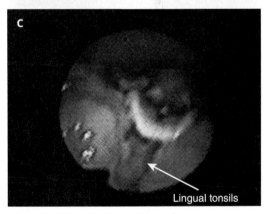

FIGURE 16-19 Tonsillar hypertrophy. **(A)** Note both tonsils in the oropharynx as seen from above through nasopharyngoscopy. **(B)** Note that the patient's left tonsil (on the right side of the view) is in the airway. **(C)** Note large lingual tonsils.

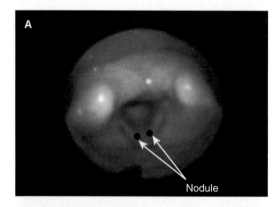

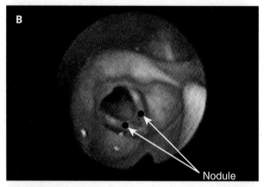

FIGURE 16-20 Bilateral vocal fold nodules.

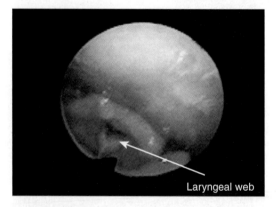

FIGURE 16-21 A laryngeal web in a patient with velocardiofacial/22q11.2 deletion syndrome.

laryngeal web (**FIGURE 16-21**), or thickening or edema of the folds. Any other anomalies of the vocal folds or their movement should also be noted.

Results of VPI Surgery

Nasopharyngoscopy is an excellent procedure for a postoperative assessment of surgery for VPI, such as a pharyngeal flap, a sphincter pharyngoplasty, or pharyngeal augmentation (see the chapter *Surgical Management* for details regarding each type of surgery) (Abdel-Aziz, 2007). This is usually done only if there is persistent hypernasality or nasal emission, despite the surgical procedure. Nasopharyngoscopy helps to determine the location and cause of the remaining velopharyngeal leak, which is important for planning surgical revision. **FIGURE 16-22** shows sphincter pharyngoplasties that fail to close during speech and therefore require revision. **FIGURE 16-23A–F** shows pharyngeal flaps. Figures 16-23A and B show pharyngeal flaps that function normally for both nasal breathing and speech. Figures 16-23C–F show pharyngeal flaps that require revision.

It should be kept in mind when performing nasopharyngoscopy that if the patient is still using compensatory productions (e.g., pharyngeal fricatives and glottal stops), there will still be an opening on these sounds because they are produced in the pharynx. In addition to evaluating velopharyngeal function for speech, nasopharyngoscopy is helpful in the assessment of the nasopharyngeal airway in patients with postoperative airway obstruction. If a port is too narrow for nasal breathing or production of nasal sounds, it should be reported.

Reporting the Results

As with videofluoroscopic speech studies, some centers report nasopharyngoscopy results with a narrative report. Several authors have suggested using either a numeric scale or a particular form to rate various parameters of structure and function (D'Antonio, Marsh, Province, Muntz, & Phillips, 1989; D'Antonio et al., 1988; Karnell, Ibuki, Morris, & Van Demark, 1983; Sinclair, Davies, & Bracka, 1982; Zwitman, Sonderman, & Ward, 1974). See Appendix 16B for

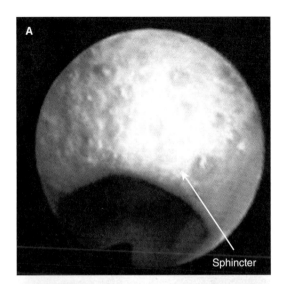

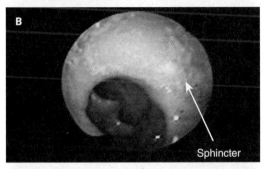

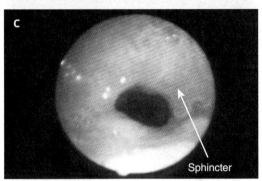

FIGURE 16-22 Sphincter pharyngoplasty.
(A) This shows a sphincter pharyngoplasty during speech with maximum closure. A large gap remains in midline despite the presence of the sphincter.
(B) This sphincter is too low (note the epiglottis below) and caused sleep apnea, yet it does not close the port during speech. **(C)** Sphincter that leaves a large midline opening during speech.

an example of a nasopharyngoscopy examination form.

As noted in the chapter on videofluoroscopy, a multidisciplinary group of clinicians was assembled in 1990 by the American Cleft Palate–Craniofacial Association to address the question of standardizing reporting techniques for multiview videofluoroscopy and nasopharyngoscopy (Golding-Kushner et al., 1990). As with videofluoroscopy, the proposed system was to rate the movement of the velum, the posterior pharyngeal wall, and each lateral wall in relation to the structure that it is moving toward. The resting position of the structure is rated as 0.0, and the resting position of the opposing structure is 1.0. Using a ratio, the movement of the structure is scored according to the degree of its movement toward the resting position of the opposing structure. It is unclear how many centers are currently using this system, but its use may be somewhat limited because of its considerable complexity. In addition, this type of precision is really not necessary. It is the location and cause of the opening that is important for determining treatment recommendations.

Regardless of the procedure used to report the results, it is most important that there is consistency in the observations that are made in each study and in the way that the studies are reported. In addition, the reliability of judgments from nasopharyngoscopy is greatly dependent on the experience of the evaluator (D'Antonio et al., 1989). Therefore, working with another experienced examiner initially is important to help the novice evaluator develop the necessary skills.

Although results are reported to other professionals, they must also be reported to the family. The person who counsels the family must use clear, easy-to-understand language. All medical terms should be clearly defined. When discussing the function of the velopharyngeal valve, pictures and diagrams should be used. After the initial explanation, it may also be helpful to play the video of the procedure and point out the structures and their function.

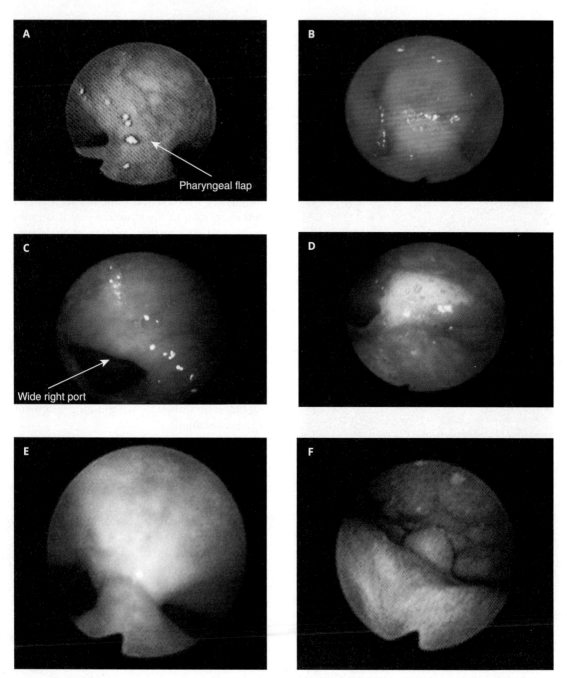

FIGURE 16-23 Nasopharyngoscopy of pharyngeal flaps. **(A)** Pharyngeal flap during nasal breathing. Note the lateral ports on each side are patent for normal breathing. **(B)** Pharyngeal flap during speech with both ports completely closed. **(C)** Pharyngeal flap with a persistent opening in the (patient's) right port during speech. **(D)** Pharyngeal flap at rest with the (patient's) right port open for normal nasal breathing, but the (patient's) left port stenosed, causing upper airway obstruction. **(E)** Narrow flap with ports that are too wide to close during speech. **(F)** Low, narrow flap that allows for persistent nasal emission.

Cleaning and Storing the Endoscope

Once the endoscope has been used, care should be taken so that the scope is not placed on a surface that will be touched by others. Instead, the scope should be taken for immediate cleaning and disinfection (McCullagh & Baker, 2000). Guidelines for disinfection of the scope have been developed by the Association for the Advancement of Medical Instrumentation (AAMI, 2015). However, each medical facility should have a specific policy on how endoscopes are reprocessed. Cleaning and high-level disinfection or sterilization is easier and more complete for endoscopes that can be immersed. Therefore, this should be considered when purchasing a new scope.

There are nine steps to reprocessing an endoscope as noted in the following list (J. Paul Willging, personal communication, May 12, 2006):

1. **Precleaning:** Before disinfection and sterilization, the scope is carefully cleaned of visible residue with a cloth and enzymatic detergent solution. "Sterile dirt" can still cause infection (Catalone & Koos, 2005).

2. **Transportation to the cleaning facility:** The scope is placed in a closed, rigid container for the protection of patients, healthcare workers, and the scope. The cleaning facility must have a separate dirty area to receive the contaminated scope.

3. **Leakage testing:** The scope is tested for leakage to ensure the integrity of the external skin. If cleaning materials leak into the core of the scope, the fiberoptic bundles will be severely damaged. If there is a leak, the scope is removed from service until it is repaired.

4. **Manual cleaning:** The scope is immersed in an enzymatic solution and cleaned manually to remove retained debris that can interfere with the capability of germicides to effectively kill microorganisms.

5. **Rinsing:** The endoscope is rinsed to remove residual debris and detergent. The endoscope is then dried to prevent dilution of the chemical germicide during disinfection.

6. **High-level disinfection:** A liquid chemical germicide is used with the required exposure time. These are toxic substances, so personal protection equipment is important (e.g., gloves, mask, eye protection, and impervious gown).

7. **Rinsing:** The scope is moved to a designated clean area and thoroughly rinsed in sterile, filtered water. It is important to remove the chemical residue to prevent injury to the skin and mucous membranes of the next patient.

8. **Drying:** The endoscope is dried with a lint-free towel, which inhibits the growth of waterborne organisms.

9. **Storage:** The scope is hung in a storage cabinet with adequate ventilation to prevent moisture buildup or physical damage (**FIGURE 16-24**). The scope should not be stored in the case provided by the manufacturer.

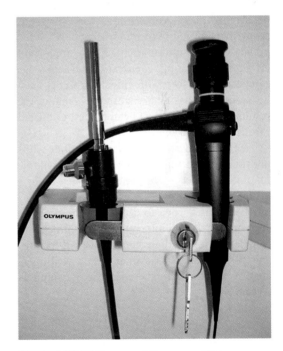

FIGURE 16-24 Storage of the scope. The scope should ideally be hung when stored for adequate ventilation to prevent moisture buildup and physical damage.

Advantages and Limitations of Nasopharyngoscopy

The most commonly used methods for direct visualization of the velopharyngeal mechanism are nasopharyngoscopy and videofluoroscopy (Rowe & D'Antonio, 2005). There are differences in opinion as to the best method of assessment in all cases. The examiner should consider what is most important to visualize in each patient's case and the relative benefits and risks of each procedure before determining which type of assessment to use. (See Table 13-2 in the chapter *Overview of Instrumental Procedures* for a comparison of the two procedures.)

One advantage of nasopharyngoscopy over videofluoroscopy is that all structures of the velopharyngeal mechanism can be seen in great detail and almost at the same time. The location, size, shape, and cause of the opening can be determined more easily through nasopharyngoscopy than through videofluoroscopy. As noted previously, this information is very important for surgical planning. Even very small openings (that cannot be seen with videofluoroscopy) can be seen with nasopharyngoscopy. Finally, the results of surgeries for VPI can be best evaluated through nasopharyngoscopy

Of course, nasopharyngoscopy is done without radiation; therefore, there is no risk of harmful physical effects to the patient. Because there is no radiation involved, the examiner can take as much time as needed to determine the problem and the appropriate intervention. The procedure can also be repeated as often as needed for pre- and post-treatment assessments. It is well tolerated by most children, even those as young as 3 years old.

Nasopharyngoscopy can be used as a biofeedback tool. The speech-language pathologist can give the individual instructions on placement, and the patient can watch the velopharyngeal results on the monitor as he tries to follow the instructions. This is a particularly powerful procedure for the treatment of certain learned causes of velopharyngeal dysfunction (Brunner et al., 1994; D'Antonio et al., 1988; Kunzel, 1982; Rich, Farber, & Shprintzen, 1988; Siegel-Sadewitz & Shprintzen, 1982; Witzel et al., 1988; Witzel, Tobe, & Salyer, 1989; Ysunza et al., 1997). For more information on the use of nasopharyngoscopy for biofeedback, please see the chapter *Speech Therapy*.

The risks or limitations associated with nasopharyngoscopy are minimal. The biggest disadvantage of nasopharyngoscopy is that the examiner cannot see the entire length of the pharyngeal wall during speech. In addition, some clinicians argue that videofluoroscopy is less invasive than nasopharyngoscopy. However, introduction of barium in the nasopharynx for videofluoroscopy is also invasive, and the large machinery can be just as frightening to a child as nasopharyngoscopy.

Nasopharyngoscopy requires cooperation from the individual to successfully complete the study. Getting the scope through to the right place is not difficult. However, getting a child to talk and repeat sentences with the scope in place and without crying can be a challenge. Although nasopharyngoscopy should not be a painful procedure, it can cause some discomfort, especially if the scope hits a nasal spur or the base of the nasal septum. However, with a good coating of topical anesthesia and previous preparation as to what to expect, the nasopharyngoscopy procedure is usually well tolerated by children as young as 3 years of age. A final disadvantage is that the nasopharyngoscopy equipment is expensive to purchase and maintain.

SUMMARY

Instrumental assessment is not required for the diagnosis of velopharyngeal dysfunction because this can be determined through a perceptual assessment alone. However, nasopharyngoscopy is a very useful tool for visualizing the structures and function of the velopharyngeal valve. Nasopharyngoscopy allows the examiner to directly visualize the size, shape, location, and cause of the velopharyngeal gap. This information is used to determine the surgical procedure that has the greatest chance of success for the individual patient.

Nasopharyngoscopy is also ideal for evaluating the effectiveness of surgery for VPI because the structures as a result of the surgery can be clearly seen. Nasopharyngoscopy can be used to determine the presence of obstruction in the vocal tract, which can also affect resonance. Finally, it is used to evaluate swallowing and vocal fold anomalies or dysfunction.

Although nasopharyngoscopy is somewhat invasive and can be scary to young children, it can be done successfully with children over the age of 3 with adequate patient preparation and the use of a topical anesthetic.

FOR REVIEW AND DISCUSSION

1. What equipment is absolutely necessary for a nasopharyngoscopy examination? What additional components are strongly recommended, and why?

2. Why is it important to do a perceptual evaluation of speech before the nasopharyngoscopy exam?

3. Discuss the methods for nasal anesthesia and decongestion.

4. Describe the procedure for passing the scope. What conditions can make passing the scope more challenging? Why is the scope passed through the middle nasal meatus rather than the inferior nasal meatus or the superior nasal meatus? What should you do if the scope lens becomes cloudy?

5. What determines the appropriate speech samples to use in the exam? Why is it preferable to obtain a sample without the child crying? What are methods to calm the child and stop the crying if it occurs?

6. What are potential complications during the exam, and how should they be handled?

7. What structures can be viewed through nasopharyngoscopy? What clinical observations can be seen that could affect resonance?

8. What are the advantages of nasopharyngoscopy? What are some of the limitations?

REFERENCES

Abdel-Aziz, M. (2007). Treatment of submucous cleft palate by pharyngeal flap as a primary procedure. *International Journal of Pediatric Otorhinolaryngology, 71*(7), 1093–1097.

American Speech-Language-Hearing Association (ASHA). (n.d.). Infection control in speech-language pathology. Retrieved from www.asha.org/slp/infectioncontrol.htm

American Speech-Language-Hearing Association (ASHA). (2004a). Knowledge and skills for speech-language pathologists with respect to vocal tract visualization and imaging. Retrieved from www.asha.org/policy/KS2004-00071.htm

American Speech-Language-Hearing Association (ASHA). (2004b). Vocal tract visualization and imaging: Technical report. Retrieved from www.asha.org/policy/TR2004-00156.htm

American Speech-Language-Hearing Association (ASHA). (2005). The role of the speech-language pathologist in the performance and interpretation of endoscopic evaluation of swallowing: Technical report. Retrieved from www.asha.org/policy/TR2005-00155.htm

Association for the Advancement of Medical Instrumentation (AAMI). (2015). ANSI/AAMI ST91: Comprehensive guide to flexible and semi-rigid endoscope processing in health care facilities. Retrieved from http://www.aami.org/productspublications/ProductDetail.aspx?ItemNumber=2477

Aviv, J. E., Kim, T., Thomson, J. E., Sunshine, S., Kaplan, S., & Close, L. G. (1998). Fiberoptic endoscopic evaluation of swallowing with sensory testing (FEESST) in healthy controls [see Comments]. *Dysphagia, 13*(2), 87–92.

Bastian, R. W. (1991). Videoendoscopic evaluation of patients with dysphagia: An adjunct to the modified barium swallow. *Otolaryngology-Head & Neck Surgery, 104*(3), 339–350.

Bastian, R. W. (1993). The videoendoscopic swallowing study: An alternative and partner to the videofluoroscopic swallowing study. *Dysphagia, 8*(4), 359–367.

Bastian, R. W. (1998). Contemporary diagnosis of the dysphagic patient. *Otolaryngology Clinics of North America, 31*(3), 489–506.

Brunner, M., Stellzig, A., Decker, W., Strate, B., Komposch, C., Wirth, C., & Verres, R. (1994). Video-feedback therapy with the flexible nasopharyngoscope: The potentials for modifying velopharyngeal closure and phonation deficiencies in cleft patients. *Fortschritte de Kieferorthopadei, 55*(4), 197–201.

Brunner, M., Stellzig-Eisenhauer, A., Proschel, U., Verres, R., & Komposch, G. (2005). The effect of nasopharyngoscopic biofeedback in patients with cleft palate and velopharyngeal dysfunction. *The Cleft Palate–Craniofacial Journal, 42*(6), 649–657.

Cain, A. J., Murray, D. P., & McClymont, L. G. (2002). The use of topical nasal anaesthesia before flexible nasendoscopy: A double-blind, randomized, controlled trial comparing cophenylcaine with placebo. *Clinical Otolaryngology & Allied Sciences, 27*(6), 485–488.

Catalone, B., & Koos, G. (2005). Beyond cleaning: Reprocessing flexible GI endoscopes successfully. *Healthcare Purchasing News, 29*(11), 38–39.

Centers for Disease Control and Prevention (CDC). (2005, May 3). Recommendations for application of standard precautions for the care of all patients in all healthcare settings. Retrieved from www.cdc.gov/sars/guidance/I-infection/app1.html

Centers for Disease Control and Prevention (CDC). (2013, September 27). Handwashing: Clean hands save lives. Retrieved from www.cdc.gov/handwashing/

Croft, C. B., Shprintzen, R. J., & Rakoff, S. J. (1981). Patterns of velopharyngeal valving in normal and cleft palate subjects: A multiview videofluoroscopic and nasendoscopic study. *Laryngoscope, 91*(2), 265–271.

D'Antonio, L. L., Achauer, B. M., & Vander Kam, V. M. (1993). Results of a survey of cleft palate teams concerning the use of nasendoscopy. *The Cleft Palate–Craniofacial Journal, 30*(1), 35–39.

D'Antonio, L. L., Chait, D., Lotz, W., & Netsell, R. (1986). Pediatric videonasoendoscopy for speech and voice evaluation. *Otolaryngology-Head & Neck Surgery, 94*(5), 578–583.

D'Antonio, L. L., & Marsh, J. L. (1987). Abnormal carotid arteries in the velocardiofacial syndrome [Letter]. *Plastic and Reconstructive Surgery, 80*(3), 471–472.

D'Antonio, L. L., Marsh, J. L., Province, M. A., Muntz, H. R., & Phillips, C. J. (1989). Reliability of flexible fiberoptic nasopharyngoscopy for evaluation of velopharyngeal function in a clinical population. *Cleft Palate Journal, 26*(3), 217–225; discussion 225.

D'Antonio, L. L., Muntz, H. R., Marsh, J. L., Marty-Grames, L., & Backensto-Marsh, R. (1988). Practical application of flexible fiberoptic nasopharyngoscopy for evaluating velopharyngeal function. *Plastic and Reconstructive Surgery, 82*(4), 611–618.

Donzelli, J., Brady, S., Wesling, M., & Theisen, M. (2005). Effects of the removal of the tracheotomy tube on swallowing during the fiberoptic endoscopic exam of the swallow (FEES). *Dysphagia, 20*(4), 283–289.

Douglas, R., Hawke, L., & Wormald, P. J. (2006). Topical anaesthesia before nasendoscopy: A randomized controlled trial of co-phenylcaine compared with lidocaine. *Clinical Otolaryngology, 31*(1), 33.

Finkelstein, Y., Berger, G., Nachmani, A., & Ophir, D. (1996). The functional role of the adenoids in speech. *International Journal of Pediatric Otorhinolaryngology, 34*(1/2), 61–74.

Finkelstein, Y., Lerner, M. A., Ophir, D., Nachmani, A., Hauben, D. J., & Zohar, Y. (1993). Nasopharyngeal profile and velopharyngeal valve mechanism. *Plastic and Reconstructive Surgery, 92*(4), 603–614.

Finkelstein, Y., Nachmani, A., & Ophir, D. (1994). The functional role of the tonsils in speech. *Archives of Otolaryngology-Head & Neck Surgery, 120*(8), 846–851.

Finkelstein, Y., Talmi, Y. P., Kravitz, K., Bar-Ziv, J., Nachmani, A., Hauben, D. J., & Zohar, Y. (1991). Study of the normal and insufficient velopharyngeal valve by the "Forced Sucking Test." *Laryngoscope, 101*(11), 1203–1212.

Finkelstein, Y., Zohar, Y., Nachmani, A., Talmi, Y. P., Lerner, M. A., Hauben, D. J., & Frydman, M. (1993). The otolaryngologist and the patient with velocardiofacial syndrome. *Archives of Otolaryngology-Head & Neck Surgery, 119*(5), 563–569.

Frosh, A. C., Jayaraj, S., Porter, G., & Almeyda, J. (1998). Is local anaesthesia actually beneficial in flexible fibreoptic nasendoscopy? *Clinics in Otolaryngology, 23*(3), 259–262.

Georgalas, C., Sandhu, G., Frosh, A., & Xenellis, J. (2005). Cophenylcaine spray vs. placebo in flexible nasendoscopy: A prospective double-blind randomized controlled trial. *International Journal of Clinical Practice, 59*(2), 130–133.

Gereau, S. A., & Shprintzen, R. J. (1988). The role of adenoids in the development of normal speech following palate repair. *Laryngoscope, 98*(3), 299–303.

Golding-Kushner, K. J., Argamaso, R. V., Cotton, R. T., Grames, L. M., Henningsson, G., Jones, D. L., . . . Marsh J. L. (1990). Standardization for the reporting of nasopharyngoscopy and multiview videofluoroscopy: A report from an International Working Group. *Cleft Palate Journal, 27*(4), 337–347; discussion 347–348.

Gosain, A. K., Conley, S. F., Marks, S., & Larson, D. L. (1996). Submucous cleft palate: Diagnostic methods and outcomes of surgical treatment. *Plastic and Reconstructive Surgery, 97*(7), 1497–1509.

HCPro. (2008). Coding tip: Learn the difference between nasopharyngoscopy and endoscopy procedures. *Ambulatory Surgery Reimbursement Update.* Retrieved from www.hcpro.com/HOM-204089 -2949/Coding-tip-Learn-the-difference-between -nasopharyngoscopy-and-endoscopy-procedures .html

Henningsson, G., & Isberg, A. (1988). Influence of tonsils on velopharyngeal movements in children with craniofacial anomalies and hypernasality. *American Journal of Orthodontics and Dentofacial Orthopedics, 94*(3), 253–261.

Henningsson, G., & Isberg, A. (1991). Comparison between multiview videofluoroscopy and nasendoscopy of velopharyngeal movements. *The Cleft Palate-Craniofacial Journal, 28*(4), 413–417; discussion 417–418.

Hung, C. H., & Cheng, S. Y. (1989). Application of nasopharyngoscopy and videofluoroscopy in the fabrication of a speech aid for soft palate defects. *Journal of the Formosan Medical Association, 88*(8), 812–818.

Igawa, H. H., Nishizawa, N., Sugihara, T., & Inuyama, Y. (1998). A fiberscopic analysis of velopharyngeal movement before and after primary palatoplasty in cleft palate infants. *Plastic and Reconstructive Surgery, 102*(3), 668–674.

Jonas, N. E., Visser, M. F., Oomen, A., Albertyn, R., van Dijk, M., & Prescott, C. A. (2007). Is topical local anaesthesia necessary when performing paediatric flexible nasendoscopy? A double-blind randomized controlled trial. *International Journal of Pediatric Otorhinolaryngology, 71*(11), 1687–1692.

Karnell, M. P. (1994). *Videoendoscopy: From velopharynx to larynx.* San Diego, CA: Singular Publishing Group.

Karnell, M. P., Ibuki, K., Morris, H. L., & Van Demark, D. R. (1983). Reliability of the nasopharyngeal fiberscope (NPF) for assessing velopharyngeal function: Analysis by judgment. *Cleft Palate Journal, 20*(3), 199–208.

Karnell, M. P., & Langmore, S. (1998). Videoendoscopy in speech and swallowing for the speech-language pathologist. In A. F. Johnson & B. H. Jacobson (Eds.), *Medical speech-language pathology: A practitioner's guide* (pp. 563–584). New York, NY: Thieme.

Karnell, M. P., Rosenstein, H., & Fine, L. (1987). Nasal videoendoscopy in prosthetic management of palatopharyngeal dysfunction. *Journal of Prosthetic Dentistry, 58*(4), 479–484.

Kuehn, D. P., & Henne, L. J. (2003). Speech evaluation and treatment of patients with cleft palate. *American Journal of Speech-Language Pathology, 12,* 103–109.

Kummer, A. W. (2016). Evaluation of speech and resonance for children with craniofacial anomalies. *Facial Plastic Surgery Clinics of North America, 24*(4), 445–451.

Kummer, A. W., Billmire, D. A., & Myer, C. M. (1993). Hypertrophic tonsils: The effect on resonance and velopharyngeal closure. *Plastic and Reconstructive Surgery, 91*(4), 608–611.

Kummer, A. W., Clark, S. L., Redle, E. E., Thomsen, L. L., & Billmire, D. A. (2011). Current practice in assessing and reporting speech outcomes of cleft palate and velopharyngeal surgery: A survey of cleft palate/craniofacial professionals. *The Cleft Palate-Craniofacial Journal, 49*(2), 146–152.

Kummer, A. W., Curtis, C., Wiggs, M., Lee, L., & Strife, J. L. (1992). Comparison of velopharyngeal gap size in patients with hypernasality, hypernasality and nasal emission, or nasal turbulence (rustle) as the primary speech characteristic. *The Cleft Palate-Craniofacial Journal, 29*(2), 152–156.

Kunzel, H. J. (1982). First applications of a biofeedback device for the therapy of velopharyngeal incompetence. *Folia Phoniatrica, 34*(2), 92–100.

Lam, D. J., Starr, J. R., Perkins, J. A., Lewis, C. W., Eblen, L. E., Dunlap, J., & Sie, K. C. (2006). A comparison of nasendoscopy and multiview videofluoroscopy in assessing velopharyngeal insufficiency. *Otolaryngology-Head & Neck Surgery, 134*(3), 394–402.

Langmore, S. E., Schatz, K., & Olsen, N. (1988). Fiberoptic endoscopic examination of swallowing safety: A new procedure. *Dysphagia, 2*(4), 216–219.

Leder, S. B., Acton, L. M., Lisitano, H. L., & Murray, J. T. (2005). Fiberoptic endoscopic evaluation of swallowing (FEES) with and without blue-dyed food. *Dysphagia, 20*(2), 157–162.

Lertsburapa, K., Schroeder, J. W., Jr., & Sullivan, C. (2010). Assessment of adenoid size: A comparison of lateral radiographic measurements, radiologist assessment, and nasal endoscopy. *International Journal of Pediatric Otorhinolaryngology, 74*(11), 1281–1285.

Lewin, M. L., Croft, C. B., & Shprintzen, R. J. (1980). Velopharyngeal insufficiency due to hypoplasia of the musculus uvulae and occult submucous cleft palate. *Plastic and Reconstructive Surgery, 65*(5), 585–591.

Lewis, J. R., Andreassen, M. L., Leeper, H. A., Macrae, D. L., & Thomas, J. (1993). Vocal characteristics of children with cleft lip/palate and associated velopharyngeal incompetence. *Journal of Otolaryngology, 22*(2), 113–117.

Lotz, W. K., D'Antonio, L. L., Chait, D. H., & Netsell, R. W. (1993). Successful nasoendoscopic and aerodynamic examinations of children with speech/voice disorders. *International Journal of Pediatric Otorhinolaryngology, 26*(2), 165–172.

MacKenzie-Stepner, K., Witzel, M. A., Stringer, D. A., & Laskin, R. (1987). Velopharyngeal insufficiency due to hypertrophic tonsils: A report of two cases. *International Journal of Pediatric Otorhinolaryngology, 14*(1), 57–63.

MacKenzie-Stepner, K., Witzel, M. A., Stringer, D. A., Lindsay, W. K., Munro, I. R., & Hughes, H. (1987). Abnormal carotid arteries in the velocardiofacial syndrome: A report of three cases. *Plastic and Reconstructive Surgery, 80*(3), 347–351.

McCullagh, L., & Baker, K. (2000). Endoscope reprocessing: Taking the mystery out of high-level disinfection. *ORL-Head and Neck Nursing, 18*(1), 6–10.

Miyazaki, T., Matsuya, T., & Yamaoka, M. (1975). Fiberscopic methods for assessment of velopharyngeal closure during various activities. *Cleft Palate Journal, 12,* 107–114.

Nacci, A., Ursino, F., La Vela, R., Matteucci, F., Mallardi, V., & Fattori, B. (2008). Fiberoptic endoscopic evaluation of swallowing (FEES): Proposal for informed consent. *ACTA Otorhinolaryngologica Italica, 28*(4), 206–211.

Nankivell, P. C., & Pothier, D. D. (2008). Nasal and instrument preparation before rigid and flexible nasendoscopy: A systematic review. *The Journal of Laryngology & Otology, 122*(10), 1024–1028.

Osberg, P. E., & Witzel, M. A. (1981). The physiologic basis for hypernasality during connected speech in cleft palate patients: A nasendoscopic study. *Plastic and Reconstructive Surgery, 67*(1), 1–5.

Perry, J., & Schenck, G. (2013). Instrumental assessment in cleft palate care. *SIG 5 Perspectives on Speech Science and Orofacial Disorders, 23*(2), 49–61.

Peterson-Falzone, S. J. (1985). Velopharyngeal inadequacy in the absence of overt cleft palate. *Journal of Craniofacial Genetics and Developmental Biology, 1,* 97–124.

Peterson-Falzone, S. J., & Graham, M. S. (1990). Phoneme-specific nasal emission in children with and without physical anomalies of the velopharyngeal mechanism. *Journal of Speech and Hearing Disorders, 55*(1), 132–139.

Pigott, R. W., Bensen, J. F., & White, F. D. (1969). Nasendoscopy in the diagnosis of velopharyngeal incompetence. *Plastic and Reconstructive Surgery, 43*(2), 141–147.

Pigott, R. W., & Makepeace, A. P. (1982). Some characteristics of endoscopic and radiological systems used in elaboration of the diagnosis of velopharyngeal incompetence. *British Journal of Plastic Surgery, 35*(1), 19–32.

Pothier, D. D., Awad, Z., Whitehouse, M., & Porter, G. C. (2005). The use of lubrication in flexible fibreoptic nasendoscopy: A randomized controlled trial. *Clinical Otolaryngology, 30*(4), 353–356.

Pothier, D. D., Raghava, N., Monteiro, P., & Awad, Z. (2006). A randomized controlled trial: Is water better than a standard lubricant in nasendoscopy? *Clinical Otolaryngology, 31*(2), 134–137.

Ramamurthy, L., Wyatt, R. A., Whitby, D., Martin, D., & Davenport, P. (1997). The evaluation of velopharyngeal function using flexible nasendoscopy. *Journal of Laryngology & Otology, 111*(8), 739–745.

Rich, B. M., Farber, K., & Shprintzen, R. J. (1988). Nasopharyngoscopy in the treatment of palatopharyngeal insufficiency. *International Journal of Prosthodontics, 1*(3), 248–251.

Ross, D. A., Witzel, M. A., Armstrong, D. C., & Thomson, H. G. (1996). Is pharyngoplasty a risk in velocardiofacial syndrome? An assessment of medially displaced carotid arteries. *Plastic and Reconstructive Surgery, 98*(7), 1182–1190.

Rowe, M. R., & D'Antonio, L. L. (2005). Velopharyngeal dysfunction: Evolving developments in evaluation. *Current Opinion in Otolaryngology & Head & Neck Surgery, 13*(6), 366–370.

Sadek, S. A., De, R., Scott, A., White, A. P., Wilson, P. S., & Carlin, W. V. (2001). The efficacy of topical anaesthesia in flexible nasendoscopy: A double-blind randomized controlled trial. *Clinical Otolaryngology & Allied Sciences, 26*(1), 25–28.

Shetty, S., Frampton, S., & Patel, N. (2009). Flexible nasendoscopy. [Letter]. *Clinical Otolaryngology, 34*(2), 169–171.

Shprintzen, R. J. (1979). The use of multiview videofluoroscopy and flexible fiberoptic nasopharyngoscopy as a predictor of success with pharyngeal flap surgery. In R. Ellis & F. C. Flack (Eds.), *Diagnosis and treatment of palato-glossal malfunction* (pp. 6–14). London: College of Speech Therapists.

Shprintzen, R. J. (1995). Instrumental assessment of velopharyngeal valving. In R. J. Shprintzen & J. Bardach (Eds.), *Cleft palate speech management: A multidisciplinary approach* (vol. 4, pp. 221–256). St. Louis, MO: Mosby.

Shprintzen, R. J. (1996). Nasopharyngoscopy. In K. R. Bzoch (Ed.), *Communicative disorders related to cleft lip and palate* (vol. 4, pp. 387–409). Austin, TX: Pro-Ed.

Shprintzen, R. J., & Golding-Kushner, K. J. (1989). Evaluation of velopharyngeal insufficiency. *Otolaryngology Clinics of North America, 22*(3), 519–536.

Shprintzen, R. J., Lewin, M. L., Croft, C. B., Daniller, A. L., Argamaso, R. V., Ship, A. G., & Strauch, B. (1979). A comprehensive study of pharyngeal flap surgery: Tailor-made flaps. *Cleft Palate Journal, 16*(1), 46–55.

Shprintzen, R. J., Rakof, S. J., Skolnick, M. L., & Lavorato, A. S. (1977). Incongruous movements of the velum and lateral pharyngeal walls. *Cleft Palate Journal, 14*(2), 148–157.

Siegel-Sadewitz, V. L., & Shprintzen, R. J. (1982). Nasopharyngoscopy of the normal velopharyngeal sphincter: An experiment of biofeedback. *Cleft Palate Journal, 19*(3), 194–200.

Siegel-Sadewitz, V. L., & Shprintzen, R. J. (1986). Changes in velopharyngeal valving with age. *International Journal of Pediatric Otorhinolaryngology, 11*(2), 171–182.

Sinclair, S. W., Davies, D. M., & Bracka, A. (1982). Comparative reliability of nasal pharyngoscopy and videofluorography in the assessment of velopharyngeal incompetence. *British Journal of Plastic Surgery, 35*(2), 113–117.

Skolnick, M. L., Shprintzen, R. J., McCall, G. N., & Rakoff, S. (1975). Patterns of velopharyngeal closure in subjects with repaired cleft palate and normal speech: A multi-view videofluoroscopic analysis. *Cleft Palate Journal, 12,* 369–376.

Smith, B. E., & Kuehn, D. P. (2007). Speech evaluation for velopharyngeal dysfunction. *The Journal of Craniofacial Surgery, 18*(2), 251–261; quiz 266–267.

Smith, J. C., & Rockley, T. J. (2002). A comparison of cocaine and "co-phenylcaine" local anaesthesia in flexible nasendoscopy. *Clinical Otolaryngology & Allied Sciences, 27*(3), 192–196.

Strauss, R. A. (2007). Flexible endoscopic nasopharyngoscopy. *Atlas of the Oral and Maxillofacial Surgery Clinics of North America, 15*(2), 111–128.

Taub, S. (1966). The Taub oral panendoscope: A new technique. *Cleft Palate Journal, 3,* 328–346.

Willging, J. P. (2003). Velopharyngeal insufficiency. *Current Opinion in Otolaryngology & Head & Neck Surgery, 11*(6), 452–455.

Williams, R. G., Preece, M., Rhys, R., & Eccles, R. (1992). The effect of adenoid and tonsil surgery on nasalance. *Clinics in Otolaryngology, 17*(2), 136–140.

Witt, P. D., Miller, D. C., Marsh, J. L., Muntz, H. R., & Grames, L. M. (1998). Limited value of preoperative cervical vascular imaging in patients with velocardiofacial syndrome. *Plastic and Reconstructive Surgery, 101*(5), 1184–1195; discussion 1196–1199.

Witzel, M. A., & Posnick, J. C. (1989). Patterns and location of velopharyngeal valving problems: Atypical findings on video nasopharyngoscopy. *Cleft Palate Journal, 26*(1), 63–67.

Witzel, M. A., Tobe, J., & Salyer, K. (1988). The use of nasopharyngoscopy biofeedback therapy in the correction of inconsistent velopharyngeal closure.

International Journal of Pediatric Otorhinolaryngology, 15(2), 137–142.

Witzel, M. A., Tobe, J., & Salyer, K. E. (1989). The use of videonasopharyngoscopy for biofeedback therapy in adults after pharyngeal flap surgery. *Cleft Palate Journal, 26*(2), 129–134; discussion 135.

Ysunza, A., Pamplona, M., Femat, T., Mayer, L., & Garcia-Velasco, M. (1997). Videonasopharyngoscopy as an instrument for visual biofeedback during speech in cleft palate patients. *International Journal of Pediatric Otorhinolaryngology, 41*(3), 291–298.

Zajac, D. J., & Linville, R. N. (1989). Voice perturbations of children with perceived nasality and hoarseness. *Cleft Palate Journal, 26*(3), 226–231; discussion 231–232.

Zwitman, D. H., Sonderman, J. G., & Ward, P. H. (1974). Variations in velopharyngeal closure assessed by endoscopy. *Journal of Speech and Hearing Disorders, 39*(3), 366–372.

CREDITS

Coloring Book Pages

Coloring book pages to help prepare the child for a nasopharyngoscopy examination:

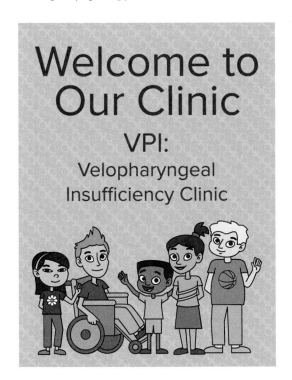

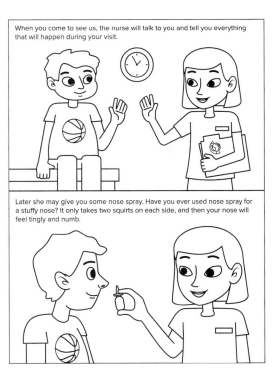

When you come to see us, the nurse will talk to you and tell you everything that will happen during your visit.

Later she may give you some nose spray. Have you ever used nose spray for a stuffy nose? It only takes two squirts on each side, and then your nose will feel tingly and numb.

Next it will be time to see your nose on TV. The doctor will put a long, skinny tube inside your nose. This is called a scope and it looks like a piece of black spaghetti.

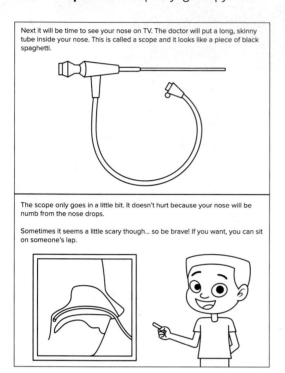

The scope only goes in a little bit. It doesn't hurt because your nose will be numb from the nose drops.

Sometimes it seems a little scary though... so be brave! If you want, you can sit on someone's lap.

Once the scope is in your nose, the speech pathologist will ask you to repeat some sentences again.

When you are talking, you can watch the inside of your nose on TV. There are parts in there that move... almost like magic!

It is very important to hold very still so the tube doesn't bump around inside.

What do you think the inside of your nose looks like?

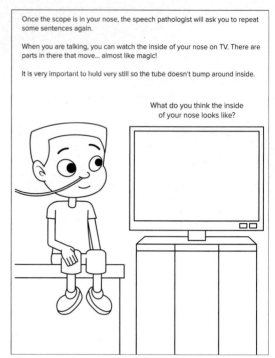

CREDITS

Appendix opener photo: PeopleImages/Getty Images

Courtesy of the Cleft and Craniofacial Center at Cincinnati Children's Hospital Medical Center.

Nasopharyngoscopy Examination Form

NASOPHARYNGOSCOPY EXAMINATION FORM

Velopharyngeal Function

☐ **Normal** ☐ **Abnormal:** ☐ borderline ☐ mild ☐ moderate ☐ severe ☐ very severe

Velopharyngeal Opening

Size: ☐ pinhole ☐ small ☐ medium ☐ large ☐ very large

Shape: ☐ circular ☐ sagittal ☐ coronal ☐ bowtie

Location: ☐ midline ☐ R of midline ☐ R corner ☐ L of midline ☐ L corner ☐ both corners

Consistency: ☐ consistent ☐ inconsistent

☐ phoneme-specific sounds affected: _____

Additional Findings: _____

(e.g., occult submucous cleft, bubbling of secretions, tonsils in pharynx, irregular adenoids, medialized carotid arteries, Passavant's ridge, fistula, vocal nodules, laryngeal web)

Probable Cause

☐ VP insufficiency ☐ VP incompetence ☐ poor lateral pharyngeal wall movement

☐ irregular adenoids ☐ phoneme-specific misarticulation ☐ other _____

Previous Secondary Surgery: ☐ None

Type: ☐ pharyngeal flap ☐ sphincter pharyngoplasty ☐ pharyngeal augmentation ☐ Furlow

Status: ☐ intact ☐ too low ☐ too narrow

(continues)

Ports During Speech:

Left port:	☐ open ☐ stenosed	**Right port:**	☐ open ☐ stenosed
Both ports:	☐ open ☐ stenosed	**Central (sphincter) port:**	☐ open ☐ stenosed

Recommendation

☐ Surgical intervention

   ☐ pharyngeal flap   ☐ sphincter pharyngoplasty

   ☐ pharyngeal augmentation   ☐ Furlow palatoplasty

   ☐ adenoidectomy   ☐ tonsillectomy

☐ **Prosthetic intervention:** ☐ palatal lift   ☐ palatal obturator   ☐ speech bulb

☐ **Speech therapy:** Target sounds:_____

CREDITS

Appendix opener photo: PeopleImages/Getty Images

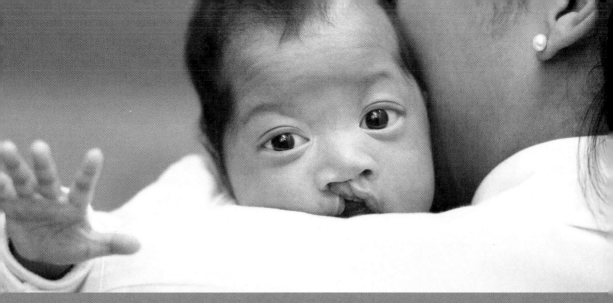

Treatment Procedures: Speech, Resonance, and Velopharyngeal Dysfunction

CHAPTER 17

Surgical Management

With acknowledgment to David A. Billmire, Deepak Krishnan, Julia Corcoran, and Haithem Elhadi Babiker for their contributions to this chapter.

CHAPTER OUTLINE

INTRODUCTION

Cleft lip and/or palate (CLP) occurs on a spectrum, from the abortive form, such as a forme fruste of the lip, a bifid uvula, or an asymptomatic submucous cleft palate, to a bilateral complete cleft of the lip and palate. Regardless of the degree of involvement, the surgical principles remain the same. For example, in an incomplete cleft of the lip, although a portion of the lip may be intact, the underlying muscle, nasal cartilage, and oral sphincter function are usually significantly affected. Therefore, correction requires a complete lip repair. For the same reason, correction of a symptomatic submucous cleft of the palate requires the same type of repair as if it were a complete cleft.

In addition to the obvious defect of the lip and roof of the mouth, CLP affects other areas, such as the nose, upper jaw, teeth, oral sphincter, and velopharyngeal valve. In addition, CLP often affects the functional areas of breathing, speech, voice, resonance, hearing, feeding, and even the psychological aspects that involve the individual's identity. As much as possible, the surgeon attempts to normalize both the anatomy and physiology, which usually improves the psychological state as well.

Structural defects that cause velopharyngeal insufficiency require physical management, usually in the form of surgery. In addition, surgical management can also improve velopharyngeal incompetence (due to abnormal neurophysiology) in some cases. Although surgical concepts and approaches have become more standardized in the past few years, there is a wide range of interpretation of these "standards" throughout the world, across the country, and even within a single treatment team. Treatment options, surgical techniques, timing, and philosophies are presented in this chapter purely as broad general guidelines.

Cleft Lip Repair

The technique used for cleft lip repair, known as a cheilorraphy, depends on whether the cleft is unilateral or bilateral. In addition, there are variations in the specific techniques chosen, based on the surgeon's training, previous experience, and bias. The goals of the cleft lip repair are to bring the skin, muscle (orbicularis oris), and mucous membrane together; to achieve symmetry of the nostrils and Cupid's bow; to achieve a natural border (white roll) between the vermilion and the skin of the upper lip; and to minimize the appearance of the scars. The continuity of the lip after the repair helps to mold the underlying bony structures, particularly the premaxilla.

Presurgical Management

Presurgical management is sometimes necessary to align the lip and maxillary segments prior to the formal lip repair. This is typically needed for a wide cleft or a bilateral complete cleft, especially if the premaxilla is significantly protruded and/or the two lateral segments of the maxilla are collapsed behind the premaxilla. Overall, presurgical management can result in a more successful initial result and an improved long-term aesthetic outcome.

Presurgical management may include taping the lip, performing a temporary lip adhesion, or using a nasoalveolar molding device (Bhuskute & Tollefson, 2016). If the premaxilla and/or lateral maxillary segments need to be aligned, premaxillary orthopedics is done. Presurgical management is usually done around 6 weeks of age and followed by a formal lip repair at the age of 3 to 4 months.

Unilateral Cleft Lip Repair Techniques

Currently, there are two primary methods for repairing the unilateral cleft lip: the Millard technique (Paranaiba et al., 2009; Trier, 1985b) and the Tennison-Randall technique (or a modification thereof) (Brauer & Cronin, 1983; Lazarus, Hudson, van Zyl, Fleming, & Fernandes, 1998; Leon-Valle, 1980; Tan & Atik, 2007) (**FIGURE 17-1**). With both techniques, the lip is repaired in three layers from inside out: mucosa, muscle, and skin. In addition, the shortened philtral ridge is lengthened by inserting a "patch" of tissue. In the Millard repair, it is inserted at the top of the lip, just beneath the nose. In the Tennison-Randall repair, it is inserted just above the vermilion border of the lip. This brings the ridge down to match the unaffected side.

The Millard technique (or rotation advancement flap) is used in approximately 80% of cases and is perhaps the most anatomical of the repairs. It is described as a "cut as you go technique."

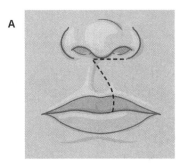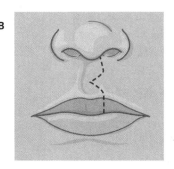

FIGURE 17-1 Unilateral cleft lip repairs. **(A)** Millard repair. **(B)** Tennison-Randall repair.

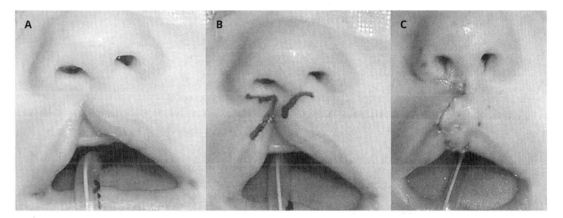

FIGURE 17-2 Millard lip repair.

Figure 17-1A shows the basic technique for the Millard lip repair, and **FIGURE 17-2** is a photograph of this type of repair. **FIGURE 17-3A** shows a patient preoperatively, **FIGURE 17-3B** shows the patient 1 day after a Millard repair, and **FIGURE 17-3C** shows the patient 6 months postoperatively. In contrast, the Tennison-Randall technique (or triangular flap procedure) is used in about 20% of cases. This procedure is precise and measured; therefore, it is often referred to as a "cookie cutter" technique.

Regardless of the type of lip repair chosen, it is important to reconstruct the oral sphincter. This is because when there is a cleft lip, the orbicularis oris muscles, which create the oral sphincter around the lips, are discontinuous, and the divided ends are abnormally inserted. Therefore, these abnormal insertions have

to be taken down surgically and the muscles realigned into the correct orientation. Failure to do so results in distortion of the lip on animation, noticeable depressions, bulges on the side of the philtrum, and an overall poor aesthetic result.

Bilateral Cleft Lip Repair Techniques

Repair of a bilateral cleft lip is more challenging than repair of a unilateral cleft lip because of the magnitude of the lip and nasal deformities. The major methods of bilateral cleft lip repair include the modified Broadbent-Manchester repair, the Millard repair, and the Mulliken repair (Mulliken, 2009; Tan, Greene, & Mulliken, 2012) (**FIGURE 17-4**). As with the unilateral cleft, the

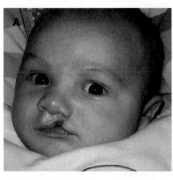
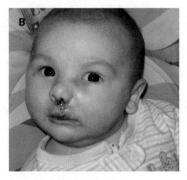
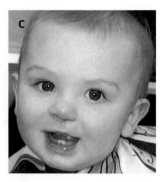

FIGURE 17-3 Unilateral cleft lip repair. **(A)** Patient preoperatively. **(B)** Patient 1 day postoperatively following a Millard repair. **(C)** Patient 6 months postoperatively.

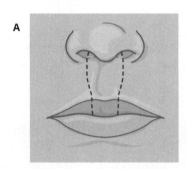
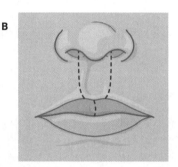

FIGURE 17-4 Bilateral cleft lip repairs. **(A)** Modified Manchester repair. **(B)** Millard bilateral cleft repair.

bilateral cleft surgery includes repair of the mucosa and muscle and then the skin.

In the bilateral cleft, the prolabium is prominently located just in front of the premaxilla. Because of the discontinuity of the orbicularis oris, the prolabium has no muscle in it. Instead, the orbicularis oris muscles insert abnormally.

Potential Complications

There are few complications associated with cleft lip surgery other than a less-than-desirable aesthetic result. Infrequently, however, the lip repair can result in stenosis of the nasal vestibule. When this occurs, the nasal obstruction can cause problems with nasal breathing and sleep and can even cause abnormal resonance.

Timing of Cleft Lip Repair

At one time, the cleft lip repair was done shortly after birth and before the child was sent home. Although a few cleft palate centers are reintroducing the concept of repair within the first week of life, most centers advocate delaying the lip repair until between 10 and 12 weeks of age.

There are several reasons for delaying surgery. For example, a delay allows time for investigation of other associated abnormalities or medical conditions, which may not be readily apparent at birth, and for presurgical treatment for the best outcomes. Finally, it gives the infant time to develop feeding skills and gain weight before undergoing extensive surgery. For these reasons, most centers follow some variation of the **rule of 10s**. This guideline suggests that the infant should be at least 10 weeks of age, weigh at least 10 pounds, and have hemoglobin of 10 grams before the lip repair.

Cleft Palate Repair

Cleft palate repair, also called palatoplasty, is done to close off the oral cavity from the nasal cavity for the benefit of feeding and middle ear function but most of all for speech. Although the cleft lip repair dates back to antiquity, successful palate repair dates from only the early 19th century. With the advent of anesthesia and specialized instrumentation, success rates of palate repair have improved dramatically over the years. The goals of palate repair are to establish a normal velopharyngeal mechanism, minimize the occurrence of fistulas, and optimize facial growth (Woo, 2017).

Presurgical Management

Depending on the center and the surgeon, there may be a recommended change in the feeding technique used with the infant prior to the palatoplasty. Although some surgeons will allow bottle feeding postoperatively, others prefer the child to be off the bottle prior to the palatoplasty. Therefore, the infant may need to be transitioned to either syringe or cup feeding. The postoperative feeding precautions can vary in length from just a few days to as long as 3 weeks depending on the center and the surgeon's preferences.

Cleft Palate Repair Techniques

The palate is closed in three layers: nasal mucosa, muscle layer (reorientation of the levator to create the sling), and oral mucosa. There are several techniques for cleft palate repair. The commonly used techniques are described as follows.

von Langenbeck

The von Langenbeck repair, illustrated in **FIGURE 17-5**, is one of the oldest and most successful means of palatal closure and is still popular today (Murison & Pigott, 1992; Trier & Dreyer, 1984). In this repair, an incision is made just inside the gum line, starting behind the area of the molars and extending up to the area of the canine tooth. The mucoperiosteum is carefully raised off the bone and, in conjunction with the velum, separated in one large layer. The cleft margin is incised, and the raw edges are brought together and sewn down the middle. The incisions along the gum line are usually left open and fill in naturally with time. With this operation, the levator muscle was typically not addressed (although it can easily be reconstructed), and there was a high incidence of velopharyngeal insufficiency. This set off a search for a procedure that not only closed the opening but also actively lengthened the palate.

Wardill–Kilner V–Y Pushback

A number of approaches for lengthening the palate have been tried (Bae, Kim, Lee, Hwang, & Kim, 2002). Some approaches have caused problems with maxillary growth, wound healing, and airway obstruction. One technique that is commonly used however is the Wardill–Kilner V–Y pushback procedure, which is illustrated in **FIGURE 17-6**. In this procedure, the initial incisions are similar to those of the von Langenbeck procedure except instead of leaving the mucoperiosteum attached in the front of the mouth, it is cut across as a V. The resulting open area is Y shaped. This frees up the mucoperiosteum of the whole palate and allows it to be pushed back in an attempt to lengthen it. With this procedure, the levator muscle is still not addressed, although it could be, and a high incidence of anterior fistulas has been reported (Moore, Lawrence, Ptak, & Trier, 1988).

Intravelar Veloplasty (IVVP)

A cleft palate causes the levator veli palatini muscles to insert onto the back of the hard

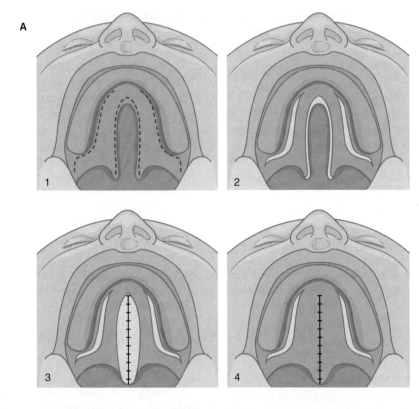

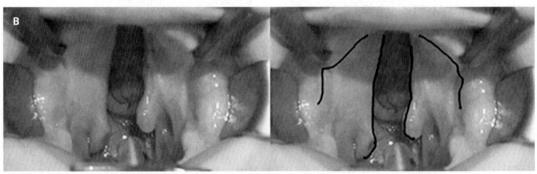

FIGURE 17-5 von Langenbeck repair. **(A)** Note lateral relaxing incisions, which are left open. **(B)** Photograph of the palate marked for von Langenbeck repair. Anterior palate remains attached, forming a bipedicle flap.

palate instead of interdigitating in the midline of the velum. As noted above, the original palate repair techniques do not address the orientation of the muscles. Therefore, some surgeons have advocated doing an intravelar veloplasty (IVVP), which

normalizes the velopharyngeal sling and can be done in conjunction with any type of palate repair (Brown, Cohen, & Randall, 1983; Dreyer & Trier, 1984). Unfortunately, intravelar veloplasty has not been as successful as was initially hoped (Brothers,

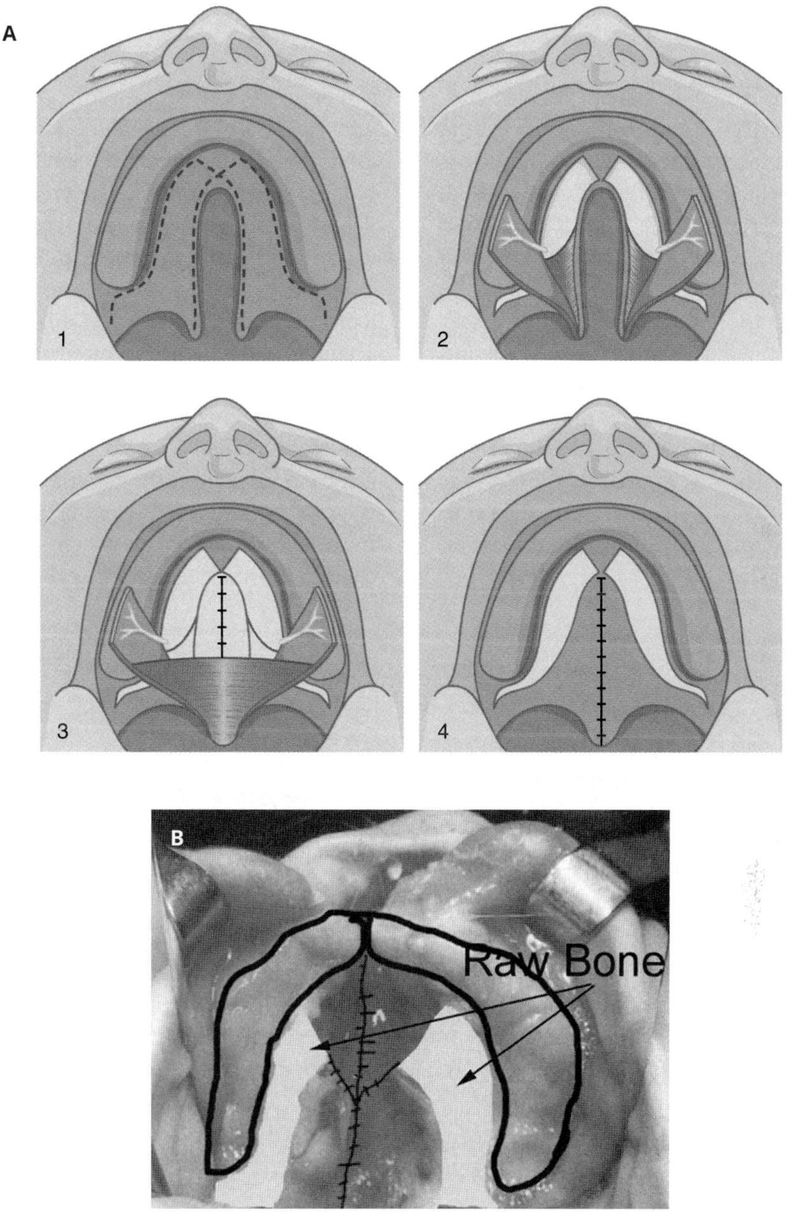

FIGURE 17-6 Wardill–Kilner repair. **(A)** The palate is lengthened by "pushing" back the mucoperiosteum. The raw area is allowed to fill by secondary healing (scarring). **(B)** Photograph of the Wardill–Kilner repair.

Dalston, Peterson, & Lawrence, 1995; Coston, Hagerty, Jannarone, McDonald, & Hagerty, 1986; Jarvis & Trier, 1988). In fact, some surgeons have found no difference in velopharyngeal function between palatoplasty with or without intravelar veloplasty (Marsh, Grames, & Holtman, 1989). Therefore, if there is a beneficial effect of intravelar veloplasty, it is likely to be minimal.

Furlow Z-Palatoplasty

A *Z-plasty* is a plastic surgery technique that is used to lengthen tissue. The Furlow Z-palatoplasty involves reconstruction of the levator sling and lengthening the velum by closing it with opposing Z-plasties (Furlow, 1986; Furlow, 1990; Furlow, 2009; Gunther, Wisser, Cohen, & Brown, 1998) (**FIGURE 17-7**). This is done by borrowing tissue from the width of the velum to add to the length. The resulting scar looks like a Z. To avoid possible breakdown and development of a fistula, the procedure is done so that the Z on the oral surface goes in the opposite direction of the Z on the nasal side of the velum. The levator muscles are carried on the Zs, one on each side, so that when they are moved into position, they automatically overlap and form an intravelar veloplasty.

Potential Complications

Although it may appear that a palate repair is simple in comparison to a lip repair, palate surgery can be quite challenging for several reasons. First, it is technically more demanding than a lip repair. In addition, there is a greater risk of postoperative problems, such as *dehiscence*, which is a breakdown in the surgical repair that causes a fistula or excessive scarring. If these problems occur, they are very difficult to correct. There is a potential for airway compromise or excessive bleeding, which may put the patient's life in jeopardy. Finally, merely closing the palate is not enough. The palate not only serves as a physical barrier between the mouth and nose, but the velum must also function dynamically for speech. In some cases, the palate repair alone is not sufficient for normal velopharyngeal function.

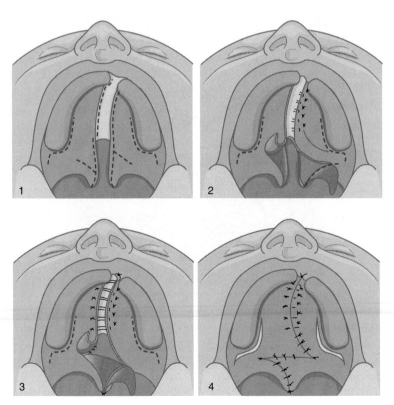

FIGURE 17-7 Furlow Z-palatoplasty. Note the Z-plasty closure of both the nasal side and mirror image on the oral side.

Timing of Cleft Palate Repair

The appropriate timing of the cleft palate repair has been debated over the years. Some surgeons have advocated early palate repair within the first year, whereas others have advocated delaying the palate repair until as late as 5 years of age. Most centers now do the palate repair between 9 and 12 months of age unless there are significant airway issues resulting from mandibular micrognathia as seen in Pierre Robin sequence.

It is generally acknowledged that early palate repair results in better speech, with a lower incidence of velopharyngeal insufficiency (Hardin-Jones & Jones, 2005; Murthy, Sendhilnathan, & Hussain, 2010). However, some surgeons have argued in the past that early palate repair (rather than inherent dysplasia of the bones) is the primary cause of restricted maxillary growth in patients with CLP.

Because of that belief, Schweckendiek (1955) advocated closing the velum at around 6 months, using an obturator for the hard palate, and finally repairing the hard palate around 4 or 5 years of age. His theory was that this procedure promoted velopharyngeal closure while avoiding restriction in maxillary growth, which causes midface deficiency and class III malocclusion (Blocksma, Leuz, & Mellerstig, 1975; Dingman & Grabb, 1971; Liao, Yang, Wang, Yun, & Huang, 2010; Perko, 1979; Schweckendiek, 1966; Schweckendiek, 1968; Schweckendiek, 1983; Schweckendiek & Doz, 1978). However, studies of the results of this two-stage approach have not proved this theory (Holland et al., 2007; Pradel et al., 2009). Several studies showed a high percentage of the patients treated with this method failed to develop acceptable speech and required pharyngeal flaps (Bardach, Morris, & Olin, 1984; Cosman & Falk, 1980; Fara & Brousilova, 1988; Fara, Brousilova, Hrivnakova, & Tvrdek, 1992; Jackson, McLennan, & Scheker, 1983). Other studies found that with the delayed palatoplasty, the hard palate is actually more difficult to close and greater orthodontic effort is needed to achieve an aligned dentoalveolar arch (Cosman & Falk, 1980; Fara et al., 1992; Jackson et al., 1983; Smahel & Horak, 1993).

SPEECH NOTES

Timing of Cleft Palate Repair

Overall, early palate repair (within the first year) can reduce the incidence of velopharyngeal insufficiency and the development of compensatory speech productions. In fact, after the palatoplasty, most children are able to catch up to their unaffected peers in speech sound development.

If the patient has not had an early palate repair, a pharyngeal flap is often done in conjunction with the repair, and speech therapy is usually needed. Once the palate repair is done, the parents should be instructed on how to actively stimulate the imitation of oral sounds, beginning with plosives.

Finally, studies showed that there is virtually no difference in facial growth between patients who have early palate repair and those who have the two-stage procedure with delayed palate repair (Fara et al., 1992; Smahel & Horak, 1993).

Surgery for Velopharyngeal Insufficiency/ Incompetence (VPI)

Velopharyngeal insufficiency following a palatal repair can be caused by a number of factors. Scarring from the initial palatoplasty can shorten the velum, making it impossible to reach the posterior pharyngeal wall during speech. In addition, there may be muscular dysfunction, resulting in poor movement of the velum. Despite the best palatoplasty procedures, most centers report a 20% to 30% rate of velopharyngeal insufficiency in patients with cleft palate despite the surgical repair (Naran, Ford, & Losee, 2017).

Velopharyngeal insufficiency is not just caused by cleft palate; it can be caused by a variety of other structural causes (see the chapter *Speech/Resonance Disorders and Velopharyngeal*

Dysfunction). In addition, some patients have velopharyngeal incompetence because of neuromuscular dysfunction. Both forms of VPI (due to abnormal anatomy or abnormal neurophysiology) require surgical correction or prosthetic management if surgery is not an option.

There are several surgical procedures that are designed to correct VPI. All of them are considered a type of pharyngoplasty. All pharyngoplasty procedures involve introducing something into the velopharyngeal opening to reduce the size of the gap. As a result, there is always a risk of compromising the upper airway.

The goals of VPI surgery are to "normalize" velopharyngeal closure for speech while avoiding symptomatic airway compromise. As such, the surgeon tries to ensure that the velopharyngeal port not only closes completely for oral speech but also opens adequately for nasal breathing and the production of nasal sounds.

Presurgical Management

Before considering surgery for VPI, it is important to obtain a speech evaluation that includes an assessment of velopharyngeal function. This is necessary to confirm the diagnosis of VPI and to rule out velopharyngeal mislearning as the cause of the speech characteristics. It is important to ensure that the surgery will make a sufficient difference in the child's speech and communication skills to warrant the surgical risks.

The patient should also undergo an evaluation to rule out airway obstruction. Enlarged tonsils, adenoid hypertrophy, or micrognathia (as is common with Pierre Robin sequence) may portend airway obstruction in the immediate postoperative period as well as long-term problems with obstructive sleep apnea (OSA). Some centers advocate routine tonsillectomy before pharyngoplasty, although this is usually not necessary unless the tonsils are enlarged (bigger than 2+). If tonsillectomy is indicated, it should precede the pharyngoplasty by at least 6 weeks so that the raw surfaces

are well healed. Although adenoidectomy is usually not recommended for patients with repaired cleft palate, an adenoidectomy prior to pharyngoplasty may allow the surgeon to position the flap higher in the nasopharynx for better speech results and to avoid port obstruction postoperatively. Therefore, a conservative adenoidectomy (excising the upper portion only) at the time of tonsillectomy is often appropriate, although it may worsen the VPI until the pharyngoplasty is done.

Patients with velocardiofacial/22q11.2 deletion syndrome (VCFS/22q deletion syndrome) often have carotid arteries that course medially so that they are beneath the posterior pharyngeal wall rather than in their normal lateral position (D'Antonio & Marsh, 1987; Finkelstein et al., 1993; MacKenzie-Stepner et al., 1987; Ross, Witzel, Armstrong, & Thomson, 1996). These displaced carotid arteries can often be seen pulsating on the posterior pharyngeal wall through nasopharyngoscopy (Ysunza et al., 2004). Some surgeons order a magnetic resonance imaging (MRI) or magnetic resonance angiography (MRA) before the pharyngoplasty to identify the position of the arteries (Krugman & Brant-Zawadski, 1997; Lai, Lo, Wong, Wang, & Yun, 2004; Mitnick, Bello, Golding-Kushner, Argamaso, & Shprintzen, 1996). Others feel that imaging is unnecessary because the vessels can be found by palpating the pharyngeal walls when the patient is in surgery (Mehendale & Sommerlad, 2004; Witt, Miller, Marsh, Muntz, & Grames, 1998).

Following the presurgical evaluation, some patients are found to be poor candidates for surgical intervention of VPI. In fact, surgery may not be appropriate for patients with the following conditions: significant airway obstruction that is not well managed; neurological conditions, particularly those that are progressive; significant cognitive disability; severe hearing loss or deafness; previous oropharyngeal radiation; a bleeding disorder; and in rare cases, a carotid artery that is medialized in the posterior pharynx.

Correction Techniques for VPI

There are several pharyngoplasty techniques for the correction of VPI. The choice of technique is often determined by the size, location, and cause of the opening; the history of airway obstruction; and the surgeon's experience and preference. These techniques are described in the following sections.

Furlow Z-Palatoplasty

Because of its success as a primary cleft palate repair procedure, the Furlow Z-plasty technique is now being used as a secondary technique to redo the palate when the original repair was a different approach (see Figure 17-7) (Deren et al., 2005; Lindsey & Davis, 1996; Perkins, Lewis, Gruss, Eblen, & Sie, 2005; Por, Tan, Chang, & Chen, 2010; Sie & Gruss, 2002; Sie, Tampakopoulou, Sorom, Gruss, & Eblen, 2001). This repair has two advantages: lengthens the palate with the Z-plasty technique and guarantees reconstruction of the levator sling. This is effective in correcting cases of mild VPI where there is a very narrow velopharyngeal opening of 5 mm or less. The Furlow procedure has also become the typical technique used to repair a submucous cleft palate that results in velopharyngeal insufficiency. Disadvantages of this technique include the fact that it is not effective for larger openings and is somewhat prone to fistula development in patients with cleft palate.

Pharyngeal Wall Augmentation

When the velopharyngeal opening is small (10 mm in diameter or less) and localized, some surgeons use posterior pharyngeal wall augmentation (Witt et al., 1997). With this procedure, a substance is injected in the posterior pharyngeal wall in the area of the velopharyngeal opening. The injection is placed deep in the superior pharyngeal constrictors but superficial to the prevertebral fascia. The augmentation can even be done in the posterior border of the velum. Initially, over-correction is required in anticipation of some resorption. In addition, more than one injection may be necessary

to achieve the desired results. **FIGURE 17-8** illustrates velopharyngeal insufficiency prior to the implant and then the closure that occurs with the augmented posterior pharyngeal wall.

Various materials have been previously used for augmentation, including calcium hydroxylapatite, cartilage, fascia, silicone, porous polyethylene, proplast, and even Teflon™ (Brigger, Ashland, & Hartnick, 2010; Cantarella, Mazzola, Mantovani, Baracca, & Pignataro, 2011; Dejonckere & van Wijngaarden, 2001; Denny, Marks, & Oliff-Carneol, 1993; Gray, Pinborough-Zimmerman, & Catten, 1999; Leuchter, Schweizer, Hohlfeld, & Pasche, 2009; Remacle, Bertrand, Eloy, & Marbaix, 1990; Terris & Goode, 1993; Trigos, Ysunza, Gonzalez, & Vazquez, 1988; Ulkur et al., 2008; Witt et al., 1997; Wolford, Oelschlaeger, & Deal, 1989). Currently, the main materials used for pharyngeal augmentation are fat and Deflux, which is a gel-like substance.

Sphincter Pharyngoplasty

The sphincter pharyngoplasty, also called Orticochea sphincteroplasty (Orticochea, 1970; Orticochea, 1983; Orticochea, 1997; Orticochea, 1999), was designed to create a sphincter that

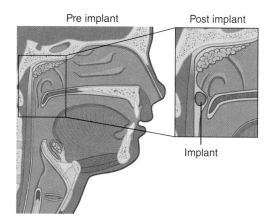

FIGURE 17-8 Pharyngeal augmentation. Note velopharyngeal insufficiency prior to the implant and then the closure that occurs with the augmentation of the posterior pharyngeal wall.

encircles the velopharyngeal port (**FIGURE 17-9**). In this procedure, bilateral, superiorly based myomucosal flaps are raised from the posterior faucial pillars, which include the palatopharyngeus muscles (Marsh, 2009). These flaps are rotated posteriorly and inset into a transverse incision in the nasopharynx, just at the level of velopharyngeal closure. This effectively narrows the lateral aspects of the pharynx. A small, superiorly based

pharyngeal flap can then be raised and attached to the lateral flaps. This leaves a single round port (opening) of about 1 cm in diameter in the center of the pharynx for nasal breathing, nasal drainage, and the production of nasal sounds.

Initially, it was felt that this procedure would create a dynamic sphincter that would completely close for oral sounds because of the muscles that were transposed in the flaps. However,

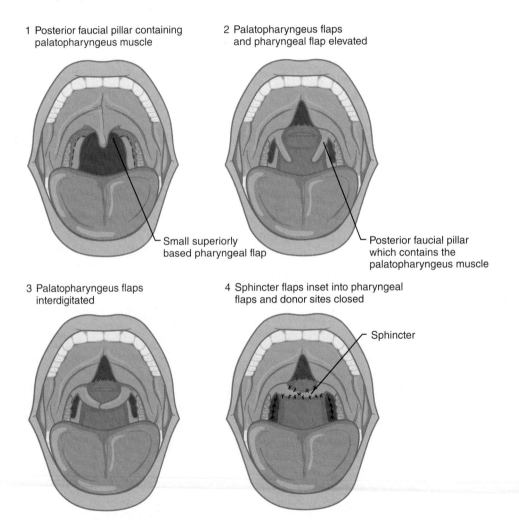

FIGURE 17-9 Sphincter pharyngoplasty. Bilateral myocutaneous flaps are raised from the posterior faucial pillars, which include the palatopharyngeus muscles. These muscles are rotated posteriorly and inset into a transverse incision on the posterior pharyngeal wall, just at the level of velopharyngeal closure. A small, superiorly based flap may also be raised and attached to the lateral flaps. This effectively narrows the velopharyngeal port for speech.

recent studies have shown that the muscle fibers in the sphincter are actually passive and that all movements seen postoperatively are caused by the contraction of the superior constrictor muscles and the movement of the velum. Therefore, it actually serves as a partial obturator for the port. The sphincter pharyngoplasty procedure has undergone a series of modifications. In its most current and widely used form, it now exists with the Jackson modification (Jackson, 1985; Jackson, McGlynn, Huskie, & Dip, 1980; Jackson & Silverton, 1977; Losken, Williams, Burstein, Malick, & Riski, 2003; Marsh, 2009; Sie et al., 1998).

Because the sphincter pharyngoplasty narrows the lateral borders of the velopharyngeal sphincter, it has been advocated for use with narrow coronal gaps that include poor lateral pharyngeal wall motion or for corner gaps caused by deep lateral pharyngeal recesses. The sphincter pharyngoplasty can be done unilaterally if the opening is in just one corner. It is also appropriate for treatment of velopharyngeal incompetence secondary to unilateral palatal paralysis or unilateral velar dysplasia as is commonly seen in hemifacial microsomia (Lin, Wang, Cheong, & Lo, 2010).

Pharyngeal Flap

The pharyngeal flap is the most commonly used procedure for correction of VPI (Cable, Canady, Karnell, Karnell, & Malick, 2004). It is designed to be a passive, soft-tissue obturator that is placed in the middle of the velopharyngeal port (Tharanon, Stella, & Epker, 1990; Trier, 1985a; Vedung, 1995; Wu & Epker, 1990; Yoshida, Stella, Ghali, & Epker, 1992).

The pharyngeal flap procedure is done by making an incision in the posterior pharyngeal wall beginning at the top of the nasopharynx, down to the area near the base of the tongue, then transversely, and finally, up again. This forms a superiorly based pharyngeal flap that includes the mucosal surface and the underlying musculature all the way down to the prevertebral fascia of the spinal column. Next, the velum is split up to the hard palate. The flap from the posterior pharyngeal wall is elevated and then sutured into the velum, forming a bridge between the posterior pharyngeal wall and the velum. The pharyngeal flap is lined with mucosal flaps from the nasal side of the velum to prevent the natural tendency of a flap to tube and narrow. A port is left on each side of the flap to allow for normal nasal breathing, drainage of nasal secretions, and production of nasal sounds. To keep the ports patent, stents are sometimes placed in the ports and kept there overnight. They are then removed the next day.

Because the pharyngeal flap is placed in the middle of the nasopharynx, it is effective in the treatment of midline gaps (which are most common following a cleft repair) and large gaps in the anterior–posterior dimension (Saman & Tatum, 2012). **FIGURE 17-10A** shows a lateral view of a pharyngeal flap as would be seen by lateral videofluoroscopy. **FIGURE 17-10B** shows a diagram of a superior view of the pharynx before and after placement of the pharyngeal flap as would be seen through nasopharyngoscopy. Note the pharyngeal flap in the midline and the open lateral ports on either side. **FIGURE 17-10C** is a lateral radiograph showing the pharyngeal flap connecting the velum and posterior pharyngeal wall. **FIGURE 17-11** shows pharyngeal flaps as viewed through nasopharyngoscopy. In these examples, the ports are open for nasal breathing. During oral speech production, the lateral pharyngeal walls move medially to close against the flap, thus completely closing the lateral ports (Forrest, Klaiman, & Mason, 2009).

There are several factors that determine the success of a pharyngeal flap in correcting VPI. One factor is the vertical position of the flap in the nasopharynx (Skolnick & McCall, 1972). For best results, the flap should be set as high as possible, preferably at the level of the skull base and hard palate because this is the area of maximum lateral pharyngeal wall movement. In correct position, the flap should be too high to be visible through an intraoral examination.

A

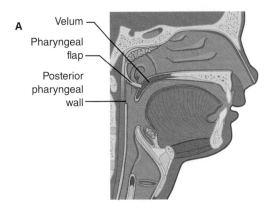

Velum

Pharyngeal flap

Posterior pharyngeal wall

A

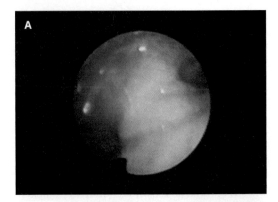

B

Pharynx prior to a pharyngeal flap

Pharynx with a pharyngeal flap

Posterior pharyngeal wall

Lateral port

Lateral pharyngeal wall

Velum (nasal surface)

Pharyngeal flap

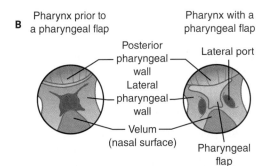

B

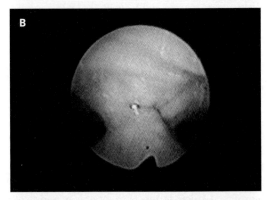

C

Pharyngeal flap

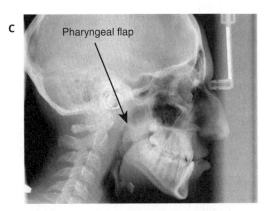

C

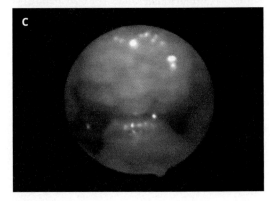

FIGURE 17-10 Pharyngeal flap. **(A)** A lateral view of a pharyngeal flap as would be seen through lateral videofluoroscopy. The flap is raised from the posterior pharyngeal wall and then sutured into the velum. **(B)** A superior view of the pharyngeal flap, as would be seen through nasopharyngoscopy. On the right is a view of the pharynx with a pharyngeal flap during nasal breathing. **(C)** A lateral radiograph showing the pharyngeal flap connecting the velum and posterior pharyngeal wall.

FIGURE 17-11 Pharyngeal flaps as viewed through nasopharyngoscopy during nasal breathing. In each example, note the pharyngeal flap is in midline and the lateral ports are open on each side.

Another important factor in the success of a flap is its width. A wide flap is preferable to a narrow flap because it increases the possibility of lateral port closure during speech. In addition, the wider the base of the flap, the greater the blood supply will be, which lowers the chance of flap dehiscence.

Finally, flaps should be as long as possible because if they are too short, they will be under tension. Tension or limited blood supply can result in more scarring and contraction, which adversely affects the function of the flap. In general, a pharyngeal flap should be wide and set as high as possible in the pharynx for best speech outcomes.

In addition to these surgical factors, the function of the velopharyngeal mechanism following the placement of the flap is affected by the patient's lateral pharyngeal wall movement (Argamaso et al., 1980). Patients with a sagittal pattern of closure or good lateral pharyngeal wall movement preoperatively have the best prognosis for total correction of VPI with a pharyngeal flap. Patients with poor lateral wall motion require a wider flap for total correction. A topic of some debate is whether the extent of lateral wall movement changes with the introduction of the pharyngeal flap. Some researchers have found no change in lateral wall motion postoperatively (Lewis & Pashayan, 1980), whereas others have reported adaptation of lateral pharyngeal wall adduction to different flap widths (Karling, Henningsson, Larson, & Isberg, 1999).

Regardless, the challenge for the surgeon is to make the flap wide enough for speech yet not so wide that it causes upper airway obstruction with hyponasality and OSA (Ysunza et al., 1993). When there is hypotonia, as in VCFS/22q deletion syndrome, or a compromised airway caused by retrognathia, the surgeon may need to compromise perfect speech results for a functional airway.

Choice of Procedure

The choice of a surgical procedure to treat VPI is usually dependent on the cause, the size, and the location of the opening. It can also be dependent on the patient's medical condition, the size of the airway, and previous surgeries. Finally, the selected procedure is influenced by the surgeon's experience,

skill, and surgical preference (Abdel-Aziz, El-Hoshy, & Ghandour, 2011; Armour, Fischbach, Klaiman, & Fisher, 2005; Seagle, Mazaheri, Dixon-Wood, & Williams, 2002; Witt & D'Antonio, 1993; Ysunza et al., 2002).

For small openings, treatment may involve augmentation of the posterior pharyngeal wall or a Furlow Z-palatoplasty. Larger gaps require a sphincter or a pharyngeal flap. If the velopharyngeal opening is in one or both sides, a unilateral or bilateral sphincter pharyngoplasty should be considered. If the opening is in midline, then a pharyngeal flap would work best.

Because any of these procedures may fail, it is important that surgical correction be performed with this possibility in mind. For instance, a posterior wall augmentation can usually be "upgraded" to either a pharyngeal flap or sphincter pharyngoplasty operation. Although the superiorly based pharyngeal flap is the gold standard and provides the highest chance of success, particularly for children with cleft palate, it carries a higher incidence of airway obstruction and OSA (Cole, Banerji, Hollier, & Stal, 2008). However, if a flap needs to be taken down because of airway obstruction, it can easily be converted to a simple augmentation, a redo palatoplasty, or a sphincter pharyngoplasty. On the other hand, if a sphincter pharyngoplasty fails to correct VPI, it is not as easy to convert to a pharyngeal flap.

Further research on the outcomes of each procedure for different patient populations is greatly needed. One issue that complicates this research is that centers vary in their criteria for determining success. In some centers (including ours at Cincinnati Children's), the surgery is considered a success only when there is normal resonance and no audible nasal emission postoperatively (aside, that is, from articulation errors). In other centers, success is defined as either "acceptable" speech or "improved" speech (Kummer, Clark, Redle, Thomsen, & Billmire, 2012; Lauck, Lee, Kummer, Billmire, & Bandaranayake, 2006). Centers also vary in who determines success (the surgeon, the speech-language pathologist, or the family) and the procedures for measuring success (perceptual judgment and/or instrumental assessment). Until there is standardization of the measurement of success, it will be impossible to compare studies of surgical efficacy.

Potential Complications

Regardless of the type of VPI surgery, there is always a risk of unwanted complications. Complications from pharyngeal augmentation include infections, extrusion, reabsorption, and even migration of the material after insertion. Granuloma formation and migration of the material leading to embolus have been associated with Teflon implantation, so it is no longer used. These implants are not always effective because they are often too small or in the wrong location to completely fill the opening and totally correct VPI. A Furlow Z-plasty can cause an oronasal fistula. All of these procedures may result in over-correction (which causes airway obstruction, OSA, and hyponasality) or under-correction (which results in persistent VPI).

Immediately after placement of the pharyngeal flap or sphincter, there is significant edema (swelling) in the pharynx. As a result, most patients exhibit hyponasality and loud snoring during the immediate postoperative period. Temporary sleep apnea is also common and usually resolves within 2 to 6 weeks postoperatively after the swelling has gone down.

Snoring is the most common consequence of pharyngoplasty, and many patients will snore to some extent for the rest of their lives. However, chronic OSA is a risk following both a pharyngeal flap and sphincterpharyngoplasty. Some authors have reported a prevalence of sleep apnea as high as 10% following pharyngeal flap surgery, but a prevalence of 5% or less is probably more common (personal unpublished data). The prevalence of sleep apnea may be less following a sphincter pharyngoplasty, but it does occur, particularly if the sphincter is low in the pharynx (Witt, Marsh, Muntz, Marty-Grames, & Watchmaker, 1996). Regardless of procedure,

sleep apnea is the greatest risk for patients who have micrognathia, such as those with Pierre Robin sequence, or for patients with neurological impairment.

Sleep apnea cannot be ignored because it can cause serious health problems if left untreated. Therefore, if OSA is suspected postoperatively, it is usually evaluated with polysomnography (a sleep study). If sleep apnea is confirmed, an evaluation is done to determine the actual cause of the obstruction. For example, the source of the obstruction in a patient with a pharyngeal flap might actually be micrognathia, glossoptosis, or even hypotonia rather than the flap. Nasopharyngoscopy can be helpful in identifying the source of obstruction. For complex cases, however, a sleep MRI is often needed.

The treatment of sleep apnea usually involves the use of continuous positive air pressure (CPAP) through a mask. This positive air pressure keeps the pharynx patent during sleep. Patients with sleep apnea are restudied about every 6 months, and in most cases the problem resolves within 1 to 2 years. In refractory cases, however, the flap needs to be taken down. Fortunately, taking down the flap does not necessarily cause deterioration in speech because the bulk of tissue from the flap, which remains in the posterior pharyngeal wall, continues to provide a pad to assist with velopharyngeal closure. The speech patterns that were learned with the flap in place are often maintained after flap division (Agarwal et al., 2003).

In addition to over-correcting VPI and causing airway obstruction, the pharyngoplasty can under-correct velopharyngeal insufficiency. One of the most common causes of persistent VPI after surgery is low placement of the pharyngeal flap or sphincter flaps. **FIGURE 17-12** shows examples of low-set sphincter pharyngoplasties, and **FIGURE 17-13** shows examples of low-set pharyngeal flaps. If the flaps can be viewed from an intraoral perspective, they are almost always too low to eliminate VPI. In addition, a low sphincter or pharyngeal flap is more

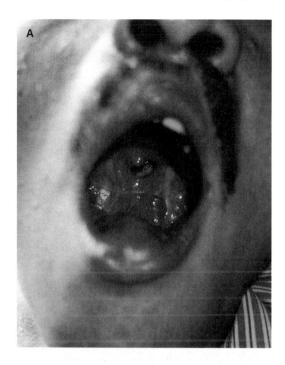

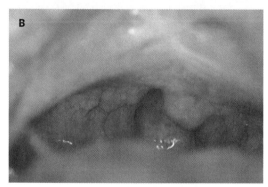

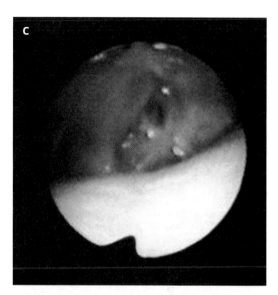

FIGURE 17-12 Unsuccessful sphincter pharyngoplasties. In each case, evidence of the sphincter can be seen intraorally, which means it is too low to assist with velopharyngeal closure. A low sphincter is also more likely to cause airway obstruction, particularly if it is at the level of the tongue base. Note in (A), the central port is very narrow, which also causes airway obstruction.

likely to cause airway obstruction, particularly if it is at the level of the tongue base.

Persistent postoperative VPI can also be caused by flaps that are too narrow to adequately obturate the nasopharyngeal port during speech (Figure 17-13D). It can even be caused by inadequate lateral pharyngeal wall motion to close the central port of a sphincter or lateral ports of a pharyngeal flap. Patients with VCFS/22q deletion syndrome often have less-than-ideal

postoperative results because of generalized hypotonicity of the velopharyngeal mechanism, which results in poor lateral pharyngeal wall movement (Kasten, Buchman, Stevenson, & Berger, 1997; Witt, Marsh, Marty-Grames, & Muntz, 1995). Finally, there may be partial or total dehiscence of the flap or sphincter days or weeks after the surgery. **FIGURE 17-14** shows an example of a dehisced pharyngeal flap. Remnants of the flap can be seen on the posterior border of the velum.

With pharyngeal flaps, secondary revisions are relatively uncommon. An appropriately placed pharyngeal flap has a greater than 90% chance for normal speech when accompanied by speech therapy. Our personal (unpublished) data shows a revision rate of 5% to 10% in pharyngeal flaps. The overall success rate of the sphincter pharyngoplasty for the elimination of hypernasality and nasal air emission is reported to be only 60% to 85% (James, Twist, Turner, & Milward,

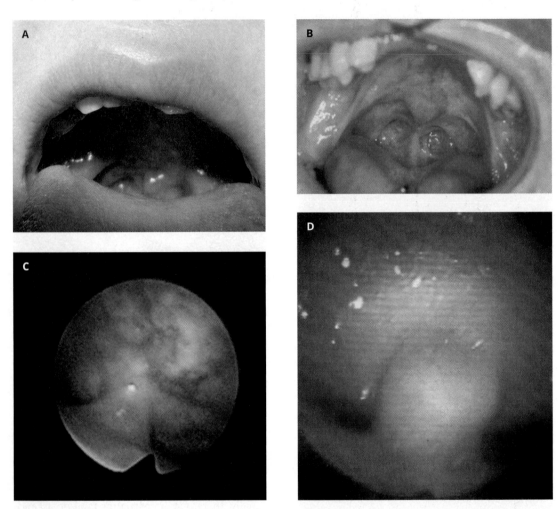

FIGURE 17-13 Unsuccessful pharyngeal flaps. **(A)** and **(B)** In each case, the pharyngeal flap can be seen intraorally, which means it is too low to assist with velopharyngeal closure. A low pharyngeal flap is also more likely to cause airway obstruction, particularly if it is at the level of the tongue base. **(C)** and **(D)** A narrow pharyngeal flap as noted through nasopharyngoscopy. Note that the lateral ports are wide in comparison to the width of the pharyngeal flap. If the lateral ports do not close completely for oral sounds, hypernasality and/or nasal emission will persist.

1996; Kasten et al., 1997; Riski, Ruff, Georgiade, & Barwick, 1992; Riski, Ruff, Georgiade, Barwick, & Edwards, 1992; Roberts & Brown, 1983; Sie et al., 1998; Witt, D'Antonio, Zimmerman, & Marsh, 1994; Yin et al., 2010). One reason for this may be patient selection. The sphincter pharyngoplasty narrows the lateral borders of the velopharyngeal port but leaves a midline opening in the anterior–posterior dimension (Ren & Wang, 1993). Therefore, it is likely to be less successful than the pharyngeal flap in correcting VPI caused by cleft palate or short velum where the gap is usually in the midline.

Evaluation of postoperative results should begin with a perceptual speech evaluation. If this evaluation reveals hypernasality and/or nasal emission or hyponasality and/or evidence of airway obstruction, a nasopharyngoscopy assessment should be done. The nasopharyngoscopy gives essential information regarding the location of a persistent gap, the function of the port(s), the function of the velum, the position and integrity of the flap or sphincter, and the airway. Armed with this information, the surgeon can do a revision as needed.

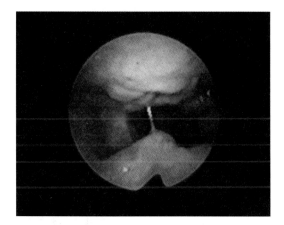

FIGURE 17-14 A dehisced pharyngeal flap. Remnants of the flap can be seen on the posterior border of the velum. The breakdown of the flap has left a large velopharyngeal opening.

If the flap or sphincter is too low to be maximally effective, the surgeon may attempt to raise the existing flap(s) to a more appropriate position. In other cases, the flap(s) may need to be completely taken down and redone. Surgical revisions may also include opening a port for better breathing if the port is too narrow or has become stenosed from scarring. More commonly, a port needs to be augmented or closed down further to correct persistent hypernasality or nasal air emission. An auxiliary flap can be raised to augment the primary flap(s) to further close a leaking port.

Regardless of the pharyngoplasty procedure chosen, the surgery must be followed by a reassessment of the speech so that an appropriate plan of speech therapy can be instituted. Because it takes about 3 months for most of the swelling to resolve and the flap or sphincter to begin to function, this is the best time for the reevaluation. Patients and parents must realize that treating VPI is a two-stage process. The surgery is done first to correct the anatomical defect. Following the surgery, speech therapy is required to help the child to eliminate compensatory productions and learn how to use the new mechanism effectively.

SPEECH NOTES

Pharyngoplasties and Speech

Regardless of the pharyngoplasty procedure chosen, best speech results are obtained if the flap(s) is placed high in the nasopharynx (at the level of the skull base). If the flap can be seen during an intraoral evaluation, it is probably too low to be effective for speech and is much more likely to cause sleep apnea because it is at the level of the tongue base.

The challenge with pharyngoplasty surgery is that it needs to result in a good balance between total obstruction of the velopharyngeal port for oral speech and a sufficiently open port for nasal breathing and production of nasal sounds. Over-correction, resulting in a small or collapsed port(s), can cause significant upper airway obstruction and OSA. It can also result in hyponasality or even denasality during speech. Under-correction, resulting in a lack of port closure during production of oral sounds, can result in persistent hypernasality and/or nasal emission. Ironically, a decrease in the size of the velopharyngeal port during speech can actually make the speech sound worse by increasing the audibility of the nasal emission/nasal rustle.

When either over-correction or under-correction occurs, surgical revision can be done to further open the port(s) or further close the remaining gap. Nasopharyngoscopy is usually done before the revision to determine the source of the obstruction or opening, which is important for the surgeon in planning the revision.

Timing of VPI Surgery

Pharyngoplasty procedures can technically be performed at a very young age. In fact, one surgical group used to advocate for simultaneous palatal repair and pharyngeal flap before the first birthday. This is no longer an acceptable practice because it often resulted in significant morbidity and the procedure was done before it was determined that it was really needed for speech.

Currently, a diagnosis of VPI must be made before considering a pharyngoplasty. This cannot be done definitively until the child begins to produce connected speech and can cooperate with the speech-language pathologist for stimulability testing. In most cases, this is around the age of 3 to 4 years. Some children with cleft palate have normal velopharyngeal function in the preschool years but develop velopharyngeal insufficiency from a growth spurt or shrinkage of the adenoid pad around puberty. Therefore, longitudinal follow-up of these patients through adolescence is very important.

In addition to the perceptual examination, evaluation of velopharyngeal function may include nasopharyngoscopy and/or videofluoroscopy. The speech-language pathologist's perceptual evaluation is the most critical, however, because surgical decisions are based on the auditory perception of the speech rather than on instrumental measures.

Once the patient has been diagnosed with VPI, surgical intervention should be done as soon as possible to avoid the development of strongly habituated compensatory productions, which are harder to correct as the child becomes older. By adulthood, the chance of success, or even improvement, with pharyngoplasty is significantly reduced and the risk of complications, such as OSA, is increased. Therefore, the risks and benefits of pharyngoplasty for adults must be carefully considered.

Although it is generally accepted that early intervention for VPI results in the best speech outcomes, surgical correction must be delayed in some cases. For example, if the child has signs of OSA, pharyngoplasty should not be done until the airway issues are resolved. In particular, patients with a history of Pierre Robin sequence with micrognathia and upper airway obstruction may not be candidates for pharyngoplasty surgery until the mandible grows and the size of the airway increases. This may require a mandibular advancement procedure (mandibular distraction), a tongue base reduction, removal of enlarged lymphoid tissue in the nasopharyngeal area, or any combination of these procedures.

Alveolar Bone Grafting

Despite the lip and palate repairs, the alveolar cleft is not repaired during these initial surgical procedures. Instead, the cleft is left open to allow anterior maxillary growth without restriction from a surgical closure or scarring. If left untreated, however, over time the gap in the arch can lead to a loss of the permanent lateral incisor and/or canine because of lack of supporting bone to secure the teeth within the alveolus. In addition, the alveolar cleft leaves the palatine segments unattached, which usually leads to lateral crossbite on the lesser segment (the side of the cleft) (**FIGURE 17-15**).

One of the greatest improvements in cleft care has been the routine implementation of alveolar bone grafting (El-Sayed & Khalil,

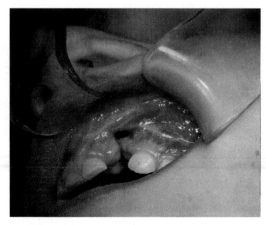

FIGURE 17-15 Nasolabial fistula. The bony cleft in the alveolus can be seen as the dark gap between the teeth.

2010; Eppley & Sadove, 2000; van Aalst, Eppley, Hathaway, & Sadove, 2005). The purpose of the alveolar bone graft is to surgically insert bone into the alveolar cleft at an appropriate time. This allows eruption and retention of the permanent dentition through the bony support from the graft and completes the dental arch.

Alveolar Bone Grafting Techniques

Primary alveolar bone grafting (at the time of lip repair) has been described in the past but has largely been abandoned. Currently, secondary alveolar bone grafting is the universally performed method.

To correct an alveolar cleft, the two alveolar segments are surgically placed in a normal arch alignment and then secured with a bone graft. The bone graft can be harvested from the hip (iliac crest), or allograft bone (obtained from a donor) can be used. With this procedure, the edges of the cleft are opened. Then, the floor of the nose is sewn closed, and the bone graft is packed into the alveolar space. Finally, the gingiva is repaired over the bone graft. This approach helps build up the bone deficiency in both the nasal base and para-alar areas. About 3 months later, when the bone is solidly healed, the orthodontist can then direct the teeth into the appropriate positions along a complete maxillary alveolar arch.

Once healed, the bone graft provides a stable scaffold for the permanent dentition and the upper lip. **FIGURE 17-16A** is an intraoperative photo of a patient just before the bone graft. The picture shows the gingival and periosteal tissues reflected off the alveolar cleft. Note how the cleft extends to the floor of the nose. **FIGURE 17-16B** is another intraoperative photo of the same patient following the bone graft insertion and filling of the alveolar cleft with the graft material. **FIGURE 17-16C** shows a picture of the grafted cleft alveolus following orthodontic therapy that aligned the erupted teeth into perfect form.

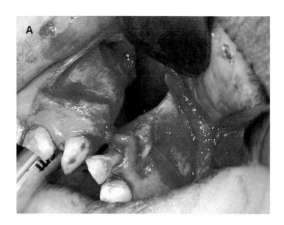

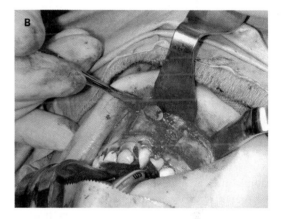

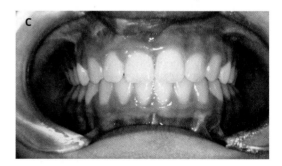

FIGURE 17-16 Bone graft for an alveolar cleft. **(A)** An intraoperative photo of a patient just before the bone graft. Note how the cleft extends to the floor of the nose. **(B)** An intraoperative photo of the same patient following the bone graft insertion and filling of the alveolar cleft with the graft material. **(C)** The grafted cleft alveolus following orthodontic therapy that aligned the erupted teeth into perfect form.

Potential Complications

Certain complications can occur with bone grafting. Bleeding and infection are the most common adverse circumstances. Infrequently, the bone graft does not take, causing a breakdown of the repair and persistence of the fistula.

Timing of Alveolar Bone Grafting

Secondary bone grafting is done when the roots of the permanent lateral incisor or canine (both located at the edges of the cleft) are about two-thirds developed and ready to erupt. Bone grafting is specific to the patient and depends on the child's dental development. It is done just in time to provide support for the eruption of these teeth, which usually occurs sometime between 6 and 11 years of age (Cohen, Polley, & Figueroa, 1993; Walia, 2011). The pediatric dentist or orthodontist uses serial radiographs to determine when the tooth roots are mature. The lateral incisor erupts earlier than the cuspid. Therefore, the actual timing of the bone graft depends on which tooth is more at risk for that child.

While waiting for maturation, the orthodontist uses an expanding device to put the arch segments into correct alignment. Once aligned, a holding device (a retainer or a lingual arch wire) is used for retention.

Oronasal Fistula Repair

A fistula is an abnormal opening between two hollow organs in the body. As noted above, the alveolus under the lip is not repaired at the time of the primary palatoplasty, thus leaving a cleft or nasolabial fistula (often called an intentional fistula) until the time of the bone graft. There may also be an unintentional oronasal fistula, which is an opening between the oral and nasal cavities that occurs when the palate fails to heal after a palatoplasty (Waite & Waite, 1996). This fistula is usually closed at the time of alveolar bone grafting.

Unintentional fistulas in the palate have been reported to occur in 5% to 30% of cases. These fistulas are often blamed on growth of the patient or expansion of the dental arch. However, growth and expansion do not actually cause fistulas. Instead, they can cause existing fistulas to get bigger and become symptomatic.

Oronasal Fistula Repair Techniques

Closure of a fistula can be a daunting task. Closure is usually attempted with the use of local autogenous (the individual's own) tissue first. If there is no adequate local tissue or the use of local tissue has failed in a previous closure attempt, a more complex procedure may be necessary.

Methods of closing a fistula include the use of flaps of tissue from the turbinates, the buccal (cheek) mucosa, and even the tongue (**FIGURE 17-17**) (Argamaso, 1990; Assuncao, 1993; Barone & Argamaso, 1993; Busic, Bagatin, & Boric, 1989; Coghlan, O'Regan, & Carter, 1989; Penna, Bannasch, & Stark, 2007; Pigott, Rieger, & Moodie, 1984; Posnick & Getz, 1987; Thind, Singh, & Thind, 1992).

With the tongue flap procedure, the dorsum of the tongue is sutured into the fistula and left for 2 to 3 weeks to develop its blood supply. At that point, the tongue flap is severed from the rest of the tongue

Potential Complications

Closure of an oronasal fistula can be very difficult, especially if autogenous tissue is used

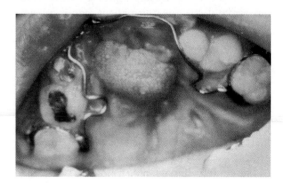

FIGURE 17-17 Fistula repair with a tongue flap. Note the tongue tissue in the anterior portion of the palate.

SPEECH NOTES

Oronasal Fistula

The effect of an oronasal fistula on speech depends on its size and location.

As a general rule, the bigger the fistula, the more it will affect speech. Actually, small fistulas can be relatively asymptomatic. They can cause slight regurgitation of food and fluids into the nasal cavity but no problem with speech. However, if the fistula is 5 mm or larger, it can cause a leak of airflow into the nasal cavity. A fistula of 1 cm or larger can cause audible nasal emission, and a fistula of 2 cm or larger can cause both audible nasal emission and hypernasality.

The effect of the fistula on speech also depends on its location. Overall, the farther posterior the fistula is on the hard palate, the less likely it will affect speech. This is because on velar sounds (/k/, /g/), the airflow is stopped by the back of the tongue against the velum and then released. The airflow then travels across the fistula, not perpendicular to it, so unless the fistula is very large, there will be no audible nasal emission. In contrast, a fistula in the anterior part of the oral cavity is more likely to cause nasal emission. A fistula in the area of the incisive foramen (a common location because this is where the three bones of the palate join) is just above the tongue tip. As the tongue tip elevates for lingual-alveolar and sibilant sounds or is blocked for bilabial plosives, the airstream may be pushed directly into the fistula, causing audible nasal emission.

Some patients compensate for a fistula by holding the tip or dorsum of the tongue against the opening to prevent the loss of airflow. This results in palatal–dorsal productions, which cause a lateral distortion.

because the mucosa on the palate is very thin. Even tongue flaps and buccal flaps can be challenging. As a result, there is about a 37% or more recurrence risk, which gets higher with subsequent repairs (Cohen, Kalinowski, LaRossa, & Randall, 1991). At times, total surgical correction is not possible, and the use of a palatal obturator is recommended instead.

Timing of Oronasal Fistula Repair

The timing of fistula repair varies. It is often done in conjunction with the bone graft to the alveolar arch (around age 7 to 9). If it is large and affecting speech, the closure may be done earlier, or a temporary speech obturator is used until the fistula can be surgically repaired.

Maxillary Advancement

Patients with craniofacial conditions, including cleft lip and palate, hemifacial microsomia, and craniosynostosis syndromes, often have maxillary growth deficiency that leads to midface retrusion. This causes a concave profile and Class III malocclusion. These patients are therefore candidates for orthognathic surgery (surgery that involves one or both of the jaws). Orthognathic surgery with maxillary advancement can result in a significant improvement in facial aesthetics and dental occlusion for this population of patients.

The purpose of maxillary advancement is to bring the maxilla into proper alignment with the mandible, thus correcting the facial profile and the malocclusion. This improves both the aesthetics and functional problems with chewing and speech production.

Maxillary Advancement Techniques

Maxillary advancement is done through a surgical approach using a Le Fort I osteotomy with or without distraction osteogenesis. These techniques are described in the following sections.

SPEECH NOTES

Tongue Flap

Although a tongue flap leaves scarring on the top of the tongue, it does not adversely affect the movement of the tongue for speech or feeding. The scar on the tongue is usually not well received by patients, however. In addition, the tongue flap can be large and bulky, thus interfering with speech. In these cases, the tongue flap can be shaved down in a later procedure.

SPEECH NOTES

Effects of Maxillary Retrusion on Speech

Maxillary retrusion with Class III malocclusion usually affects articulation of the tongue tip and lips. Although the tongue is in its normal position in the mandible, the maxillary retrusion causes the tongue tip to rest in an anterior position relative to the alveolar ridge. This can lead to fronting of lingual-alveolar and sibilant sounds, which is an obligatory distortion. If the child attempts to compensate for this misalignment of the jaws, he may use a palatal–dorsal placement for these same sounds, which results in lateral distortion. When Class III malocclusion is severe, it can even affect bilabial and labiodental sounds, often leading to the use of reverse labiodental production (upper lip against the mandibular teeth) as a substitution for both (see the chapter *Psychosocial Aspects* for more information). Finally, the posterior displacement of the maxilla leads to a small pharyngeal space, which can cause hyponasality and OSA (Demetriades, Chang, Laskarides, & Papageorge, 2010).

Le Fort Osteotomies

René Le Fort (1901) originally described the naturally occurring fracture planes in the facial skeleton. These lines of natural weakness collapse or break during trauma and are used to describe midfacial fracture patterns. Le Fort's three fracture planes are now used by surgeons when they create an osteotomy (planned surgical cut) in the facial skeleton to position the facial bones in their appropriate functional and pleasing position. **FIGURE 17-18** illustrates the levels of the three Le Fort osteotomies. **FIGURE 17-19A** shows maxillary retrusion and the cuts for a Le Fort I osteotomy. **FIGURE 17-19B** shows the position of the maxilla after the surgery.

The most common osteotomy is the Le Fort I, which includes the maxilla only. The maxilla is cut transversely, just above the tooth roots and the base of the nose. This allows the surgeon to move the alveolar arch and palate as a single unit. In addition to bringing the midface forward, the maxilla can be rotated to match midlines and tilted to correct a cant. A narrow maxilla can also be widened by further osteotomizing it into segments.

FIGURES 17-20A and **B** show a young woman with severe midface retrusion caused by maxillary deficiency. **FIGURES 17-20C** and **D** demonstrate the dramatic results of moving this segment of maxilla forward through a Le Fort I advancement. **FIGURE 17-21** shows a dramatic improvement in both profile and dental occlusion as a result of a Le Fort I advancement.

If the surgeon needs to reposition the bridge of the nose as well as the teeth (which is commonly needed for patients with Treacher Collins), a Le Fort II osteotomy is done because it includes both the maxilla and the nasal pyramid. If the cheeks have to be brought forward to correct proptosis (protrusion of the eye), which is common in

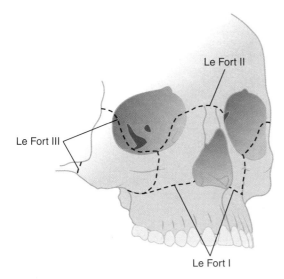

FIGURE 17-18 Le Fort osteotomies. This line drawing demonstrates the level of the various Le Fort osteotomies. The Le Fort II osteotomy also includes the territory of the Le Fort I osteotomy. The Le Fort III osteotomy also includes the territory of the Le Fort I and Le Fort II osteotomies.

patients with Crouzon and Apert syndromes, a Le Fort III osteotomy is done because it includes the maxilla, nasal pyramid, zygomas, and orbital rims. **FIGURES 17-22A** and **B** show preoperative proptosis, an open bite, and maxillary hypoplasia. **FIGURES 17-22C** and **D** show the postoperative improvement after Le Fort III advancement was done with this patient. The ultimate goals of maxillary repositioning include normal occlusion, normal-sized oral and pharyngeal cavities for resonance and breathing, and improved facial proportions.

Orthognathic surgery requires careful planning and communication between the orthodontist and surgeon. They compare the patient's current maxillary position against known normative values to determine how far and at what angle the maxilla must be moved to achieve the desired result. The orthodontist then places the teeth into correct position within the arch. Once the orthodontia is completed, the surgeon performs the procedure on plaster cast models.

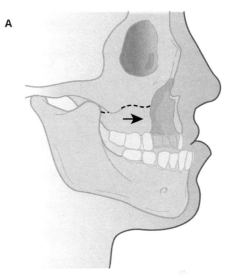

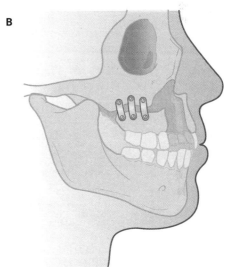

FIGURE 17-19 Maxillary advancement surgery. **(A)** Maxillary retrusion and the cuts for a Le Fort I. **(B)** The position of the maxilla after Le Fort I surgery.

Guiding surgical stents are made from these models and used in the operating room to replicate the proposed maxillary position intraoperatively. More recently, surgical planning can be done virtually on a computer instead of in the laboratory. This is more accurate and increasingly

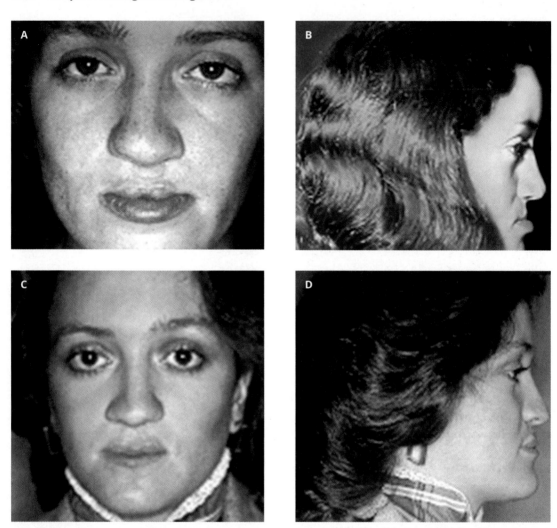

FIGURE 17-20 Le Fort I. **(A)** and **(B)** Preoperative photos that show a young girl with severe midface retrusion caused by maxillary deficiency. **(C)** and **(D)** Postoperative photos that show a remarkable change in profile and facial harmony after the Le Fort I procedure.

becoming the standard of care, especially in double jaw surgeries.

During the surgical procedure, the osteotomies are made to release the bone. The surgeon then fixes the maxilla into the advanced position with metal plates and screws. If the advancement is greater than a few millimeters, bone grafts are used to support the maxilla and prevent relapse into its original position. Postoperatively, the jaws

are held in occlusion with elastic bands, and the patient is placed on a soft pureed diet for 6 weeks.

Maxillary Distraction

Distraction osteogenesis is a method of gradually lengthening a bone by taking advantage of the fact that the body heals a fracture by laying down new bone. If the ends of a fracture are

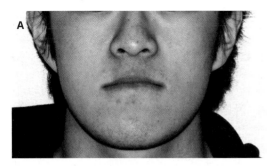

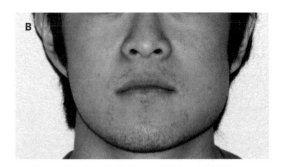

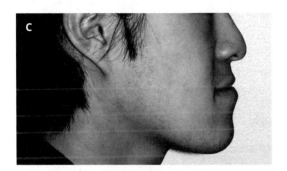

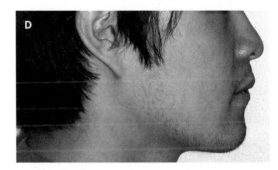

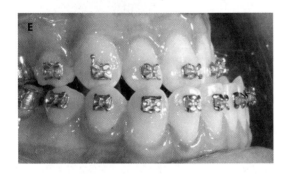

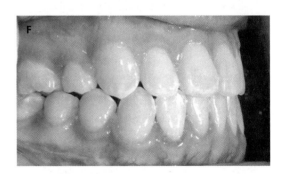

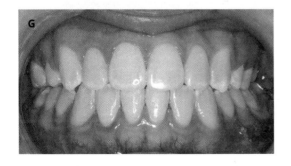

FIGURE 17-21 Le Fort I. **(A)–(D)** Preoperative photos of a young man with maxillary retrusion and dental malocclusion. **(E)–(G)** Dramatic improvement in profile, facial harmony, and dental occlusion as a result of a Le Fort I.

gradually separated, the body will create new bone to fill the gap. Distraction osteogenesis has been used relatively recently in orthognathic surgery (Cheung & Chua, 2006; Cohen, Burstein, & Williams, 1999; Denny, Kalantarian, & Hanson, 2003; Imola & Tatum, 2002; Mofid et al., 2001;

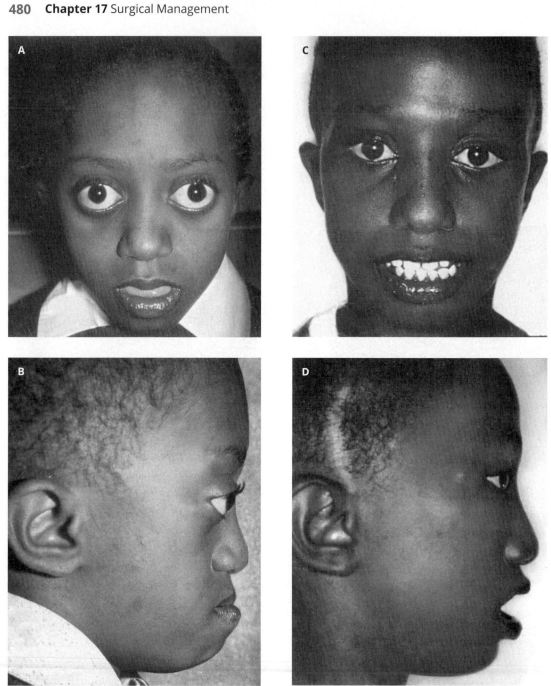

FIGURE 17-22 Le Fort III. **(A)** and **(B)** Preoperative photos of a boy with Crouzon's syndrome. **(C)** and **(D)** Postoperative pictures after Le Fort III advancement. The changes in the orbits and occlusion are dramatic.

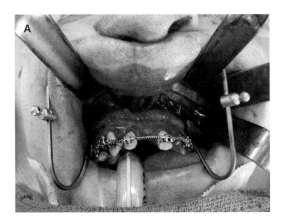

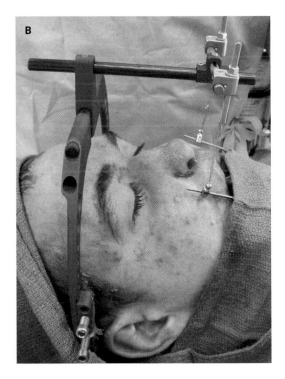

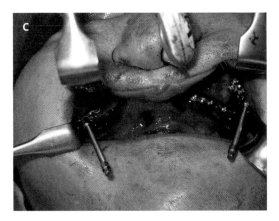

FIGURE 17-23 Maxillary distraction. **(A)** An intraoperative view of a patient who has had a maxillary osteotomy so that the maxillary device can be placed in position. **(B)** Shows how an external maxillary distraction device attaches to the skull. **(C)** An internal maxillary distractor in situ following maxillary osteotomy.

frame that supports the device and its extensions into the maxilla. An internal device is smaller and concealed within the mouth.

After several days of rest (the latent period), the distraction device is activated (the activation period) to expand and stretch the immature callus over a period of time until the maxillary segment is moved into the desired position. This stretched callus is then allowed to mature and consolidate over time to become normal bone (consolidation period). This slow, deliberate advancement allows the body to lay down new bone growth, which solidly bolsters the maxilla in its new position and eliminates the need for bone grafts to fill the large gaps (Takigawa, Uematsu, & Takada, 2010). **FIGURE 17-23A** shows an intraoperative view of a patient who has had a maxillary osteotomy so that the maxillary device can be placed in position. **FIGURE 17-23B** demonstrates how an external maxillary distraction device attaches to the skull. **FIGURE 17-23C** shows an internal maxillary distractor in situ following maxillary osteotomy. **FIGURE 17-24** shows a patient preoperatively in the distraction device and then postoperatively.

Swennen, Schliephake, Dempf, Schierle, & Malevez, 2001).

Distraction for maxillary advancement involves making a planned Le Fort osteotomy and then the placement of either an external or internal distraction device. An external device anchors onto stable cranial bone and has a large

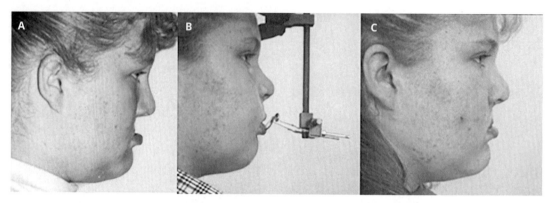

FIGURE 17-24 Distraction osteogenesis as applied to the midface. The left panel demonstrates the preoperative profile, the middle panel shows the patient at the end of distraction in her halo device, and the right panel shows the postoperative results.

Advantages of distraction over traditional surgery include a shorter surgical procedure with less blood loss and postoperative swelling. New bone is generated in the process of distraction, eliminating the need for bone grafting. Because the advancement is gradual, it can be adjusted somewhat as needed, unlike in the traditional technique. The gradual nature of the bone repositioning allows soft-tissue adaptation to occur over time, which often increases the amount of advancement that can be achieved. Finally, the living bone formation in the distraction path helps to prevent relapse.

Disadvantages of distraction include the obvious nature of the hardware and the cumbersome prolonged period of activation that involves the patient wearing the device as well as its daily activation. There may be pain, difficulty sleeping, speech distortion, eating problems, and disruption in the patient's recreational activities (Primrose et al., 2005). There is the potential for hardware to fail and require replacement during the distraction period. The majority of external devices can be removed in the office setting, but internally based hardware requires surgical removal in the operating room.

Anterior Maxillary Distraction

The traditional Le Fort I osteotomy to correct maxillary retrusion in CLP patients (with or without distraction osteogenesis) may worsen the speech because the velum moves forward with the advanced maxilla. Therefore, patients may develop velopharyngeal insufficiency postoperatively, or have a worsening of preoperative velopharyngeal insufficiency, thus requiring surgical intervention.

A new and promising technique is anterior maxillary distraction. In this technique, only the anterior maxilla is moved forward while the velum and soft palate are left intact. It involves making osteotomies horizontally in the maxilla, but instead of carrying the osteotomy all the way posteriorly (like in a traditional Le Fort I), this horizontal osteotomy is connected to two vertical osteotomies between the first and second molar teeth. This way, the posterior maxilla (with the attached soft palate and velum) is left intact; thus, there is no adverse effect on velopharyngeal function. A small distraction device (Hyrax device) is then applied to the palate, and the anterior maxillary segment is slowly distracted using the standard distraction principles.

In addition to the fact that velopharyngeal function is not affected with this procedure, other advantages are that the surgery is simpler than the traditional Le Fort I and also has less morbidity. The disadvantages are that it is not appropriate for severe cases of maxillary retrusion and does not correct hypoplasia in the malar region. As with other orthognathic surgeries, good orthodontic care is also required (Richardson, Agni, & Selvraj, 2011).

Timing of Maxillary Advancement

Orthognathic surgery of the maxilla in patients with cleft lip and palate is usually done when the patient reaches skeletal maturity. At this age, the jaws have reached their maximum growth, and all permanent teeth have erupted, allowing safe performance of the osteotomies without damage to the tooth roots. Because the mandible is the last bone to mature in the facial skeleton, waiting until mandibular growth is complete assures that the new maxillary placement will be appropriate for the mature facial bones. Consequently, this type of surgery is usually not done until age 14 to 16 in girls and 16 to 18 in boys. If the malformation is severe and the child is experiencing psychological trauma, however, corrective jaw surgery can be done at an early skeletal maturity stage (14 to 16 years).

For patients with craniosynostosis syndromes, a Le Fort III advancement is commonly done during the mixed dentition stage. This surgery helps to improve the airway, close the anterior open bite, increase the oral cavity size, and most importantly, protect the proptotic globes (relative protrusion of the eyes). Maxillary distraction for midface advancement is well suited to the younger patient because of the shorter operation time and lower blood loss as compared to traditional surgery (Cheung & Chua, 2006). Any surgery done at this age will not hold up to future growth, however. Therefore, these patients usually need a Le Fort I advancement or possibly a repeat Le Fort III advancement in the teenage years to balance the occlusion, improve facial harmony, and create a convex profile.

Potential Complications

Potential complications associated with maxillary advancement include major blood loss requiring massive transfusion, infection of the facial soft tissues, relapse of the maxilla, decreased sensation in the upper lip and midface, loss of teeth, loss of gingiva, persistent malocclusion (not correctable with orthodontia) from relapse (Kramer et al., 2004), and very rarely, blindness and stroke. There is also a risk of postoperative velopharyngeal insufficiency, particularly for those with cleft palate or submucous cleft.

To correct a relapsed maxilla, advancement must be performed again, with additional presurgical orthodontia. Loss of gingiva can be improved by periodontal correction. Loss of teeth can be masked with prosthetic replacement. Changes in sensation may correct over time, or the patient is no longer bothered by reduced sensation. Finally, an additional surgery may be needed to correct postoperative velopharyngeal insufficiency.

SPEECH NOTES

Effect of Maxillary Advancement on Speech Sound Production

A primary purpose of maxillary advancement is to normalize the occlusal relationship between the maxillary and mandibular arches. Because malocclusion is a common cause of speech sound distortion, it stands to reason that the correction of the malocclusion could improve the clarity of speech. In fact, many studies have reported improved speech following maxillary advancement without intervening speech therapy (Guyette, Polley, Figueroa, & Smith, 2001; Janulewicz et al., 2004; Kummer, Strife, Grau, Creaghead, & Lee, 1989; Lee, Whitehill, Ciocca, & Samman, 2002; Maegawa, Sells, & David, 1998; McCarthy, Coccaro, & Schwartz, 1979; Vallino, 1990; Ward, McAuliffe, Holmes, Lynham, & Monsour, 2002). It should be noted that this improvement occurs only with obligatory distortions where tongue position (articulation) was normal during production before the surgery, but the structure was abnormal, causing speech sound distortion. When there are compensatory errors resulting in abnormal tongue position, the maxillary advancement improves the potential for correction of these errors, but speech therapy is required.

SPEECH NOTES

Effect of Maxillary Advancement on Airway and Resonance

Advancement of the maxilla, and thus the velum, increases the anterior–posterior dimension of the pharyngeal cavity. This can be beneficial for patients with craniosynostosis syndromes, who often have restriction of the nasopharynx. These patients often have hyponasality and upper airway obstruction that can be improved or eliminated with the increased diameter of the pharynx and the reduction of nasal airway resistance (Dalston, 1996; Maegawa et al., 1998; Sharshar & El-Bialy, 2012; Trindade, Yamashita, Suguimoto, Mazzottini, & Trindade, 2003).

SPEECH NOTES

Effect of Maxillary Advancement on Velopharyngeal Function

For patients with a repaired cleft palate or submucous cleft, maxillary advancement can have a negative effect on velopharyngeal function even if done gradually through distraction. With the anterior movement of the maxilla and corresponding anterior movement of the velum, there is an increase in the anterior–posterior depth of the velopharyngeal port. If the velum is unable to stretch sufficiently to make up the difference, this will cause development or worsening of velopharyngeal insufficiency (Dalston, 1996; Dalston & Vig, 1984; Haapanen, Kalland, Heliovaara, Hukki, & Ranta, 1997; Heliovaara, Hukki, Ranta, & Haapanen, 2004; Heliovaara, Ranta, Hukki, & Haapanen, 2002; Janulewicz et al., 2004; Kummer et al., 1989; Maegawa et al., 1998; Niemeyer, Gomes Ade, Fukushiro, & Genaro, 2005; Okazaki et al., 1993; Satoh et al., 2004; Watzke, Turvey, Warren, & Dalston, 1990). It would seem that the gradual nature of maxillary advancement through distraction might allow for the velopharyngeal mechanism to adapt to its new situation and minimize post-advancement hypernasality. Studies have shown, however, that there is no significant difference in the risk for velopharyngeal insufficiency between traditional surgical advancement and advancement through distraction (Chanchareonsook, Whitehill, & Samman, 2007; Chua, Whitehill, Samman, & Cheung, 2010; Guyette et al., 2001; Ko, Figueroa, Guyette, Polley, & Law, 1999; Trindade et al., 2003).

Postoperative velopharyngeal insufficiency is most likely to occur in patients with cleft palate or submucous cleft, tenuous velopharyngeal closure preoperatively, or a maxillary advancement that is 10 mm or greater. Some patients have a temporary period of hypernasality and/or nasal emission postoperatively that corrects itself as the velopharyngeal structures accommodate to their new anatomic relationships. If it does not resolve within a few weeks, a pharyngoplasty is needed for correction.

Patients who have already had a pharyngeal flap for correction of velopharyngeal insufficiency pose particular challenges with maxillary advancement. Nasal intubation for the procedure is more difficult with the flap in situ. In addition, the tethering of the flap on the velum can make it more difficult to physically mobilize the maxilla forward. Finally, patients with a pharyngeal flap before maxillary advancement seem to have an increased incidence of relapse (retro positioning of the maxilla toward its original location) over time, which is presumably caused by the pull of the flap. For these reasons, if a patient has borderline velopharyngeal insufficiency and will later undergo maxillary advancement, it is advisable to perform the maxillary advancement first and the pharyngeal flap later.

Some surgeons advocate taking the pharyngeal flap down to minimize maxillary relapse, but in general this is not necessary. Fortunately, if the flap has been in place for some time, division of the flap does not always cause deterioration in velopharyngeal function. This is probably because of the residual flap tissue and possibly changes in the inclination of the pharyngeal wall that would have occurred with growth. However, the patient may be at increased risk for a recurrence of velopharyngeal insufficiency after the maxillary advancement surgery.

Before maxillary advancement surgery, it is important to counsel patients and parents regarding the risk of postoperative velopharyngeal insufficiency and the treatment if it occurs. If the patient and family are interested, a preoperative speech pathology assessment can be done to predict the probable effect of maxillary advancement on the patient's speech (Phillips, Klaiman, Delorey, & MacDonald, 2005). Otherwise, for patients with no history of cleft who are undergoing elective surgery to improve facial harmony, a simple disclosure of the risk by the surgeon is sufficient.

SUMMARY

The goals of surgical correction of cleft lip and palate are to normalize the structure for normal feeding, speech, dentition, facial profile, and aesthetics. There are several surgical approaches that can be used to correct each type of cleft. The success of the surgery is dependent upon many factors, including the location, size, and severity of the cleft; type of procedure used; and experience of the surgeon. With the improvement in surgical techniques in recent years, the functional and aesthetic outcomes of surgery have also improved.

Velopharyngeal insufficiency continues to be a risk for patients with cleft palate even after successful palate repair. The treatment requires close cooperation and teamwork between the surgeon and the speech-language pathologist for the best outcomes. Failure to work cooperatively as a team may result in unnecessary additional surgery, unnecessary speech therapy, or both. It should be remembered that VPI (both kinds) always requires surgery for correction of the structures first and then speech therapy afterward in many cases to correct the abnormal function.

Orthognathic surgery can improve aesthetic and functional problems that occur from malocclusion of the jaws. Improvement of the jaw relationship, and thus dental occlusion, can have a positive effect on speech if there were speech distortions or articulation errors caused by the malocclusion. In addition, maxillary advancement can improve airway obstruction and eliminate hyponasality in some cases. However, there is a risk of postoperative velopharyngeal insufficiency following maxillary advancement, particularly in patients with cleft palate or submucous cleft. If desired, the speech-language pathologist can help to predict that risk and also help with the management of it if it actually occurs postoperatively. Fortunately, anterior maxillary distraction is a new and promising technique to achieve the objectives of maxillary advancement without adversely affecting velopharyngeal function.

Overall, patients with CLP and other craniofacial conditions often require a series of surgeries beginning in infancy and finally ending after skeletal growth is complete. See TABLE 17-1 for a summary of the timeline of surgical procedures for patients with CLP. Although it is a journey through time, most patients and families can expect greatly improved aesthetics and normal function as a result of these procedures.

TABLE 17-1 **Timetable of Surgeries for Patients with Cleft Lip and Palate**		
Approximate Age	**Surgery**	**Type of Cleft**
Newborn	Premaxillary orthopedics Lip adhesion (optional)	Bilateral cleft lip Cleft lip
3 months	Lip repair	Cleft lip
10–12 months	Palate repair	Cleft palate
3–5 years	Surgery for velopharyngeal insufficiency if necessary	Cleft palate
School age	Lip and/or nose revision if needed	Cleft lip
7–9 years	Bone graft to the maxilla Nasolabial fistula repair	Cleft lip Cleft lip and palate
14–15 for girls 17–18 for boys	Le Fort I maxillary advancement if needed	Cleft lip and palate

FOR REVIEW AND DISCUSSION

1. What is the rule of 10s, and how does it relate to cleft lip repair?

2. What are the reasons for aligning the maxillary segments before cleft lip surgery? Why is this not done in all cases? What are the different methods?

3. Describe the differences among the von Langenbeck, the Wardill-Kilner V-Y pushback, and the Furlow Z-palatoplasty as if you were explaining it to a parent.

4. Discuss the general timing of cleft palate repair. What are the potential advantages and disadvantages of early versus late repair of the palate?

5. Discuss the reason for alveolar bone grafting, and describe how and when it is done as if you were explaining it to a parent.

6. List the types of surgeries that can be done for VPI (both kinds), and describe the basic procedures for each as if you were explaining it to a parent. What factors influence the choice of procedure for the patient?

7. Where should a pharyngeal flap be placed for best speech results and a decreased risk of sleep apnea?

8. Discuss the potential complications of surgery for velopharyngeal insufficiency. Which patients may be at particular risk?

9. What are the problems that can occur with pharyngoplasty surgery if there is overcorrection? What changes in speech production could occur with a sphincter or pharyngeal flap that improves velopharyngeal closure but does not completely close the port during oral speech?

10. What is orthognathic surgery? What is the goal of this type of surgery?

11. Explain the origin of the Le Fort classification system. What is the difference between Le Fort I, Le Fort II, and Le Fort III osteotomies?

12. Why do children with a history of CLP often benefit from maxillary advancement? Discuss the appropriate timing of this surgery. What are the potential risks and benefits of maxillary advancement on speech and resonance?

REFERENCES

Abdel-Aziz, M., El-Hoshy, H., & Ghandour, H. (2011). Treatment of velopharyngeal insufficiency after cleft palate repair depending on the velopharyngeal closure pattern. *The Journal of Craniofacial Surgery, 22*(3), 813–817.

Agarwal, T., Sloan, G. M., Zajac, D., Uhrich, K. S., Meadows, W., & Lewchalermwong, J. A. (2003). Speech benefits of posterior pharyngeal flap are preserved after surgical flap division for obstructive sleep apnea: Experience with division of 12 flaps. *Journal of Craniofacial Surgery, 14*(5), 630–636.

Argamaso, R. V. (1990). The tongue flap: Placement and fixation for closure of postpalatoplasty fistulae. *Cleft Palate Journal, 27*(4), 402–110.

Argamaso, R. V., Shprintzen, R. J., Strauch, B., Lewin, M. L., Daniller, A. L., Ship, A. G., & Croft, C. B. (1980). The role of lateral pharyngeal wall movement in pharyngeal flap surgery. *Plastic and Reconstructive Surgery, 66*(2), 214–219.

Armour, A., Fischbach, S., Klaiman, P., & Fisher, D. M. (2005). Does velopharyngeal closure pattern affect the success of pharyngeal flap pharyngoplasty? *Plastic and Reconstructive Surgery, 115*(1), 45–52; discussion 53.

Assuncao, A. G. (1993). The design of tongue flaps for the closure of palatal fistulas. *Plastic and Reconstructive Surgery, 91*(5), 806–810.

Bae, Y. C., Kim, J. H., Lee, J., Hwang, S. M., & Kim, S. S. (2002). Comparative study of the extent of palatal lengthening by different methods. *Annals of Plastic Surgery, 48*(4), 359–364.

Bardach, J., Morris, H. L., & Olin, W. H. (1984). Late results of primary veloplasty: The Marburg Project. *Plastic and Reconstructive Surgery, 73*(2), 207–218.

Barone, C. M., & Argamaso, R. V. (1993). Refinements of the tongue flap for closure of difficult palatal fistulas. *Journal of Craniofacial Surgery, 4*(2), 109–111.

Bhuskute, A. A., & Tollefson, T. T. (2016). Cleft lip repair, nasoalveolar molding, and primary cleft rhinoplasty. *Facial Plastic Surgery Clinics of North America, 24*(4), 453–466.

Blocksma, R., Leuz, C. A., & Mellerstig, K. E. (1975). A conservative program for managing cleft palates without the use of mucoperiosteal flaps. *Plastic and Reconstructive Surgery, 55*(2), 160–169.

Brauer, R. O., & Cronin, T. D. (1983). The Tennison lip repair revisited. *Plastic and Reconstructive Surgery, 71*(5), 633–642.

Brigger, M. T., Ashland, J. E., & Hartnick, C. J. (2010). Injection pharyngoplasty with calcium hydroxylapatite for velopharyngeal insufficiency: Patient selection and technique. *Archives of Otolaryngology-Head & Neck Surgery, 136*(7), 666–670.

Brothers, D. B., Dalston, R. W., Peterson, H. D., & Lawrence, W. T. (1995). Comparison of the Furlow double-opposing Z-palatoplasty with the Wardill-Kilner procedure for isolated clefts of the soft palate. *Plastic and Reconstructive Surgery, 95*(6), 969–977.

Brown, A. S., Cohen, M. A., & Randall, P. (1983). Levator muscle reconstruction: Does it make a difference? *Plastic and Reconstructive Surgery, 72*(1), 1–8.

Busic, N., Bagatin, M., & Boric, V. (1989). Tongue flaps in repair of large palatal defects. *International Journal of Oral Maxillofacial Surgery, 18*(5), 291–293.

Cable, B. B., Canady, J. W., Karnell, M. P., Karnell, L. H., & Malick, D. N. (2004). Pharyngeal flap surgery: Long-term outcomes at the University of Iowa. *Plastic and Reconstructive Surgery, 113*(2), 475–478.

Cantarella, G., Mazzola, R. F., Mantovani, M., Baracca, G., & Pignataro, L. (2011). Treatment of velopharyngeal insufficiency by pharyngeal and velar fat injections. *Otolaryngology-Head & Neck Surgery, 145*(3), 401–403.

Chanchareonsook, N., Whitehill, T. L., & Samman, N. (2007). Speech outcome and velopharyngeal function in cleft palate: Comparison of Le Fort I maxillary osteotomy and distraction osteogenesis: Early results. *The Cleft Palate-Craniofacial Journal, 44*(1), 23–32.

Cheung, L. K., & Chua, H. D. (2006). A meta-analysis of cleft maxillary osteotomy and distraction osteogenesis. *International Journal of Oral & Maxillofacial Surgery, 35*(1), 14–24.

Chua, H. D., Whitehill, T. L., Samman, N., & Cheung, L. K. (2010). Maxillary distraction versus orthognathic surgery in cleft lip and palate patients: Effects on speech and velopharyngeal function. *International Journal of Oral and Maxillofacial Surgery, 39*(7), 633–640.

Coghlan, K., O'Regan, B., & Carter, J. (1989). Tongue flap repair of oronasal fistulae in cleft palate patients: A review of 20 patients. *Journal of Craniomaxillofacial Surgery, 17*(6), 255–259.

Cohen, M., Polley, J. W., & Figueroa, A. A. (1993). Secondary (intermediate) alveolar bone grafting. *Clinics in Plastic Surgery, 20*(4), 691–705.

Cohen, S. R., Burstein, F. D., & Williams, J. K. (1999). The role of distraction osteogenesis in the management of craniofacial disorders. *Annals of the Academy of Medicine, Singapore, 28*(5), 728–738.

Cohen, S. R., Kalinowski, J., LaRossa, D., & Randall, P. (1991). Cleft palate fistulas: A multivariate statistical analysis of prevalence, etiology, and surgical management. *Plastic and Reconstructive Surgery, 87*(6), 1041–1047.

Cole, P., Banerji, S., Hollier, L., & Stal, S. (2008). Two hundred twenty-two consecutive pharyngeal flaps: An analysis of postoperative complications. *Journal of Oral & Maxillofacial Surgery, 66*(4), 745–748.

Cosman, B., & Falk, A. S. (1980). Delayed hard palate repair and speech deficiencies: A cautionary report. *Cleft Palate Journal, 17*(1), 27–33.

Coston, G. N., Hagerty, R. F., Jannarone, R. J., McDonald, V., & Hagerty, R. C. (1986). Levator muscle reconstruction: Resulting velopharyngeal competence—A preliminary report. *Plastic and Reconstructive Surgery, 77*(6), 911–918.

Dalston, R. M. (1996). Velopharyngeal impairment in the orthodontic population. *Seminars in Orthodontics, 2*(3), 220–227.

Dalston, R. M., & Vig, P. S. (1984). Effects of orthognathic surgery on speech: A prospective study. *American Journal of Orthodontics, 86*(4), 291–298.

D'Antonio, L. D., & Marsh, J. L. (1987). Abnormal carotid arteries in the velocardiofacial syndrome. *Plastic and Reconstructive Surgery, 80*(3), 471–472.

Dejonckere, P. H., & van Wijngaarden, H. A. (2001). Retropharyngeal autologous fat transplantation for congenital short palate: A nasometric assessment of functional results. *Annals of Otology, Rhinology, & Laryngology, 110*(2), 168–172.

Demetriades, N., Chang, D. J., Laskarides, C., & Papageorge, M. (2010). Effects of mandibular repositioning, with or without maxillary advancement, on the oro-naso-pharyngeal airway and development of sleep-related breathing disorders. *Journal of Oral and Maxillofacial Surgery, 68*(10), 2431–2436.

Denny, A. D., Kalantarian, B., & Hanson, P. R. (2003). Rotation advancement of the midface by distraction osteogenesis. *Plastic and Reconstructive Surgery, 111*(6), 1789–1799; discussion 1800–1803.

Denny, A. D., Marks, S. M., & Oliff-Carneol, S. (1993). Correction of velopharyngeal insufficiency by pharyngeal augmentation using autologous cartilage: A preliminary report. *The Cleft Palate–Craniofacial Journal, 30*(1), 46–54.

Deren, O., Ayhan, M., Tuncel, A., Görgü, M., Altuntaş, A., Kutlay, R., & Erdoğan, B. (2005). The correction of velopharyngeal insufficiency by Furlow palatoplasty in patients older than 3 years undergoing Veau-Wardill-Kilner palatoplasty: A prospective clinical study. *Plastic and Reconstructive Surgery, 116*(1), 85–93; discussion 94–96.

Dingman, R. O., & Grabb, W. C. (1971). A rational program for surgical management of bilateral cleft lip and cleft palate. *Plastic and Reconstructive Surgery, 47*(3), 239–242.

Dreyer, T. M., & Trier, W. C. (1984). A comparison of palatoplasty techniques. *Cleft Palate Journal, 21*(4), 251–253.

El-Sayed, K. M., & Khalil, H. (2010). Transpalatal distraction osteogenesis prior to alveolar bone grafting in cleft lip and palate patients. *International Journal of Oral and Maxillofacial Surgery, 39*(8), 761–766.

Eppley, B. L., & Sadove, A. M. (2000). Management of alveolar cleft bone grafting: State of the art. *The Cleft Palate–Craniofacial Journal, 37*(3), 229–233.

Fara, M., & Brousilova, M. (1988). Long-term experience with 2-stage surgery of cleft palate in total unilateral and bilateral clefts from the aspect of maxillary development. *Rozhledy V Chirugii, 67*(11), 729–741.

Fara, M., Brousilova, M., Hrivnakova, J., & Tvrdek, M. (1992). Long-term experiences with the two-stage palatoplasty with regard to the development of maxillary arch. *Acta Chirurgiae Plasticae, 34*(3), 138–142.

Finkelstein, Y., Zohar, Y., Nachmani, A., Talmi, Y. P., Lerner, M. A., Hauben, D. J., & Frydman, M. (1993). The otolaryngologist and the patient with velocardiofacial syndrome. *Archives of Otolaryngology-Head & Neck Surgery, 119*(5), 563–569.

Forrest, C. R., Klaiman, P. M., & Mason, A. C. (2009). Posterior pharyngeal flaps. In J. E. Lossee & R. E. Kirschner (Eds.), *Comprehensive cleft care* (pp. 649–664). New York, NY: McGraw-Hill.

Furlow, L. T., Jr. (1986). Cleft palate repair by double opposing Z-plasty. *Plastic and Reconstructive Surgery, 78*(6), 724–738.

Furlow, L. T., Jr. (1990). Flaps for cleft lip and palate surgery. *Clinics in Plastic Surgery, 17*(4), 633–644.

Furlow, L. T., Jr. (2009). Correction of velopharyngeal insufficiency by a double-opposing Z-plasty. In J. E. Lossee & R. E. Kirschner (Eds.), *Comprehensive cleft care* (pp. 641–647). New York, NY: McGraw-Hill.

Gray, S. D., Pinborough-Zimmerman, J., & Catten, M. (1999). Posterior wall augmentation for treatment of velopharyngeal insufficiency. *Otolaryngology-Head & Neck Surgery, 121*(1), 107–112.

Gunther, E., Wisser, J. R., Cohen, M. A., & Brown, A. S. (1998). Palatoplasty: Furlow's double reversing Z-plasty versus intravelar veloplasty. *The Cleft Palate–Craniofacial Journal, 35*(6), 546–549.

Guyette, T. W., Polley, J. W., Figueroa, A., & Smith, B. E. (2001). Changes in speech following maxillary distraction osteogenesis. *The Cleft Palate–Craniofacial Journal, 38*(3), 199–205.

Haapanen, M. L., Kalland, M., Heliovaara, A., Hukki, J., & Ranta, R. (1997). Velopharyngeal function in cleft patients undergoing maxillary advancement. *Folia Phoniatrica et Logopedica, 49*(1), 42–47.

Hardin-Jones, M. A., & Jones, D. L. (2005). Speech production of preschoolers with cleft palate. *The Cleft Palate–Craniofacial Journal, 42*(1), 7–13.

Heliovaara, A., Hukki, J., Ranta, R., & Haapanen, M. L. (2004). Cephalometric pharyngeal changes after Le Fort I osteotomy in different types of clefts. *Scandinavian Journal of Plastic and Reconstructive Surgery and Hand Surgery, 38*(1), 5–10.

Heliovaara, A., Ranta, R., Hukki, J., & Haapanen, M. L. (2002). Cephalometric pharyngeal changes after Le Fort I osteotomy in patients with unilateral cleft lip and palate. *Acta Odontologica Scandinavica, 60*(3), 141–145.

Holland, S., Gabbay, J. S., Heller, J. B., O'Hare, C., Hurwitz, D., Ford, M. D., . . . Bradley, J. P. (2007). Delayed closure of the hard palate leads to speech problems and deleterious maxillary growth. *Plastic and Reconstructive Surgery, 119*(4), 1302–1310.

Imola, M. J., & Tatum, S. A. (2002). Craniofacial distraction osteogenesis. *Facial Plastic Surgery Clinics of North America, 10*(3), 287–301.

Jackson, I. T. (1985). Sphincter pharyngoplasty. *Clinics in Plastic Surgery, 12*(4), 711–717.

Jackson, I. T., McGlynn, M. J., Huskie, C. F., & Dip, I. P. (1980). Velopharyngeal incompetence in the absence of cleft palate: Results of treatment in 20 cases. *Plastic and Reconstructive Surgery, 66*(2), 211–213.

Jackson, I. T., McLennan, G., & Scheker, L. R. (1983). Primary veloplasty or primary palatoplasty: Some preliminary findings. *Plastic and Reconstructive Surgery, 72*(2), 153–157.

Jackson, I. T., & Silverton, J. S. (1977). The sphincter pharyngoplasty as a secondary procedure in cleft palates. *Plastic and Reconstructive Surgery, 59*(4), 518–524.

James, N. K., Twist, M., Turner, M. M., & Milward, T. M. (1996). An audit of velopharyngeal incompetence treated by the Orticochea pharyngoplasty. *British Journal of Plastic Surgery, 49*(4), 197–201.

Janulewicz, J., Costello, B. J., Buckley, M. J., Ford, M. D., Close, J., & Gassner, R. (2004). The effects of Le Fort I osteotomies on velopharyngeal and speech functions in cleft patients. *Journal of Oral & Maxillofacial Surgery, 62*(3), 308–314.

Jarvis, B. L., & Trier, W. C. (1988). The effect of intravelar veloplasty on velopharyngeal competence following pharyngeal flap surgery. *Cleft Palate Journal, 25*(4), 389–394.

Karling, J., Henningsson, G., Larson, O., & Isberg, A. (1999). Adaptation of pharyngeal wall adduction after pharyngeal flap surgery. *The Cleft Palate–Craniofacial Journal, 36*(2), 166–172.

Kasten, S. J., Buchman, S. R., Stevenson, C., & Berger, M. (1997). A retrospective analysis of revision sphincter pharyngoplasty. *Annals of Plastic Surgery, 39*(6), 583–589.

Ko, E. W., Figueroa, A. A., Guyette, T. W., Polley, J. W., & Law, W. R. (1999). Velopharyngeal changes after maxillary advancement in cleft patients with distraction osteogenesis using a rigid external distraction device: A 1-year cephalometric follow-up. *Journal of Craniofacial Surgery, 10*(4), 312–320; discussion 321–322.

Kramer, F., Baethge, C., Swennen, G., Teltzrow, T., Schulze, A., Berten, J., & Brachvogel, P. (2004). Intra- and perioperative complications of the LeFort 1 osteotomy: A prospective evaluation of 1000 patients. *Journal of Craniofacial Surgery, 15*(6), 971–977.

Krugman, M. E., & Brant-Zawadski, M. (1997). Magnetic resonance angioplasty for prepharyngoplasty assessment in velocardiofacial syndrome. *The Cleft Palate–Craniofacial Journal, 34*(3), 266–267.

Kummer, A. W., Clark, S. L., Redle, E. E., Thomsen, L. L., & Billmire, D. A. (2012). Current practice in assessing and reporting speech outcomes of cleft palate and velopharyngeal surgery: A survey of cleft palate/craniofacial professionals. *The Cleft Palate–Craniofacial Journal, 49*(2), 146–152.

Kummer, A. W., Strife, J. L., Grau, W. H., Creaghead, N. A., & Lee, L. (1989). The effects of Le Fort I osteotomy with maxillary movement on articulation, resonance, and velopharyngeal function. *Cleft Palate Journal, 26*(3), 193–199.

Lai, J. P., Lo, L. J., Wong, H. F., Wang, S. R., & Yun, C. (2004). Vascular abnormalities in the head and neck area in velocardiofacial syndrome. *Chang Gung Medical Journal, 27*(8), 586–593.

Lauck, L., Lee, L. Kummer, A. W., Billmire, D., & Bandaranayake, D. (2006, April). Speech outcomes following surgical management of velopharyngeal dysfunction. Paper presented at the Annual Meeting of the American Cleft Palate–Craniofacial Association, Vancouver, Canada.

Lazarus, D. D., Hudson, D. A., van Zyl, J. E., Fleming, A. N., & Fernandes, D. (1998). Repair of unilateral cleft lip: A comparison of five techniques. *Annals of Plastic Surgery, 41*(6), 587–594.

Lee, A. S., Whitehill, T. L., Ciocca, V., & Samman, N. (2002). Acoustic and perceptual analysis of the sibilant sound /s/ before and after orthognathic surgery. *Journal of Oral & Maxillofacial Surgery, 60*(4), 364–372; discussion 372–373.

Le Fort, R. (1901). Étude experimental sur les fractures de la machoire superieure. Parts I, II, III. *Revue de Chirurgie de Paris, 23,* 201, 360, 479.

Leon-Valle, C. (1980). The use of a cutaneous-muscular flap for primary naso-labial repair with a modified Tennison-Randall technique. *British Journal of Plastic Surgery, 33*(2), 266–269.

Leuchter, I., Schweizer, V., Hohlfeld, J., & Pasche, P. (2009). Treatment of velopharyngeal insufficiency by autologous fat injection. *European Archives of Oto-Rhino-Laryngology, 267*(6), 977–983.

Lewis, M. B., & Pashayan, H. M. (1980). The effects of pharyngeal flap surgery on lateral pharyngeal wall motion: A videoradiographic evaluation. *Cleft Palate Journal, 17*(4), 301–308.

Liao, Y. F., Yang, I. Y., Wang, R., Yun, C., & Huang, C. S. (2010). Two-stage palate repair with delayed hard palate closure is related to favorable maxillary growth in unilateral cleft lip and palate. *Plastic and Reconstructive Surgery, 125*(5), 1503–1510.

Lin, W. N., Wang, R., Cheong, E. C., & Lo, L. J. (2010). Use of hemisphincter pharyngoplasty in the management of velopharyngeal insufficiency after

pharyngeal flap: An outcome study. *Annals of Plastic Surgery, 65*(2), 201–205.

Lindsey, W. H., & Davis, P. T. (1996). Correction of velopharyngeal insufficiency with Furlow palatoplasty. *Archives of Otolaryngology-Head & Neck Surgery, 122*(8), 881–884.

Losken, A., Williams, J. K., Burstein, F. D., Malick, D., & Riski, J. E. (2003). An outcome evaluation of sphincter pharyngoplasty for the management of velopharyngeal insufficiency. *Plastic and Reconstructive Surgery, 112*(1), 1755–1761.

MacKenzie-Stepner, K., Witzel, M. A., Stringer, D. A., Lindsay, W. K., Munro, I. R., & Hughes, H. (1987). Abnormal carotid arteries in the velocardiofacial syndrome: A report of three cases. *Plastic and Reconstructive Surgery, 80*(3), 347–351.

Maegawa, J., Sells, R. K., & David, D. J. (1998). Speech changes after maxillary advancement in 40 cleft lip and palate patients. *Journal of Craniofacial Surgery, 9*(2), 177–182; discussion 183–184.

Marsh, J. L. (2009). Sphincter pharyngoplasty. In J. E. Lossee & R. E. Kirschner (Eds.), *Comprehensive cleft care* (pp. 665–671). New York, NY: McGraw-Hill.

Marsh, J. L., Grames, L. M., & Holtman, B. (1989). Intravelar veloplasty: A prospective study. *Cleft Palate Journal, 26*(1), 46–50.

McCarthy, J. G., Coccaro, P. J., & Schwartz, M. D. (1979). Velopharyngeal function following maxillary advancement. *Plastic and Reconstructive Surgery, 64*(2), 180–189.

Mehendale, F. V., & Sommerlad, B. C. (2004). Surgical significance of abnormal internal carotid arteries in velocardiofacial syndrome in 43 consecutive Hynes pharyngoplasties. *The Cleft Palate–Craniofacial Journal, 41*(4), 368–374.

Mitnick, R. J., Bello, J. A., Golding-Kushner, K. J., Argamaso, R. V., & Shprintzen, R. J. (1996). The use of magnetic resonance angiography prior to pharyngeal flap surgery in patients with velocardiofacial syndrome. *Plastic and Reconstructive Surgery, 97*(5), 908–919.

Mofid, M. M., Manson, P. N., Robertson, B. C., Tufaro, A. P., Elias, J. J., & Vander Kolk, C. A. (2001). Craniofacial distraction osteogenesis: A review of 3,278 cases. *Plastic and Reconstructive Surgery, 108*(5), 1103–1114; discussion 1115–1117.

Moore, M. D., Lawrence, W. T., Ptak, J. J., & Trier, W. C. (1988). Complications of primary palatoplasty: A twenty-one-year review. *Cleft Palate Journal, 25*(2), 156–162.

Mulliken, J. B. (2009). Repair of bilateral cleft lip and its variants. *Indian Journal of Plastic Surgery, 42*(Suppl.), S79–S90.

Murison, M. S., & Pigott, R. W. (1992). Medial Langenbeck: Experience of a modified von Langenbeck repair of the cleft palate. A preliminary report. *British Journal of Plastic Surgery, 45*(6), 454–459.

Murthy, J., Sendhilnathan, S., & Hussain, S. A. (2010). Speech outcome following late primary palate repair. *The Cleft Palate–Craniofacial Journal, 47*(2), 156–161.

Naran, S., Ford, M., & Losee, J. E. (2017). What's new in cleft palate and velopharyngeal dysfunction management? *Plastic and Reconstructive Surgery, 139*(6), 1343e–1355e.

Niemeyer, T. C., Gomes Ade, O., Fukushiro, A. P., & Genaro, K. F. (2005). Speech resonance in orthognathic surgery in subjects with cleft lip and palate. *Journal of Applied Oral Science, 13*(3), 232–236.

Okazaki, K., Satoh, K., Kato, M., Iwanami, M., Ohokubo, F., & Kobayashi, K. (1993). Speech and velopharyngeal function following maxillary advancement in patients with cleft lip and palate. *Annals of Plastic Surgery, 30*(4), 304–311.

Orticochea, M. (1970). Results of the dynamic muscle sphincter operation in cleft palates. *British Journal of Plastic Surgery, 23*(2), 108–114.

Orticochea, M. (1983). A review of 236 cleft palate patients treated with dynamic muscle sphincter. *Plastic and Reconstructive Surgery, 71*(2), 180–188.

Orticochea, M. (1997). Physiopathology of the dynamic muscular sphincter of the pharynx. *Plastic and Reconstructive Surgery, 100*(7), 1918–1923.

Orticochea, M. (1999). The timing and management of dynamic muscular pharyngeal sphincter construction in velopharyngeal incompetence. *British Journal of Plastic Surgery, 52*(2), 85–87.

Paranaiba, L. M., Almeida, H., Barros, L. M., Martelli, D. R., Orsi, J. D., Jr., & Martelli, H., Jr. (2009). Current surgical techniques for cleft lip-palate in Minas Gerais, Brazil. *Brazilian Journal of Otorhinolaryngology, 75*(6), 839–843.

Penna, V., Bannasch, H., & Stark, G. B. (2007). The turbinate flap for oronasal fistula closure. *Annals of Plastic Surgery, 59*(6), 679–681.

Perkins, J. A., Lewis, C. W., Gruss, J. S., Eblen, L. E., & Sie, K. C. (2005). Furlow palatoplasty for management of velopharyngeal insufficiency: A prospective study of 148 consecutive patients. *Plastic and Reconstructive Surgery, 116*(1), 72–80; discussion 81–84.

Perko, M. A. (1979). Two-stage closure of cleft palate (progress report). *Journal of Maxillofacial Surgery, 7*(1), 46–80.

Phillips, J. H., Klaiman, P., Delorey, R., & MacDonald, D. B. (2005). Predictors of velopharyngeal insufficiency in cleft palate orthognathic surgery. *Plastic and Reconstructive Surgery, 115*(3), 681–686.

Pigott, R. W., Rieger, F. W., & Moodie, A. F. (1984). Tongue flap repair of cleft palate fistulae. *British Journal of Plastic Surgery, 37*(3), 285–293.

Por, Y. C., Tan, Y. C., Chang, F. C., & Chen, P. K. (2010). Revision of pharyngeal flaps causing obstructive airway symptoms: An analysis of treatment with three different techniques over 39 years. *Journal of Plastic, Reconstructive, & Aesthetic Surgery, 63*(6), 930–933.

Posnick, J. C., & Getz, S. B., Jr. (1987). Surgical closure of end-stage palatal fistulas using anteriorly based dorsal tongue flaps. *Journal of Oral Maxillofacial Surgery, 45*(11), 907–912.

Pradel, W., Senf, D., Mai, R., Ludicke, G., Eckelt, U., & Lauer, G. (2009). One-stage palate repair improves speech outcome and early maxillary grown in patients with cleft lip and palate. *Journal of Physiology and Pharmacology, 60*, 37–41.

Primrose, A. C., Broadfoot, E., Diner, P. A., Molina, F., Moos, K. F., & Ayoub, A. F. (2005). Patients' responses to distraction osteogenesis: A multicentre study. *International Journal of Oral & Maxillofacial Surgery, 34*(3), 238–242.

Remacle, M., Bertrand, B., Eloy, P., & Marbaix, E. (1990). The use of injectable collagen to correct velopharyngeal insufficiency. *Laryngoscope, 100*(3), 269–274.

Ren, Y. F., & Wang, G. H. (1993). A modified palatopharyngeous flap operation and its application in the correction of velopharyngeal incompetence. *Plastic and Reconstructive Surgery, 91*(4), 612–617.

Richardson, S., Agni, N., & Selvraj, D. (2011). Anterior maxillary distraction using a tooth-borne device for hypoplastic cleft maxillas: A pilot study. *Journal of Oral Maxillofacial Surgery, 69*, 542–548.

Riski, J. E., Ruff, G. L., Georgiade, G. S., & Barwick, W. J. (1992). Evaluation of failed sphincter pharyngoplasties. *Annals of Plastic Surgery, 28*(6), 545–553.

Riski, J. E., Ruff, G. L., Georgiade, G. S., Barwick, W. J., & Edwards, P. D. (1992). Evaluation of the sphincter pharyngoplasty. *The Cleft Palate–Craniofacial Journal, 29*(3), 254–261.

Roberts, T. M., & Brown, B. S. (1983). Evaluation of a modified sphincter pharyngoplasty in the treatment of speech problems due to palatal insufficiency. *Annals of Plastic Surgery, 10*(3), 209–213.

Ross, D. A., Witzel, M. A., Armstrong, D. C., & Thomson, H. G. (1996). Is pharyngoplasty a risk in velocardiofacial syndrome? An assessment of medially displaced carotid arteries. *Plastic and Reconstructive Surgery, 98*(7), 1182–1190.

Saman, M., & Tatum, S. A., III. (2012). Recent advances in surgical pharyngeal modification procedures for the treatment of velopharyngeal insufficiency in patients with cleft palate. *Archives of Facial Plastic Surgery, 14*(2), 85–88.

Satoh, K., Nagata, J., Shomura, K., Wada, T., Tachimura, T., Fukuda, J., & Shiba, R. (2004). Morphological evaluation of changes in velopharyngeal function following maxillary distraction in patients with repaired cleft palate during mixed dentition. *The Cleft Palate–Craniofacial Journal, 41*(4), 355–363.

Schweckendiek, W. (1955). Zur zweiphasigen Gaumenspalten-operation bei primarem Velumerschluss. *Fortschritte Kiefer-und Gesichtschtschirurgie, 1,* 73–76.

Schweckendiek, W. (1966). The technique of early veloplasty and its results. *Acta Chirurgiae Plasticae, 8*(3), 188–194.

Schweckendiek, W. (1968). Early veloplasty and its results. *Acta Oto-Rhino-Laryngologica Belgica, 22*(6), 697–703.

Schweckendiek, W. (1983). Primary closure of cleft lip and cleft palate. *Zahnarztl Prax, 34*(8), 317–320.

Schweckendiek, W., & Doz, P. (1978). Primary veloplasty: Long-term results without maxillary deformity. A twenty-five year report. *Cleft Palate Journal, 15*(3), 268–274.

Seagle, M. B., Mazaheri, M. K., Dixon-Wood, V. L., & Williams, W. N. (2002). Evaluation and treatment of velopharyngeal insufficiency: The University of Florida experience. *Annals of Plastic Surgery, 48*(5), 464–470.

Sharshar, H. H., & El-Bialy, T. H. (2012). Cephalometric evaluation of airways after maxillary anterior advancement by distraction osteogenesis in cleft lip and palate patients: A systematic review. *The Cleft Palate–Craniofacial Journal, 49*(3), 255–261.

Sie, K. C., & Gruss, J. S. (2002). Results with Furlow palatoplasty in the management of velopharyngeal insufficiency. *Plastic and Reconstructive Surgery, 109*(7), 2588–2589; author reply 2590–2591.

Sie, K. C., Tampakopoulou, D. A., de Serres, L. M., Gruss, J. S., Eblen, L. E., & Yonick, T. (1998). Sphincter pharyngoplasty: Speech outcome and complications. *Laryngoscope, 108*(8, Pt. 1), 1211–1217.

Sie, K. C., Tampakopoulou, D. A., Sorom, J., Gruss, J. S., & Eblen, L. E. (2001). Results with Furlow palatoplasty in management of velopharyngeal insufficiency. *Plastic and Reconstructive Surgery, 108*(1), 17–25; discussion 26–29.

Skolnick, M. L., & McCall, G. N. (1972). Velopharyngeal competence and incompetence following pharyngeal flap surgery: Videofluoroscopic study in multiple projections. *Cleft Palate Journal, 9*(1), 1–12.

Smahel, Z., & Horak, I. (1993). The effect of two-stage palatoplasty on facial development in unilateral cleft lip and palate. *Acta Chirurgiae Plasticae, 35*(1/2), 67–72.

Swennen, G., Schliephake, H., Dempf, R., Schierle, H., & Malevez, C. (2001). Craniofacial distraction osteogenesis: A review of the literature. Part 1: Clinical studies. *International Journal of Oral & Maxillofacial Surgery, 30*(2), 89–103.

Takigawa, Y., Uematsu, S., & Takada, K. (2010). Maxillary advancement using distraction osteogenesis with intraoral device. *The Angle Orthodontist, 80*(6), 1165–1175.

Tan, O., & Atik, B. (2007). Triangular with ala nasi (TAN) repair of unilateral cleft lips: A personal technique and early outcomes. *The Journal of Craniofacial Surgery, 18*(1), 186–197.

Tan, S. P., Greene, A. K., & Mulliken, J. B. (2012). Current surgical management of bilateral cleft lip in North America. *Plastic & Reconstructive Surgery, 129*(6), 1347–1355.

Terris, D. J., & Goode, R. L. (1993). Costochondral pharyngeal implants for velopharyngeal insufficiency. *Laryngoscope, 103*(5), 565–569.

Tharanon, W., Stella, J. P., & Epker, B. N. (1990). The modified superior-based pharyngeal flap. Part III. A retrospective study. *Oral Surgery, Oral Medicine, Oral Pathology, and Endodontics, 70*(3), 256–267.

Thind, M. S., Singh, A., & Thind, R. S. (1992). Repair of anterior secondary palate fistula using tongue flaps. *Acta Chirurgiae Plasticae, 34*(2), 79–91.

Trier, W. C. (1985a). The pharyngeal flap operation. *Clinics in Plastic Surgery, 12*(4), 697–710.

Trier, W. C. (1985b). Repair of bilateral cleft lip: Millard's technique. *Clinics in Plastic Surgery, 12*(4), 605–625.

Trier, W. C., & Dreyer, T. M. (1984). Primary von Langenbeck palatoplasty with levator reconstruction: Rationale and technique. *Cleft Palate Journal, 21*(4), 254–262.

Trigos, L., Ysunza, A., Gonzalez, A., & Vazquez, M. C. (1988). Surgical treatment of borderline velopharyngeal insufficiency using homologous cartilage implantation with videonasopharyngoscopic monitoring. *Cleft Palate Journal, 25*(2), 167–170.

Trindade, I. E., Yamashita, R. P., Suguimoto, R. M., Mazzottini, R., & Trindade, A. S., Jr. (2003). Effects of orthognathic surgery on speech and breathing of subjects with cleft lip and palate: Acoustic and aerodynamic assessment. *The Cleft Palate–Craniofacial Journal, 40*(1), 54–64.

Ulkur, E., Karagoz, H., Uygur, F., Celikoz, B., Cincik, H., Mutlu, H., . . . Ciyiltepe, M. (2008). Use of porous polyethylene implant for augmentation of the posterior pharynx in young adult patients with borderline velopharyngeal insufficiency. *Journal of Craniofacial Surgery, 19*(3), 573–579.

Vallino, L. D. (1990). Speech, velopharyngeal function, and hearing before and after orthognathic surgery. *Journal of Oral and Maxillofacial Surgery, 48*(12), 1274–1281; discussion 1281–1282.

van Aalst, J. A., Eppley, B. L., Hathaway, R. R., & Sadove, A. M. (2005). Surgical technique for primary alveolar bone grafting. *Journal of Craniofacial Surgery, 16*(4), 706–711.

Vedung, S. (1995). Pharyngeal flaps after one- and two-stage repair of the cleft palate: A 25-year review of 520 patients. *The Cleft Palate–Craniofacial Journal, 32*(3), 206–215; discussion 215–216.

Waite, P. D., & Waite, D. E. (1996). Bone grafting for the alveolar cleft defect. *Seminars in Orthodontics, 2*(3), 192–196.

Walia, A. (2011). Secondary alveolar bone grafting in cleft of the lip and palate patients. *Contemporary Clinical Dentistry, 2*(3), 146–154.

Ward, E. C., McAuliffe, M., Holmes, S. K., Lynham, A., & Monsour, F. (2002). Impact of malocclusion and orthognathic reconstruction surgery on resonance and articulatory function: An examination of variability in five cases. *British Journal of Oral & Maxillofacial Surgery, 40*(5), 410–417.

Watzke, L., Turvey, T. A., Warren, D. W., & Dalston, R. (1990). Alterations in velopharyngeal function after maxillary advancement in cleft palate patients. *Journal of Oral and Maxillofacial Surgery, 48*(7), 685–689.

Witt, P. D., & D'Antonio, L. L. (1993). Velopharyngeal insufficiency and secondary palatal management: A new look at an old problem. *Clinics in Plastic Surgery, 20*(4), 707–721.

Witt, P. D., D'Antonio, L. L., Zimmerman, G. J., & Marsh, J. L. (1994). Sphincter pharyngoplasty: A preoperative and postoperative analysis of perceptual speech characteristics and endoscopic studies of velopharyngeal function. *Plastic and Reconstructive Surgery, 93*(6), 1154–1168.

Witt, P. D., Marsh, J. L., Marty-Grames, L., & Muntz, H. R. (1995). Revision of the failed sphincter pharyngoplasty: An outcome assessment. *Plastic and Reconstructive Surgery, 96*(1), 129–138.

Witt, P. D., Marsh, J. L., Muntz, H. R., Marty-Grames, L., & Watchmaker, G. P. (1996). Acute obstructive sleep apnea as a complication of sphincter pharyngoplasty. *The Cleft Palate–Craniofacial Journal, 33*(3), 183–189.

Witt, P. D., Miller, D. C., Marsh, J. L., Muntz, H. R., & Grames, L. M. (1998). Limited value of preoperative cervical vascular imaging in patients with velocardiofacial syndrome. *Plastic and Reconstructive Surgery, 101*(5), 1184–1195; discussion 1196–1199.

Witt, P. D., O'Daniel, T. G., Marsh, J. L., Grames, L. M., Muntz, H. R., & Pilgram, T. K. (1997). Surgical management of velopharyngeal dysfunction: Outcome analysis of autogenous posterior pharyngeal wall augmentation. *Plastic and Reconstructive Surgery, 99*(5), 1287–1296; discussion 1297–1300.

Wolford, L. M., Oelschlaeger, M., & Deal, R. (1989). Proplast as a pharyngeal wall implant to correct velopharyngeal insufficiency. *Cleft Palate Journal, 26*(2), 119–126; discussion 126–128.

Woo, A. S. (2017). Evidence-based medicine: Cleft palate. *Plastic and Reconstructive Surgery, 139*(1), 191e–203e.

Wu, J., & Epker, B. N. (1990). The modified superiorly based pharyngeal flap technique. Part II. An anatomic study. *Oral Surgery, Oral Medicine, Oral Pathology, 70*(3), 251–255.

Yin, H., Zhao, S. F., Zheng, G. N., Li, S., Wang, Y., Zheng, Q., & Shi, B. (2010). Investigation of the optimized surgical procedure for the cleft palate patients over six years old. *West China Journal of Somatology, 28*(3), 294–297.

Yoshida, H., Stella, J. P., Ghali, G. E., & Epker, B. N. (1992). The modified superiorly based pharyngeal flap. Part IV. Position of the base of the flap. *Oral Surgery, Oral Medicine, Oral Pathology, 73*(1), 13–18.

Ysunza, A., Garcia-Velasco, M., Garcia-Garcia, M., Haro, R., & Valencia, M. (1993). Obstructive sleep apnea secondary to surgery for velopharyngeal insufficiency. *The Cleft Palate–Craniofacial Journal, 30*(4), 387–390.

Ysunza, A., Pamplona, M. C., Molina, F., Drucker, M., Felemovicius, J., Ramirez, E., & Patiño, C. (2004). Surgery for speech in cleft palate patients. *International Journal of Pediatric Otorhinolaryngology, 68*(12), 1499–1505.

Ysunza, A., Pamplona, G., Ramirez, E., Molina, F., Mendoza, M., & Silva, A. (2002). Velopharyngeal surgery: A prospective randomized study of pharyngeal flaps and sphincter pharyngoplasties. *Plastic and Reconstructive Surgery, 110*(6), 1401–1407.

CREDITS

CHAPTER 18

Prosthetic Management

CHAPTER OUTLINE

INTRODUCTION

Individuals with a history of cleft lip, cleft palate, or other craniofacial anomalies often have anatomical problems that affect facial aesthetics, dental arch stability, speech, mastication, and swallowing. These physical and functional problems can also affect the social, emotional, and psychological well-being of the patient in a very negative way.

Historically, patients with cleft lip and palate underwent multiple surgical and habilitative procedures to achieve an acceptable aesthetic and functional outcome. Surgical repairs were done later in life than they are today, and the success of the surgical procedures was not as high as it is currently. Despite the best efforts of the surgeon, the patient often had remaining dental and maxillary arch deficiencies and speech problems from occlusal anomalies and velopharyngeal insufficiency. Because of these residual problems, prosthetic management was often the most effective form of treatment and therefore was commonly used. In recent years, however, there has been an increase in the understanding of the nature of craniofacial growth and development. In addition, advancements and improvements in surgical techniques have resulted in greatly improved aesthetic and speech outcomes. Therefore, prosthetic devices are no longer needed to achieve optimum results in most patients with cleft lip/palate, particularly those who receive early and appropriate surgical intervention (Delgado, Schaaf, & Emrich, 1992; Reisberg, 2000).

Although surgery is usually the option of choice for correction or improvement of many of these structural and functional problems, there still is a need for prosthetic treatment in certain cases. Prosthetic treatment is an excellent option for patients when surgery is not desired or possible for a variety of reasons.

The overall goal of management, whether through surgical or prosthetic treatment, is to obtain the optimum results. Therefore, in choosing a treatment option, it is important to consider not only the preferences of the patient and the expected outcome but also the total amount of time necessary to achieve results, the risks to the patient, and the cost of treatment. A successful treatment option is one that meets the particular needs and expectations of the patient and the family with the least amount of time and the lowest cost.

The purpose of this chapter is to discuss the various types of prosthetic devices available for individuals with a history of cleft lip/palate or other craniofacial conditions. Speech-language pathologists should be well informed about the options for prosthetic management and when it is appropriate for the patient.

Prosthetic Devices

A **prosthesis**, also called a **prosthetic device** or appliance, is a fabricated substitute for a body part that is missing or malformed. This substitute may be fixed so that it is essentially permanent, or it can be removable so the patient can take it out for eating, sleeping, and cleaning. Prosthetic management can be done on a temporary basis before surgical correction or on a permanent basis if surgical correction is not possible or desired by the patient.

Construction of a prosthetic device may be done by an orthodontist or pediatric dentist. However, this work is most often done by a prosthodontist who specializes in the construction of these devices. A **prosthodontist** is a dental professional who not only deals with the restoration of teeth but also with the fabrication of appliances to improve the appearance of missing or malformed oral and facial structures. These devices improve the aesthetics and assist the patient with certain functions, such as feeding and velopharyngeal closure. The prosthodontist is a very important member of a craniofacial team because she can often further improve the speech and appearance of individuals with significant anomalies following the best surgical attempts at correction.

Dental Appliances

Patients who have had a cleft of the entire primary palate often have missing teeth, particularly in the line of the cleft. Patients with other craniofacial anomalies are also at risk for missing and malformed teeth in addition to malocclusion. In these cases, prosthetic management can improve facial aesthetics, mastication, and even speech by the replacement of missing teeth or correction of malocclusion.

There are significant challenges when attempting to replace teeth for individuals with a history of cleft of the primary palate. These challenges may include a shortened upper lip, decreased upper lip mobility from scarring, protrusion of the premaxilla, spaces created by missing teeth, and supernumerary teeth. Additional problems include jaw discrepancies, an occlusal cant, distortion of the midline of the dentition and face, and scar tissue in the alveolar or palatal areas (Ramstad, 1998). Added to these challenges may be poor dental hygiene from neglect as a result of psychological factors, which is common in this population.

Replacement of teeth can be done in several ways. A fixed bridge is typically used to replace dental segments, and complete dentures are used when all of the teeth in an arch must be replaced. If some of the teeth are to be retained but are not functional, overlay dentures are often used. Overlay dentures fit over the existing teeth and usually provide more vertical dimension, which improves both function and appearance for individuals who have over closure of the vertical dimension and thus a deep bite. These dental appliances can be combined with any type of speech appliance if needed. The long-term use of this type of denture can place the underlying teeth at risk for decay and periodontal disease, however.

Although misaligned teeth can make the fabrication of dentures a challenge, tooth extractions are typically avoided unless required for orthodontic purposes. Even a misaligned tooth may serve a purpose in the future, such as providing an anchor for a prosthetic device. Tooth extraction in the cleft area of the dental arch is especially avoided because it usually results in resorption of the alveolar bone, which widens and deepens the cleft. This tissue and bone loss may exceed that which can be replaced by a fixed partial prosthesis. Therefore, correction would result in a more complex reconstruction than if the tooth is preserved (McKinstry, 1998a).

Facial Prostheses

Individuals with craniofacial anomalies can demonstrate significant facial defects that affect the person's overall appearance to such a degree that his quality of life is greatly affected. Although surgical intervention often leads to significant improvement, this is not always the case. Acquired facial defects caused by injury or ablative surgery for cancer can be even more challenging if not impossible to improve with surgery. Fortunately, prosthetic rehabilitation can make a major difference in the affected person's life, allowing the individual to function normally in society.

Whenever there is a severe facial defect, particularly one that cannot be significantly improved with surgery, a facial prosthesis is a very good option. Even glossectomy patients can benefit from a specially designed prosthesis for the tongue (Mueller et al., 2011).

FIGURE 18-1A shows the type of person who can benefit from a facial prosthesis. This woman had a squamous cell carcinoma, which required a resection of the anterior maxilla, the upper lip, and the nose. A facial prosthesis was used to replace missing parts of the facial anatomy, resulting in a dramatic improvement in appearance (Grisius, 1991; Lundgren, Moy, Beumer, & Lewis, 1993) (**FIGURE 18-1B–D**). In addition to replacing facial parts, individuals with aural atresia can benefit from the fabrication of a prosthetic ear. Although the ear will not be functional, it appears very much like a real ear, and thus the anomaly is not noted by others. The same can be done for the eyes or nose and even for the cheek (Singh, Bharadwaj, & Nair, 1997).

A skilled prosthodontist is able to match skin color, tone, and texture so that the prosthesis blends in with the natural tissue. The prosthodontist is also able to shape structures in a way that makes them very realistic in appearance.

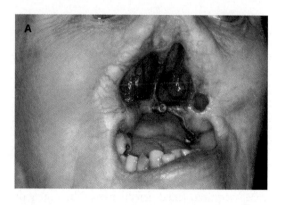
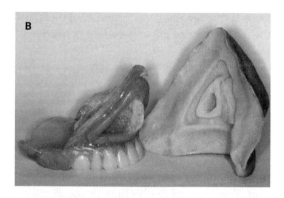
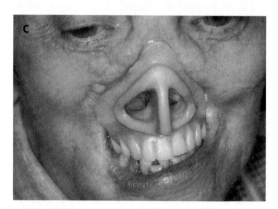
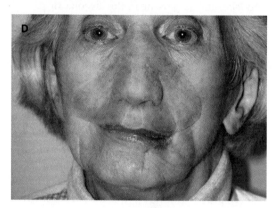

FIGURE 18-1 Facial prostheses. **(A)** Patient with a history of squamous cell carcinoma who underwent a midface resection that included the anterior maxilla, the upper lip, and the nose. A gold bar spans across the defect and is secured and stabilized by dental implants. When in place, the prosthesis attaches to this bar through the use of two retentive pins. **(B)** Prosthesis that includes a maxillary obturator and a nasal extension. On the nasal portion, there is a retentive ridge where the silicone prosthesis (nose, cheek, and lip) snaps on for retention. **(C)** Maxillary and nasal prosthesis in place. The nose prosthesis attaches to this base. **(D)** Both the maxillary and soft-tissue prostheses in position.

In addition to using the conventional manual sculpturing techniques, some prosthodontists use optical three-dimensional imaging and computer-aided design and manufacturing systems to fabricate facial prostheses more precisely (Ahmed, Farshad, & Yazdanie, 2011; Feng et al., 2010; Mueller et al., 2011).

Retention of the prosthesis is often accomplished through the use of osseointegrated implants (implants that are drilled in the bone) (Beumer, Roumanas, & Nishimura, 1995; dos Santos et al., 2010; Goiato, dos Santos, Haddad, & Moreno, 2012; Parel, Holt, Branemark, & Tjellstrom, 1986). With the implants in place, the prosthesis can be secured through the use of mechanical clips, magnetic bars, or implants (Chang, Garrett, Roumanas, & Beumer, 2005).

Because of what is involved to secure the device, facial prostheses work best for adults who are responsible and motivated. They do not work as well for young children, who may be less motivated and are less responsible. In addition, periodic modifications and replacement are necessary for children as they grow.

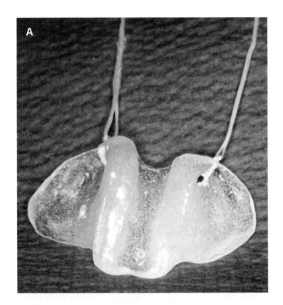

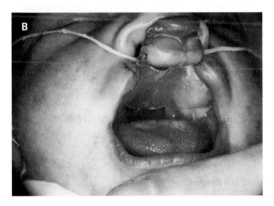

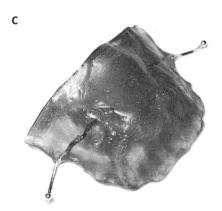

FIGURE 18-2 Feeding obturators.

Feeding Obturators

A feeding obturator is a prosthetic appliance that can be used in the first few months of life to assist the infant with cleft palate in feeding (**FIGURE 18-2**) (Goyal, Chopra, Bansal & Marwaha, 2014; Hansen, Cook, & Ahmad, 2016; Nagda, Deshpande, & Mhatre, 1996; Osuji, 1995; Savion & Huband, 2005; Sultana, Rahman, Nessa, & Alam, 2011). The obturator covers a portion of the infant's unrepaired cleft palate. As such, it keeps the tongue from resting inside the cleft and provides a solid surface so the tongue can achieve compression of the nipple to express the milk. It also helps to eliminate the regurgitation of liquids into the nose. The appliance occludes the hard palate but does not obturate the soft palate. Therefore, it does not help the infant achieve suction, which would require complete velopharyngeal closure (McKinstry, 1998b).

The feeding obturator is made of light-cured resins or acrylic and is fabricated using plaster molds (Sultana et al., 2011). It is made so that it fits tightly against the roof of the mouth during feeding. Because the infant does not have teeth to anchor the appliance in place, suction against the palate and a tight fit are particularly important. One or two holes are drilled in the appliance, and dental floss is then tied to the appliance through the holes. These strings are attached to the appliance to make it easy for the caregiver to remove it following the feeding.

Although feeding obturators are still used in some centers, most craniofacial centers now feel that they are unnecessary. In fact, there are some obvious disadvantages of using feeding obturators, including the expense, the need to frequently redo the obturator because of growth, and the effort needed to train parents in their use. Fortunately, with only simple modifications, most infants with cleft palate can feed adequately and gain weight appropriately without the use of an obturator (see the chapter *Early Feeding Problems*). Perhaps obturators are more useful for infants with multiple structural anomalies of the airway or certain types of neurological dysfunction (Sidoti & Shprintzen, 1995).

Speech Appliances

When surgical correction of velopharyngeal insufficiency/incompetence (VPI) or a symptomatic fistula is not an option, prosthetic management is a good alternative (Gallagher, 1982; Gardner & Parr, 1996). Typically, an interdisciplinary team does an assessment to determine whether the patient is a good candidate for an appliance. The role of the speech-language pathologist is to identify the aspects of speech that may be affected by the appliance and determine the potential benefit on speech intelligibility. The speech-language pathologist may also participate in the designing of the appliance to achieve the best speech outcomes. In a position statement by the American Speech-Language-Hearing Association (ASHA), it was stated that "[P]articipation in the evaluation and treatment of individuals being considered for oral and oropharyngeal prostheses to facilitate speech and swallowing is within the scope of practice of the certified speech-language pathologist" (ASHA, 1993). The knowledge and skills necessary for the speech-language pathologist to assist in the design of a speech prosthesis are outlined in this position statement. Overall, it is important for the speech-language pathologist and prosthodontist to work together for the best speech outcomes (Dhakshaini, Pushpavathi, Garhnayak, & Dhal, 2015).

Three types of speech appliances can be used to assist with speech production: a palatal obturator, a palatal lift, and a speech bulb obturator. The palatal obturator is used to close defects of the hard palate or velum, the palatal lift is used to raise the velum for velopharyngeal incompetence, and the speech bulb obturator is used for velopharyngeal insufficiency. Each of these speech appliances is described separately in the following sections.

Palatal Obturator

A palatal obturator is a removable prosthetic device that is used to cover an open palatal defect

that is symptomatic during speech or is causing nasal regurgitation during feeding (Walter, 2005). The most common use of palatal obturators is to occlude a palatal (oronasal) fistula (**FIGURE 18-3**). Although palatal fistulas do not occur as frequently as in the past, they are still a problem for some patients. When a fistula is present, the surgical closure is often delayed so that it can be done as part of another surgery. With either a delay in surgical correction or a decision not to surgically correct the fistula, obturation can be considered for temporary or permanent correction (Pinborough-Zimmerman, Canady, Yamashiro, & Morales, 1998).

At one time, obturators were used to temporarily occlude hard palate clefts, which were not repaired until facial growth was complete (around age 14 for girls and age 18 for boys). This practice was done by a few treatment centers that subscribed to the theory that early cleft palate closure contributed to a reduction in midfacial growth, causing the high incidence of maxillary deficiency in this population (Schweckendiek, 1966; Schweckendiek, 1968). To counter this effect, these centers opted to close only the velum at an early age and leave the hard palate open until the teenage years. More recent research has suggested that it is not the early repair that affects maxillary growth but rather the inherent deficiency in the maxilla. As a result, surgical correction of the hard palate and velum are now done at the same time, usually at around 10 months of age.

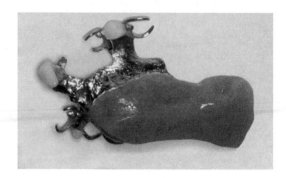

FIGURE 18-3 A palatal obturator. This obturator is designed to fit tightly in the palatal defect. Note the addition of teeth.

SPEECH NOTES

Palatal Obturator

A palatal obturator appliance functions by filling an oronasal opening to close off the nasal cavity from the oral cavity. This allows the patient to be able to impound intraoral pressure for the production of speech sounds. When appropriate and implemented at an early age, an obturator can help the child to develop normal articulation placement instead of compensatory productions (Dorf, Reisberg, & Gold, 1985; Raju, Padmanabhan, & Narayan, 2009). This is particularly true if the child receives focused speech stimulation or speech therapy at the same time (Lohmander-Agerskov, Soderpalm, Friede, & Lilja, 1990). If the palatal opening is very large, an obturator can also reduce or eliminate hypernasality.

A palatal obturator consists of an acrylic body that looks similar to a dental retainer. However, it has additional acrylic on the top of the appliance, which fits tightly into the area of deficiency. This prevents a leak of air or fluid into the nasal cavity. If the obturator has to be large to fill in the defect, it can be hollowed out so that its weight does not cause a problem with retention (Blair & Hunter, 1998).

Palatal Lift

A palatal lift prosthesis is a removable device that elevates a passive velum and holds it in place against the posterior pharyngeal wall for speech. Therefore, a palatal lift is indicated in cases of velopharyngeal incompetence where the velum is of normal length but has inadequate and/or inconsistent velar elevation for closure of the valve. Ideally, there should be adequate velar length and thickness and even good lateral pharyngeal wall movement. A palatal lift can be used in some cases of velopharyngeal insufficiency if there is sufficient length of the velum beyond the natural level of velar elevation. However, if the entire length of the velum is too short to reach the posterior pharyngeal wall, a palatal lift will not be effective.

The palatal lift consists of an anterior base that is retained and stabilized by the teeth and a fingerlike tailpiece that extends to the velum. When treatment is first initiated, the tailpiece may reach to the anterior portion of the velum only (**FIGURE 18-4A**). As the patient learns to tolerate the device, this extension is gradually widened and lengthened until it reaches the area of the velar dimple at the very least (**FIGURE 18-4B**). The extension exerts an upward force against the velum to move it in a superior and posterior direction (**FIGURE 18-4C**).

It is important that this tailpiece be positioned correctly so that it can push the velum against the posterior pharyngeal wall in the area of maximum lateral pharyngeal wall movement. With the palatal lift in place, the velum is held against the posterior pharyngeal wall at all times. Because this is the appropriate position for speech, additional velar movement during speech is unnecessary. If the patient has little lateral wall movement, the lift can be widened to further close the lateral borders of the port.

There are some challenges to using a palatal lift. For example, this type of prosthesis works best if the velum is very flaccid so there is no resistance to the lift. In addition, natural elevation of the velum can cause the prosthesis to become dislodged (Reisberg, 2000). Individuals who have a hyperactive gag reflex or who are hypersensitive to touch in the area of the soft palate may require desensitization in the area before a palatal lift can be effective. This can be done by gentle massage of the soft palate with the index finger to increase the person's tolerance for touch in this area. The finger should massage the velum from side to side and then gradually move posteriorly (Daniel, 1982).

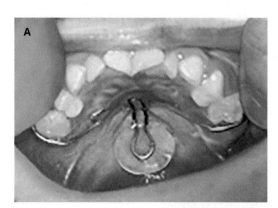
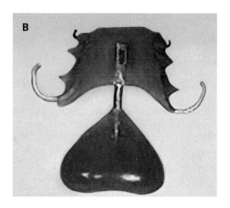
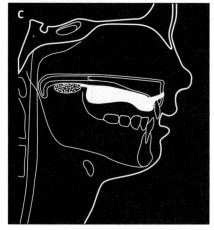

FIGURE 18-4 A palatal lift. **(A)** This lift is in the early stages of development. It will gradually be lengthened as the patient learns to tolerate the device. **(B)** This device is long enough to be positioned in the mouth so that it elevates the velum at the point of its natural bend. **(C)** The palatal lift is in place as can be seen through this X-ray tracing.

SPEECH NOTES

Palatal Lift

A palatal lift can be very effective in the treatment of individuals with velopharyngeal incompetence, which is a neurological impairment that impairs the movement, timing, and coordination of velopharyngeal structures. Velopharyngeal incompetence can be caused by a variety of neurophysiological causes (e.g., cerebral palsy, neuromuscular disorders, brain tumors, strokes, traumatic brain injury), and it accounts for most acquired conditions causing velopharyngeal dysfunction.

Velopharyngeal incompetence typically causes moderate to severe hypernasality and is often associated with dysarthria. **Dysarthria** is a motor speech disorder that affects all the subsystems of speech, including respiration, phonation, articulation, and velopharyngeal function. There is usually weakness or poor movement of the speech articulators (tongue, lips, jaw, and velopharyngeal valve). Typical speech characteristics include slurred or imprecise articulation, slow rate, abnormal prosody, low volume, breathiness, short utterance length, and hypernasality.

A palatal lift can be useful for dysarthric patients when hypernasality due to velopharyngeal incompetence is the primary contributor to the unintelligibility of speech and articulation and phonation are not severely compromised (Bedwinek & O'Brien, 1985; Esposito, Mitsumoto, & Shanks, 2000; Koidis & Topouzelis, 2003; Shifman, Finkelstein, Nachmani, & Ophir, 2000; Yorkston et al., 2001). A palatal lift can reduce or eliminate hypernasality and improve breath support by closing the leak of air through the nose. It can even improve volume by directing sound into the mouth so that it is not absorbed by tissues of the pharynx and nasal cavity. A palatal lift may even be considered for individuals with severe apraxia that affects velopharyngeal coordination (Hall, Hardy, & LaVelle, 1990).

One disadvantage of a palatal lift is that because the velum is held against the posterior pharyngeal wall at all times, it can potentially interfere with the production of nasal sounds and nasal breathing, particularly if the lift has to be made wide for adequate velopharyngeal closure. Therefore, hyponasality is often a necessary side effect of forced velopharyngeal closure for adequate oral speech. Because the palatal lift can be removed during speech, obstructive sleep apnea (OSA) is not a concern.

Speech Bulb Obturator

A speech bulb obturator, also known as a speech aid appliance, is a removable device that is used for the treatment of velopharyngeal insufficiency (Rieger et al., 2009; Tuna, Pekkan, Gumus, & Aktas, 2010). It has even been used for velopharyngeal incompetence in severe cases (Dutka, Uemeoka, Aferri, Pegoraro-Krook, & Marino, 2011; Shifman et al., 2000; Sun, Li, & Sun, 2002).

The speech bulb obturator usually has an oral base section that clasps on to the teeth and a posterior tail with the speech bulb on the end. When in place, the bulb is positioned in the nasopharynx, just behind the velum. Therefore, the speech bulb is not visible from an intraoral perspective. The bulb sits high in the nasopharynx to occlude the velopharyngeal port for speech.

FIGURES 18-5A and **B** show two typical speech bulb obturators. **FIGURE 18-5C** shows a patient with a very short velum. **FIGURE 18-5D** shows the same patient with a speech bulb in place. Finally, **FIGURE 18-5E** shows the position of the speech bulb obturator in the nasopharynx.

As with other types of appliances, a speech bulb obturator can be combined with partial or complete dentures (Abreu, Levy, Rodriguez, & Rivera, 2007). Note that the patient has dental implants in Figure 18-5B. This patient's speech bulb was made with maxillary arch dental overlays as can be seen in Figure 18-5D.

Although speech bulbs are used infrequently with children, they are an important method of treatment for adult patients who have undergone ablative surgery or radiation for treatment of oropharyngeal cancer or other maxillary tumors (Arigbede, Dosumu, Shaba, & Esan, 2006; Bohle et al., 2005; Chambers, Lemon, & Martin, 2004; Keyf, Sahin, & Aslan, 2003; Rieger, Tang, Wolfaardt, Harris, & Seikaly, 2011; Yenisey, Cengiz, & Sarikaya, 2011). They also can be used for those who have had traumatic injuries to the palate where surgical correction is not an option. **FIGURE 18-6A** shows a patient who underwent a maxillectomy and removal of most of the velum. A palatal obturator combined with a speech bulb obturator was used for correction as can be seen in **FIGURE 18-6B**.

SPEECH NOTES

Speech Bulb Obturator

A speech bulb obturator fills a nasopharyngeal gap to close off the nasal cavity from the oral cavity for speech. As with a palatal obturator, this allows the patient to be able to impound intraoral pressure for the production of speech sounds. It can also reduce or eliminate hypernasality.

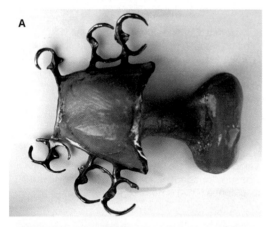

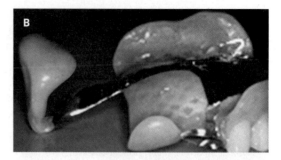

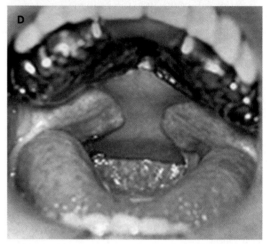

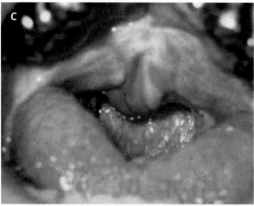

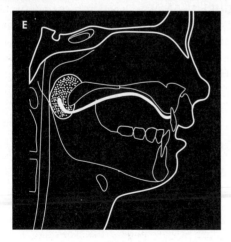

FIGURE 18-5 A speech bulb. **(A)** and **(B)** A speech bulb with the obturator at the end of the tail. **(C)** A patient with a very short velum and dental implants. **(D)** The speech bulb obturator and dental overlays in place. **(E)** The placement of the speech bulb in the pharynx as can be seen through this X-ray tracing.

Speech bulb appliances are removed at night, which allows an open airway for normal breathing and reduces the risk of sleep apnea. Although the appliance can help to eliminate nasal regurgitation, many individuals prefer to remove the appliance during meals.

Fabrication of a Speech Appliance

Speech appliances are individually designed to meet the specific needs of the patient. In addition, dental professionals may differ in the techniques and materials that they prefer to use. Although there is considerable variation among speech devices, there are also many commonalties in the way that they are designed.

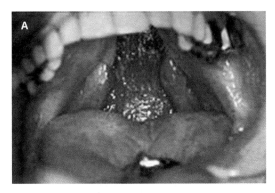
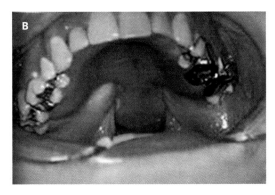

FIGURE 18-6 Palatal obturator and speech bulb obturator. **(A)** This is a patient with a large palatal defect following a maxillectomy and removal of the velum for a malignancy. **(B)** A combination palatal obturator and speech bulb in place.

Most speech appliances have an anterior palatal section (of a prosthesis), which is the body portion of the appliance. The purpose of this section is to hold the appliance in place against the roof of the mouth. It can also serve as an obturator to close off a defect in the palate. This part of the prosthesis may appear similar to a common orthodontic retainer.

The palatal section is usually made of either acrylic resins or metal. This part of the appliance must be made thick enough to avoid easy breakage but not so thick as to interfere with speech production. The appliance is formed from a plaster model of the roof of the mouth. It is designed to fit snugly against the contours of the individual's teeth and hard palate so that there is good retention during oral activity. Artificial palatal rugae can be added to assist with tongue tip orientation and articulation (Gitto, Esposito, & Draper, 1999).

The palatal section is held in place by metal wires, which are attached around the teeth for anchorage. The teeth may need to be prepared with buccal lugs on soldered bands, special caps, crowns, or undercuts to adequately retain the wires and the appliance. Retention and stability of an appliance can be a significant challenge for the prosthodontist in patients who do not have adequate maxillary teeth for use as anchors.

Fortunately, recent advances in the use of osseointegrated implants have greatly increased the ability to rehabilitate individuals with intraoral anomalies and even those with an edentulous maxillary arch (Grisius, 1991; Hudson & Russell, 1994; Lundqvist & Haraldson, 1992; Lundqvist, Haraldson, & Lindblad, 1992; Parel et al., 1986).

Osseointegrated implants are small cylinders (5 to 6 mm in diameter) that are usually made of titanium. They are fitted into a carefully prepared channel that is drilled into the alveolar bone. At least four implants of a minimum of 10 mm in length are usually recommended in the maxilla of patients with clefts (Ramstad, 1998). Once in place, the bone grows directly around the implant, resulting in osseointegration (direct connection between the implant and the bone) and a pseudo root. With these implants embedded in the bone, a speech appliance can be attached and retained. Implants can also be used to support dental restorations. A single implant can support a crown to replace an individual tooth. Multiple implants can be used to support restorations of a row of missing teeth or to secure dentures for an entire dental arch.

In addition to the palatal section, the palatal lift and speech bulb appliances have an extension, or tailpiece, that projects posteriorly to close the velopharyngeal port during speech.

Prior to constructing the tailpiece, the palatal section is fabricated because it forms the basis of the rest of the prosthesis. In fabricating the tailpiece, the prosthodontist starts with a small bulb and then slowly adds a thin layer of thermoplastic wax compound until the appropriate size and shape are achieved. This is usually done by putting it in the individual's mouth, testing it with speech, and then making modifications as needed. For a speech bulb, the device is inserted, and the patient is asked to move his head up and down and then back and forth to mold the bulb appropriately. Wax is gradually added to the bulb until it fits comfortably and works effectively in the pharynx for speech. The challenge is to make the bulb fill the space while keeping it from causing undue pressure against the soft tissue of the pharynx. The individual must be able to move his head without discomfort or irritation of the pharyngeal mucosa. Once the form is finalized, the permanent lift or bulb is made of acrylic. Sometimes speech bulbs must be large, and therefore they become too heavy for the teeth to bear. When this is the case, the bulb can be hollowed out to make it lighter and more stable.

Depending on the needs of the patient, various combinations of appliances can be constructed. For example, the speech appliance may have an oral base section with partial or complete dentures. A palatal obturator can be combined with a palatal lift or speech bulb (Alpine, Stone, & Badr, 1990) (Figure 18-6), or it can be used with a maxillary expansion appliance (Hobson & Clasper, 1995). Although these combinations are very beneficial to the patient, the mechanical design of prosthetic appliances should be kept as simple as possible.

Wear and tear on the device should be expected, and breakage will occasionally occur. Hence, devices that are simple and easy to repair are better in the long term (Mazahari, 1996). It is also important that the device be designed so that oral hygiene can be maintained.

Some children and adults learn to accept and tolerate the prosthetic appliance quickly and easily, especially those who are motivated to work for aesthetic or speech improvement. Other patients, particularly young children, are less compliant and even resist wearing a prosthetic device. In these cases, working with the family is the best avenue for achieving compliance and the inherent benefits of the device.

Procedures for Assessment and Modification of a Speech Appliance

A palatal obturator is relatively easy to fit because it includes only the palatal section and the palatal opening or fistula is not dynamic. In contrast, the palatal lift and speech bulb appliances are used to improve the closure of a dynamic opening in the velopharyngeal port. Therefore, fine adjustments must be made to these appliances so that the velopharyngeal port is closed enough for speech but not overly closed so that upper airway problems occur.

The speech-language pathologist can be very helpful to the prosthodontist in providing information on speech and resonance changes that occur as fine adjustments are made to the device. To assess the effectiveness of the speech appliance, the examiner should test the production of pressure-sensitive phonemes (plosives, fricatives, and affricates) in syllable repetition tasks and sentences (see Table 11-3 in the chapter *Speech and Resonance Assessment*). The examiner could use a simple listening tube or straw to detect subtle changes in velopharyngeal closure as the modifications to the device are made. If pressure-sensitive sounds can be produced without nasal air emission and there is no evidence of hypernasality, then the velopharyngeal port is adequately closed for speech. The speech-language pathologist should then assess the ease of nasal breathing with the appliance in place and test the production of nasal sounds (/m/, /n/, /ŋ/) in repetitive syllables and sentences. Again, a listening tube or straw can help to detect the amount of sound or air that is passing through the nasopharynx. Based on this assessment, the appliance can be modified until an appropriate balance is achieved between closure for oral speech and patency for nasal breathing and the production of nasal phonemes (Rosen & Bzoch, 1997).

In addition to a perceptual assessment, indirect instrumental measures (which provide objective data but no visualization of the velopharyngeal port) can be used to evaluate the effectiveness of a prosthetic appliance. For example, nasometry can provide objective information regarding the extent of improvement with the appliance and the relative normalcy of speech as a result (Pinborough-Zimmerman et al., 1998; Scarsellone, Rochet, & Wolfaardt, 1999). It can also provide information regarding the patency of the airway while the appliance is in place.

Although a perceptual assessment and indirect instrumental assessment techniques are helpful in evaluating the effect of an appliance on speech and airway, these procedures do not give the prosthodontist necessary information if adjustments have to be made. For this information, a direct instrumental approach (where the velopharyngeal valve can be visualized) is needed so that the prosthodontist knows where the appliance should

be augmented and where it should be reduced. The best procedure for assessment of an appliance is nasopharyngoscopy.

By performing nasopharyngoscopy with the device in place, the extent of velopharyngeal closure can be easily determined as a result of the device (D'Antonio, Muntz, Marsh, Marty-Grames, & Backensto-Marsh, 1988; Karnell, Rosenstein, & Fine, 1987; Rich, Farber, & Shprintzen, 1988; Rieger, Zalmanowitz, & Wolfaardt, 2006). In addition, the effect of the device on nasal sounds and the patency of the airway during nasal breathing can be viewed. **FIGURE 18-7A** shows the nasopharyngoscopy exam of a patient with velopharyngeal incompetence, resulting in a midline opening. **FIGURE 18-7B** shows greatly improved velopharyngeal closure as a result of a palatal lift.

An optimal fit often requires trial and error and several adjustments to the appliance. If there is still a leak in velopharyngeal closure, then the appliance can be augmented for that specific area. At times, the airway must be compromised slightly for the best speech benefit. At other times, perfect speech must be compromised for the sake of the airway. However, with the benefit

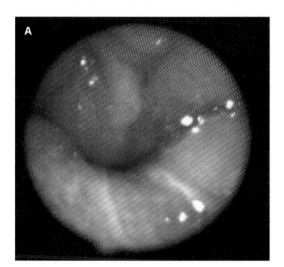
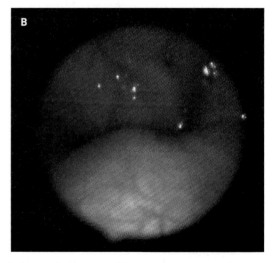

FIGURE 18-7 (A) A velopharyngeal opening during speech from velopharyngeal incompetence as can be seen through nasopharyngoscopy. **(B)** Greatly improved velopharyngeal competence as a result of placement of a palatal lift.

of a nasopharyngoscopy view, the device can be modified until it appears to be optimal for both speech and the airway.

Advantages and Disadvantages of Prosthetic Management

Although surgical correction is usually considered the best option for the treatment of structural defects from cleft lip/palate, there are cases where prosthetic management is more appropriate or necessary. These cases include patients for whom surgery must be delayed because of a medical condition or the need to do other procedures first. Prosthetic devices can be used effectively in the management of large soft palate perforations or palatal fistulas that are very difficult if not impossible to repair. They are appropriate for patients with persistent VPI after several unsuccessful surgical repairs (Hoffman, 1985). For example, if a pharyngeal flap was done but the lateral ports do not close sufficiently, a device can be made that has a bulb on one or both sides to fill in the area of the port(s) (McKinstry, 1998a). Prosthetic devices are sometimes used on a trial basis in cases where the outcome of surgical correction is unclear. If the prosthodontist is routinely consulted in the initial treatment planning, alternatives to surgical management might be considered for patients with high potential for postsurgical failure (McKinstry & Aramany, 1985).

Speech appliances are sometimes appropriate for patients with structural disorders not related to cleft palate. For example, a uvulopalatopharyngoplasty (UPPP), which is done to alleviate snoring and sleep apnea, can cause velopharyngeal insufficiency in rare cases. When this occurs, prosthetic management is often appropriate because there is no risk of causing further sleep problems with this form of correction (Finkelstein, Shifman, Nachmani, & Ophir, 1995).

Prosthetic management is particularly useful following cancer treatment, especially if the treatment involved ablative surgery of the maxilla or velum. Patients with oral carcinomas often require resection of other parts of the mouth as well, including the tongue, the floor of the mouth, or the bone of the mandible. In these cases, prosthetic treatment may include a tongue prosthesis, a palatal device, and other types of prostheses to improve articulation, resonance, and swallowing (Pinto & Pegoraro-Krook, 2003).

Patients who exhibit normal velopharyngeal anatomy but demonstrate velopharyngeal incompetence secondary to neuromotor disorders may not be appropriate surgical candidates. However, as mentioned before, individuals with dysarthria (Bedwinek & O'Brien, 1985) or apraxia (Hall et al., 1990) may derive significant benefit from a palatal lift. This allows the individual to concentrate on anterior articulation and not be concerned about velopharyngeal articulation.

Prosthetic management is usually most successful with individuals who have adequate dentition for retention of the device and good oral hygiene. Another consideration when trying to fit a palatal lift or speech bulb is the gag reflex. Although the prosthodontist can work to gradually desensitize the patient to the device, a strong gag reflex or oral sensitivity makes successful prosthetic management very difficult if not impossible to achieve. Finally, successful prosthetic management is somewhat dependent on good articulation because corrected velopharyngeal function for speech will not improve intelligibility significantly if the articulation is poor.

Although prosthetic devices have been used successfully by many patients for closure of a fistula or management of VPI, they have some distinct disadvantages. Unlike surgery, these devices do not result in a permanent correction. When they are removed, the speech symptoms recur. Prosthetic appliances are expensive and often are not covered by insurance. The cost is greater for children because their appliance needs to be modified or completely redone as they grow and dentition changes. Appliances can be easily lost or damaged. They need to be removed for daily cleaning and sleep, so there is a need for manual dexterity or the assistance of others. They may be uncomfortable to wear and can cause ulceration of the surrounding mucosa. Retention of appliances can be a challenge for patients with irregularities in the dentition or missing teeth. Finally, there may be poor compliance, especially with young children.

Because of these limitations, removable prosthetic devices are not well suited for patients who are very young or developmentally delayed or have significant physical handicaps. They do not work well for patients who have difficulty managing secretions, a strong gag reflex, or significant upper airway obstruction. When they are offered as a temporary treatment, most patients who are able to undergo surgical correction usually do opt for surgery after a period of prosthetic management (Marsh & Wray, 1980). Despite their limitations, prosthetic devices should always be considered for correction of a palatal defect or VPI when surgery is not an option for medical reasons (McKinstry, 1998a).

Prosthetic Management and Speech Therapy

A prosthetic device (e.g., palatal lift or speech bulb obturator) can greatly improve velopharyngeal closure and therefore give the individual the ability to impound intraoral air pressure for production of oral sounds (Gallagher, 1982). This makes speech therapy much more effective in eliminating any compensatory articulation productions that developed prior to prosthetic management (Pinto, da Silva Dalben, & Pegoraro-Krook, 2007).

Prosthetic devices have also been used as a form of therapy to attempt to improve velopharyngeal function, although this is very controversial. This type of therapy, called reduction therapy, is done in hopes of stimulating increased movement of the velopharyngeal structures to avoid surgery or reduce the extent of the surgery that is needed.

When a palatal lift has been used in reduction therapy, the length of the lift is gradually reduced, or the wearing time of the lift is gradually decreased in hopes of stimulating velar movement. However, it has been shown that the passive elevation of the velum actually reduces levator veli palatini muscle activity (Nohara et al., 2010; Tachimura, Nohara, Fujita, Hara, & Wada, 2001). Therefore, this use of a lift may ultimately be more harmful than beneficial in increasing velar movement.

Reduction therapy has also been done with a speech bulb in the nasopharynx. The size of the bulb is gradually reduced in hopes of gradually increasing velar and lateral wall movement. Some authors have reported some success in improving lateral wall motion with this procedure (Golding-Kushner, Cisneros, & LeBlanc, 1995). However, these results do not seem to be maintained, and most individuals still require surgical intervention for correction despite this therapy (Witt et al., 1995; Wolfaardt, Wilson, Rochet, & McPhee, 1993). Considering the lack of evidence for real and lasting benefit with reduction therapy and the time and expense of the prosthesis and speech therapy, this does not seem to be a viable treatment method at this time.

SUMMARY

With the advances in surgical procedures and improvement in the timing of surgery, prosthetic management of cleft lip/palate and VPI is not done as frequently as in years past. However, there is a definite need for prosthetic management in certain cases, particularly in cases where surgical intervention is not an option. Prosthetic management can be very effective in improving the individual's appearance and speech. Speech appliances can be effective in improving or eliminating hypernasality and nasal emission from either a fistula or VPI. When fabricating a palatal lift or a speech bulb, it is important to balance the need to close off the nasal cavity for oral speech sounds while leaving an adequate opening for nasal breathing. The ultimate goal of prosthetic management is to help the patient achieve the best possible outcome with the device.

FOR REVIEW AND DISCUSSION

1. Why do you think prosthetic devices are actually used less than they were 20 years ago?

2. What types of patients could benefit from a facial or oral prosthetic device? What professionals are trained to construct these devices?

3. What is the purpose of a dental appliance? What are the different types? How do you think a dental appliance could affect speech?

4. How does a feeding obturator improve an infant's feeding when there is a cleft palate? Why is it now used infrequently for children with cleft palate?

5. Describe the three types of speech appliances that are used for improvement of speech and resonance. What is the appropriate indication for each?

6. What are the components of most speech appliances? What materials are used? How are they retained?

7. Describe ways that the speech-language pathologist should work with the prosthodontist (or dental professional) to achieve the best outcome with a speech appliance.

8. What are the clinical indications and contraindications for the use of prosthetic devices for speech?

9. How have prosthetic devices been used as part of the speech therapy process? Discuss the controversy regarding the use of reduction therapy.

REFERENCES

Abreu, A., Levy, D., Rodriguez, E., & Rivera, I. (2007). Oral rehabilitation of a patient with complete unilateral cleft lip and palate using an implant-retained speech-aid prosthesis: Clinical report. *The Cleft Palate–Craniofacial Journal, 44*(6), 673–677.

Ahmed, B., Farshad, A. F., & Yazdanie, N. (2011). Rehabilitation of a large maxillo-facial defect using acrylic resin prosthesis. *Journal of College of Physicians and Surgeons Pakistan, 21*(4), 254–256.

Alpine, K. D., Stone, C. R., & Badr, S. E. (1990). Combined obturator and palatal-lift prosthesis: A case report. *Quintessence International, 21*(11), 893–896.

American Speech-Language-Hearing Association (ASHA). (1993). Position statement and guidelines for oral and oropharyngeal prostheses. *ASHA, 35*(Suppl. 10), 14–16.

Arigbede, A. O., Dosumu, O. O., Shaba, O. P., & Esan, T. A. (2006). Evaluation of speech in patients with partial surgically acquired defects: Pre and post prosthetic obturation. *Journal of Contemporary Dental Practice, 7*(1), 89–96.

Bedwinek, A. P., & O'Brien, R. L. (1985). A patient selection profile for the use of speech prostheses in adult dysarthria. *Journal of Communication Disorders, 18*(3), 169–182.

Beumer, J., III, Roumanas, E., & Nishimura, R. (1995). Advances in osseointegrated implants for dental and facial rehabilitation following major head and neck surgery. *Seminars in Surgical Oncology, 11*(3), 200–207.

Blair, F. M., & Hunter, N. R. (1998). The hollow box maxillary obturator. *British Dental Journal, 184*(10), 484–487.

Bohle, G., III, Rieger, J., Huryn, J., Verbel, D., Hwang, F., & Zlotolow, I. (2005). Efficacy of speech aid prostheses for acquired defects of the soft palate and velopharyngeal inadequacy: Clinical assessments and cephalometric analysis. *Head & Neck, 27*(3), 195–207.

Chambers, M. S., Lemon, J. C., & Martin, J. W. (2004). Obturation of the partial soft palate defect. *Journal of Prosthetic Dentistry, 91*(1), 75–79.

Chang, T. L., Garrett, N., Roumanas, E., & Beumer, J., III. (2005). Treatment satisfaction with facial prostheses. *Journal of Prosthetic Dentistry, 94*(3), 275–280.

Daniel, B. (1982). A soft-palate desensitization procedure for patients requiring palatal lift prostheses. *Journal of Prosthetic Dentistry, 48*(5), 565–566.

D'Antonio, L. L., Muntz, H. R., Marsh, J. L., Marty-Grames, L., & Backensto-Marsh, R. (1988). Practical application of flexible fiberoptic nasopharyngoscopy for evaluating velopharyngeal function. *Plastic and Reconstructive Surgery, 82*(4), 611–618.

Delgado, A. A., Schaaf, N. G., & Emrich, L. (1992). Trends in prosthodontic treatment of cleft palate patients at one institution: A twenty-one year review. *The Cleft Palate–Craniofacial Journal, 29*(5), 425–428.

Dhakshaini, M.R., Pushpavathi M., Garhnayak, M., & Dhal, A. (2015). Prosthodontic management in conjunction with speech therapy in cleft lip and palate: A review and case report. *Journal of International Oral Health, 7*(Suppl. 2), 106–111.

Dorf, D. S., Reisberg, D. J., & Gold, H. O. (1985). Early prosthetic management of cleft palate. Articulation development prosthesis: A preliminary report. *Journal of Prosthetic Dentistry, 53*(2), 222–226.

dos Santos, D. M., Goiato, M. C., Pesqueira, A. A., Bannwart, L. C., Rezende, M. C., Magro-Filho, O., & Moreno, A. (2010). Prosthesis auricular with osseointegrated implants and quality of life. *Journal of Craniofacial Surgery, 21*(1), 94–96.

Dutka, J. C., Uemeoka, E., Aferri, H. C., Pegoraro-Krook, M. I., & Marino, V. C. (2011). Total obturation of the velopharynx for treatment of velopharyngeal hypodynamism: Case report. *The Cleft Palate–Craniofacial Journal, 49*(4), 488–493.

Esposito, S. J., Mitsumoto, H., & Shanks, M. (2000). Use of palatal lift and palatal augmentation prostheses to improve dysarthria in patients with amyotrophic lateral sclerosis: A case series. *Journal of Prosthetic Dentistry, 83*(1), 90–98.

Feng, Z. H., Dong, Y., Bai, S. Z., Wu, G. F., Bi, Y. P., Wang, B., & Zhao, Y. M. (2010). Virtual transplantation in designing a facial prosthesis for extensive maxillofacial defects that cross the facial midline using computer-assisted technology. *International Journal of Prosthodontics, 23*(6), 513–520.

Finkelstein, Y., Shifman, A., Nachmani, A., & Ophir, D. (1995). Prosthetic management of velopharyngeal insufficiency induced by uvulopalatopharyngoplasty. *Otolaryngology–Head & Neck Surgery, 113*(5), 611–616.

Gallagher, B. (1982). Prosthesis in velopharyngeal insufficiency: Effect on nasal resonance. *Journal of Communication Disorders, 15*(6), 469–473.

Gardner, L. K., & Parr, G. R. (1996). Prosthetic rehabilitation of the cleft palate patient. *Seminars in Orthodontics, 2*(3), 215–219.

Gitto, C. A., Esposito, S. J., & Draper, J. M. (1999). A simple method of adding palatal rugae to a complete denture. *Journal of Prosthetic Dentistry, 81*(2), 237–239.

Goiato, M. C., dos Santos, D. M., Haddad, M. F., & Moreno, A. (2012). Rehabilitation with ear prosthesis linked to osseointegrated implants. *Gerodontology, 29*(2), 150–154.

Golding-Kushner, K. J., Cisneros, G., & LeBlanc, E. (1995). Speech bulbs. In R. J. Shprintzen & J. Bardach (Eds.), *Cleft palate speech management* (pp. 352–363). St. Louis, MO: Mosby.

Goyal, M., Chopra, R., Bansal, K., & Marwaha, M. (2014). Role of obturators and other feeding interventions in patients with cleft lip and palate: A review. *European Archives of Paediatric Dentistry, 15*(1), 1–9.

Grisius, R. J. (1991). Maxillofacial prosthetics. *Current Opinions in Dentistry, 1*(2), 155–159.

Hall, P. K., Hardy, J. C., & LaVelle, W. E. (1990). A child with signs of developmental apraxia of speech with whom a palatal lift prosthesis was used to manage palatal dysfunction. *Journal of Speech and Hearing Disorders, 55*(3), 454–460.

Hansen, P. A., Cook, N. B., & Ahmad, O. (2016). Fabrication of a feeding obturator for infants. *The Cleft Palate Craniofacial Journal, 53*(2), 240–244.

Hobson, R. S., & Clasper, R. (1995). A combined obturator and expansion appliance for use in patients with patent oral-nasal fistula. *British Journal of Orthodontics, 22*(4), 357–359.

Hoffman, S. (1985). Correction of lateral port stenosis following a pharyngeal flap operation. *Cleft Palate Journal, 22*(1), 51–55.

Hudson, J. W., & Russell, R., Jr. (1994). Contributions within dental science to cleft lip/palate management: A literature review. *Compendium, 15*(1), 116, 118–120, 122; quiz 126.

Karnell, M. P., Rosenstein, H., & Fine, L. (1987). Nasal videoendoscopy in prosthetic management of palatopharyngeal dysfunction. *Journal of Prosthetic Dentistry, 58*(4), 479–484.

Keyf, F., Sahin, N., & Aslan, Y. (2003). Alternative impression technique for a speech-aid prosthesis. *The Cleft Palate–Craniofacial Journal, 40*(6), 566–568.

Koidis, P. T., & Topouzelis, N. (2003). Palatal lift prosthesis for palatopharyngeal closure in Wilson's disease. *Orthodontics & Craniofacial Research, 6*(2), 101–103.

Lohmander-Agerskov, A., Soderpalm, E., Friede, H., & Lilja, J. (1990). Cleft lip and palate patients prior to delayed closure of the hard palate: Evaluation of maxillary morphology and the effect of early stimulation on pre-school speech. *Scandinavian Journal of Plastic and Reconstructive Surgery and Hand Surgery, 24*(2), 141–148.

Lundgren, S., Moy, P. K., Beumer, J., III, & Lewis, S. (1993). Surgical considerations for endosseous implants in the craniofacial region: A 3-year report. *International Journal of Oral and Maxillofacial Surgery, 22,* 272–277.

Lundqvist, S., & Haraldson, T. (1992). Oral function in patients wearing fixed prosthesis on osseointegrated implants in the maxilla: A 3-year follow-up study. *Scandinavian Journal of Dental Research, 100*(5), 279–283.

Lundqvist, S., Haraldson, T., & Lindblad, P. (1992). Speech in connection with maxillary fixed prostheses on osseointegrated implants: A three-year follow-up study. *Clinics in Oral Implants Research, 3*(4), 176–180.

Marsh, J. L., & Wray, R. C. (1980). Speech prosthesis versus pharyngeal flap: A randomized evaluation of the management of velopharyngeal incompetency. *Plastic and Reconstructive Surgery, 65*(5), 592–594.

Mazahari, M. (1996). Prosthetic speech appliances for patients with cleft palate. In S. Berkowitz (Ed.), *Cleft lip and palate with introduction to other craniofacial abnormalities: Perspectives in management* (vol. 2, pp. 177–194). San Diego, CA: Singular Publishing Group.

McKinstry, R. E. (1998a). Cleft palate prosthetics. In R. E. McKinstry (Ed.), *Cleft palate dentistry* (pp. 206–235). Arlington, VA: ABI Professional Publications.

McKinstry, R. E. (1998b). Presurgical management of cleft lip and palate patients. In R. E. McKinstry (Ed.), *Cleft palate dentistry* (pp. 33–66). Arlington, VA: ABI Professional Publications.

McKinstry, R. E., & Aramany, M. A. (1985). Prosthodontic considerations in the management of surgically compromised cleft palate patients. *Journal of Prosthetic Dentistry, 53*(6), 827–831.

Mueller, A. A., Paysan, P., Schumacher, R., Zeilhofer, H. F., Berg-Boerner, B. I., Maurer, J., . . . Schwenzer-Zimmerer, K. (2011). Missing facial parts computed by a morphable model and transferred directly to a polyamide laser-sintered prosthesis: An innovation study. *British Journal of Oral & Maxillofacial Surgery, 49*(8), e67–e71.

Nagda, S., Deshpande, D. S., & Mhatre, S. W. (1996). Infant palatal obturator. *Journal of the Indian Society of Pedodontics & Preventive Dentistry, 14*(1), 24–25.

Nohara, K., Kotani, Y., Sasao, Y., Ojima, M., Tachimura, T., & Sakai, T. (2010). Effect of a speech aid prosthesis on reducing muscle fatigue. *Journal of Dental Research, 89*(5), 478–481.

Osuji, O. O. (1995). Preparation of feeding obturators for infants with cleft lip and palate. *Journal of Clinical Pediatric Dentistry, 19*(3), 211–214.

Parel, S. M., Holt, G. R., Branemark, P. I., & Tjellstrom, A. (1986). Osseointegration and facial prosthetics. *International Journal of Oral and Maxillofacial Implants, 1*(1), 27–29.

Pinborough-Zimmerman, J., Canady, G., Yamashiro, D. K., & Morales, L., Jr. (1998). Articulation and nasality changes resulting from sustained palatal fistula obturation. *The Cleft Palate–Craniofacial Journal, 35*(1), 81–87.

Pinto, J. H., da Silva Dalben, G., & Pegoraro-Krook, M. I. (2007). Speech intelligibility of patients with cleft lip and palate after placement of speech prosthesis. *The Cleft Palate–Craniofacial Journal, 44*(6), 635–641.

Pinto, J. H., & Pegoraro-Krook, M. I. (2003). Evaluation of palatal prosthesis for the treatment of velopharyngeal dysfunction. *Journal of Applied Oral Science, 11*(3), 192–197.

Raju, H., Padmanabhan, T. V., & Narayan, A. (2009). Effect of a palatal lift prosthesis in individuals with velopharyngeal incompetence. *International Journal of Prosthodontics, 22*(6), 579–585.

Ramstad, T. (1998). Fixed prosthodontics. In R. E. McKinstry (Ed.), *Cleft palate dentistry* (pp. 236–262). Arlington, VA: ABI Professional Publications.

Reisberg, D. J. (2000). Dental and prosthodontic care for patients with cleft or craniofacial conditions. *The Cleft Palate–Craniofacial Journal, 37*(6), 534–537.

Rich, B. M., Farber, K., & Shprintzen, R. J. (1988). Nasopharyngoscopy in the treatment of palatopharyngeal insufficiency. *International Journal of Prosthodontics, 1*(3), 248–251.

Rieger, J., Bohle, G., III, Huryn, J., Tang, J. L., Harris, J., & Seikaly, H. (2009). Surgical reconstruction versus prosthetic obturation of extensive soft palate defects: A comparison of speech outcomes. *International Journal of Prosthodontics, 22*(6), 566–572.

Rieger, J. M., Tang, J. A., Wolfaardt, J., Harris, J., & Seikaly, H. (2011). Comparison of speech and aesthetic outcomes in patients with maxillary reconstruction versus maxillary obturators after maxillectomy. *Otolaryngology-Head & Neck Surgery, 40*(1), 40–47.

Rieger, J. M., Zalmanowitz, J. G., & Wolfaardt, J. F. (2006). Nasopharyngoscopy in palatopharyngeal prosthetic rehabilitation: A preliminary report. *International Journal of Prosthodontics, 19*(4), 383–388.

Rosen, M. S., & Bzoch, K. R. (1997). Prosthodontic management of the individual with cleft lip and palate for speech habilitation needs. In K. R. Bzoch (Ed.), *Communicative disorders related to cleft lip and palate* (vol. 4, pp. 153–168). Austin, TX: Pro-Ed.

Savion, L., & Huband, M. L. (2005). A feeding obturator for a preterm baby with Pierre Robin sequence. *Journal of Prosthetic Dentistry, 93*(2), 197–200.

Scarsellone, J. M., Rochet, A. P., & Wolfaardt, J. F. (1999). The influence of dentures on nasalance values in speech. *The Cleft Palate–Craniofacial Journal, 36*(1), 51–56.

Schweckendiek, W. (1966). The technique of early veloplasty and its results. *Acta Chiruriae Plasticae, 8*(3), 188–194.

Schweckendiek, W. (1968). Early veloplasty and its results. *Acta Oto-Rhino-Laryngologica Belgica, 22*(6), 697–703.

Shifman, A., Finkelstein, Y., Nachmani, A., & Ophir, D. (2000). Speech-aid prostheses for neurogenic velopharyngeal incompetence. *Journal of Prosthetic Dentistry, 83*(1), 99–106.

Sidoti, E. J., & Shprintzen, R. J. (1995). Pediatric care and feeding of the newborn with a cleft. In R. J. Shprintzen & J. Bardach (Eds.), *Cleft palate speech management* (pp. 63–74). St. Louis, MO: Mosby.

Singh, V. P., Bharadwaj, G., & Nair, K. C. (1997). Direct observation of tongue positions in speech: A patient study. *International Journal of Prosthodontics, 10*(3), 231–234.

Sultana, A., Rahman, M. M., Nessa, J., & Alam, M. S. (2011). A feeding aid prosthesis for a preterm baby with cleft lip and palate. *Mymensingh Medical Journal, 20*(1), 22–27.

Sun, J., Li, N., & Sun, G. (2002). Application of obturator to treat velopharyngeal incompetence. *Chinese Medical Journal (English), 115*(6), 842–845.

Tachimura, T., Nohara, K., Fujita, Y., Hara, H., & Wada, T. (2001). Change in levator veli palatini muscle activity of normal speakers in association with elevation of the velum using an experimental palatal lift prosthesis. *The Cleft Palate–Craniofacial Journal, 38*(5), 449–454.

Tuna, S. H., Pekkan, G., Gumus, H. O., & Aktas, A. (2010). Prosthetic rehabilitation of velopharyngeal insufficiency: Pharyngeal obturator prostheses with different retention mechanisms. *European Journal of Dentistry, 4*(1), 81–87.

Walter, J. D. (2005). Obturators for cleft palate and other speech appliances. *Dental Update, 32*(4), 217–218.

Witt, P. D., Rozelle, A. A., Marsh, J. L., Marty-Grames, L., Muntz, H. R., Gay, W. D., & Pilgram, T. K. (1995). Do palatal lift prostheses stimulate velopharyngeal neuromuscular activity? *The Cleft Palate–Craniofacial Journal, 32*(6), 469–475.

Wolfaardt, J. F., Wilson, F. B., Rochet, A., & McPhee, L. (1993). An appliance-based approach to the management of palato-pharyngeal incompetency: A clinical pilot project. *Journal of Prosthetic Dentistry, 69*(2), 186–195.

Yenisey, M., Cengiz, S., & Sarikaya, I. (2011). Prosthetic treatment of congenital hard and soft palate defects: A clinical report. *The Cleft Palate–Craniofacial Journal, 49*(5), 618–621.

Yorkston, K. M., Spencer, K., Duffy, J., Beukelman, D., Golper, L. A., & Miller, R. (2001). Evidence-based practice guidelines for dysarthria: Management of velopharyngeal function. *Journal of Medical Speech Language Pathology, 9*(4), 257–274.

CREDITS

Chapter opener photo: © PeopleImages/Getty Images

Figure 18-5A and 18-7 (A–B): Courtesy of the Cleft and Craniofacial Center at Cincinnati Children's Hospital Medical Center.

All other photos courtesy of Gordon Huntress, DDS, Cincinnati Children's Hospital Medical Center & University of Cincinnati College of Medicine.

CHAPTER 19

Speech Therapy

CHAPTER OUTLINE

INTRODUCTION

Children with cleft lip/palate or craniofacial anomalies are at risk for certain speech and resonance disorders secondary to velopharyngeal insufficiency or incompetence (VPI), oral anomalies, and dental malocclusion. Even with early surgical repair, the majority of preschoolers with cleft palate will demonstrate some difficulties with speech sound development (Hardin-Jones & Jones, 2005). In addition to cleft palate, velopharyngeal dysfunction can occur for a variety of other reasons.

As has been discussed in other chapters, when the velopharyngeal valve is defective, speech may be characterized by hypernasality and/or nasal air emission. In addition, inadequate intraoral pressure as a result of nasal emission can cause weak consonant production, short utterance length, and the development of compensatory articulation productions. It is important to determine the underlying cause of these speech characteristics through perceptual and instrumental methods because the cause has a direct effect on the selection of the appropriate treatment method (e.g., speech therapy and/or surgery).

It is very important to understand that speech therapy does not correct hypernasality or nasal emission caused by either form of VPI. Speech therapy is effective in correcting only abnormal speech sound placement that may result from these disorders. It is also important to know that oral-motor exercises (blowing, sucking, or any other nonspeech activities) are completely ineffective in correcting resonance or velopharyngeal function and therefore should not be used for this purpose. Instead, speech therapy techniques to change abnormal articulation placement are most appropriate and effective.

The purpose of this chapter is to discuss when speech therapy is indicated for children with structural anomalies that affect speech and resonance. In addition, speech therapy techniques for abnormal articulation placement will be described in detail.

Timetable for Intervention and Goals

Involvement of the speech-language pathologist in the care of the child with a cleft or other craniofacial condition begins soon after birth and may extend into adulthood. The intensity of involvement is greatest in the preschool years between ages 3 and 5. However, adolescents and even adults will sometimes need speech therapy.

Infants and Toddlers

During the first few weeks of life, the airway and ability to adequately feed are priorities. Once effective feeding has been established, the next priority for a speech-language pathologist is language development. The parents should be counseled that during the first 3 years, they should concentrate on the *quantity* of speech (how much the child can understand, how many different words the child uses, and how many words are used in utterances) and not worry as much about the *quality* of speech (articulation, resonance, and intelligibility).

The speech-language pathologist on the cleft palate/craniofacial team should counsel families on methods of both speech sound stimulation and language stimulation during this critical period of time. Because the parents are the primary instructors of speech and language for the child, they should be advised on how to be most effective in that job (Amorosa & Endres, 2004; O'Gara & Logemann, 1990; Pamplona & Ysunza, 2000; Phillips, 1990; Skeat, Eadie, Ukoumunne, & Reilly, 2010; Stevens, Watson, & Dodd, 2001). Families should be given both verbal instructions and a printed home program on speech and language stimulation because children with clefts are especially at greater risk (Antonarakis & Kiliaridis, 2009; Hardin, 1991). If language does not develop normally or there are feeding problems, therapy should be initiated immediately.

Although articulation and resonance are not the primary focus of the first 3 years, there are some things that parents can do to stimulate early phonemic development. Parents should be shown how to encourage vocalizations by imitating the child's cooing and babbling. If there is a cleft palate, they should be instructed on how to encourage the production of plosives once the cleft is repaired. By teaching parents how to work with the child on normal sound production, the development of compensatory articulation productions may be prevented (Golding-Kushner, 2001). If there is hypernasality or nasal air emission during production, the parents can be shown how to gently pinch the child's nostrils during sound imitation to allow for more normal production.

Preschool Children

By the age of 3, most children are communicating with complete sentences, although errors in syntax and morphology are common. The child should be using nasal and plosive sounds, some fricatives, and even affricate phonemes. Therefore, this is an appropriate time to evaluate speech, resonance, and velopharyngeal function and if indicated begin treatment. If it is determined that secondary surgical intervention is needed, it is best done between the ages of 3 and 5. Although speech therapy can be initiated to work on placement errors before surgery for VPI, the therapy will be easier and less frustrating for the child if the surgery is done first. In addition, progress will be much faster, and as a result, the therapy will be more cost effective.

Parents and even older siblings should be active in the treatment process for the best results. Therefore, they should be encouraged to observe therapy. Progress is much faster if the parents are involved and there is frequent practice between the therapy sessions (Pamplona & Ysunza, 2000; Pamplona, Ysunza, & Jimenez-Murat, 2001; Pamplona, Ysunza, & Uriostegui, 1996).

The goal of physical management and speech therapy in the preschool years is to attain age-appropriate speech or close to it by the time the child enters kindergarten. This is important because preschool children are more receptive to acquiring new speech patterns and correcting abnormal speech patterns than older children because of the neural plasticity (Dowling, 2004). Also, speech patterns are not strongly habituated and are therefore easier to change. Finally, early

correction avoids the social and emotional problems that come from teasing in the school-age years.

There are several practical reasons for early intervention in a specialty hospital. One reason is that funding for private speech therapy through medical insurance is more available for preschool children than for school-age children. In addition, individual therapy with frequent collaboration with parents can be offered in a hospital or specialty center. Finally, there are usually specialists in craniofacial anomalies and VPI to provide the therapy.

School-Age Children

School-age children who continue to have speech problems typically receive therapy through their school system. At this point, VPI should have been corrected if it was present. If there is still hypernasality or nasal emission, the child should be referred to the craniofacial team for evaluation (or reevaluation) of velopharyngeal function and consideration of physical management.

Children in this age group often have malocclusion or dental anomalies that cause obligatory distortions or compensatory errors. If orthognathic surgery is required, this will not be done until after facial growth is complete around age 14 for girls and 18 for boys. Therefore, the child with speech distortions may be in a "holding pattern" until the surgical correction. It is important to help parents, teachers, and healthcare professionals understand why speech therapy is not appropriate when this occurs. The speech-language pathologist should not be pressured into providing speech therapy if there is no reasonable expectation that improvement can be made because this would be an ethical violation.

Adolescents and Adults

Speech therapy is sometimes required after the patient undergoes orthognathic surgery. In addition, adolescents or adults with a cleft or craniofacial condition occasionally decide to seek speech improvement. If the primary problem is uncorrected VPI, surgical or prosthetic intervention should be done first. If the person's articulation is essentially normal, then there should be significant improvement in speech with physical management alone.

If there are many compensatory productions (with or without VPI), the prognosis for correction with speech therapy is uncertain because of the strong habit strength of the current speech productions (Wang, Jiang, Wu, Chen, & Li, 2003). The person should be counseled that speech therapy will not be effective unless there is consistent daily practice at home. Overall, the severity of the speech and the individual's motivation must be considered before recommending surgical intervention and speech therapy at an older age.

Speech Therapy versus Physical Management

Whenever there are structural anomalies in the cavities of the vocal tract, there is a risk for speech distortions and/or placement errors in speech sound production in addition to a risk for abnormal resonance. In some cases, speech therapy is appropriate for correction. In other cases, physical management (surgery or a prosthetic device) is indicated. It is very important to determine the appropriate form of management for the child based on the existing structural anomalies and the characteristics of the speech.

Obligatory Distortions

Obligatory distortions are those that occur when function (e.g., articulation) is normal, but the structure is abnormal. Resonance disorders and nasal emission are obligatory distortions unless they are phoneme specific, which indicates that they are caused by abnormal articulation placement.

Because obligatory distortions are caused by abnormal structure, they can be eliminated only by correcting the structure. Speech therapy is not indicated for obligatory distortions because

articulation placement is normal (Kummer, 2011; Trost-Cardamone, 1997). In fact, for ethical reasons, the speech-language pathologist must refuse to offer speech therapy for an individual whose speech distortion is caused by a structural abnormality. The only exception to this rule is if the structure cannot (or will not) be corrected. In that case, speech therapy may be appropriate to help the person develop compensatory strategies to improve the intelligibility of speech.

When there is slight and/or inconsistent nasal emission caused by a small and/or inconsistent velopharyngeal opening, it may be tempting to try speech therapy for correction. Although the child may be able to achieve closure and eliminate nasal emission with conscious thought and extra effort (as in the therapy session), it is unlikely that he will be able to maintain this closure throughout the day. Therefore, even with a small, inconsistent opening, surgical management is more appropriate. The decision to consider surgical management for a small opening should be made based on how much the nasal emission affects the quality and intelligibility of speech. Only the family and child can determine whether its effect on speech warrants the surgical procedure.

Compensatory Errors

Compensatory errors are those that occur when articulation placement is altered in response to abnormal structure, such as velopharyngeal insufficiency or dental malocclusion. Compensatory speech productions are functional errors and therefore require speech therapy for correction. The therapy procedures are based on achieving normal placement for the intended sound, not the compensatory production. Therefore, the same therapy techniques are used for compensatory productions as for substitution errors from other causes.

Oronasal Fistula

The effect of an oronasal fistula on speech is determined by its size and location. If the oronasal fistula is symptomatic for speech, the child may compensate by either backing to valve the airflow behind the fistula before the air escapes through it or holding the tongue against the fistula to prevent nasal escape. These errors cannot be easily corrected with speech therapy as long as the fistula remains.

Ideally, surgical correction of a symptomatic oronasal fistula is needed before speech therapy should be initiated. However, the oronasal fistula closure is often done in conjunction with the bone graft, at around age 6 or 7, so that it does not require a separate procedure. If the child is much younger and speech is affected, it is often worth using a palatal obturator to occlude the fistula for normal speech development and/or for speech therapy. The obturator is used only until the fistula is surgically closed.

Before VPI Surgery

Some surgeons (and even some speech-language pathologists) advocate speech therapy to try to correct articulation placement of compensatory errors before surgical correction of the VPI. (Ironically, these professionals would never suggest speech therapy to correct compensatory productions before repairing the cleft palate.)

Although changing placement before correction of VPI may be possible in some cases, it does not obviate the need for surgical correction of VPI. In addition, speech therapy in the presence of an inadequate velopharyngeal valve is very difficult, time-consuming, and therefore expensive. Even if successful, the change in placement usually results in a loss of intelligibility given the fact that compensatory errors are developed to increase intelligibility. Therefore, if the child has VPI, it is usually best to start speech therapy for compensatory productions after surgical correction so the child has the physical ability to produce sounds normally. Once structure is normalized, correction of the compensatory productions is much faster, easier, and less frustrating for both the child and the speech-language pathologist.

Typically, VPI surgery is done as soon as it is a confirmed diagnosis and it is safe from an airway perspective. This is usually around age 3 or 4. Unfortunately, the surgery is delayed for some patients, particularly those with upper airway obstruction (often secondary to Pierre Robin sequence), cardiac issues or other complicating medical conditions, and neurological conditions that may predispose the child to central sleep apnea. If the surgery is on hold and there is concern that the child is developing compensatory productions, speech therapy can still be done with certain modifications.

For speech therapy to be effective, the child needs to have enough airflow in the oral cavity to work on normal placement of pressure-sensitive consonant sounds. If there is not enough airflow to work on placement, the speech-language pathologist should plug the child's nose during therapy either manually or preferably with a nose clip (**FIGURE 19-1**). In addition, the child should wear the nose clip at home as much as possible, not just during practice. This allows the child to feel the airflow and oral pressure with speech, which can shorten or eliminate the need for speech therapy once the velopharyngeal valve is corrected with surgery.

After VPI Surgery

As noted previously, hypernasality and nasal emission are usually obligatory distortions that cannot be corrected with speech therapy. One notable exception is when there is continued nasality following surgical correction of VPI.

It should be remembered that surgery changes structure and the potential to achieve velopharyngeal closure. It does not change abnormal function, however, such as faulty articulation placement. Therefore, if the child used compensatory productions in the pharynx prior to surgery, the child will continue to do so after the surgery, resulting in phoneme-specific nasal emission. Speech therapy to eliminate the abnormal pharyngeal placement will eliminate the nasal

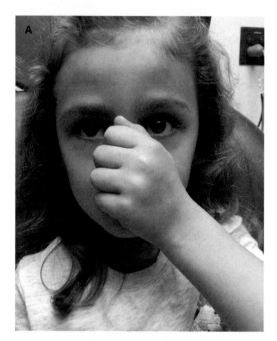
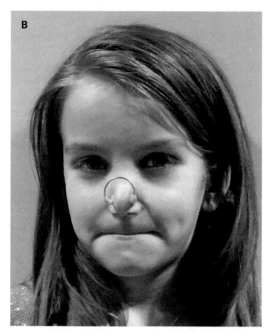

FIGURE 19-1 Closing off the nose to eliminate the nasal emission and increase oral airflow for oral articulation placement. This is helpful if the child has VPI and surgery is being delayed because of airway obstruction or other medical reasons. **(A)** The child is asked to pinch his nostrils while working on placement of oral sounds. The child is told to notice the oral airflow during production. **(B)** A nose clip is even better and can be used during therapy and practice at home.

emission, assuming the velopharyngeal valve is fully functional as a result of the surgery.

Continued hypernasality following VPI surgery may also occur if there was a large velopharyngeal opening preoperatively. With a large opening, the velum is short. As a result, there is little or no lateral pharyngeal wall movement because the velum is not there to close against. Once a pharyngeal flap is placed in the midline, it may take a while for the lateral walls to begin to function normally by moving medially to close against the flap. Sometimes, the lateral walls begin to function spontaneously after the surgery. In other cases, speech therapy (particularly with auditory feedback) is needed.

Finally, there may be residual hypernasality or nasal emission because the surgery was not totally successful. If this persists for more than a few months despite normal articulation placement and auditory feedback, the child should be sent back for further evaluation and consideration of a surgical revision.

For Velopharyngeal Mislearning

Velopharyngeal mislearning is a cause of developmental misarticulations. Certain misarticulations can cause phoneme-specific hypernasality, and other misarticulations can cause phoneme-specific nasal emission despite normal velopharyngeal structure and physiology. For example, the substitution of ŋ/l and ŋ/r can cause the perception of hypernasality in connected speech. In addition, the production of a pharyngeal fricative as a substitution for certain sibilants can lead to phoneme-specific nasal emission. Changing the place and/or manner of production of these sounds leads to an elimination of the perception of "nasality."

Speech therapy is also appropriate when there is hypernasality or nasal emission because of oral-motor dysfunction, particularly apraxia. With inconsistent articulation of the anterior structures, there is also inconsistent articulation of the velopharyngeal valve. This results in variable resonance. Articulation therapy is therefore effective in improving the coordination of velopharyngeal movement for speech sound production.

When in Doubt

There are times when the cause of hypernasality or nasal emission is uncertain, particularly when the speech-language pathologist is inexperienced in this area. In these cases, it is always best to do a trial period of speech therapy (Golding-Kushner, 2001; Hardin, 1991; Tomes, Kuehn, & Peterson-Falzone, 1996; Ysunza, Pamplona, & Toledo, 1992; Ysunza-Rivera, Pamplona-Ferreira, & Toledo-Cortina, 1991). It usually takes only a few weeks to determine whether the therapy will be effective. It should be noted that if either hypernasality or nasal air emission is noted with most speech sounds or is noted despite normal articulation placement, surgical management will be needed.

Biofeedback for Nasality

Biofeedback is a technique for making unconscious or autonomic physiological processes perceptible to the senses to manipulate them by conscious mental control. Biofeedback techniques are based on the principle that a desired response can be learned when it is determined that a specific thought process can produce that physiological response.

Different types of biofeedback techniques have been used in medicine for years and found to be effective for certain uses, such as reducing tension, decreasing heart rate, and even decreasing pain. In recent years, biofeedback techniques have been applied in speech pathology, particularly in the areas of voice (Cavalli & Hartley, 2010; Maryn, De Bodt, & Van Cauwenberge, 2006; Rossiter, Howard, & DeCosta, 1996; Van Lierde, Claeys, De Bodt, & Van Cauwenberge,

2004), fluency (Saltuklaroglu, Dayalu, Kalinowski, Stuart, & Rastatter, 2004), and dysarthria (Marchant, McAuliffe, & Huckabee, 2008; Murdoch, Pitt, Theodoros, & Ward, 1999).

There are several ways to provide biofeedback hypernasality or nasal emission. The feedback can be auditory, visual, or tactile-kinesthetic. The biofeedback can be low tech or high tech, using sophisticated instrumentation. The clinician must keep in mind however that biofeedback will be successful only if the individual is anatomically and physiologically capable of achieving normal velopharyngeal closure. In addition, the child needs to be old enough to actively participate and understand the feedback and then determine what needs to be done to achieve a desired result.

Low-Tech Therapy Tools

There are several low-tech tools that can help to provide sensory feedback when working to correct misarticulations through therapy (Kummer, 2011). Although all forms of sensory feedback are helpful, auditory feedback is usually most effective because this is how speech is normally learned.

See-Scape™

The See-Scape is a pneumatic device that is sold by several distributors (e.g., Pro-Ed, Mayer Johnson, Slosson Educational Publications, and AliMed). A "nasal olive" is placed in the child's nostril. The nasal olive is attached to a flexible tube that is connected to a rigid plastic vertical tube. The child is asked to produce pressure-sensitive consonants (plosives, fricatives, and affricates) without allowing the Styrofoam® float to rise in the tube (**FIGURE 19-2**). (Note that the float will rise during the production of nasal phonemes and with nasal breathing at the end of the utterance.)

There are several significant problems with this device. First, it is very expensive! The retail cost of over $100 is significant. In addition, this device should be thoroughly cleaned

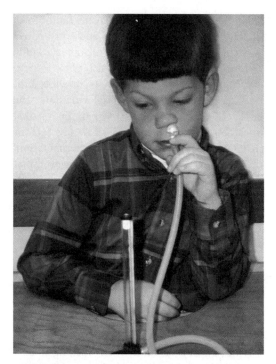

FIGURE 19-2 Use of the See-Scape. The child is instructed to put the nasal olive in one nostril. He is then asked to try to produce the consonants that have phoneme-specific nasal emission without allowing the foam stopper to rise in the tube. Note that the floater cannot be sanitized, so the device can be used by only one person.

and disinfected between uses, which is virtually impossible because of the Styrofoam float. Therefore, this device should be used only one time with one patient, making it very impractical.

Air Paddle

A little paddle can be cut from a piece of paper and serve as a visual feedback device for oral airflow and pressure. The air paddle is placed in front of the child's mouth during the production of pressure-sensitive phonemes (**FIGURE 19-3**). The child is asked to produce the sound with enough air pressure to force the air paddle to move. This works best for plosives but is not very effective for fricatives.

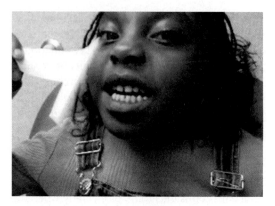

FIGURE 19-3 Use of an air paddle to encourage an increase in oral airflow during production of plosives. The child is instructed to try to make the paper move with each plosive production.

Straw or Listening Tube

A simple bending straw can serve as the most useful therapy tool in a speech-language pathologist's toolbox. Fortunately, it is cheap (less than a penny each), widely available (even in a school cafeteria), and disposable (so you do not have to clean it!). The benefit of a straw is the same as that of a stethoscope in that it amplifies sound. In speech therapy, it can amplify the sound of the airstream (nasal or oral) and the phonated sound (oral and nasal) (**FIGURE 19-4A**).

A listening tube can be used in exactly the same way as a straw. It also amplifies sound for auditory feedback. A listening tube can consist of virtually any kind of flexible tubing. Suction tubing works particularly well (**FIGURE 19-4B**). In addition, tube (or snake) whistles, which can be purchased on the Internet, are effective and double as a prize for the child at the end of the session (**FIGURE 19-4C**). The advantage of a tube is that it is longer and therefore a little easier to use than a straw when the child is using it for feedback. The disadvantage is that it is less available and must be either disinfected for further use or used by only one child.

To provide the child with feedback regarding hypernasality or nasal emission, the child puts one end of the straw or tube at the entrance

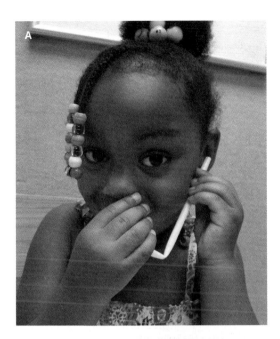

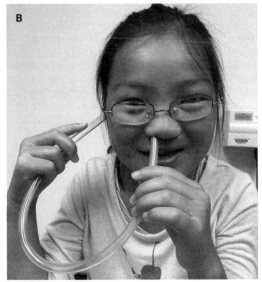

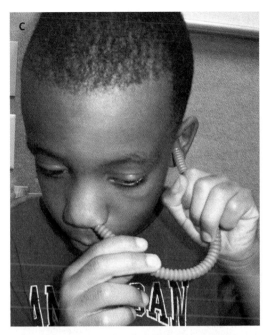

FIGURE 19-4 Amplification of hypernasality and/or nasal emission through a tube to provide the child with feedback. The child puts one end of the tube at the entrance of a nostril and the other end in or near his ear. This is useful in working on compensatory productions and other misarticulations that cause phoneme-specific nasal emission or phoneme-specific hypernasality. **(A)** Use of a straw. **(B)** Use of a simple tube (in this case, a suction tube). **(C)** Use of a snake whistle, which can be bought online.

of a nostril and the other end near his ear. (The straw will need to be bent one more time.) When hypernasality or nasal emission occurs on a sound, it is heard loudly through the straw or tube. The child is then instructed to produce the sound with correct placement in the mouth to eliminate the sound going to the ear. He will know if he is successful because there will be no sound coming through the tube during the sound or word production.

To provide the child with feedback regarding oral airstream, the child should put one end of the straw or tube in front of her lips or incisors (depending on the target sound). During normal production of oral airflow sounds, the child will hear the airflow going through the straw (**FIGURE 19-5A**). If there is lateral distortion, the straw can be moved to the side of the dental arch until the airstream can be heard through the straw (**FIGURE 19-5B**). When using a tube, it is best to put the other end of the tube near the child's

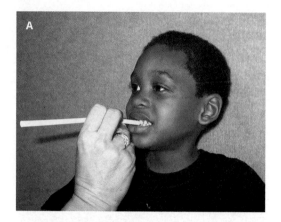

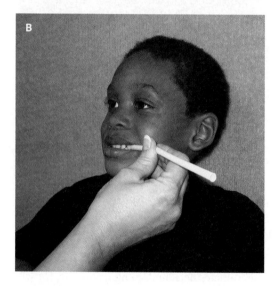

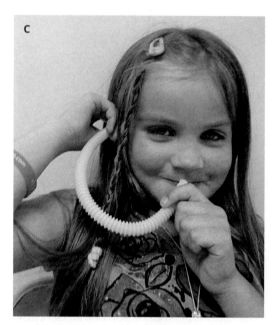

FIGURE 19-5 (A) To promote anterior airflow during production of /s/ and other sibilants, put a straw in front of the child's incisors and have the child try to produce the sound until he can hear the airflow through the straw. (This also works for correction of a lateral lisp.) **(B)** To eliminate a lateral distortion, put a straw on the side of the dental arch until you hear air going through the straw during a sustained /s/. Then, place the straw in the front of the child's dental arch and note that there is no air going through the straw. Have the child produce a /t/ sound and push the air into the straw. Then, have the child do the same with the teeth closed until it produces an /s/. **(C)** Use of a tube to provide feedback of oral airflow. The child is asked to produce the sound so that it is loud in her ear.

ear (**FIGURE 19-5C**). During therapy, the child should be told to push the airstream through the straw or tube in front of her mouth. Then, the child should push the airstream through the straw or tube in front of her incisors for a normal frontal production.

Oral & Nasal Listener™ (ONL)

Although a straw or a simple listening tube provides the child with feedback regarding resonance and nasal emission, the placement of the tubing in one of the nostrils makes it harder for the clinician to hear the sound at the same time. This affects the clinician's ability to provide appropriate feedback and instruction. To solve this problem, the Oral & Nasal Listener (ONL) (Super Duper® Publications, Inc., at www.superduperinc .com/products/view.aspx?stid=188&s=the-voral -nasal-listener) was developed at Cincinnati Children's Hospital Medical Center. It is basically a dual stethoscope, which allows both the child and the speech-language pathologist to hear the nasality and oral airflow at the same time and at the same volume (**FIGURE 19-6A**).

As with a straw or listening tube, the end of the tube is placed in the child's nostril. When both the child and the speech-language pathologist wear the earpieces, the child receives

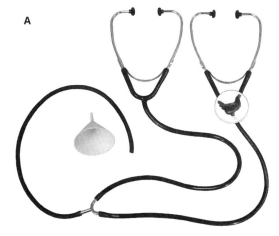

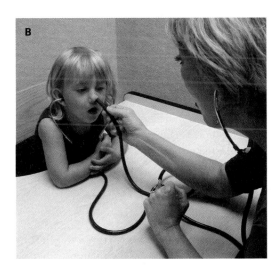

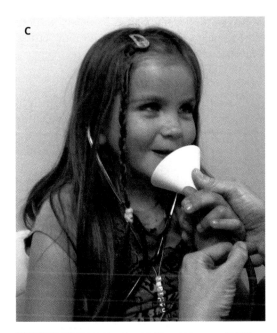

FIGURE 19-6 (A) The Oral & Nasal Listener (ONL). **(B)** The Oral & Nasal Listener was designed to allow the child and the speech-language pathologist (or the parent) to hear the nasal emission and/or hypernasality in an amplified manner at the same time. With this device, the adult is able to give the child appropriate feedback. Otherwise, it is hard for the adult to hear the nasal emission with the tube in the child's nose. **(C)** With the funnel, the oral sound is amplified for the child. Again, the adult can hear what the child hears. This device is useful for not only work on resonance and nasal emission, but it can also be used for working on articulation, particularly for children who need amplified feedback. (The Oral & Nasal Listener was developed by Jonathon Cross, Jessica Link, and Ann Kummer at Cincinnati Children's Hospital Medical Center and is patented under the name Nasoscope, 12/2/03, patent number 6656128.)

feedback, and the speech-language pathologist can give instructions and monitor progress (**FIGURE 19-6B**).

The ONL also has a funnel, which is used to amplify oral sound production and oral airflow. This allows the child to easily hear the difference between weak consonants or hypernasal vowels and those that are oral. With the ONL, the child can better compare her own productions with the models provided by the clinician (**FIGURE 19-6C**). (This also works very well for children who have hearing problems or are easily distracted in therapy.)

Although practice at home is critically important for progress and ultimate carryover, parents are often unsure about what they are hearing and how to give feedback. With the ONL, the parents can easily hear nasal emission and hypernasality, so they can provide more effective coaching for the child and also know when the child is making progress.

High-Tech Therapy Tools

Speech therapy, even with children, requires minimal resources and virtually no equipment.

However, when equipment is available, particularly equipment that is found in a hospital setting, there are some benefits to its use in treatment.

Digital Recording Equipment

Video recordings with good audio clarity can be helpful in the therapeutic process. The speech-language pathologist could first have the child listen to recorded samples of normal versus abnormal productions of the target sound. The child could then listen to recordings of his good and "not so good" productions of this sound. This can increase the child's attention to his speech and help him learn to self-evaluate and eventually self-correct his errors.

Nasometer

The Nasometer™ (PENTAX Medical, Montvale, NJ) provides the child with visual feedback that can help in eliminating compensatory errors that cause phoneme-specific nasal air emission and nasal substitutions for oral sounds. It may also help to modify resonance in certain cases of velopharyngeal incompetence caused by neuromotor dysfunction (Bae, Kuehn, & Ha, 2007; Heppt, Westrich, Strate, & Mohring, 1991). The clinician can set a threshold line to serve as the child's visual target. The target can be adjusted downward as the child becomes more proficient in reaching the goal.

The Nasometer software includes lists of sentences that can be used in therapy. These sentences are grouped according to phoneme and degree of difficulty in achieving velopharyngeal closure. Statistics regarding performance can help the clinician to track the child's progress over time with serial records. See Chapter 14 for more information.)

Nasopharyngoscopy

Nasopharyngoscopy provides visual information regarding the actions of the velopharyngeal mechanism during speech (Brunner, Stellzig-Eisenhauer, Proschel, Verres, & Komposch, 2005; Rich, Farber, & Shprintzen, 1988; Siegel-Sadewitz & Shprintzen, 1982; Witzel, Tobe, & Salyer, 1988; Witzel, Tobe, & Salyer 1989; Ysunza, Pamplona, Femat, Mayer, & Garcia-Velasco, 1997). As such, nasopharyngoscopy is commonly used as a diagnostic procedure. When it is determined through nasopharyngoscopy that the function of the velopharyngeal valve is normal, yet there is incomplete closure on certain sounds, the clinician may extend the examination to provide the patient with visual biofeedback as the first step toward correction (Brunner et al., 2005; Neumann & Romonath, 2011; Witzel et al., 1988). Biofeedback through nasopharyngoscopy may also help the child increase lateral pharyngeal wall movement following a pharyngeal flap procedure (Paal, Reulbach, Strobel-Schwarthoff, Nkenke, & Schuster, 2005; Siegel-Sadewitz & Shprintzen, 1982; Witzel et al., 1989; Ysunza et al., 1997). Unlike videofluoroscopy, nasopharyngoscopy is the only practical method of biofeedback using direct visualization because it does not involve radiation and is well tolerated by most children (O'Sullivan, Finger, & Zwerdling, 2004; Santos, Cipolotti, D'Avila, & Gurgel, 2005). (See the chapter *Videofluoroscopy* for more information.)

Speech Therapy Techniques

Speech therapy is effective in correcting misarticulations that lead to nasal emission or hypernasality. Therapy is not appropriate or effective in correcting overall hypernasality or nasal emission.

General Principles

Treating misarticulations that are the functional sequelae of velopharyngeal valving disorders and/or malocclusion is done through standard articulation therapy. The goal of therapy is correct placement (and sometimes manner) of production (Kummer, 2011).

The speech therapy techniques used with this population are not very different from the techniques that are used in therapy for other speech sound disorders. The following basic steps for correction are suggested:

- **Determine the phonemes to target first.** Consider the following when selecting phonemes to target:
  - **Select sounds in which the child is most stimulable.** If the child is stimulable for correct production, the sound will be easiest to correct. Therefore, working on this sound will give the child early success.
  - **Select sounds that will have the greatest effect on intelligibility.** In some cases, a developmental sequence may not be the best approach. For example, you may want to start with the /s/ sound when working with a 3-year-old to promote the development of the other sibilants rather than starting with an /f/ sound, which would have less effect on intelligibility.
  - **Select anterior sounds before posterior sounds.** Anterior sounds are more visible than other sounds and therefore easier for the child to correct.
  - **Select continuant cognates before movement sounds.** With a continuant sound, the child can hold the placement. Therefore, /n/ is easier than /d/, and /ʃ/ is easier than /ʧ/.
  - **For voiced plosives, achieve placement on the nasal cognate first.** Nasal sounds are continuants; therefore, it is easier to achieve and hold placement than a plosive. Once placement is established, have the child produce the nasal sound in a syllable and then repeat it with the nose closed. This turns the consonant into a voiced plosive (e.g., /na/ with the nose closed turns into /da/).
  - **For fricatives, select the voiceless sound in isolation before the voiced cognate (which requires a vowel).** Voiceless fricatives (e.g., /f/, /s/, /ʃ/) are continuants and have one less feature than the voiced sound.

- **Be sure the child can discriminate between the correct and incorrect sounds.** Work on auditory; visual; and if possible, tactile–kinesthetic identification of the correct and incorrect productions. This will help the child to pay attention to the difference and eventually self-monitor and self-correct.
- **Establish placement of production first.** Establish correct placement and then manner of production (including voicing).
- **Work on continuants and voiceless phonemes first in isolation.** In contrast to voiced plosives, continuants and voiceless sounds can be produced in isolation, without the vowel. Therefore, work on these sounds in isolation.
- **Work on voiced plosives in syllables.** For voiced plosives (e.g., /b/, /d/, /g/), work on the sound in a simple syllable with an easy vowel (e.g., /ba/).
- **Once placement is obtained, work on the sound in consonant–vowel (CV) syllables.** Work on the sound in syllables with a variety of vowels. Then, work on single syllable words.
- **Use /h/ to transition the consonant to the vowel.** If there is difficulty transitioning from the new placement of the consonant to the vowel, add an /h/ before the vowel (e.g., /p/ . . . /ha/). Gradually, close the time gap between the two to achieve the syllable (e.g., /pa/).
- **Begin with the sound in the initial word position.** When working at the word level, begin with the sound in the initial position of a word unless the child is more stimulable for the final position. The opposite is true for /r/, however. Always begin with the final position because the final /ɚ/ is a continuant. Then, move to the initial position, which requires movement.
- **Next, determine whether the medial or final position is easier.** Once the speech sound is produced correctly in the initial position, determine whether the child is more stimulable for production of that sound

in the medial or final position. Choose the position that is easier for the child, and make that the next step.

- **For the medial position, break up the word into syllables.** For example, if the target is /k/ and the word is "baker," have the child produce each syllable individually but in sequence. For example, she should say "ba . . . ker." Gradually, bring the two syllables closer together. The use of visuals (e.g., a red block for the first syllable and a blue block for the second syllable) can be helpful.
- **The phonemic context of a medial sound can change its production.** It is important to work on the sound and not the letter of medial phonemes. For example, in Standard American English, the /t/ in words that end with /n/ (e.g., "kitten," "button," "mitten," etc.) is usually not aspirated but instead is co-articulated with a glottal stop. In addition, the word "butter" is produced with a medial /d/, not a /t/, sound.
- **When working on the final position, break up the word.** Introduce the final word position of the sound by first breaking up the syllable or word. For example, if the target sound is /k/ and the work is "bake," the child should say "baaaa . . . k."
- **When working on the final word position, combine it with a word that starts with a vowel.** If the word following the final consonant starts with a vowel, the final consonant becomes similar to an initial sound. For example, you could have the child say "Ba*ke* it."
- **Work on sounds in categories.** If there are several errors in a class of speech sounds, work on sounds in phonological categories based on place or manner of production. This usually results in faster progress because several sounds can be corrected at once (Pamplona, Ysunza, & Espinosa, 1999).
- **When moving to the next sound in a category, change one feature at a time.** When

the sound is in a related group of phonemes (e.g., plosives or bilabials), be sure to take small steps when moving to the next sound by changing only one feature at a time (e.g., placement, manner, or voicing).

- **For consonant blends, divide the clusters into individual components.** If the first sound is a continuant, that sound should be prolonged before moving on to the next sound. For example, for the word "snake," the child should say "ssss . . . nake." For the word "flag," the child should say "fffff . . . lag." If the first sound is a plosive, the plosive should be made into a syllable. For example, for the word "play," the child should say "pa . . . lay."
- **When /s/ is combined with a typically voiceless consonant, the voiceless consonant becomes voiced.** When the /s/ is combined with a /p/, /t/, or /k/, these plosives are produced as their voiced cognates. It is important to work on the speech sound, not the written letter. Examples of this include the following:
  - spell =   s . . . bell
  - stop =   s . . . dop
  - skate =   s . . . gate
- **Work on the sound in carrier phrases.** When working on carrier phrases, it is helpful to start with the sound at the beginning of the carrier phrase. For example, when working on /l/, the carrier phrase may be "Let me . . ." or "Look at the . . ." To make it harder, the target sound may be within the carrier phrase, such as "I like . . ." or "I love . . ." or "I like . . . , but I don't like . . ." The sound can even complete the carrier phrase, such as "I have a [ladder]."
- **Work on the sound in novel sentences.** Have the child produce a word with the sound in novel sentences. Correct only the targeted sound or sounds.
- **Obtain as many correct productions of the sound in a session as possible.** Correcting abnormal speech sound production requires

motor learning, which occurs through many repetitions (e.g., practice). Therefore, once the child is able to produce the sound accurately, speech therapy should incorporate drill work to achieve as many correct productions as possible in the session.

- **Work on carryover using unstructured speech.** While trying to produce the target sound correctly, have the child tell a story, relay an incident, describe a picture, give instructions, and so on. Also, have the child read aloud while trying to produce each word with the target sound correctly. Correct errors only on the targeted sound or sounds.
- **Involve the parents and caregivers (including babysitters) in the process.** Success of therapy, and particularly of carryover, depends on the frequency of practice at home. The parents should be given instructions for incorporating practice in their daily lives.

Specific Therapy Techniques

Whenever possible, clinical decision making should incorporate the principles of evidence-based practice (EBP) (American Speech-Language-Hearing Association [ASHA], 2005). EBP is the integration of practitioner expertise with current research to provide quality clinical care. Unfortunately, research on specific therapy techniques is limited at best. Therefore, the therapy techniques that are offered in this text are based primarily on this author's expertise in phonology and extensive experience.

APPENDIX 19A contains lists of specific speech therapy techniques in a "cookbook" type of format. These strategies can be used for correction of misarticulations that are produced in the pharynx, either as compensatory productions or merely from mislearning. Because these therapy techniques focus on obtaining correct oral placement, regardless of the error, they are equally effective when used with children who have other types of substitution errors.

Oral-Motor Exercises . . . That Do Not Work!

In the past, clinicians used a variety of oral-motor "exercises" (i.e., blowing, sucking, gagging, etc.) in hopes of strengthening the muscles of the velopharyngeal valve to improve function for speech (Berry & Eisenson, 1956; Kanter, 1947; Massengill, Quinn, Pickrell, & Levinson, 1968; Muttiah, Georges, & Brackenbury, 2011; Van Riper, 1963). Several investigators even tried to stimulate velopharyngeal movement through the use of electrical "exercisers" (Cole, 1971; Cole, 1979; Lubit & Larsen, 1969; Lubit & Larsen, 1971; Massengill, Quinn, & Pickrell, 1971; Peterson, 1974; Tash, Shelton, Knox, & Michel, 1971; Weber, Jobe, & Chase, 1970; Yules & Chase, 1969). However, none of these exercises were effective (Kuehn & Henne, 2003; Powers & Starr, 1974; Ruscello, 1982; Ruscello, 2008a; Ruscello, 2008b).

Later research showed significant differences in the velopharyngeal closure patterns of speech and nonspeech activities, suggesting that nonspeech "exercises" could not possibly be effective in improving velopharyngeal function for speech (Flowers & Morris, 1973; Golding-Kushner, 2001; Moll, 1965; Peterson, 1973; Peterson-Falzone, Trost-Cardamone, Karnell, & Hardin-Jones, 2006; Shprintzen, Lencione, McCall, & Skolnick, 1974). In addition, children with cleft palate have a structural abnormality, not weakness of the musculature that would respond to exercise. Even if exercises could improve velopharyngeal function, the child would have to continue the exercises for the rest of his life to maintain that improvement!

Given current knowledge and the need to adhere to an evidence-based practice, procedures that should NOT be used in the treatment of speech disorders related to VPI include blowing, sucking, whistling, gagging, swallowing, cheek puffing, icing, stroking, palatal massage, electrical stimulation, playing wind instruments, or any type of oral-motor exercises (Golding-Kushner, 2001; Kummer, 2011; Lof, 2008; Lof, 2011; McCauley, Strand, Lof, Schooling, & Frymark, 2009; Ruscello, 2008a;

Ruscello, 2008b; Watson & Lof, 2008). Unfortunately, even though there is a total lack of evidence in the literature to support the efficacy of nonspeech exercises in improving velopharyngeal function (or even speech) and it does not make sense to use exercises for structural abnormalities, some clinicians continue to incorporate these exercises in their treatment (Lof & Watson, 2008; Watson & Lof, 2009).

Other Treatment Methods

There are two other treatment procedures that warrant mention. These procedures are controversial and require additional research.

Continuous Positive Airway Pressure

A continuous positive airway pressure (CPAP) device is an instrument that consists of a flow generator, a valve mechanism, a hose, and a nasal mask. Pressurized airflow is delivered to the nasal cavity, and thus the pharynx, through the hose and nasal mask. CPAP has been found to be useful in the treatment of individuals with obstructive sleep apnea (OSA) because the positive pressure prevents the collapse of the pharyngeal airway during sleep.

Kuehn (1991, 1997) suggested the use of CPAP for the treatment of hypernasality secondary to velopharyngeal insufficiency. He suggested that CPAP could provide resistance training for the velopharyngeal muscles by having them work actively against the positive air pressure. Based on the principles of exercise physiology, CPAP therapy is designed to overload the muscles by subjecting them to a greater level of resistance than usual during velar elevation for speech. Once the muscles adapt to a certain level of pressure, the pressure is increased. Through this progressive resistance training, it is theorized that the muscles gain strength and become more resistant to

fatigue. An important difference between this procedure and other muscle training procedures is that this is done during speech and for speech activities only.

Kuehn, Moon, and Folkins (1993) compared electromyographic activity of the levator veli palatini during the use of CPAP and with atmospheric air pressure only. There was a significant increase in the activity of the levator muscle with an increase in the intranasal pressure, suggesting that this muscle actively reacts to the resistance and possibly increases in strength. One study found a reduction in the degree of hypernasality in some children (Kuehn et al., 2002).

Some caveats of this form of treatment include the fact that child selection is very important. Perhaps this form of treatment is best suited for cases with mild velopharyngeal incompetence where there is poor velar movement as in the traumatic brain injury population (Cahill et al., 2004). It is unlikely to be successful if there is more than mild velopharyngeal incompetence or if there is a structural defect. In cases where improvement from CPAP therapy is noted, another unknown is whether it is sustained when the exercises are no longer done. Further research is needed to determine the short-term and long-term efficacy of this technique.

Prosthesis Reduction Therapy

Some authors have described the use of a temporary speech prosthesis as a means of improving velopharyngeal function (Golding-Kushner, Cisneros, & LeBlanc, 1995; Israel, Cook, & Blakeley, 1993; McGrath & Anderson, 1990; Sell, Mars, & Worrell, 2006; Wolfaardt, Wilson, Rochet, & McPhee, 1993). The procedure is to use a palatal lift or speech bulb for a period of time and then gradually reduce its size in hopes of promoting an increase in velopharyngeal movement. However, research has not shown that the lift promotes an increase in muscle function. In fact, it actually negates the need for velopharyngeal function so that it could be argued that the velar muscles could actually be negatively affected. Neither device has been found to eliminate the need for further surgery (Tachimura, Nohara, Fujita, Hara, & Wada, 2001; Yorkston et al., 2001). Therefore, this type of management is still controversial especially because prosthetic devices are expensive and compliance with children is difficult (see the chapter *Prosthetic Management* for more information).

Motor Learning and Motor Memory

Speech requires a sequence of oral-motor movements that are fast, complex, automatic, and effortless. This ability is developed through both motor learning and motor memory. As a new motor program is learned, new connections and pathways are formed in the brain, thus enhancing the ability to execute the new motor skills easily and automatically (Maas et al., 2008; Schmidt, Lee, Winstein, Wulf, & Zelaznik, 2019).

Motor Learning

Motor learning is the acquisition of new motor skills through a combination of the following: instructions, trial and error, and then feedback. Feedback helps with both the development and ultimate refinement of the motor program. Motor learning is necessary for an individual to be able to execute complex motor movements and motor sequences without conscious thought. Examples of skills that require motor learning include playing a musical instrument (e.g., the piano); learning a dance (e.g., salsa); learning to play a sport (e.g., kicking the ball in soccer); and, of course, learning to produce speech sounds in sequence for connected speech.

If a child has not learned to produce certain speech sounds correctly on his own, speech therapy is necessary to change the incorrect motor pattern. During speech therapy, the child is first taught how to produce the sound correctly through instruction. The child then goes through

a period of trial and error. While the child is trying to produce the sound, the speech-language pathologist gives constant feedback. This cycle continues until the child is able to produce the sound correctly on his own.

Motor Memory

Motor memory is what develops the automaticity of a newly learned motor movement so that the movement can be done without conscious thought. It also makes the new learning relatively permanent, although this learning can degrade with a lack of use. Motor memory is dependent on constant repetition, in other words, practice! Practice results in the development and reinforcement of new neural pathways so that ultimately the movement can be done without conscious thought. As with other types of motor learning, speech learning (or relearning, which is often the case with speech disorders) is also greatly dependent on practice. In fact, practice is what ultimately results in carryover into conversational speech.

So how much practice is necessary for a carryover of a learned speech sound into conversational speech? The answer is, it depends on the child and many other factors. However, there is no debate about the fact that, with motor learning, the more a new motor skill is practiced, the faster it will be acquired into motor memory. Therefore, it can be assumed that children will make significantly greater gains when provided with a higher "dose" of practice (Allen, 2013).

The term dose has been borrowed from pharmacology. When it comes to medication as a treatment modality, it is important to know the optimum dose (or dose range) for the patient to achieve maximal benefit with minimal harm. In speech therapy, dose refers to the number of learning opportunities experienced by the child, not to the number of therapy sessions or the length of a practice session (Strand, Stoeckel, & Baas, 2006; Warren, Fey, & Yoder, 2007). In speech sound disorders, the number of correct productions obtained of the target phoneme during a session is particularly important (Edeal & Gildersleeve-Neumann, 2011). Therefore, drill work should be an integral part of therapy to maximize the dose.

The use of tokens (i.e., little teddy bears, poker chips, pennies, etc.) can be very helpful in a drill. A token is held up to the side of the speech-language pathologist's (SLP's) face to direct the child's visual attention to her mouth. The SLP then poduces a stimulus (e.g., a sound, syllable, word or sentence) for the child to imitate. If the child is reasonably successful in imitating the stimulus correctly, the SLP can say "Good talking" or Good job." The token should then be dropped in a closed container, preferably one in which the child can see the earned tokens, but cannot reach into it to play with them. **FIGURE 19-7** shows little teddy bears, which can

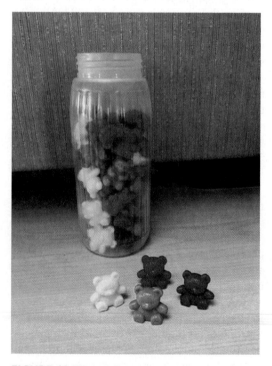

FIGURE 19-7 For drill work, the speech-language pathologist can use small teddy bears as tokens and a plastic bottle as a container.

be used as the tokens, and a tall, plastic bottle, which can be used as the container. Although this type of drill can greatly increase the number of correct responses achieved in the session, the SLP must also consider the potential harm of an "overdose," which could include burnout or resistance from the child. Therefore, drill work needs to be made interesting with variable tokens, and interspersed with other activities.

In addition to the dose (or intensity) of practice, the frequency of practice can also affect progress. In motor learning, it has been found that distributed practice can facilitate both short-term performance and long-term memory. Therefore, it is better to have frequent short practice sessions than infrequent longer sessions (Strand & Debertine, 2000; Strand et al., 2006). A practice session can be as short as a minute or less, particularly if it is done frequently throughout the day.

Of course, there is always some practice that takes place in a therapy session after motor learning has taken place. However, if the child is able to produce the speech sound easily in the therapy session, the majority of the practice can and should take place at home. In fact, practice is not considered "skilled work" by payers. Given the cost of speech therapy (to the parents, insurance providers, and taxpayers), each therapy session should be geared primarily toward learning new skills.

To ensure that practice takes place at home, it is important to convince family members that they are integral to the treatment process. It can be said that speech therapy is like taking piano lessons: If you do not practice the piano at home, you will not learn to play the piano. Other analogies can be used, but the family needs to understand that practice at home is critically important to the success of therapy. In fact, even with severe disorders, most children do not need "intense therapy." Instead, they need intense practice, which should take place at home.

Parents are more likely to be successful in practicing with the child if they are instructed on how to incorporate short sessions into their daily activities. For example, a few minutes of practice can be done during a meal or while giving the child a bath, playing a game, or doing daily chores around the house. Practice can be done while riding in the car, where the child has nothing else to do. For older children, practice can be incorporated into homework by having the child read aloud. Parents should be told that one minute can count as a practice session; however, they should do one minute several times a day, every day of the week.

Successful carryover of new speech productions into conversational speech is the measure of the true success of therapy. However, carryover is often the most frustrating aspect of therapy because it can be the most difficult to achieve in a therapy session. Carryover success depends on several factors. First, the new speech production must be very easy for the child to produce in connected speech. Again, this is why frequent daily practice at home is so important. Second, the child must be able to self-monitor and self-correct. Finally, the family members need to monitor the child's speech and correct the child periodically when necessary. If the family members have been

helping the child with practice from the beginning, they will be very aware of the child's speech goals and therefore more successful in monitoring the child's speech during the carryover stage.

The Ultimate Goal

In past generations, the goal of treatment for individuals with cleft palate was acceptable or intelligible speech because normal speech was usually not obtainable. Over the past few decades, however, there has been an increase in knowledge of the nature of the velopharyngeal mechanism. In addition, there have been advances in evaluation and surgical techniques and instrumentation. Therefore, most children born with cleft palate at this time ultimately attain normal speech. If there are additional craniofacial anomalies or neurological issues, then the prognosis for perfect speech is more guarded. Regardless, all efforts should be made to achieve normal speech (without nasal emission) and resonance (without hypernasality or hyponasality) through appropriate treatment whenever possible.

SUMMARY

Speech therapy is appropriate for the correction of articulation errors that are caused by VPI (compensatory errors), particularly after correction of the structure. Therapy is also appropriate for misarticulations from mislearning, which cause phoneme-specific hypernasality or phoneme-specific nasal emission. Therapy is not appropriate for obligatory distortions, including consistent hypernasality or nasal emission, which is usually caused by VPI. These distortions self-correct with normalization of the structure. When in doubt regarding the cause of the speech characteristics and appropriate recommendations, a short trial period of speech therapy can be done to determine the individual's response to therapy.

The therapy procedures for compensatory speech errors are no different than those used

for other placement errors. Oral-motor exercises, including those that involve blowing and sucking, are totally inappropriate for a variety of reasons, including the fact that they do not work.

Therapy should continue as long as the child is making progress. If the child is not responding to therapy, referral to a craniofacial team for further evaluation (or reevaluation) of velopharyngeal function should be done. Surgical intervention or revision may be necessary.

Finally, progress is much faster if a high dose of correct responses is elicited in each therapy session and there are frequent short practice sessions every day at home. A practice session can be as little as a minute and incorporated into daily activities at home. This makes it more doable for parents and greatly helps with the carryover process.

FOR REVIEW AND DISCUSSION

1. Discuss the appropriate focus and intervention strategies for the following developmental stages: infants and toddlers, preschool children, school-age children, and adolescents and adults. Explain why early intervention and stimulation are important.

2. In what cases is speech therapy appropriate for children with a cleft palate? When is speech therapy inappropriate for correction of abnormal speech in this population?

3. Why is speech therapy almost always ineffective in correcting hypernasality or nasal emission? Why do you think that clinicians still keep children in speech therapy for these problems? If a physician refers a child to you for correction of consistent hypernasality, what would you do and why?

4. Under what circumstances is speech therapy appropriate for nasal emission or hypernasality? What would you do if no progress had been made after 2 months of therapy?

5. Discuss methods of auditory, visual, and tactile feedback that can be used as part of therapy. Which methods would be the most effective and why?

6. Discuss the following case: The child has a history of velopharyngeal insufficiency that was corrected by a pharyngeal flap. Speech is now characterized by ŋ/l and nasal emission on s/z only. All other speech sounds are produced normally without hypernasality or nasal emission. Why is there still nasality on the /l/ sound and nasal emission on s/z? What speech therapy techniques might be used for these misarticulations?

7. What would you do if a 6-year-old boy was referred to you for a lateral lisp and you found the problem is caused by the placement of the teeth relative to the tongue?

8. How can a straw be used to correct inconsistent nasal emission? How can it be used to correct a lateral lisp?

9. Describe therapy approaches for correction of a glottal stop, a pharyngeal fricative, lateral distortion, phoneme-specific nasal emission, and ŋ/l substitution.

10. Describe low-tech methods of providing biofeedback as part of the therapy process. What are the advantages and disadvantages of each?

11. Why are oral-motor exercises, including blowing and sucking exercises, ineffective in the treatment of velopharyngeal dysfunction? Why do you think some clinicians still use them?

12. How would you explain to parents why their involvement is critically important to the success of therapy?

REFERENCES

Allen, M. M. (2013). Intervention efficacy and intensity for children with speech sound disorder. *Journal of Speech and Language Research, 53*(3), 865–877.

American Speech-Language-Hearing Association (ASHA). (2005). *Evidence-based practice in communication disorders.* Retrieved from http://www.asha.org/policy/PS2005-00221/

Amorosa, H., & Endres, R. (2004). Group training for parents of young children with specific developmental speech and language disorder (SDLD). *Psychiatrische Praxis, 31*(Suppl. 1), S129–S131.

Antonarakis, G. S., & Kiliaridis, S. (2009). Internet-derived information on cleft lip and palate for families with affected children. *The Cleft Palate–Craniofacial Journal, 46*(1), 75–80.

Bae, Y., Kuehn, D. P., & Ha, S. (2007). Validity of the Nasometer measuring the temporal characteristics of nasalization. *The Cleft Palate–Craniofacial Journal, 44*(5), 506–517.

Berry, M. F., & Eisenson, J. (1956). *Speech disorders: Principles and practices of therapy.* New York, NY: Appleton-Century-Crofts.

Brunner, M., Stellzig-Eisenhauer, A., Proschel, U., Verres, R., & Komposch, G. (2005). The effect of nasopharyngoscopic biofeedback in patients with cleft palate and velopharyngeal dysfunction. *The Cleft Palate–Craniofacial Journal, 42*(6), 649–657.

Cahill, L. M., Turner, A. B., Stabler, P. A., Addis, P. E., Theodoros, D. C., & Murdoch, B. E. (2004). An evaluation of continuous positive airway pressure (CPAP) therapy in the treatment of hypernasality following traumatic brain injury: A report of 3 cases. *Journal of Head Trauma Rehabilitation, 19*(3), 241–253.

Cavalli, L., & Hartley, B. E. (2010). The clinical application of electrolaryngography in a tertiary children's hospital. *Logopedics, Phoniatrics, Vocology, 35*(2), 60–67.

Cole, R. M. (1971). Direct muscle training for the improvement of velopharyngeal function. In K. Bzoch (Ed.), *Communicative disorders related to cleft lip and palate* (pp. 250–256). Boston, MA: Little, Brown and Company.

Cole, R. M. (1979). Direct muscle training for the improvement of velopharyngeal activity. In K. Bzoch (Ed.), *Communicative disorders related to cleft lip and palate* (2nd ed., pp. 328–340). Boston, MA: Little, Brown and Company.

Dowling, J. E. (2004). *The great brain debate: Nature or nurture?* Washington, DC: Joseph Henry Press.

Edeal, D. M., & Gildersleeve-Neumann, C. E. (2011). The importance of production frequency in therapy

Flowers, C. R., & Morris, H. L. (1973). Oral-pharyngeal movements during swallowing and speech. *Cleft Palate Journal, 10*, 181–191.

Golding-Kushner, K. J. (2001). *Therapy techniques for cleft palate & related disorders.* Englewood Cliffs, NJ: Thomson Delmar Learning.

Golding-Kushner, K. J., Cisneros, G., & LeBlanc, E. (1995). Speech bulbs. In R. J. Shprintzen & J. Bardach (Eds.), *Cleft palate speech management* (pp. 352–375). St. Louis, MO: Mosby.

Hardin, M. A. (1991). Cleft palate: Intervention. *Clinics in Communication Disorders, 1*(3), 12–18.

Hardin-Jones, M. A., & Jones, D. L. (2005). Speech production of preschoolers with cleft palate. *The Cleft Palate–Craniofacial Journal, 42*(1), 7–13.

Heppt, W., Westrich, M., Strate, B., & Mohring, L. (1991). Nasalance: A new concept for objective analysis of nasality. *Laryngorhinootologie, 70*(4), 208–213.

Israel, J. M., Cook, T. A., & Blakeley, R. W. (1993). The use of a temporary oral prosthesis to treat speech in velopharyngeal incompetence. *Facial and Plastic Surgery, 9*(3), 206–212.

Kanter, C. E. (1947). The rationale for blowing exercises for patients with repaired cleft palates. *Journal of Speech Disorders, 12*, 281.

Kuehn, D. P. (1991). New therapy for treating hypernasal speech using continuous positive airway pressure (CPAP). *Plastic and Reconstructive Surgery, 88*(6), 959–966; discussion 967–969.

Kuehn, D. P. (1997). The development of a new technique for treating hypernasality: CPAP. *American Journal of Speech-Language Pathology, 6*(4), 5–8.

Kuehn, D. P., & Henne, L. J. (2003). Speech evaluation and treatment for patients with cleft palate. *American Journal of Speech-Language Pathology, 12*, 103–109.

Kuehn, D. P., Imrey, P. B., Tomes, L., Jones, D. L., O'Gara, M. M., Seaver, E. J., . . . Watchel, J. M. (2002). Efficacy of continuous positive airway pressure for treatment of hypernasality. *The Cleft Palate–Craniofacial Journal, 39*(3), 267–276.

Kuehn, D. P., Moon, J. B., & Folkins, J. W. (1993). Levator veli palatini muscle activity in relation to intranasal air pressure variation. *The Cleft Palate–Craniofacial Journal, 30*(4), 361–368.

Kummer, A. W. (2011). Speech therapy for errors secondary to cleft palate and velopharyngeal dysfunction. *Seminars in Speech and Language, 32*(2), 191–199.

Lof, G. L. (2008). Controversies surrounding nonspeech oral motor exercises for childhood speech disorders. *Seminars in Speech and Language, 29*(4), 253–255.

Lof, G. L. (2011). Science-based practice and the speech-language pathologist. *International Journal of Speech-Language Pathology, 13*(3), 189–196.

Lof, G. L., & Watson, M. M. (2008). A nationwide survey of nonspeech oral motor exercise use: Implications for evidence-based practice. *Language Speech Hearing Services Schools, 39*(3), 392–407.

Lubit, E. C., & Larsen, R. E. (1969). The Lubit palatal exerciser: A preliminary report. *Cleft Palate Journal, 6*, 120–133.

Lubit, E. C., & Larsen, R. E. (1971). A speech aid for velopharyngeal incompetency. *Journal of Speech and Hearing Disorders, 36*(1), 61–70.

Maas, E., Robin, D. A., Austermann Hula, S. N., Freedman, S. E., Wulf, G., & Ballard, K. J. (2008). Principles of motor learning in treatment of motor speech disorders. *American Journal of Speech-Language Pathology, 17,* 277–298.

Marchant, J., McAuliffe, M. J., & Huckabee, M. L. (2008). Treatment of articulatory impairment in a child with spastic dysarthria associated with cerebral palsy. *Developmental Neurorehabilitation, 11*(1), 81–90.

Maryn, Y., De Bodt, M., & Van Cauwenberge, P. (2006). Effects of biofeedback in phonatory disorders and phonatory performance: A systematic literature review. *Applied Psychophysiology and Biofeedback, 31*(1), 65–83.

Massengill, R., Jr., Quinn, G. W., & Pickrell, K. L. (1971). The use of a palatal stimulator to decrease velopharyngeal gap. *Annals of Otology, Rhinology, and Laryngology, 80,* 135–137.

Massengill, R., Jr., Quinn, G. W., Pickrell, K. L., & Levinson, C. (1968). Therapeutic exercise and velopharyngeal gap. *Cleft Palate Journal, 5,* 44–47.

McCauley, R. J., Strand, E., Lof, G., Schooling, T., & Frymark, T. (2009). Evidence-based systematic review: Effects of nonspeech oral motor exercises on speech. *American Journal of Speech-Language Pathology 18*(4), 343–360.

McGrath, C. O., & Anderson, M. W. (1990). Prosthetic treatment of velopharyngeal incompetence. In J. Bardach & H. L. Morris (Eds.), *Multidisciplinary management of cleft lip and palate* (pp. 809–815). Philadelphia, PA: W. B. Saunders.

Moll, K. L. (1965). A cinefluorographic study of velopharyngeal function in normals during various activities. *Cleft Palate Journal, 2,* 112.

Murdoch, B. E., Pitt, G., Theodoros, D. G., & Ward, E. C. (1999). Real-time continuous visual biofeedback in the treatment of speech breathing disorders following childhood traumatic brain injury: Report of one case. *Pediatric Rehabilitation, 3*(1), 5–20.

Muttiah, N., Georges, K., & Brackenbury, T. (2011). Clinical and research perspectives on nonspeech oral motor treatments and evidence-based practice. *American Journal of Speech-Language Pathology, 20*(1), 47–59.

Neumann, S., & Romonath, R. (2011). Effectiveness of nasopharyngoscopic biofeedback in clients with cleft palate speech: A systematic review. *Logopedics Phoniatrics Vocology, 37*(3), 95–106.

O'Gara, M. M., & Logemann, J. A. (1990). Early speech development in cleft palate babies. In J. Bardach & H. L. Morris (Eds.), *Multidisciplinary management of cleft lip and palate* (pp. 717–726). Philadelphia, PA: W. B. Saunders.

O'Sullivan, B. P., Finger, L., & Zwerdling, R. G. (2004). Use of nasopharyngoscopy in the evaluation of children with noisy breathing. *Chest, 125*(4), 1265–1269.

Paal, S., Reulbach, U., Strobel-Schwarthoff, K., Nkenke, E., & Schuster, M. (2005). Evaluation of speech disorders in children with cleft lip and palate. *Journal of Orofacial Orthopedics, 66*(4), 270–278.

Pamplona, M. C., & Ysunza, A. (2000). Active participation of mothers during speech therapy improved language development of children with cleft palate. *Scandinavian Journal of Plastic and Reconstructive Surgery and Hand Surgery, 34*(3), 231–236.

Pamplona, M. C., Ysunza, A., & Espinosa, J. (1999). A comparative trial of two modalities of speech intervention for compensatory articulation in cleft palate children, phonologic approach versus articulatory approach. *International Journal of Pediatric Otorhinolaryngology, 49*(1), 21–26.

Pamplona, M. C., Ysunza, A., & Jimenez-Murat, Y. (2001). Mothers of children with cleft palate undergoing speech intervention change communicative interaction. *International Journal of Pediatric Otorhinolaryngology, 59*(3), 173–179.

Pamplona, M. C., Ysunza, A., & Uriostegui, C. (1996). Linguistic interaction: The active role of parents in speech therapy for cleft palate patients. *International Journal of Pediatric Otorhinolaryngology, 37*(1), 17–27.

Peterson, S. J. (1973). Velopharyngeal closure: Some important differences. *Journal of Speech and Hearing Disorders, 38,* 89.

Peterson, S. J. (1974). Electrical stimulation of the soft palate. *Cleft Palate Journal, 11,* 72–86.

Peterson-Falzone, S. J., Trost-Cardamone, J. E., Karnell, M. P., & Hardin-Jones, M. A. (2006). *The clinician's guide to treating cleft palate speech.* St. Louis, MO: Mosby Elsevier.

Phillips, B. J. (1990). Early speech management. In J. Bardach & H. L. Morris (Eds.), *Multidisciplinary management of cleft lip and palate* (pp. 732–736). Philadelphia, PA: W. B. Saunders.

Powers, G. L., & Starr, C. D. (1974). The effect of muscle exercises on velopharyngeal gap and nasality. *Cleft Palate Journal, 11,* 28.

Rich, B. M., Farber, K., & Shprintzen, R. J. (1988). Nasopharyngoscopy in the treatment of palatopharyngeal insufficiency. *International Journal of Prosthodontics, 1*(3), 248–251.

Rossiter, D., Howard, D. M., & DeCosta, M. (1996). Voice development under training with and without the influence of real-time visually presented biofeedback. *Journal of the Acoustical Society of America, 99*(5), 3253–3256.

Ruscello, D. M. (1982). A selected review of palatal training procedures. *Cleft Palate Journal, 19*(3), 181–193.

Ruscello, D. M. (2008a). An examination of non-speech oral motor exercises for children with velopharyngeal inadequacy. *Seminars in Speech and Language, 29*(4), 293–303.

Ruscello, D. M. (2008b). Nonspeech oral motor treatment issues related to children with developmental speech sound disorders. *Language Speech and Hearing Services in Schools, 39*(3), 380–391.

Saltuklaroglu, T., Dayalu, V. N., Kalinowski, J., Stuart, A., & Rastatter, M. P. (2004). Say it with me: Stuttering inhibited. *Journal of Clinical and Experimental Neuropsychology, 26*(2), 161–168.

Santos, R. S., Cipolotti, R., D'Avila, J. S., & Gurgel, R. Q. (2005). Schoolchildren submitted to video nasopharyngoscopy examination at school: Findings and tolerance. *Jornal de Pediatria (Rio J), 81*(6), 443–446.

Schmidt, R. A., Lee, T. D., Winstein, C. J., Wulf, G., & Zelaznik, H. N. (2019). *Motor control and learning: A behavior emphasis* (6th ed.). Champaign, IL: Human Kinetics.

Sell, D., Mars, M., & Worrell, E. (2006). Process and outcome study of multidisciplinary prosthetic treatment for velopharyngeal dysfunction. *International Journal of Language Communication Disorders, 41*(5), 495–511.

Shprintzen, R. J., Lencione, R. M., McCall, G. N., & Skolnick, M. L. (1974). A three-dimensional cinefluoroscopic analysis of velopharyngeal closure during speech and nonspeech activities in normals. *Cleft Palate Journal, 11*, 412–428.

Siegel-Sadewitz, V. L., & Shprintzen, R. J. (1982). Nasopharyngoscopy of the normal velopharyngeal sphincter: An experiment of biofeedback. *Cleft Palate Journal, 19*(3), 194–200.

Skeat, J., Eadie, P., Ukoumunne, O., & Reilly, S. (2010). Predictors of parents seeking help or advice about children's communication development in the early years. *Child: Care, Health and Development, 36*(6), 878–887.

Stevens, L., Watson, K., & Dodd, K. (2001). Supporting parents of children with communication difficulties: A model. *International Journal of Language Communication Disorders, 36*(Suppl.), 70–74.

Strand, E. A., & Debertine, P. (2000). The efficacy of integral stimulation intervention with developmental apraxia of speech. *Journal of Medical Speech-Language Pathology, 8*, 295–300.

Strand, E. A., Stoeckel, R., & Baas, B. (2006). Treatment of severe childhood apraxia of speech: A treatment efficacy study. *Journal of Medical Speech-Language Pathology, 14*, 297–306.

Tachimura, T., Nohara, K., Fujita, Y., Hara, H., & Wada, T. (2001). Change in levator veli palatini muscle activity of normal speakers in association with elevation of the velum using an experimental palatal lift prosthesis. *The Cleft Palate–Craniofacial Journal, 38*(5), 449–454.

Tash, E. L., Shelton, R. L., Knox, A. W., & Michel, J. F. (1971). Training voluntary pharyngeal wall movements in children with normal and inadequate velopharyngeal closure. *Cleft Palate Journal, 8*, 277–290.

Tomes, L., Kuehn, D., & Peterson-Falzone, S. (1996, April). Behavioral therapy for speakers with velopharyngeal impairment. *NCVS Status and Progress Report, 9*, 159–180.

Trost-Cardamone, J. E. (1997). Diagnosis of specific cleft palate speech error patterns for planning therapy of physical management needs. In K. R. Bzoch (Ed.), *Communicative disorders related to cleft lip and palate* (vol. 4, pp. 313–330). Austin, TX: Pro-Ed.

Van Lierde, K. M., Claeys, S., De Bodt, M., & Van Cauwenberge, P. (2004). Outcome of laryngeal and velopharyngeal biofeedback treatment in children and young adults: A pilot study. *Journal of Voice, 18*(1), 97–106.

Van Riper, C. (1963). *Speech correction: Principles and methods* (4th ed.). New York, NY: Prentice Hall.

Wang, G. M., Jiang, L. P., Wu, Y. L., Chen, Y., & Li, Q. Y. (2003). A preliminary study on speech therapy for adult cleft palate patients. *Shanghai Kou Qiang Yi Xue, 12*(2), 81–84.

Warren, S. F., Fey, M. E., & Yoder, P. J. (2007). Differential treatment intensity research: A missing link to creating optimally effective communication interventions. *Mental Retardation and Developmental Disabilities Research Reviews, 13*, 70–77.

Watson, M. M., & Lof, G. L. (2008). Epilogue: What we know about nonspeech oral motor exercises. *Seminars in Speech and Language, 29*(4), 339–344.

Watson, M. M., & Lof, G. L. (2009). A survey of university professors teaching speech sound disorders: Nonspeech oral motor exercises and other topics. *Language, Speech, and Hearing Services in Schools, 40*(3), 256–270.

Weber, J., Jobe, R. P., & Chase, R. A. (1970). Evaluation of muscle stimulation in the rehabilitation of patients with hypernasal speech. *Plastic and Reconstructive Surgery, 46,* 173–174.

Witzel, M. A., Tobe, J., & Salyer, K. (1988). The use of nasopharyngoscopy biofeedback therapy in the correction of inconsistent velopharyngeal closure. *International Journal of Pediatric Otorhinolaryngology, 15*(2), 137–142.

Witzel, M. A., Tobe, J., & Salyer, K. E. (1989). The use of videonasopharyngoscopy for biofeedback therapy in adults after pharyngeal flap surgery. *Cleft Palate Journal, 26*(2), 129–134; discussion 135.

Wolfaardt, J. F., Wilson, F. B., Rochet, A., & McPhee, L. (1993). An appliance-based approach to the management of palatopharyngeal incompetency: A clinical pilot project. *Journal of Prosthetic Dentistry, 69*(2), 186–195.

Yorkston, K. M., Spencer, K. A., Duffy, J. R., Beukelman, D. R., Golper, L. A., Miller, R. M., . . . Sullivan, M. (2001). Evidence-based practical guidelines for dysarthria: Management of velopharyngeal function. *Journal of Medical Speech-Language Pathology, 9*(4), 257–273.

Ysunza, A., Pamplona, M., Femat, T., Mayer, L., & Garcia-Velasco, M. (1997). Video-nasopharyngoscopy as an instrument for visual biofeedback during speech in cleft palate patients. *International Journal of Pediatric Otorhinolaryngology, 41*(3), 291–298.

Ysunza, A., Pamplona, C., & Toledo, E. (1992). Change in velopharyngeal valving after speech therapy in cleft palate patients. A videonasopharyngoscopic and multiview videofluoroscopic study. *International Journal of Pediatric Otorhinolaryngology, 24*(1), 45–54.

Ysunza-Rivera, A., Pamplona-Ferreira, M. C., & Toledo-Cortina, E. (1991). Changes in valvular movements of the velopharyngeal sphincter after speech therapy in children with cleft palate: A videonasopharyngoscopic and videofluoroscopic study of multiple incidence. *Boletin Medico del Hospital Infantil de Mexico, 48*(7), 490–501.

Yules, R. B., & Chase, R. A. (1969). A training method for reduction of hypernasality in speech. *Plastic and Reconstructive Surgery, 43*(2), 180–185.

CREDITS

APPENDIX 19A

Speech Therapy "Cookbook"

This appendix serves as a "cookbook" of specific therapy techniques that are helpful for correction of articulation productions that are produced in the pharynx either as compensatory productions or merely from mislearning. It should be noted that all therapy techniques to achieve appropriate placement are based on the target sound, not the abnormal placement. Therefore, these therapy techniques are appropriate for other misarticulations or oral sounds regardless of causality or the particular substitution.

It is important to note that the techniques described are effective only if the child has the physical ability (adequate structure and neurophysiological abilities) to produce the speech sounds. If hypernasality and/or nasal emission persists despite normal articulation placement, velopharyngeal function should be evaluated (or reevaluated) by specialists associated with a craniofacial team. Speech therapy should be discontinued if there has been no demonstrable progress over the past 2 months.

Correction of Plosives (/p/, /b/, /t/, /d/, /k/, /g/)	
Common substitutions	Glottal stops
Awareness	Tell the child that you are going to eliminate the "jerk" in her neck during the sound production.
Feedback	• **Visual feedback:** Have the child watch her neck in a mirror during production of the glottal stop. The child will notice an obvious jerk in the neck area in front of the larynx. Then, have the child produce a prolonged vowel or a nasal–vowel syllable (e.g., /mɑ/), and have her notice the difference. Have the child watch your neck as you produce the plosive without the glottal stop.

(continues)

Correction of Plosives (/p/, /b/, /t/, /d/, /k/, /g/) *(continued)*

- **Tactile feedback:** Have the child place her hand on her neck, over the larynx, during the production of a syllable where she would normally produce a glottal stop (**FIGURE 19A-1**). Tell her to feel the "jerk" during production. Then, have her feel her neck during a prolonged vowel or a nasal–vowel syllable to feel the difference. Have the child feel your neck as you produce the plosive without the glottal stop.
- **Auditory feedback:** Have the child listen to your productions of plosives without the glottal stop and then plosives with co-articulation of the glottal stop. Perhaps have the child point to a happy face or sad face to indicate the correct versus incorrect production.

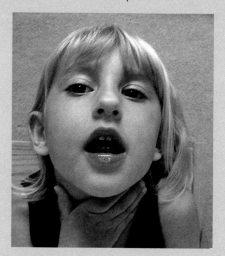

FIGURE 19A-1 To eliminate glottal stops, have the child feel her neck for the "jerk" during production. Then, have the child feel the difference with the production of an /m/ or voiceless /p/ (without a vowel).

Instructions:
Plosives without glottal stop

1. Have the child produce a voiceless plosive (e.g., /p/) without the vowel. (A glottal stop is voiced. Therefore, the glottal stop does not occur until transition from a voiceless phoneme to the voiced vowel.)
2. Have the child produce the voiceless plosive and then the vowel preceded by an /h/ (e.g., /p . . . hɑ/ for /pɑ/ and /p . . . ho/ for /po/). The /h/ is voiceless and therefore keeps the vocal folds open and prevents the production of a glottal stop before the vowel. Gradually, decrease the transition time from the consonant to the /h/ and then the vowel. As the transition is decreased, the /h/ essentially disappears so that the syllable is produced normally without a glottal stop.
3. Once syllables beginning with voiceless plosives are produced easily, move to voiced plosives, which necessarily include the vowel. Have the child "whisper" the syllable and produce it slowly. Gradually, increase the rate and volume. At the same time, have the child feel or watch her neck in a mirror for feedback.

Correction of Velars (/ŋ/, /k/, /g/)

Common substitutions	Pharyngeal plosives
Awareness	Tell the child that her current sound is produced in her throat. The goal is to make the sound in the back of her mouth with the back of her tongue.
Feedback	• **Visual feedback:** Have the child watch her mouth in a mirror during production of the pharyngeal plosive. Then, have the child watch your mouth as you produce a velar sound (/k/ or /g/). • **Tactile feedback:** Have the child place her hand at the top of her neck, just under her chin, during the production of a syllable where she would normally produce a pharyngeal plosive (same as in Figure 19A-1). Tell her to feel the "jerk" during production. Then, have her feel your neck during production of a velar sound to feel the difference. • **Auditory feedback:** Have the child listen to your productions of velars. If you can imitate a pharyngeal plosive, have the child indicate the correct versus incorrect production.
Instructions: /k/ and /g/	1. Establish velar placement by starting with an /ŋ/, which is a continuant, making it easier to produce. 2. If the child cannot produce an /ŋ/, put a tongue blade on the mid part of the tongue. Push down and back slightly until she produces the sound. If this does not work, put your thumb under her chin, which is under the base of the tongue, and press up firmly while the child phonates. Have the child produce the sound with the help of this manipulation and then without it. 3. Once placement for the /ŋ/ has been obtained, have the child produce an /ŋ/ and then drop the tongue. This should be done repetitively to work on an up-and-down, rather than a back-and-forth, movement of the back of the tongue, which occurs with the pharyngeal plosive. Then, have the child produce the /ŋ/ with a vowel as in /ŋɑ/. 4. Have the child produce the /ŋɑ/ syllable with her nose closed. This will turn it into /gɑ/. Have the child repeat this until she can do it without the nose closed. 5. One the child is able to produce /gɑ/ easily, have her whisper the syllable to elicit the /k/ sound.

Correction of Lingual-Alveolars (/n/, /t/, /d/)

Abnormal placement	Palatal–dorsal production
Awareness	Tell the child that her current sound is produced with the middle of the tongue. The goal will be to make the sound with the tongue tip instead.
Feedback	• **Visual feedback:** Have the child watch her tongue tip movement in a mirror during production of the /t/ sound. Then, have the child watch your mouth as you produce a /t/ sound. Note that the child's tongue tip will be down instead of up during production. • **Tactile feedback:** Have the child produce the sound as she normally does. Use a tongue blade to touch the part of the tongue that incorrectly articulates against the palate. Then, touch the tongue tip, which will be used for the new articulation. • **Auditory feedback:** Put the end of a straw just in front of your central incisors (see Figure 19-5A). Produce a /t/ sound, making sure that the airstream is audible as it goes through the straw. Have the child listen to the sound of airflow through the straw.

(continues)

Correction of Lingual-Alveolars (/n/, /t/, /d/) *(continued)*

Instructions:
/n/, /t/, and /d/

1. Have the child bite on a tongue blade (**FIGURE 19A-2**).
2. Tell the child to put her tongue tip on the tongue blade and then back down.
3. Then, have the child produce an /n/ sound using her tongue tip and hold the sound. Have her note the placement.
4. Have the child produce the /n/ sound and then drop the tongue several times. Then, have the child produce the /n/ with a vowel (e.g., /nɑ/).
5. Because the /n/ is voiced, the next target sound should be the /g/, which is also voiced. Have the child produce the /nɑ/ syllable with her nose closed. This will turn it into /dɑ/. Have the child repeat this until she can do it without the nose closed.
6. Once the child is able to produce /dɑ/ easily, have her whisper the syllable to elicit the /t/ sound.
7. Place a straw in front of the child's incisors. Tell the child to use the tongue tip to push the air through the straw during the production of /t/.

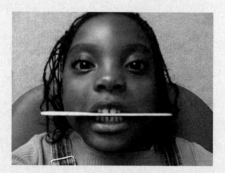

FIGURE 19A-2 To eliminate palatal–dorsal articulation of lingual-alveolar sounds, have the child bite on a tongue blade. Have the child try to produce the sounds with the tongue tip articulating on the tongue blade.

A. Correction of Sibilant Fricatives (/s/, /z/, /ʃ/)

Common substitutions	Pharyngeal/posterior nasal fricative with nasal emission
Awareness	Tell the child that his current sound is produced in his throat. The goal is to make the sound in the front of the mouth with his tongue tip instead.
Feedback	• **Visual feedback:** Have the child watch his tongue tip movement in a mirror during production of the /t/ sound. Tell the child that for the /s/ sound, the air goes just between the tongue tip and the ridge that the tongue touches when producing a /t/. • **Tactile feedback:** Have the child produce the sound as he normally does while you pinch his nostrils closed. The child will feel the nasal blockage. Then, ask the child to place his hand in front of your mouth as you produce the /t/ sound and then an /s/ sound. Tell the child to note the feel of the airstream as a result of this sound production. Then, have the child put his hand in front of his own mouth while he tries to produce a /t/ and /s/ and feel the airstream. (The child should wash his hands or use a waterless disinfectant on his hands immediately after this procedure.)

- **Auditory feedback (posterior nasal fricative [PNF]):** Put the end of a straw or tube in the child's nostril and the other end in the child's ear. Have the child produce the sound as he normally does. The child will hear significant nasal air emission through the tube. Have the child produce another oral sound that he produces correctly. Have the child notice that there is no audible nasal emission during production of the sound. Then, put the end of a straw or tube in your nostril and the other end in the child's ear. Produce the /s/ sound and have the child note that there is no nasal audible emission through the tube.

Instructions: Sibilant fricatives: /s/, /z/, and /ʃ/	**Pharyngeal/posterior nasal fricative (PNF):**
	1. Make sure the child produces the /t/ sound with correct placement. If he does not, work on the /t/ sound first.
	2. Have the child try to produce the /s/ sound with the nostrils occluded and then open to get the feel for oral versus nasal airflow.
	3. Place a straw at the front of the child's closed central incisors during production of the /s/, and note the lack of audible airstream through the straw (see Figure 19-5A).
	4. Have the child produce a /t/ sound while feeling the tongue tip movement.
	5. Put a straw just in front of the child's incisors again. Have the child produce a /t/ while pushing the airstream into the straw.
	6. Then, have the child produce the /t/ with the teeth closed, which results in /ts/.
	7. Have the child increase the duration of the production until it becomes /tssss/.
	8. Have the child produce a /tssss/ sound while consciously trying to push air into the straw. At the same time, have the child feel the airstream flowing over his tongue tip during production.
	9. Put one end of a straw or tube in the child's nostril and the other end in the child's ear for auditory feedback.
	10. Have the child produce the /tssss/ with his teeth closed. Tell the child to be sure he does not hear anything coming through the tube.
	11. For the /ʃ/, have the child produce the /tssss/ with the lips rounded.

B. Correction of Sibilant Fricatives (/s/, /z/, /ʃ/)

Common substitutions	Lateral lisp for sibilant fricatives, often caused by a palatal-dorsal placement
Awareness	Tell the child that his current sound is produced with the tongue touching something in the mouth (e.g., the teeth, alveolar ridge, or palate). This causes air to go out the sides of the mouth. The goal is to make the sound so the air goes over the tip of the tongue and out the front of the mouth instead.
Feedback	• **Visual feedback:** Have the child watch his tongue tip movement in a mirror during production of the /t/ sound. Tell the child that for the /s/ sound, the air goes just between the tongue tip and the ridge that the tongue touches when producing a /t/. • **Tactile feedback:** Have the child produce the sound as he normally does. Then, have the child use a tongue blade to touch the part of the tongue that articulates against the palate. Have the child then touch his tongue tip and tell him that with the new production, he will feel air going over that part of his tongue. • **Auditory feedback:** Put the end of a straw just in front of your central incisors. Produce an /s/ sound, making sure that the airstream is heard as it goes through the straw. Then, produce the /s/ sound with a lateral lisp by having your tongue block the airstream. Point out that the air is no longer heard through the straw. Move the straw to the side of your dental arch until you find where the airstream is actually being emitted.

(continues)

B. Correction of Sibilant Fricatives (/s/, /z/, /ʃ/) *(continued)*

Instructions:
Sibilant fricatives: /s/, /z/, and /ʃ/

1. Make sure the child produces the /t/ sound with correct placement. If he does not, work on the /t/ sound first.
2. Move a straw to the side of the child's dental arch during production of the /s/ to find the place where the airstream can be heard through the straw (see Figure 19-5B).
3. Place a straw at the front of the child's closed incisors during production of the /s/, and note the lack of audible airstream through the straw (see Figure 19-5A).
4. Have the child produce a /t/ sound while feeling the tongue tip movement.
5. Put a straw just in front of the child's incisors. Have the child produce a /t/ while pushing the airstream into the straw.
6. Then, have the child produce the /t/ with the teeth closed, which results in /ts/.
7. Have the child increase the duration of the production until it becomes /tssss/.
8. Have the child produce a /tssss/ sound while consciously trying to push air into the straw. At the same time, have the child feel the airstream flowing over his tongue tip during production.
9. Finally, eliminate the tongue tip movement for the /t/ component for the /s/.
10. To achieve placement for /ʃ/, have the child produce the /tssss/ sound with the lips rounded. Have the child prolong this production, which will turn into an /ʃ/.
11. Have the child find the same tongue position to produce an /ʃ/ without starting with a /t/.

Correction of Affricates (/tʃ/ and /dʒ/)

Abnormal placement	Pharyngeal/posterior nasal fricative with nasal emission or a lateral lisp
Awareness	Using letters if the child can read, write out the following for the child: ch = t + sh and j = d + zh (as in "measure").
Feedback	See Correction of Sibilant Fricatives (A and/or B).
Instructions: Affricates: /tʃ/ and /dʒ/	1. Make sure the child can produce both the /t/ and the /ʃ/ or /s/ in isolation. 2. Start with /tʃ/ because this sound contains a /t/ and is voiceless. Follow the same procedures as noted above for /s/, but have the child round his lips during production. Tell the child that this is a sneeze sound with the teeth closed. 3. Once the /tʃ/ sound is mastered, work on the /dʒ/ in the same way, but start with a /d/ sound. Alternatively, have the child produce the /tʃ/ sound with his voice. 4. Once /tʃ/ is mastered, have the child prolong the sound and note the position of the tongue and feel the airstream flowing over the tongue tip during production. 5. Finally, eliminate the tongue tip movement for the /t/ component.

Correction of /ɚ/ and /r/

Abnormal placement	The final /ɚ/ sound is produced by articulating the sides of the posterior tongue against the gum under the molars. The middle portion of the tongue forms a groove through which sound resonates. If the child raises the entire back of the tongue, the sound becomes an /ŋ/ sound, which results in nasal resonance. Of course, another common error is when the back of the tongue does not raise on each side. Regardless of the error, the following techniques help to achieve appropriate placement.
Awareness	Tell the child that the /ɚ/ sound is produced with the sides of the tongue touching the roof of the mouth. Using your hand, show the child how the shape of the tongue forms a boat. In addition, the back of the tongue must touch the gums near the back teeth (**FIGURE 19A-3A**).
Feedback	• **Tactile feedback:** Using a tongue blade, lightly scratch the sides of the child's tongue toward the back. This causes the tongue to tingle for a few seconds. Have the child produce the sound as usual. Ask the child to determine whether the tingly part of his tongue is down or up or whether the middle part of the tongue is up. • **Auditory feedback:** Auditory training and discrimination is particularly important when working on /ɚ/ so that the child can ultimately achieve the right acoustic quality. Have the child listen to your correct production of /ɚ/ and then your incorrect production of /ɚ/. Have the child listen carefully and indicate correct versus incorrect productions. • **Visual feedback:** Produce the /ɚ/ sound. Using a flashlight, have the child note that the back of your tongue is up on both sides.
Instructions: Final /ɚ/	The final /ɚ/ is a continuant. The initial /r/ requires achieving the /ɚ/ placement first and then moving the tongue forward. Therefore, it is important to establish normal production of /ɚ/ before working on initial /r/. 1. Have the child stick out his tongue. With a tongue blade, stimulate one side of the back of the tongue and then the other side (**FIGURE 19A-3B**). Then, stimulate the gum ridge just under the maxillary molars on both sides. This causes tingling of both. Tell the child that these parts need to come together for the /ɚ/ sound. 2. Manually assist the child with placement. Put your thumb under the chin, which is under the base of the tongue, and press up firmly while the child attempts to produce the sound. If you feel resistance from the tongue, have the child "make it loose" until you can push up easily. To achieve lip placement at the same time, use your middle finger to push under the chin while squeezing the cheeks with your thumb and forefinger to obtain lip rounding (**FIGURE 19A-3C**). 3. Tell the child to move his entire tongue (not the tip) backward until the sides are touching under his teeth.
Instructions: Initial /r/	1. Once the final /ɚ/ is established, demonstrate with your hand how the tongue moves forward for the initial /r/. 2. Tell the child that the /r/ is produced with the tongue, not the lips. Demonstrate the difference in the lips when producing /r/ and /w/. 3. Have the child place his hands on his cheeks and watch his lips in a mirror. Have the child produce a /w/ sound. He should feel the movement of the cheeks from the movement of the lips and see the movement of the lips in a mirror. Tell the child that /r/ is a tongue sound, not a lip sound. Therefore, there should be no movement of the face or lips when producing the /r/.

(continues)

Correction of /ɚ/ and /r/   *(continued)*

4. While watching in a mirror and with his hands on his cheeks, have the child begin by producing the final /ɚ/. Then, have the child move the tongue forward for initial /r/ while making sure that there is no movement felt in the cheeks or seen with his lips.
5. If the child is substituting an /ŋ/ for /ɚ/, close the child's nose during his attempts to produce the sound. That will make the /ŋ/ (which is a nasal sound) impossible to produce.

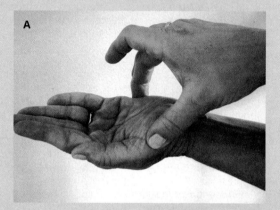

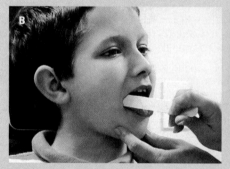
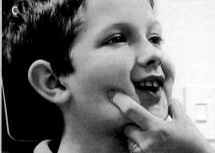

FIGURE 19A-3 Working on the /r/ and /ɚ/ phonemes. **(A)** Show the child with your hands how the tongue makes a boat shape with a groove in the back and how the back of the tongue must articulate on the gums near the upper molars. **(B)** Using a tongue blade, stimulate the back of the tongue on both sides and then the upper gums on both sides, just behind the molars. **(C)** To encourage appropriate placement for final /ɚ/, use your middle finger to push up firmly under the child's chin, near the neck. This pushes against the base of the tongue. With the index finger and thumb, squeeze the cheeks to achieve lip rounding.

Correction of ŋ/l

Abnormal placement	ŋ/l
Awareness	Tell the child that the /l/ is produced with the front of the tongue, not the back of the tongue.
Feedback	• **Visual feedback:** Using a flashlight, have the child look in your mouth as you produce the /l/ sound. Then, have the child observe her tongue position during production through a mirror. • **Tactile feedback:** Lightly scratch the tip of the child's tongue and the alveolar ridge with a tongue blade. Explain that the tongue tip needs to touch the ridge during production. • **Auditory feedback:** Produce the targeted sound for the child. Then, close your nose while you produce the sound. Point out that there is no difference in the sound when the nose is closed. Have the child produce the sound as she normally does and then do it again with the nose closed. Point out that there is a change in the sound because it is coming out of the nose.
Instructions: /l/	1. Tell the child to produce a big yawn. This causes the back of the tongue to go down and the velum to go up. 2. Have the child notice the "stretch" in the back of her mouth. 3. Have the child co-articulate the /l/ sound with a yawn. 4. Gradually, have the child make the co-articulated yawn a little smaller. 5. Have the child produce the new sound with the nose open and then closed. If there is a difference, have the child try to make the sound the same with the nose open and with it closed. 6. Place a straw or tube in the child's nostril and the other end near her ear. Have the child produce the sound without allowing sound to come through the nose.

Correction of Nasalization of a Vowel

Abnormal placement	Abnormally high posterior tongue position, causing phoneme-specific nasalization of a vowel, usually /i/
Awareness	Tell the child that the back of her tongue is blocking the sound from coming out of her mouth on certain sounds. The goal is to open up the back of the mouth.
Feedback	• **Visual feedback:** Using a flashlight, have the child look in your mouth as you say /æ/ with your tongue out as far as possible. Have the child note how the back of your tongue is down so that all the sound can come out. • **Tactile feedback:** Have the child place her fingers on the side of her nose while producing the sound as she normally does. The child will be able to feel vibration from the hypernasality. Have the child produce an oral sound that she does not nasalize. Have the child note that there is no vibration (**FIGURE 19A-4**).

(continues)

Correction of Nasalization of a Vowel *(continued)*

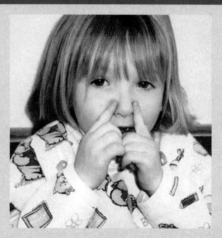

FIGURE 19A-4 Tactile feedback for nasal air emission or hypernasality. By having the child lightly touch the side of her nose, the child will often be able to feel the vibration that occurs with hypernasality and/or a nasal rustle.

- **Auditory feedback:** Produce the targeted sound for the child. Then, close your nose while you produce the sound. Point out that there is no difference in the sound when the nose is closed. Have the child produce the sound as she normally does and then do it again with the nose closed. Point out that there is a change in the sound because it is coming out of the nose.

Instructions:
Oral vowels

1. Tell the child to produce a big yawn. This causes the back of the tongue to go down and the velum to go up.
2. Have the child notice the "stretch" in the back of her mouth.
3. Have the child co-articulate the vowel sound with a yawn.
4. Gradually, have the child make the co-articulated yawn a little smaller.
5. Have the child produce the new sound with the nose open and then closed. If there is a difference, have the child try to make the sound the same with the nose open and with it closed.
6. Place a straw or tube in the child's nostril and the other end near her ear. Have the child produce the sound without allowing sound to come through the nose.

CREDITS

Appendix opener photo: PeopleImages/Getty Images

All photos courtesy of the Cleft and Craniofacial Center at Cincinnati Children's Hospital Medical Center.

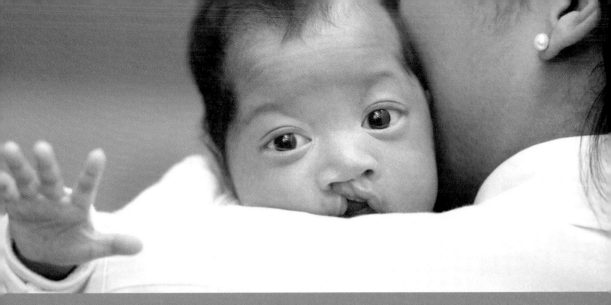

549

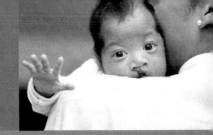

CHAPTER 20

The Team Approach

INTRODUCTION

Individuals with craniofacial anomalies, including cleft lip and palate, typically demonstrate multiple complex issues. These issues may include early feeding and nutritional problems, developmental delay or learning disabilities, hearing loss, obstructive sleep apnea, neurological problems, dentofacial and orthodontic abnormalities, aesthetic concerns, psychosocial problems, and of course, communication disorders. Because of these various concerns, these patients usually have the need for medical, surgical, dental, and allied health (including speech pathology) services. Not only do these patients require treatment from a variety of professionals, but the treatment occurs over a very long period of time. In fact, the entire habilitative process can last from infancy into adulthood.

Because of the complexity of needs, the number of professionals needed, and the length of time for treatment to be completed, team care is essential for the best treatment outcomes. In addition, most families prefer a coordinated team approach over multiple individual appointments (Jeffery & Boorman, 2001).

The purpose of this chapter is to impress upon the reader the importance of the team approach in the management of patients with cleft lip/palate or other craniofacial anomalies. This chapter includes information about various types of teams, a list of typical team members, and a description of team structure and function. The advantages of the team approach are discussed along with common problems with this type of clinical management. Finally, information is given on how to find a specialty team to refer a child for further assessment and intervention when appropriate.

Need for Team Management

There are many qualified professionals throughout the United States and the world who can care for patients with craniofacial anomalies. However, independent care by a variety of professionals with no interdisciplinary communication is not optimal care for patients with chronic needs, such as those with clefts or craniofacial conditions. This is because the treatment of one professional can have an effect on the treatment of the other professionals. In addition, the sequence of treatment from each discipline must be carefully planned for a variety of reasons. Finally, there is evidence to suggest that patients who do not receive team care are less likely to receive all the services they need (Austin et al., 2010). Therefore, for maximum benefit, services to patients with clefts and craniofacial anomalies must be provided in a coordinated and integrated manner over a period of years (Glade & Deal, 2016; Naran, Ford, & Losee, 2017).

The importance of team management for patients with cleft lip and palate was first recognized by H. K. Cooper, who founded the Lancaster Cleft Palate Clinic in the early 1930s (Krogman, 1979). Many cleft palate or craniofacial teams were formed across the United States in subsequent years.

In 1987, the Surgeon General of the United States recognized the need for a coordinated team approach in the management of patients with special healthcare needs and articulated this need in a report (Surgeon General's Report, 1987). In response to this report, the Maternal and Child Health Bureau provided funding to the American Cleft Palate–Craniofacial Association (ACPA) to develop recommended practices in the care of patients with craniofacial anomalies. To accomplish this, a large group of various professionals from around the United States was convened for a consensus conference in 1991. This meeting resulted in the publishing of a comprehensive document by the ACPA called *Parameters for Evaluation and Treatment of Patients with Cleft Lip/ Palate or Other Craniofacial Anomalies*, which has since been revised (ACPA, 2009). One of the fundamental principles contained in this document is that the management of patients with craniofacial anomalies is best provided by an interdisciplinary team of specialists who see a significant number of these patients each year and therefore develop expertise through experience (p. 7).

TABLE 20-1 Advantages of the Team Approach to Management of Care

- Patients have access to multiple professionals who specialize in their condition and can provide interdisciplinary evaluations and regular follow-up services.
- Care is more efficient and cost effective because multiple professionals can evaluate the child in one visit, usually at a lower cost than individual evaluations.
- Care is focused on the whole child and not just on one particular abnormality or functional disability.
- Care is provided in a coordinated and consistent manner with consideration for the patient's overall medical, developmental, and psychological needs.
- Decision making is shared among the team members, who work together and understand each other's disciplines. Therefore, decisions are based on more information than one professional would have compiled independently.
- There is better long-term treatment planning from birth to adulthood, proper sequencing of evaluations and treatments, and better continuity of care.
- The team coordinator can provide assistance with follow-up appointments and serve as the main contact person for the entire team of professionals.
- Teams often provide parent groups, special camps, and pamphlets and other educational materials.
- The team approach increases interprofessional communication, which increases the knowledge of each professional.
- The team approach makes it possible to keep good serial records and collect data for quality assurance and collaboration in research and publications.
- There is regular and frequent communication among all professionals involved in the patient's care. This saves time for the providers by expediting the collaboration process.

There is now general consensus among professionals regarding the importance of a team approach to the care of patients with cleft lip/palate or craniofacial anomalies (ACPA, 2010; Austin et al., 2010; Capone & Sykes, 2007; David, Anderson, Schnitt, Nugent, & Sells, 2006; Schnitt, Agir, & David, 2004; Stal, Chebret, & McElroy, 1998; Strauss, 1998; Strauss, 1999; Strohecker, 1993; Thomas, 2000; Vargervik, Oberoi, & Hoffman, 2009; Wellens & Vander Poorten, 2006; Will & Parsons, 1991). This is because there are so many advantages of the team approach to the patient, the patient's family, and even to the providers. Some of these advantages are listed in TABLE 20-1.

Characteristics of Teams

There are many cleft palate/craniofacial teams in various cities across the country. They are similar in their belief that patients with clefts and/or other craniofacial conditions require integrated care from many different professionals. They often differ, however, in many aspects, including the type and size of the team, team membership and structure, team leadership, clinical processes, and even quality.

Types of Teams

A team of professionals can be multidisciplinary or interdisciplinary depending on the working relationship of the members and the structure of the team. A multidisciplinary team is a group of professionals from various disciplines who work independently in evaluating and treating patients with complex medical needs. The members of this type of team have well-defined roles and cooperate with each other, but there is little communication and interaction among the team members (Butler, Samman, & Gollogly, 2011; Strauss, 1999; Thomas, 2000). The biggest problem with a multidisciplinary team is that the patient receives a series of evaluations and recommendations but there is little integration of the information or recommendations.

On the other hand, an interdisciplinary team is a group of professionals from various disciplines who work together to coordinate the care of the patient. With this model, there is collaboration, interaction, communication, and cooperation among the specialists who are involved in the patient's care. There may or may not be a joint evaluation, but there definitely is a joint plan of care. This is developed when all members of the team come together to discuss the findings, impressions, and recommendations. The final plan of care is negotiated and based on the integration of all recommendations (Moller, 2001; Strauss, 1999). With this approach, one person and one document can outline the sequence of procedures and approximate timelines for the entire team. Therefore, the interdisciplinary team model is felt to be most effective in the management of patients with craniofacial anomalies.

A cleft palate or craniofacial team that works together for a period of time may even evolve into a transdisciplinary team. This type of team has members who truly understand each other's disciplines and how they relate to the total care of the patient. Although transdisciplinary team members cannot perform duties across disciplines, they have enough understanding of the various disciplines to see the "big picture" and answer more questions from the family. This can certainly affect the quality of care provided to the patient and the family.

A cleft palate or craniofacial team often serves as the primary treating team for its patients. In larger centers, however, the team may also serve as a consulting team. In the role of a consulting team, the team members provide an opinion as a group regarding the total care of the patient. This opinion is forwarded to the treating professionals for consideration and follow-up. The treating professionals may be in the local community or far away. Regardless, there must be excellent communication between the consulting team and the treating practitioners.

Team Membership

To meet the complex needs of the patients and their families, cleft palate or craniofacial teams typically include medical, surgical, dental, and allied health professionals (Kasten et al., 2008) (**FIGURE 20-1**). TABLE 20-2 lists the various professionals who are often members of a cleft or craniofacial team and gives a description of each professional's role in the management of these patients.

In the *Parameters* document, ACPA has established basic standards for membership of a cleft palate team (CPT) and a craniofacial team (CFT) (ACPA, 2009). One standard requirement is that each team must have a coordinator, who is usually a nurse or other healthcare professional (see Table 20-2 for responsibilities of the coordinator). ACPA also has standards for which disciplines must be members of the team for the team to be approved and listed in the ACPA team directory. The minimum standards for team membership are as follows:

- Cleft palate team (CPT): A CPT must have a surgeon, an orthodontist, a speech-language pathologist, and at least one additional specialist. ACPA also requires this type of team to evaluate at least 50 patients per year and have at least one surgeon who operates on at least 10 primary clefts per year.

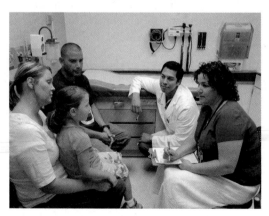

FIGURE 20-1 The team approach to assessment.

TABLE 20-2 **Professional Roles within a Cleft Palate or Craniofacial Team**

Role	Description
Audiologist	The audiologist is the person who is responsible for testing the child's hearing and middle ear function. Because individuals with craniofacial anomalies are at high risk for structural ear anomalies, middle ear disease, and hearing loss, the audiologist works with the otolaryngologist in monitoring the hearing and middle ear function of these individuals.
Craniofacial surgeon	Craniofacial surgery is a subspecialty of both oral/maxillofacial surgery and plastic surgery. The role of this surgeon is to correct the congenital deformities of the head, skull, face, neck, jaws, and associated structures for an improvement in both aesthetics and function.
Dentist (pediatric)	The role of the pediatric dentist (sometimes called a pedodontist) is to be responsible for the general care of the child's teeth and the prevention and treatment of tooth decay. The pediatric dentist ensures that despite the cleft or malocclusion, the child develops habits of good oral hygiene for the promotion of healthy teeth and gums. The pediatric dentist tries to protect and preserve even the primary teeth because they act as placeholders for the permanent teeth. The pediatric dentist may be involved in the management of misaligned cleft segments prior to the lip closure. When the child is in the primary or mixed dentition stages, the pediatric dentist is often the one who improves early malocclusion, which often includes moving the maxillary segments through palatal expansion.
Geneticist	A geneticist (also called a dysmorphologist) is responsible for assessing patients with a history of cleft, velopharyngeal dysfunction, or craniofacial anomalies for a pattern that indicates a known syndrome or cause. If a syndrome is identified, the geneticist counsels the family regarding the diagnosis, the recurrence risk for additional offspring of both the family and the patient, and the prognosis.
Nurse	The nurse's role on the team is to assess the child's overall physical development. The nurse can determine whether the child is growing normally and is in good general health. The nurse is often the professional who assists the family in developing compensatory feeding techniques. Finally, the nurse is usually the professional who counsels the family regarding surgical procedures and answers their specific questions.
Oral/maxillofacial surgeon	The oral surgeon is the specialist who usually does the bone grafts to the alveolar cleft area when there is deficient bone in the line of the cleft. This professional also performs the orthognathic surgeries to normalize the occlusion between the maxillary and mandibular arches. These surgeries include a maxillary advancement (such as a Le Fort I procedure) and/or a mandibular setback.
Orthodontist	The orthodontist is responsible for aligning misplaced teeth in addition to correcting dental and skeletal malocclusion. The orthodontist works to normalize jaw relationships to achieve normal dental function and improve facial and dental aesthetics.

(continues)

TABLE 20-2 **Professional Roles within a Cleft Palate or Craniofacial Team**	*(continued)*
Role	**Description**
Otolaryngologist	The otolaryngologist, also known as the ear, nose, and throat specialist (ENT), is responsible for monitoring middle ear function and hearing and treating middle ear disease, which is particularly common in children with a history of cleft or craniofacial anomalies. The otolaryngologist also manages upper airway obstruction, which is particularly important for infants with Pierre Robin sequence. The otolaryngologist assesses the structural aspects of the oral cavity, oropharynx, nasal cavity, and upper airway and treats conditions such as adenotonsillar hypertrophy, pharyngeal masses, and vocal fold abnormalities. The otolaryngologist may be the surgeon involved in the nasal and oral repairs and reconstruction. Finally, some otolaryngologists perform the nasopharyngoscopy evaluations, and some do surgeries for velopharyngeal insufficiency/incompetence (VPI).
Pediatrician	The pediatrician is responsible for assessing the patient's overall medical health, growth, and development. The pediatrician determines whether there are other related or unrelated medical conditions that must be addressed, particularly those that can affect plans for surgical intervention.
Plastic surgeon	The plastic surgeon is responsible for the surgical repair of the lip and palate and surgical reconstruction of facial and cranial anomalies. Surgery for correction of VPI is usually done by the plastic surgeon. The plastic surgeon may perform bone grafts and orthognathic surgery on the jaws. The aim of plastic surgery is to repair the structural defects so there is an improvement in the patient's overall facial aesthetics, function, and speech.
Prosthodontist	The prosthodontist is involved with the restoration of natural teeth or the replacement of missing teeth. The prosthodontist develops devices to replace or improve the appearance of oral and facial structures that cannot be adequately improved with surgery or dental care. The prosthodontist can manufacture and fit devices to assist with velopharyngeal closure if surgery is not an option.
Psychologist	The psychologist assesses the patient's psychosocial needs and assists the patient and family in dealing with the medical, social, and emotional challenges that occur from the patient's anomalies and other medical conditions. The psychologist often assists the physician in determining the emotional preparedness of the patient for each surgical procedure.
Pulmonologist	Because many children with clefts and craniofacial anomalies have airway issues and sleep problems, the pulmonologist evaluates and monitors the patient's airway and sleep. If obstructive sleep apnea (OSA) is suspected, the pulmonologist will order a sleep study.
Social worker	The social worker helps families deal with the many challenges and problems that they often experience when trying to manage the child's special needs. The social worker may be the one who coordinates appointments and assists the families in dealing with insurance and other funding sources. The social worker may help the family to manage their stress and emotional reactions to the many problems and issues associated with the child's treatment.

Speech-language pathologist	The speech-language pathologist counsels the parents regarding what to expect with communication development and how to work with the child at home. The speech-language pathologist evaluates feeding and swallowing, general development, speech, language, resonance, and velopharyngeal function. The speech-language pathologist provides therapy for communication problems and disorders of feeding or swallowing. Some speech-language pathologists perform nasopharyngoscopy evaluations.
Team coordinator	The team coordinator typically represents the team in any interactions with parents, other healthcare professionals, and the community. This person is typically responsible for scheduling patients for each team meeting and compiling the recommendations from each team member for comprehensive team reports. The coordinator helps to counsel the family regarding the team recommendations and ensures that there is follow-up on recommendations.

- **Craniofacial team (CFT):** A CFT must have a craniofacial surgeon, an orthodontist, a mental health professional (psychologist or social worker), and a speech-language pathologist. Other members may include a neurologist, a neurosurgeon and/or an ophthalmologist.

- VPI team: ACPA has made no specific recommendations for a team structure for the management of congenital and acquired VPI. However, these patients are often managed by a subset of the CPT members. A VPI team should include a speech-language pathologist, an otolaryngologist or a plastic surgeon, and ideally, a geneticist because many children with VPI of unknown origin have a previously unidentified syndrome.

In addition to the professionals on the team, the parents must be involved in determining the treatment plan for their child (Sharp, 1995). In fact, all decisions for treatment must be based on the patient's and family's wishes in addition to the clinical indications (Johansson & Ringsberg, 2004; Sharp, 1995; Vanz & Ribeiro, 2011). Appropriate family involvement can significantly improve compliance with recommendations, which can ultimately improve the outcomes of treatment. If the family members are not active participants in the decision-making process, compliance with the team's recommendations can be negatively affected (Pannbacker & Scheuerle, 1993; Paynter, Jordan, & Finch, 1990; Paynter, Wilson, & Jordan, 1993).

Team Leadership

The qualifications, personality, and skills of the team leader are highly important in determining the function and success of the team. There is little room for authoritarianism in clinical team leadership. Instead, the leader must be able to ensure that all team members are respected equally. A dominant team member can cause decisions to be made that are based upon that person's opinion rather than on team consensus. It is the responsibility of the team leader to be sure that this does not happen and that all members' opinions are heard and considered before decisions regarding the patient's care are made (Strauss & Broder, 1985). The most effective teams function by consensus even though each professional may view the needs of the patient differently (Noar, 1992; Strauss, 1999).

Team Responsibilities

ACPA has made a number of recommendations regarding the responsibilities of the team in its

Parameters document (ACPA, 2009). For example, it is recommended that each team should have an office with an administrative assistant or a coordinator and a designated phone number. The office should maintain all team documents and patient records. Patients should be evaluated at regular intervals, depending on the needs of the patient and the family. Although the patients may be examined individually by the professionals on the team, regularly scheduled team meetings must be held for discussion and negotiation of the plan of care. Communication of recommendations to the patient and family must be made verbally and in written form. There must be ongoing communication with the direct care providers in the patient's home community. The team should provide patients with information regarding resources for other services and financial assistance as needed. Finally, the team should provide educational programs for families, other care providers, and the general public.

In a diverse society, team members must be sensitive to the ethnographic and cultural characteristics of the families that they serve. These factors may determine the way in which families understand and view the medical issues and the way they follow the recommendations (Louw, Shibambu, & Roemer, 2006). To provide the most effective services, team intervention must be family focused and culturally sensitive.

Team Process

The cleft or craniofacial team typically becomes involved in the management of the child's needs soon after birth. The team begins with parent counseling and the management of airway problems and feeding issues in the neonatal period. Team care should then continue until the physical growth of the individual has been completed, which is usually between the ages of 18 and 21. Care can continue through adulthood if there are remaining medical, surgical, dental, psychological, or communication problems that can be improved or resolved by the team members.

The method of scheduling and evaluating team patients varies in different settings. In most cases, each professional evaluates the patient through a separate consultation or screening, but this often occurs on the same day in a clinic setting. When the evaluations are done in a clinic, there is the opportunity for several professionals to work together in evaluating the patient (**FIGURE 20-2**). The team members then meet to discuss impressions and recommendations and negotiate a plan of treatment. Treatment priorities and appropriate sequence of treatment are then determined. The coordinator is responsible for communicating the recommendations to the family and making sure that appropriate appointments are scheduled.

Although the team coordinator may be the primary contact person for the family, each person on the team is responsible for counseling the family about the plan of treatment relative to that person's discipline. It has been shown that when the family members are involved and informed regarding the healthcare decisions for their children, stress can be reduced and treatment outcomes improved (Ascha et al., 2016; Paynter, Edmonson, & Jordan, 1991; Walesky-Rainbow & Morris, 1978). The ultimate treatment plan is determined by the recommendations of the team members; the concerns, needs, and goals

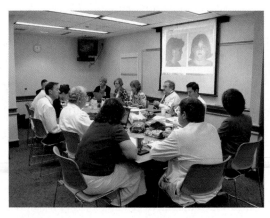

FIGURE 20-2 Team members of the Craniofacial Center at Cincinnati Children's Hospital Medical Center. Face-to-face discussions in team conferences are important for coordinated patient care.

of the patient and family; and the limitations and restrictions of the third-party payment sources.

Team Quality

The quality of the services provided by a team is difficult to measure or quantify. In many cases, quality is determined solely by the perception of the "customers." Although this is an important indicator of quality, there are other ways to assure quality of services.

First of all, the ACPA *Parameters* document includes the basic standards of team care as determined by professional consensus from around the country. These standards include regular team meetings and participation in continuing education programs about clefts or craniofacial anomalies. In addition, ACPA has a Commission on Approval of Teams (CAT), which is charged with evaluating teams around the country to ensure they meet the recommended standards.

Of course, the quality of the team's care is greatly affected by the abilities of each team member. Therefore, the team must ensure that all team members possess the requisite knowledge, experience, and skill in the specialty area of clefts and craniofacial anomalies. It is also important that team members stay current with recent developments in their respective disciplines. This can be done by keeping up with the literature or by attending continuing education meetings, particularly the annual meetings of ACPA. If the professionals are not well trained or current in their specialty area, their good intentions may not be enough to result in good decisions. As a result, they can actually do more harm than good (Sidman, 1995).

The number of patients seen per year and the number of team meetings per year have an effect on the experience base of team members and thus the quality of services provided by the team. Also, teams with a large patient base usually have more members and more disciplines represented on the team compared to teams with few patients.

Teams that use quality assurance or performance improvement methodology to evaluate

and improve their performance are likely to have better quality and outcomes (Strauss, 1999). Clinical pathways and algorithms of care have also been developed by some teams to ensure quality and consistency of services.

Finally, the extent to which the team involves the parents (and often the patient) in the decision-making process affects the overall team quality. It has been found that when parents have a high opinion of the team and the services provided, compliance with recommendations is greatest. In contrast, when parents have a low opinion of the team, compliance can be negatively affected (Paynter et al., 1990).

Team Interactions

Because teams consist of human beings, there are often problems associated with personal relationships and interactions between various team members. However, these problems can be avoided if all members decide to be good team players.

Potential Problems

One factor that can affect the function of the team is the perceived or ascribed status of various team members relative to other members. This can be based on characteristics such as age, gender, discipline, experience, or accomplishments (Cohn, 1991). If team members are not considered equals in status on the team, then the individuals with the ascribed higher status will tend to exert more influence on the decisions of the group than those members of lower status. This can have a negative effect on the quality of the group's decision making. For the team to be effective, there must be an atmosphere of equality and mutual respect among all the team members.

Problems can also occur if the individual roles are not clearly defined within the team. If the roles are not clear, there may be interdisciplinary competition or "turf issues." For example, there is often an overlap of skills among the plastic surgeon, the oral surgeon, and the otolaryngologist. As a team, it is helpful to define who does what, when it's done, and under what circumstances. This avoids conflict over such things as who does the bone graft, who does the orthognathic surgery, or who does the secondary surgery for VPI.

A different but equally disruptive problem occurs when there are members on the team who are hypersensitive to feedback. This can be a problem, for example, when a surgical procedure was not as successful as hoped and needs to be revised. Team members must be able to speak honestly without concern of "stepping on toes" or "hurting someone's feelings." They must also be able to express differences of opinion without hesitation.

Disagreements in the philosophy of care or in treatment protocols can have a major effect on the team's performance. Communication among members regarding procedures and protocols must take place so there is consensus regarding the standards of care and continuum of care within the team. If necessary, an algorithm of care can be developed to help team members reach consensus on the management of various diagnoses and patient concerns.

All potential problems of the interdisciplinary team can and should be overcome for the team to be successful. This requires ongoing communication, honesty, and mutual respect. Ultimately, the focus of the team should be on the care and well-being of the patients, not on the individual agendas and egos of the team members.

How to Be a Good Team Member

Effective interdisciplinary team members are usually those who are very competent and knowledgeable in their particular discipline. When working on an interdisciplinary team that requires specialty knowledge, such as a craniofacial team, each member must have specialty expertise in that area. At the same time, an effective team member must show a strong interest in the knowledge of other disciplines as well as a desire to learn from other disciplines.

All team members should show respect for others and their opinions, especially when there is disagreement. Each team member must feel free to express her honest opinion, without the fear of offending someone. It is important to place quality patient care and appropriate patient management first and not be willing to compromise because of concern about personal feelings or agendas. When mistakes are made, as they will be, it is important that each team member feels comfortable enough to be able to admit mistakes, without worry about undue criticism. In addition, the team members must be comfortable enough with each other to be able to admit what they don't know to further learning and professional competence.

It is important that team members be dependable and reliable because all professionals are very busy. It is not well received when one person holds up the process or lets the other members down.

Finally, the use of humor can be very effective in developing camaraderie and helps to enhance respect and working relationships among team members. Team members who use humor in their interactions with each other usually work more effectively together, and this has a positive effect on the quality of services that are ultimately provided to the patients.

Resources for Services

Finding a cleft palate/craniofacial team is a challenge for many families. Once a team is found, the next concern is funding for the services. Fortunately, resources can be found on the website for the ACPA (http://acpa-cpf.org/families).

How to Find a Cleft Palate or Craniofacial Team

There are cleft palate/craniofacial teams in most major cities and even many midsized cities around the country. There are also cleft/craniofacial teams in larger cities of developed countries and even in some developing countries. Most teams are associated within a pediatric hospital.

In general, the team has to see the patient for evaluation and consultation only once or twice a year during the active treatment process so that

CASE REPORT

The value of a team approach to clinical management is illustrated by the following case history:

Barbara was born with a bilateral complete cleft lip and cleft palate. The lip and palate repairs were done at the appropriate time. She had speech therapy in grade school but was discharged from therapy with the notation that she was "doing as well as can be expected, given her velopharyngeal mechanism." Unfortunately, she was not followed by a craniofacial team at the time, and no referral was made for further assessment and treatment.

Barbara was finally seen at the age of 16 by the craniofacial team at Cincinnati Children's. Following the team evaluation, many treatment recommendations were made:

- The orthodontist reported that the patient had a Class III malocclusion with anterior open bite and linguoverted maxillary incisors. His recommendation was to align the maxillary arch with orthodontics.
- The speech-language pathologist reported that Barbara's speech was characterized by hypernasality and significant nasal emission. Barbara also had obligatory distortions and compensatory articulation errors as a result of both the malocclusion and the VPI. A large velopharyngeal opening was noted on nasopharyngoscopy. Given those findings, the speech-language pathologist recommended a pharyngeal flap for correction of VPI. This was to be followed by postoperative speech therapy to correct the compensatory articulation errors.
- The oral surgeon reported that with the discrepancy between the position of the maxillary and mandibular arches, a Le Fort I maxillary advancement was indicated to move the maxilla to the appropriate position.
- The plastic surgeon reported that there was redundant vermilion in the line of the cleft and that the Cupid's bow needed revision with an Abbe flap.
- The psychologist reported that one of the things that really bothered Barbara about herself was her flattened nose.

Given all these concerns and recommendations, the plan of care had to be designed with the best overall results in mind. To achieve that goal, the appropriate sequencing of procedures had to be determined.

In this case, the first step was for the orthodontist to bring the teeth into alignment in preparation for the orthognathic (jaw) surgery. Bringing the teeth into proper alignment was going to make the occlusion of the jaws and profile actually worse, but doing so would yield the best ultimate results. The next step was for the oral surgeon to perform a Le Fort I maxillary advancement. This normalized the occlusion and gave more support for the upper lip and base of the nose. Once the jaws were in alignment, the plastic surgeon did a pharyngeal flap to correct the VPI and then performed the lip and nose revision. About 6 weeks after the surgery, Barbara began speech therapy to correct the remaining compensatory articulation errors. She was discharged from therapy with normal speech after less than 2 months of therapy.

With this planned sequence, Barbara had the best overall outcome for both aesthetics and speech. On the other hand, if the pharyngeal flap had been done before maxillary advancement, the position and effectiveness of the flap could have been compromised with the maxillary advancement. The maxillary advancement could also have had a detrimental effect on the lip and nose if those revisions had been done first. Hence, it can be seen that the sequence and coordination of treatment is very important for patients who require care from multiple specialists.

it is not essential that the team be located near the patient's home. Routine treatment, such as general dental care, orthodontics, speech therapy, and pediatric care, can usually be provided by professionals in the patient's own community as long as there is regular communication and consultation with the team members. The ACPA website has information for parents on team care and also maintains a list of cleft palate and craniofacial teams by geographic area.

Funding Sources

Funding for the evaluation and treatment of cleft lip, cleft palate, and other craniofacial anomalies can come from a variety of sources. Private insurance companies will usually cover most of the expenses associated with the medical care of the patient if the patient was born when the policy was in effect. Financial assistance can also be obtained through federal and state programs, such as Champus, Medicaid, the Children's Special Health Services for the state, and the Bureau of Vocational Rehabilitation, and selected Shriners' Hospitals across the country. Some private and nonprofit organizations provide funds or special services to meet the needs of children with clefts or craniofacial anomalies. Resources for financial aid can often be obtained through a social worker or team coordinator.

With changes in healthcare financing, there are some additional challenges to the team approach for the management of complex patients. Although the managed care system was designed to help control the cost of health care, many critics would argue that this is hard to do when most of the managed care organizations exist as for-profit corporations. Critics of managed care would also argue that this system discourages the use of specialists in the care of complex disorders (Strauss, 1999). In fact, there are financial disincentives for primary care providers to seek specialty care for their patients. Managed care organizations seek to control costs by limiting the number and type of professionals the patient can see and the number and type of procedures the patient can have. This certainly has an effect on the specialty team approach.

An additional concern is that some third-party payers limit access to physicians who are outside the network. If there are no specialists within the network to cover the particular medical needs, the quality of care provided to the patient may seriously be affected. This is an even greater problem when a whole team of professionals is required for quality care.

Some patients or parents are unable to move or change jobs because of a concern about changing insurance coverage. Managed care organizations often refuse to cover preexisting conditions when the policy is new. As a result, the care of patients with cleft palate or craniofacial anomalies may not be covered. In addition, there is an incentive for managed care organizations to seek to enroll groups of patients who are a low financial risk because they have few health problems. This may result in excluding individuals who really need insurance coverage for medical services.

As the healthcare system in the United States continues to evolve, it is difficult to predict the future and what it holds for specialty team care or even general medical care. With the help of the efforts of professionals and various advocacy groups, it is hoped that the system will be refined so that the specific needs of the patient are a priority.

SUMMARY

Over the past 70 years, the team approach to the management of individuals with craniofacial anomalies has evolved from a good idea to the accepted standard of care not only in this country but also internationally. Although there are some inherent difficulties that can occur when a group of professionals must work closely together, the advantages of this approach far outweigh the disadvantages. Without the team approach to management, the treatment of patients would become fragmented, and the outcomes would be negatively affected. Hopefully, as our healthcare system continues to evolve, the team approach to the care of patients with clefts, craniofacial anomalies, and all other complex medical conditions will be supported and even enhanced.

FOR REVIEW AND DISCUSSION

1. Why is team management preferable to individual management of children with craniofacial anomalies?

2. List the typical members of a cleft palate/craniofacial team and their specific roles.

3. How soon should a child be seen by a cleft team and for how long?

4. What guidelines are available for standards of team care, and where can they be found?

5. Your patient is 4 years old and has a collapsed maxillary arch, anterior crossbite, and midface retrusion. He has very poor oral hygiene and large tonsils. Speech is characterized by consistent nasal emission and compensatory productions. The child is very afraid of doctors and cries every time he comes to the hospital. Discuss the interdisciplinary management of this child. Which professionals should be involved in treatment, and how can one type of treatment affect the other treatments?

6. What are potential problems that healthcare providers might experience when providing care through an interdisciplinary team?

7. What could you do to be an effective team member?

REFERENCES

American Cleft Palate–Craniofacial Association (ACPA). (2009). *Parameters for evaluation and treatment of patients with cleft lip/palate or other craniofacial anomalies.* Retrieved from http://acpa-cpf.org/team-care/standardscat/parameters-of-care/

American Cleft Palate–Craniofacial Association (ACPA). (2010). Standards of team care for cleft palate and craniofacial teams. Revised April 13, 2016. Retrieved from http://www.acpa-cpf.org/team_care/standards/

Ascha, M., McDaniel, J., Link, I., Rowe, D., Soltanian, H., Sattar, A., . . . Lakin, G. (2016). Social and support services offered by cleft and craniofacial teams: A national survey and institutional experience. *Journal of Craniofacial Surgery, 27*(2), 356–360.

Austin, A. A., Druschel, C. M., Tyler, M. C., Romitti, P. A., West, I. I., Damiano, P. C., . . . Burnett, W. (2010). Interdisciplinary craniofacial teams compared with individual providers: Is orofacial cleft care more comprehensive and do parents perceive better outcomes? *The Cleft Palate-Craniofacial Journal, 47*(1), 1–8.

Butler, D. P., Samman, N., & Gollogly, G. (2011). A multidisciplinary cleft palate team in the developing world: Performance and challenges. *Journal of Plastic, Reconstructive & Aesthetic Surgery, 64*(11), 1540–1541.

Capone, R. B., & Sykes, J. M. (2007). The cleft and craniofacial team: The whole is greater than the sum of its parts. *Facial Plastic Surgery, 23*(2), 83–86.

Cohn, E. R. (1991). Commentary on team acceptance of recommendations by Dixon-Wood et al. *The Cleft Palate-Craniofacial Journal, 28*(3), 290–292.

David, D. J., Anderson, P. J., Schnitt, D. E., Nugent, M. A., & Sells, R. (2006). From birth to maturity: A group of patients who have completed their protocol management. Part II. Isolated cleft palate. *Plastic and Reconstructive Surgery, 117*(2), 515–526.

Glade, R. S., & Deal, R. (2016). Diagnosis and management of velopharyngeal dysfunction. *Oral and Maxillofacial Surgery Clinics of North America, 28*(2), 181–188.

Jeffery, S. L., & Boorman, J. G. (2001). Patient satisfaction with cleft lip and palate services in a regional centre. *British Journal of Plastic Surgery, 54*(3), 189–191.

Johansson, B., & Ringsberg, K. C. (2004). Parents' experiences of having a child with cleft lip and palate. *Journal of Advanced Nursing, 47*(2), 165–173.

Kasten, E. F., Schmidt, S. P., Zickler, C. F., Berner, E., Damian, L. A. K., Christian, G. M., . . . Hicks, T. L. (2008). Team care of the patient with cleft lip and palate. *Current Problems in Pediatric Adolescent Health Care, 38*(5), 139–158.

Krogman, W. M. (1979). The cleft palate team in action. In H. K. Cooper, R. L. Harding, W. M. Krogman, M. Mazaheri, & R. T. Millard (Eds.), *Cleft palate and cleft lip: A team approach to clinical management and rehabilitation of the patient* (pp. 144–161). Philadelphia, PA: W. B. Saunders.

Louw, B., Shibambu, M., & Roemer, K. (2006). Facilitating cleft palate team participation of culturally diverse families in South Africa. *The Cleft Palate–Craniofacial Journal, 43*(1), 47–54.

Moller, K. T. (2001). Interdisciplinary care for persons with cleft lip and palate in the year 2001. *Northwestern Dental Research, 80*(1), 29–36, 51.

Naran, S., Ford, M., & Losee, J. E. (2017). What's new in cleft palate and velopharyngeal dysfunction management? *Plastic and Reconstructive Surgery, 139*(6), 1343e–1355e.

Noar, J. H. (1992). A questionnaire survey of attitudes and concerns of three professional groups involved in the cleft palate team. *The Cleft Palate–Craniofacial Journal, 29*(1), 92–95.

Pannbacker, M., & Scheuerle, J. (1993). Parents' attitudes toward family involvement in cleft palate treatment. *The Cleft Palate–Craniofacial Journal, 30*(1), 87–89.

Paynter, E. T., Edmonson, T. W., & Jordan, W. J. (1991). Accuracy of information reported by parents and children evaluated by a cleft palate team. *The Cleft Palate–Craniofacial Journal, 28*(4), 329–337.

Paynter, E. T., Jordan, W. J., & Finch, D. L. (1990). Patient compliance with cleft palate team regimens. *Journal of Speech and Hearing Disorders, 55*(4), 740–750.

Paynter, E. T., Wilson, B. M., & Jordan, W. J. (1993). Improved patient compliance with cleft palate team regimes. *The Cleft Palate–Craniofacial Journal, 30*(3), 292–301.

Schnitt, D. E., Agir, H., & David, D. J. (2004). From birth to maturity: A group of patients who have completed their protocol management. Part I. Unilateral cleft lip and palate. *Plastic and Reconstructive Surgery, 113*(3), 805–817.

Sharp, H. M. (1995). Ethical decision-making in interdisciplinary team care. *The Cleft Palate–Craniofacial Journal, 32*(6), 495–499.

Sidman, J. D. (1995). The team approach to cleft and craniofacial disorders: The down side. *The Cleft Palate–Craniofacial Journal, 32*(5), 362.

Stal, S., Chebret, L., & McElroy, C. (1998). The team approach in the management of congenital and acquired deformities. *Clinics in Plastic Surgery, 25*(4), 485–491, vii.

Strauss, R. P. (1998). Cleft palate and craniofacial teams in the United States and Canada: A national survey of team organization and standards of care. The American Cleft Palate–Craniofacial Association (ACPA) Team Standards Committee. *The Cleft Palate–Craniofacial Journal, 35*(6), 473–480.

Strauss, R. P. (1999). The organization and delivery of craniofacial health services: The state of the art. *The Cleft Palate–Craniofacial Journal, 36*(3), 189–195.

Strauss, R. P., & Broder, H. (1985). Interdisciplinary team care of cleft lip and palate: Social and psychological aspects. *Clinics in Plastic Surgery, 12*(4), 543–551.

Strohecker, B. (1993). A team approach in the treatment of craniofacial deformities. *Plastic Surgery Nursing, 13*(1), 9–16.

Surgeon General's Report. (1987, June). *Children with special needs.* Washington, DC: Office of Maternal and Child Health, U.S. Department of Health and Human Services, Public Health Service.

Thomas, P. C. (2000). Multidisciplinary care of the child born with cleft lip and palate. *ORL-Head & Neck Nursing, 18*(4), 6–16.

Vanz, A. P., & Ribeiro, N. R. (2011). Listening to the mothers of individuals with oral fissures. *Revista da Escola de Enfermagem da USP, 45*(3), 596–602.

Vargervik, K., Oberoi, S., & Hoffman, W. Y. (2009). Team care for the patient with cleft: UCSF protocols and outcomes. *Journal of Craniofacial Surgery, 20* (Suppl. 2), 1668–1671.

Walesky-Rainbow, P. A., & Morris, H. L. (1978). An assessment of informative-counseling procedures for cleft palate children. *Cleft Palate Journal, 15*(1), 20–29.

Wellens, W., & Vander Poorten, V. (2006). Keys to a successful cleft lip and palate team. *Belgian ENT, Head and Neck Surgery, 2*(Suppl. 4), 3–10.

Will, L. A., & Parsons, R. W. (1991). Characteristics of new patients at Illinois cleft palate teams. *The Cleft Palate–Craniofacial Journal, 28*(4), 378–383; discussion 383–384.

CREDITS

CHAPTER 21

Cleft Care in Developing Countries

CHAPTER OUTLINE

INTRODUCTION

Cleft lip and palate (CLP) is one of the most common birth defects. It is estimated that every 3 minutes, a child is born into the world with a cleft (Operation Smile, n.d.). There are well over a quarter of a million babies born each year with cleft lip and palate. In fact, many babies will be born with a cleft during the time that it takes to read this chapter.

In developed nations, such as the United States, children born with cleft lip and/or palate typically receive surgical treatment at an early age. In fact, the visible defect (the cleft lip) is usually repaired at around 3 months of age, and the palate, around 10 months of age. In developing countries, however, individuals born with clefts often do not receive corrective surgery for a variety of reasons. As a result, they are forced to live their entire lives with the visible stigma of cleft lip and the functional problems that go along with cleft.

The purpose of this chapter is to provide information on current issues with cleft care in developing countries and how some international organizations are attempting to meet the needs of the world's population of individuals with cleft lip and palate. In addition, this chapter provides information for clinicians who are interested in helping this cause.

Clefts in Developing Countries

The prevalence of clefts varies with geography, ethnicity, and socioeconomic status (Mossey et al., 2011). Although clefts occur in all countries and all races, they occur most frequently in people of indigenous American Indian descent and second most frequently in those of Asian descent. Therefore, countries with these populations have the largest number of affected individuals. In addition, clefting is multifactorial and affected by certain exogenous factors, such as malnutrition and exposure to environmental toxins. Of course, both of them are common in developing countries that have a great deal of poverty. Because of these factors, clefts are particularly prevalent in poor countries of Central America, South America, Asia, and the Middle East.

Despite the fact that clefts are common in many developing countries, there is not always a good understanding of the cause of clefts and the fact that this is a treatable condition. Unfortunately, thousands of newborn babies with clefts have been abandoned or killed because the parents believed that the child was a curse (**FIGURE 21-1**). In fact, children with clefts in Uganda are given the name "Ajok," which literally means "cursed by God" (Smile Train, n.d.). In China, with its "one-child" social policy, children with clefts, particularly those who are girls, are commonly abandoned or put up for adoption soon after they are born.

Parents bury baby with cleft lip

DC CORRESPONDENT

ANANTAPUR

July 30: In a shocking incident, a couple buried alive their baby girl who was born with a cleft lip at Kamakkapalli in Kalyana-durgam mandal on Saturday. However, shepherds found the baby and rescued her. The child was later returned to her parents.

Lalita had delivered the baby at RDT hospital on Friday and she was discharged from the hospital on Saturday. Lalitha and her husband Shekhar felt that they would not be able to afford the cleft lip surgery for the baby. So they dug a pit and buried the baby, all the way up to her trunk. The kid was found by shepherds and was taken to the hospital. The parents were later summoned and were counselled. The baby was returned to them.

FIGURE 21-1 Article in the *Deccan Chronicle*, the largest circulated English daily in South India, Sunday, July 30, 2011.

There are millions of children and adults around the world who are currently living with an unrepaired cleft because of a variety of reasons. There is often limited access to specialized health care, particularly in remote areas. There may be a lack of hospitals that provide cleft care, a lack of trained surgeons, or even inadequate funding for equipment and technology. In many cases, the parents, who have had no formal education, may not know that clefts can be surgically repaired (Aziz, Rhee, & Redai, 2009; Gupta, Bansal, Dev, & Tyagi, 2010). It is not uncommon for a cleft palate to be left unrepaired because the parents do not understand how it affects speech and communication. Even when parents want surgical correction for their child, many families in developing countries do not have the financial resources to pay for the surgery or even transportation to go to a hospital where there is free care. Because of these problems and the fact that a cleft is not a fatal condition, many individuals in developing nations go through life with unrepaired clefts (Bermudez, 2004).

Individuals with unrepaired clefts experience all of the aesthetic and functional problems that go with this condition. Many are ostracized from society because of various superstitions, the social stigma of a cleft lip, and the speech and feeding problems with a cleft palate. In many countries, affected children are not allowed to attend school. Even if they are allowed to attend, families often do not send them to school because of the social stigma. As a result, affected individuals in developing countries are often uneducated and unemployable. In addition, because cleft lip and palate affects facial appearance and speech, these individuals suffer difficulties with social interaction and communication with others. Overall, people with unrepaired clefts often lead lives filled with isolation, shame, and heartache (Smile Train, n.d.).

International Cleft Care

To address the needs of children who are born with clefts or craniofacial conditions from around the world, several not-for-profit organizations have been formed in the United States and in other countries. Some are very large organizations (e.g., Operation Smile, ReSurge International [formerly Interplast], Rotaplast International, and Smile Train), whereas others are relatively small and go to only a few places a year (e.g., Transforming Faces, Operation of Hope/Operacion Esperanza). International care is also provided by groups of surgeons and nurses who go to the same place each year for a few weeks to donate their time. With the help of these international organizations, volunteers, and donors, millions of children born with cleft lip and/or palate in developing countries have received free cleft care.

Most organizations and international teams have two main goals in providing international care. One goal is to provide direct service for affected individuals. However, 100 surgeries will help only 100 patients (and their families). Therefore, most of these organizations recognize that to have a lasting effect, it is important to build local capacity by training and supporting in-country professionals to provide the same services. By teaching local surgeons cleft lip and palate repair techniques and empowering those who are already trained, surgeons can treat patients in their own country and train others to do the same (Hubli & Noordhoff, 2013). With this type of support, it is hoped that the need for ongoing international help will gradually be diminished and ultimately eliminated (Abenavoli, 2005; Persing, Patel, Clune, Steinbacher, & Persing, 2015; Ruiz-Razura, Cronin, & Navarro, 2000; Shrime, Sleemi, & Ravilla, 2015).

Smile Train is the largest international organization dedicated to cleft lip and palate, and it was founded in 1999 with this exact purpose of empowering in-country professionals. Smile Train's sustainable model provides training, funding, and resources to empower local professionals across 85-plus developing countries to provide 100% free cleft repair surgery and comprehensive cleft care in their own communities (Smile Train, n.d.).

As part of its training focus, Smile Train funded Virtual Surgery Videos, which was the first surgical educational tool to use virtual technology and advanced three-dimensional animation software. (Now available as a free online simulator at smiletrain.biodigital.com/#/.) To raise awareness about the plight of children with clefts in the developing world, Smile Train also funded the documentary titled *Smile Pinki*, featuring a girl from rural India whose life was dramatically changed when she received free surgery to repair her cleft lip. This documentary won an Academy Award® in 2008. It is also available for free as part of a compilation DVD on Smile Train's website.

Another large international organization is Operation Smile. Operation Smile assembles national and international teams of volunteer doctors and other professionals and then sends these teams and surgical equipment to various countries around the world. Operation Smile also donates medical equipment and provides year-round medical treatment through 13 Comprehensive Care Centers around the world. Finally, Operation Smile trains doctors and local medical professionals in its partner countries so they are empowered to treat their own local communities.

The Role of the Speech-Language Pathologist on a Mission Trip

There is a great need for speech-language pathology services in developing countries. One reason is that many countries have inexperienced, few, or no speech-language pathologists. In addition, families often do not have transportation or the financial means to access services even when they are available in their country. And finally, there is tremendous stigma around cleft lip and palate in addition to lack of community education, making it very difficult for families to recognize and prioritize speech care. Despite this great need, there

are significant challenges to providing meaningful services internationally through a cleft palate mission trip.

On a Surgical Mission Trip

The role of the speech-language pathologist on a surgical mission trip is to screen patients to determine those who have the best chance of success with a palate repair particularly because there is usually not enough time in the surgery schedule for every patient. The speech-language pathologist also works with the dentist/prosthodontist on fitting speech devices and counsels families on speech stimulation before the surgery or while the child is in surgery. Perhaps the most important role of the speech-language pathologist, however, is to train other professionals in speech therapy techniques to provide some intervention after the surgery.

It would seem that the speech-language pathologist would be a key member of a cleft palate mission team especially because the primary reason to repair a cleft palate is for speech. In fact, the role of the speech-language pathologist on most surgical missions is rather limited. One reason is that a speech evaluation is not needed to determine that an unrepaired cleft lip or palate needs to be repaired. In addition, secondary surgery for velopharyngeal insufficiency is rarely done on these trips because the focus is usually on the large number of children with unrepaired clefts. Also, secondary surgery includes risks of airway obstruction and obstructive sleep apnea that require postoperative follow-up. This is usually not available after a surgical mission. Finally, although speech therapy is usually needed following a palate repair, it cannot be done during the time of the surgical mission trip.

Providing Speech Therapy

The cleft mission concept works well for patients who require a lip repair because the surgery is done primarily for aesthetic reasons and requires little follow-up. For patients undergoing cleft palate repair however, postoperative speech therapy is usually needed for the best outcomes. This is particularly true if the child has developed compensatory articulation productions because these will not change with palate repair only. Unfortunately, under the mission model, very few children in developing countries have the opportunity to receive speech therapy following a palate repair (Kuehn & Henne, 2003). The local empowerment model is best suited for providing speech therapy services.

In an effort to resolve the lack of access to speech therapy services, some innovative models of service delivery have been developed. For example, Smile Train provides cash grants to local cleft teams that demonstrate they have a local therapist or paraprofessional able to provide effective cleft palate therapy. These grants help local teams overcome barriers to therapy supplies, therapy space, professional time, and patient travel. Pre- and post-therapy results (with videos) are recorded in Smile Train's online medical database so that the therapies are monitored and providers can be targeted for training.

Another model is based on intensive speech camps to train parents and caregivers on speech sound production and stimulation. For example, RSF-EARTHSPEAK provides weeklong training sessions for parents or caregivers. Speech sounds that are specific to the native language are presented in a developmental sequence. The child learns to imitate the production of early sounds in babbling sequences and then to produce later sounds in more complex phonemic combinations. Unfortunately, there is no way to determine those who cannot produce the sounds because of velopharyngeal insufficiency. Also, there is no published research to date to validate the outcomes of this approach. Other groups, such as ReSurge and Smile Train, provide support to local cleft teams as they use the speech camp model with their own play and group therapy practices.

There are other ways of providing speech services. One way uses local community workers who are trained to provide the basics of speech stimulation and speech sound correction (Prathanee, Dechongkit, & Manochiopinig, 2006). In addition, there is a growing, although limited, presence of speech-language pathologists in the developing world, particularly at community centers (Noordhoff, 2009). The number of trained speech-language pathologists may increase if opportunities are provided for online education and training. Some speech-language pathology programs within the United States, such as Teachers College Columbia University, have created cleft palate resources and made them available online for global use (English, www.leadersproject.org /english-cleft-palate-directory/, and Spanish, www .leadersproject.org/directorio-espanol-paladar-hendido/). Perhaps the approach that has the most potential for providing speech therapy services to underserved populations is the use of telehealth (Furr et al., 2011; Glazer et al., 2011; Whitehead et al., 2012). This model is growing significantly in the developing world, as it is in the United States. In addition to telehealth services, technology applications are also being developed to support speech and language practice at home. These services do not replace the need for speech-language pathologists but rather use songs, stories, and games to encourage children to practice their speech. For example, Smile Train worked with global cleft experts to launch a free cleft palate speech app called "Speech Games and Practice."

Providing Education and Training

The need for education is not limited to the surgical team members. Many countries do not have speech-language pathologists. However, they may have psychologists, healthcare professionals, or parent leaders who are interested in learning what they can to help children with speech disorders. Even when there are local speech-language pathologists (or similar professionals), these individuals may not be well trained in cleft management. Therefore, the most important role for the speech-language pathologist in international care is to provide education and training for other professionals regarding the evaluation and treatment of patients with clefts and velopharyngeal insufficiency. Individual and group training, seminars, lectures, handouts, and books are greatly appreciated by the local professionals.

To provide training, the speech-language pathologist must be very knowledgeable about the management of this population (Hartley & Wirz, 2002). Even with several years of clinical experience, most speech-language pathologists are at a loss when it comes to working with children with clefts unless they have had specific experience in this area. Therefore, those who are interested in working internationally should seek additional specialty training in pediatrics, cleft palate, velopharyngeal insufficiency, and resonance disorders (D'Antonio & Landis, 1994; Ducote, 1998; Ducote, 2005; Ducote & Juul, 1998; Noordhoff, 2009). The document *Parameters for Evaluation and Treatment of Patients with Cleft Lip/Palate or Other Craniofacial Anomalies*, published by the American Cleft Palate–Craniofacial Association (ACPA, 2009), should be reviewed for a basic understanding of the sequence and standards of care for individuals affected by a cleft. In addition, the speech-language pathologist should listen to and study the videos of patients with hypernasality and/or nasal emission that are associated with this book and speech samples that are on the American Cleft Palate–Craniofacial Association website (ACPA, n.d.b).

Although didactic learning is important, clinical knowledge and experience with the cleft population is also important when teaching others. Clinical experience is particularly important when a person is called upon to make decisions regarding candidates for secondary management of velopharyngeal insufficiency if that is done on cleft missions.

A sustainable way to approach education and training is to research what degree programs, if any, are already available. Often, these programs welcome visiting lecturers and may even consider adding new content to their curriculums based on how well the material is received. If cleft palate education and training materials are incorporated into these existing degree programs, more local speech-language pathologists will be available and prepared to offer ongoing care to the large population of cleft palate patients in need.

Cleft Lip/Palate Surgical Missions

As noted previously, many organizations send teams of medical professionals to countries with less-developed health care. Over a period of weeks, these teams provide services to individuals with cleft lip and palate who cannot otherwise obtain or afford the surgery.

In 1997, an International Task Force on Volunteer Cleft Missions outlined recommendations for volunteer cleft missions based on (1) mission objectives, (2) organization, (3) personal health and liability, (4) funding, (5) use of trainees in volunteer cleft missions, and (6) public relations. They agreed that the main goals for these missions are "to provide top-quality surgical service, train local doctors and staff, develop and nurture fledgling cleft programs, and finally, make new friends" (Yeow et al., 2002). More recently, the American Cleft Palate–Craniofacial Association (ACPA, n.d.a) published standards on its website for international care. These standards are "aimed towards assuring that international exchanges or mission-based cleft lip, cleft palate, and craniofacial care are delivered in a safe and high-quality manner."

Typical Team Members

A small team may consist of a few surgeons, nurses, and anesthesiologists. It may also include some professionals from the local hospital in the surgeries. Other organizations (e.g., Operation Smile) send a large group of people to the country so that there is no need for local professionals. Professional team members usually include the following:

- Anesthesiologists and/or nurse anesthetists
- Child life specialist
- Dentist and/or orthodontist and/or prosthodontist
- Intensivist and/or pediatrician
- Medical students and/or residents
- Nurses—surgical, post-anesthesia care, postoperative
- Speech-language pathologist

In addition to the clinical professionals, many people are often included to provide coordination and support, including the following:

- Biomedical technician
- Education coordinator
- Interpreters
- Medical records workers
- Team coordinator
- Volunteers

In many cases, team members do not know each other before the mission and hence have not developed over time the trust and respect that come from working on a well-established team. However, all are committed to one purpose, and that is helping as many patients as possible. This is done by working very long days under less than ideal conditions. This shared dedication and experience actually help the team to bond and work well together in a very short period of time (Fagan & Jacobs, 2009).

Typical Schedules

Surgical missions are at least a week in length, but most are 10 days or longer. During the first few days, patients are evaluated to determine which ones are candidates for surgery, dental treatment, or prosthetic devices. During this time, the nurses set up the operating and recovery rooms.

Once the screening of patients is complete and the operating rooms are ready, the rest of the days are devoted to direct treatment, including surgeries and dental or prosthodontic treatment. Some of the nurses and physicians usually stay a few extra days after others have left to provide postoperative care for the last surgical patients.

Because of the sheer volume of patients who are usually present for surgery, the majority of the surgeries tend to be primary lip and palate repairs. Therefore, if the palate is not sufficient after the primary surgery and the patient exhibits velopharyngeal insufficiency, most of these patients are not offered surgery again because of a lack of adequate resources. One mission group that was performing surgeries in the Philippines was concerned about the high rate of velopharyngeal insufficiency with their palate repairs and the difficulty of doing secondary surgery. Therefore, they began doing a simultaneous sphincter pharyngoplasty with the palate repair. They reported better speech outcomes as a result of this practice (Saboye, Chancholle, Tournier, & Maurette, 2004).

Speech Screening Procedures

On most mission trips, there are hundreds of patients who need to be evaluated for possible surgery, including older children and even some adults (**FIGURE 21-2**). These patients and their families often travel long distances to be seen and are willing to wait for hours, and even days, in hopes of receiving treatment. Parents wait in long lines for their child to be evaluated and for a determination as to whether their child will be included in the surgery schedule (**FIGURE 21-3**).

Because of the volume of patients who need to be seen, the screening has to be very quick and efficient. It is common to have to screen 100 or

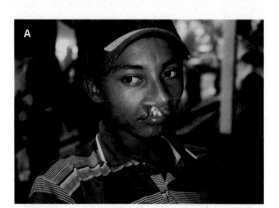

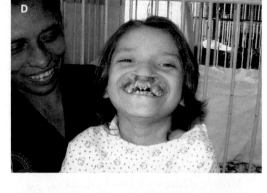

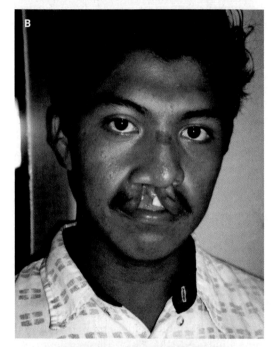

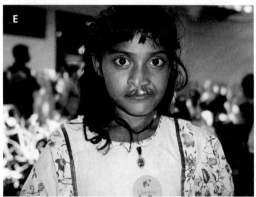

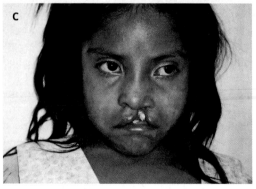

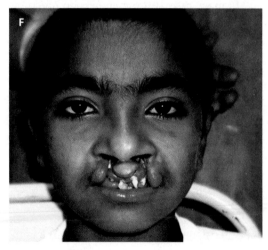

FIGURE 21-2 Examples of older patients with unrepaired clefts.

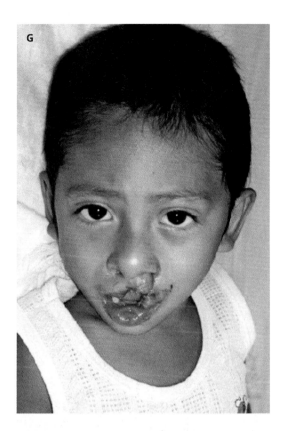

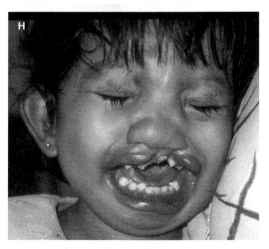

FIGURE 21-2 (CONTINUED) Examples of older patients with unrepaired clefts.

more patients in one day. Assuming a 10-hour day, this leaves 6 minutes per patient if there are no breaks for lunch or the restroom. Realistically, there may be no more than 3 to 5 minutes to do a speech assessment on each patient. This is particularly challenging if the speech-language pathologist is not fluent in the language and has to work through an interpreter.

To make the process as quick and efficient as possible, following are some suggestions:

- Before the patient comes to you, have an interpreter fill in identifying information and the answers to a few questions on a screening form.
- Have a volunteer manage the line and keep patients coming quickly, with their screening forms in hand.
- Do an intraoral examination first. With an open cleft palate or a large fistula, you do not need to assess speech because you know that the individual needs a palate or fistula repair.
- Ask the patient to count to 20 in his language. Have the patient repeat syllables with high-pressure phonemes repetitively (i.e., /pɑ, pɑ, pɑ/, /pi, pi, pi/, /sɑ, sɑ, sɑ/, /si, si, si/, etc.).
- Evaluate for the presence of hypernasality and/or nasal emission.
- Complete the screening form, and add comments as needed.
- Include recommendations for the following: surgery and type, prosthetic device and type, speech therapy, and parent counseling regarding speech-language stimulation techniques.
- For babies with open palates who are not yet candidates for a palate repair, give a handout with feeding instructions and suggestions for modifying the nipples. Have an interpreter review the instructions. Make sure the interpreter tells the parent to use boiled or bottled water for cleaning and for dry formula.

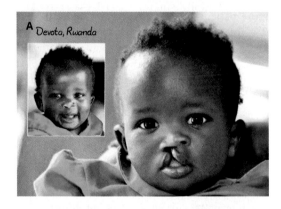

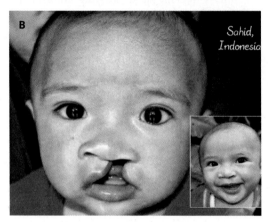

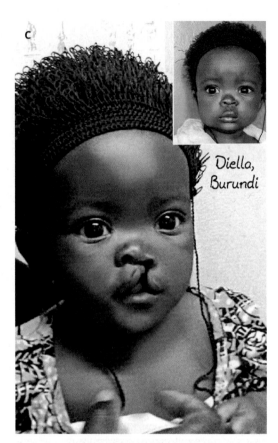

FIGURE 21-3 Before and after pictures of patients who had lip repairs done by Smile Train.

Speech Procedures during Surgery Days

Because therapy is not a quick fix and kids who are undergoing surgery cannot participate in therapy, speech therapy is not a focus during a surgical mission. Instead, the speech-language pathologist should work with a dentist, orthodontist, or prosthodontist to (1) determine those patients who are candidates for prosthetic devices, (2) make sure that the devices fit appropriately to maximize speech, and (3) help the patient learn to use the device.

Counseling families is another task to be done during surgery week (**FIGURE 21-4**). The families may have various beliefs regarding the cause of

the cleft, including God's will, past sins, becoming pregnant during a full moon, or having hiccups during pregnancy (Weatherley-White, Eiserman, Beddoe, & Vanderberg, 2005). Therefore, counseling regarding the cause and the importance of good nutrition during pregnancy can be of benefit to the families. The speech-language pathologist should also counsel parents regarding methods of speech and language stimulation for children under the age of 3 and methods of speech correction for children over the age of 3 who are undergoing palate repair. Handouts written in the parents' language are particularly helpful. Even if the parents are illiterate, they can usually find someone in their town to read for

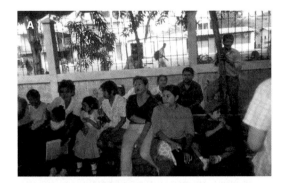

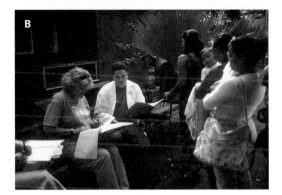

FIGURE 21-4 Patients and families waiting for screening.

them. A suggested procedure for group counseling is as follows:

- Set up a space near the surgical waiting area.
- Obtain the surgery schedule for the day.
- Talk with parents in groups of five to seven while their children are in surgery.
- Try to use the same interpreter. After doing the interpretation many times, some interpreters can then do the counseling on their own.
- The day after surgery, meet patients and their parents as a group. Repeat counseling, but direct it toward the older children. Demonstrate normal airflow and simple therapy correction techniques, using a straw for auditory feedback.

Surgery days are an appropriate time to do lectures and in-service training for local professionals. It can even be valuable to visit local schools for consultations or have an open speech clinic for children in the area with any type of speech disorders.

If there is any downtime between working on speech appliances, counseling families, and teaching, it is expected that the speech-language pathologist and all other team members will assist with other aspects of the team's work as needed (Ducote, 2005) (**FIGURE 21-5** and **FIGURE 21-6**).

Expected Costs

As a volunteer on surgical missions, the team member is usually expected to cover some of the costs of travel. This may be done by paying a set amount up front or paying directly for a portion

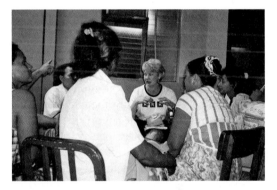

FIGURE 21-5 Counseling families in groups.

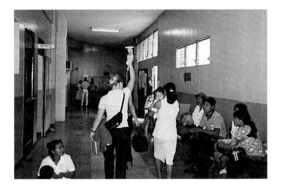

FIGURE 21-6 Helping out with other duties when necessary. In this case, the child needed someone to hold the IV bag while he walked to surgery because poles and gurneys were unavailable in the hospital.

of airfare, hotel, and food. Typically, several meals are provided by the mission organization or host country, particularly breakfast and lunch during screening and surgery days.

In addition to direct costs of travel, lodging, and food, there is also the cost of time away from work for the volunteer team members. Most employers require their employees to take vacation days for their time away for mission trips.

Concerns and Criticisms of Surgical Missions

Although most organizations subscribe to the goals of quality care and education, some achieve these goals better than others. There have been criticisms about the way some of the organizations operate (Silver, 2000). These criticisms include those listed here:

- More focus on direct care and less focus on training local professionals
- Not using qualified local surgeons, which would be far less costly than sending surgeons from outside the country
- Using volunteer professionals who are not considered experts in cleft care in the United States (e.g., using cosmetic surgeons who do not do cleft palate repairs in their practice)
- Using missions as a training ground for residents who need more surgical experience
- Doing too many surgeries to keep the numbers high
- Performing cosmetic surgery during the mission to increase the numbers
- Performing surgery on children who would not be considered healthy enough to qualify for surgery in the United States
- Not having records available for returning patients
- Not providing adequate follow-up after the team leaves
- Not providing enough training for in-country professionals
- Having a high rate of fistulas or velopharyngeal insufficiency after palate repair

- Spending too much money on administration and overhead and not enough money on direct patient care

One major issue is that about 20% to 30% of patients who undergo palate repair in the United States have velopharyngeal insufficiency following the surgery. For several reasons, this rate may actually be much higher on mission trips. Unfortunately, there is rarely a mechanism for postoperative speech evaluations or opportunities for secondary surgery for velopharyngeal insufficiency for these patients (Aziz et al., 2009).

Another concern is that there are no studies of outcomes from these missions, so the actual success rates and complication rates are unknown. Because of this, there is an urgent need for more randomized clinical trials to evaluate both the outcomes of treatment and the complications so that clinical guidelines and protocols can be developed based on strong evidence.

Because some organizations are better than others, prospective team members and donors should learn as much as possible about the organization and consider the following factors:

- Reputation of the organization
- Financial support of the organization
- Quality of procedures, policies, and structure
- Qualifications of the team members
- Experience of those who have been on other mission trips
- Method and priority systems for choosing cases
- Number of procedures typically done per surgeon
- Types of procedures done on a mission (e.g., cosmetic vs. reconstructive)
- Method of record keeping
- Method for follow-up
- Focus on teaching and training of in-country professionals for sustainability

Working with an Interpreter

If the speech-language pathologist is not fluent in the country's language, a good interpreter is

TABLE 21-1 Tips for Working with an Interpreter

- Address remarks and questions directly to the listener, not to the interpreter.
- Use simple terms and short sentences.
- Avoid technical language, idioms, expressions, and slang.
- Pause frequently so the interpreter can keep up.
- Use a positive tone and facial expression.
- Avoid body language or facial expressions that may be offensive or misconstrued.
- Periodically, check the listener's understanding. Encourage her to request clarification when something is not understood.
- Reinforce understanding with visual diagrams and information written in the listener's language.

essential when providing care on a surgical mission trip or providing direct education for local professionals. The speech-language pathologist should meet with the interpreter as soon as possible after arriving at the mission site. Spending time with the interpreter before seeing patients will help the process go more smoothly and save a great deal of time during screenings. Ideally, the interpreters should be given some written scripts of what should be asked or said during the evaluation and later during the family counseling (Ducote, 1998; Ducote, 2005; Ducote & Juul, 1998). It is important to make sure that the interpreter understands the information and the procedure that you want to follow. During the session with the family, the interpreter should convey the information in the first person as if talking directly to the person. For specific tips in working with an interpreter, see TABLE 21-1.

In addition to reviewing what the interpreters will say, it is good to learn some words and phrases from the interpreters. Knowing how to introduce yourself can enhance your interaction with the families. It helps to know the name of your profession in that country's language and to learn some basic words or sentences to use in the assessment (e.g., "How are you?" "Please sit down," "Open your mouth." "Stick out your tongue." "Say /æ/ and stick out your tongue." "Count from 1 to 20").

Interpreters are also very helpful when providing lectures or other forms of education to the local professionals. Although English is the language of medicine and thus many physicians and other healthcare providers at least understand English, certain considerations must be made when training professionals whose primary language is not English (or the language that you speak).

When giving lectures or seminars to local professionals, it is important to give the lecture slowly, pausing frequently for the interpreter. In addition, the interpreter should translate your slides and handouts for the participants before the lecture.

Preparing for International Travel

International travel requires some planning, particularly when it is to a developing country with a different language and culture. It is worth the time to learn about the country and culture before the trip. It is also important to obtain necessary vaccinations and health information. Finally, careful consideration of what to pack can make a big difference in the traveler's comfort during the trip.

Learn about the Culture and Language

Before traveling internationally whether to teach in-country professionals or to provide direct care, it is important to learn about the culture and language of the host country. As ambassadors of goodwill and humanitarian aid, professionals should make every effort to understand and respect the country's social customs and protocols (Yeow et al., 2002). It is important to know the behaviors that are considered polite and those that are considered impolite. The role of women in certain societies is important to consider when working with the families. Even if you do not speak the language, it is important to learn how to say "thank you," to memorize certain greetings and phrases, and to know the standard form of addressing children and adults (e.g., señor, señora, etc.).

On a practical note, it may be helpful to learn about the food in the host country, especially if the traveler has allergies or strong aversions to certain types of food. Knowledge about the currency and whether bargaining is expected is helpful when shopping. Tipping customs and standards are also important to know.

Basic knowledge of the language and culture can help the traveler to be more effective as an educator and/or service provider and a good representative of her home country. It can also make the trip more interesting and enjoyable.

Documents That You Need

Of course, all individuals must have a passport to travel to a foreign country. It is important to note that many countries will not accept a passport that is due to expire in 3 months or less. Some countries also require a visa. This should be determined months before the trip because it can take several months to obtain a visa. It is advisable to keep a copy of the main page of your passport and a copy of your visa in your suitcase. It is also wise to take a copy of your immunization records, written information regarding allergies or special medical issues, and the name and phone number of a contact person in case of emergency. In addition to the copies of travel documents in your suitcase, it is smart to make another set of copies to keep at home.

Protect Your Health

Different parts of the world have different health risks for the traveler. The website for the Centers for Disease Control and Prevention (CDC, 2017) provides specific information by geographic region on risks for diseases, insect bites, and food and water contamination. Recommendations for prevention and treatment are also given.

In general, the traveler should determine which vaccinations are recommended for that region of the world and receive them several weeks before the trip. Yellow fever and typhoid vaccinations are commonly recommended. Often, the vaccinations are available only through a local health department. If the travel will be in a tropical area, most authorities recommend taking malaria pills before going and using an insect repellent, particularly one containing DEET (N,N-diethyl-meta-toluamide), while there. DEET is especially important for protection against tick bites and mosquito bites, both of which can transmit disease. Clothing to cover arms and legs is also suggested.

Water is often a risk in developing countries. If this is the case, it is best to avoid drinks with ice as well as salads or raw vegetables because they are rinsed in water. Your toothbrush should be rinsed with bottled water rather than tap water. It is also wise to avoid swallowing water in the shower.

What to Pack

When packing for international travel, it is good to consider both comfort and culture. Because the days may be very long and require a lot of walking or standing, comfortable shoes are a must. Many people retain water when traveling; therefore, loose shoes and clothing are preferable.

When selecting clothing, it helps to consider the climate and the probable lack of air conditioning or adequate heating. The cultural norms of dress should also be considered. For example, in Nicaragua, women do not wear shorts. Therefore, loose-fitting, comfortable, washable, and preferably inexpensive clothes (skirts and dresses for women) should be worn.

For many countries, toilet paper is a luxury and not usually provided in public restrooms. Therefore, small packs of tissues should be taken because they fit well in a fanny pack or pocket.

On surgical mission trips, the clinicians usually need to take everything that will be needed to work with the patients (including pens and paper). A suggested list of items to take for clinical use is found in **TABLE 21-2**. A small rolling suitcase can be useful as a portable storage unit for clinical supplies. It is best to take your "supply cabinet" back to the hotel at night because things that are left unattended often disappear.

TABLE 21-2 **Items to Take for Clinical Use**
• Tongue blades
• Dental mirror
• Pen lights and batteries
• Alcohol preps or cloths
• Hand sanitizer
• Box of gloves
• Tissues
• Plastic tubing—precut
• Bending straws
• Cleft palate bottles and nipples
• Therapy tokens
• Rewards (sticker sheets, safety pops, etc.)
• Handouts and diagrams of the velopharyngeal anatomy (in the appropriate language)
• Lavaliere for pen and pen light
• Office supplies: pens, legal pad, paper clips, stapler, etc.
• Scrubs (for observing in surgery)
• Giveaway for parents (pens, hotel-sized toiletries, note cards, etc.)
• Camera
• Fanny pack
• Tote bag
• Small suitcase on rollers

SUMMARY

There are many organizations that send mission teams to do cleft repair in developing countries. Most organizations realize that educating in-country professionals is the best way to make a long-term change, and some organizations are even dedicated to the local empowerment model.

Speech-language pathologists can serve on mission teams by providing input on which patients are best candidates for surgery. In addition, they can counsel families during the mission. Speech therapy is not realistic on these trips given the limited time available. However, the speech-language pathologist can provide training for in-country professionals who can also train others. It is important for visiting speech-language pathologists to understand the level of experience and education such local professionals have in order to effectively offer training.

For those who have served on a surgical mission team, most will say that it is a remarkable experience that can change your life. You have the opportunity to work with a group of people who may come from all around the world. All have a strong sense of purpose, dedication, and compassion. They start out as strangers but quickly become friends.

Perhaps the biggest joy, however, is working with children and families who have so little but are so happy and grateful for what they have. By giving your time and efforts to them, you get so much more in return.

FOR REVIEW AND DISCUSSION

1. Why are there still millions of children and adults around the world who are living with an unrepaired cleft?

2. Describe some of the social and educational problems that individuals face in the underdeveloped countries.

3. What are the two primary goals of international not-for-profit organizations that are trying to address the needs of children who are born with clefts or craniofacial conditions? Which goal will have the greater effect for the future?

4. Describe the role of a speech-language pathologist on a surgical mission team. What are some of the limitations?

5. List the typical clinical and support team members who would be needed on a surgical mission trip. What is the primary role for each professional? What would be the

particular challenges for each professional on a surgical mission team?

6. Pretend you are planning to go on your first mission trip. What would you need to do to prepare? What would you take with you?

7. Describe what you would do to screen a large number of patients who speak a language that you do not know.

8. What is the role of the speech-language pathologist during surgery days? What can you do to maximize the long-term effect of your time and efforts?

9. What are the challenges of obtaining postoperative speech therapy for patients who have a palate repair through one of these surgical missions? What can be done in the future to provide needed postoperative speech pathology services?

REFERENCES

Abenavoli, F. M. (2005). Operation Smile humanitarian missions. *Plastic and Reconstructive Surgery, 115*(1), 356–357.

American Cleft Palate–Craniofacial Association (ACPA). (n.d.a). International treatment programs. Retrieved from http://acpa-cpf.org/wp-content/uploads/2017/06/International_Treatment_Programs.pdf

American Cleft Palate–Craniofacial Association (ACPA). (n.d.b). Speech samples. Retrieved from http://acpa-cpf.org/education/speech-samples/

American Cleft Palate–Craniofacial Association (ACPA). (2009). *Parameters for evaluation and treatment of patients with cleft lip/palate or other*

craniofacial anomalies. Retrieved from www.cleftline.org/wp-content/uploads/2012/03/Parameters.pdf

Aziz, S. R., Rhee, S. T., & Redai, I. (2009). Cleft surgery in rural Bangladesh: Reflections and experiences. *Journal of Oral and Maxillofacial Surgery, 67*(8), 1581–1588.

Bermudez, L. E. (2004). Humanitarian missions in the third world. *Plastic and Reconstructive Surgery, 114*(6), 1687–1689; author reply 1689.

Centers for Disease Control and Prevention (CDC). (2017). Travelers' health. Retrieved from https://wwwnc.cdc.gov/travel

D'Antonio, L. L., & Landis, P. (1994). *Speech-language pathology services for the individual with cleft lip/*

palate: A training manual for volunteers to developing nations. Chapel Hill, NC: American Cleft Palate–Craniofacial Association.

Ducote, C. A. (1998). Speech-language pathology services for individuals with cleft lip/palate in less developed nations: The Operation Smile approach. *Speech Science and Orofacial Disorders, 8*(1), 12–14.

Ducote, C. A. (2005). *Evaluation and treatment of cleft palate speech in developing countries: The Operation Smile approach.* Paper presented at the American Speech and Hearing Association Annual Convention, San Diego, CA.

Ducote, C. A., & Juul, A. M. (1998). *Guidelines for speech-language pathology volunteers on Operation Smile international missions.* New Orleans, LA: Operation Smile Speech Therapy Council.

Fagan, J. J., & Jacobs, M. (2009). Survey of ENT services in Africa: Need for a comprehensive intervention. *Global Health Action, 2.* doi:10.3402/gha.v2i0.1932

Furr, M. C., Larkin, E., Blakeley, R., Albert, T. W., Tsugawa, L., & Weber, S. M. (2011). Extending multidisciplinary management of cleft palate to the developing world. *Journal of Oral and Maxillofacial Surgery, 69*(1), 237–241.

Glazer, C. A., Bailey, P. J., Icaza, I. L., Valladares, S. J., Steere, K. A., Rosenblatt, E. S., & Byrne, P. J. (2011). Multidisciplinary care of international patients with cleft palate using telemedicine. *Archives of Facial Plastic Surgery, 13*(6), 436–438.

Gupta, K., Bansal, P., Dev, N., & Tyagi, S. K. (2010). Smile Train project: A blessing for population of lower socio-economic status. *Journal of Indian Medical Association, 108*(11), 723–725.

Hartley, S. D., & Wirz, S. L. (2002). Development of a "communication disability model" and its implication on service delivery in low-income countries. *Social Science Medicine, 54*(10), 1543–1557.

Hubli, E. H., & Noordhoff, M. S. (2013). Smile train: Changing the world one smile at a time. *Annals of Plastic Surgery, 71*(1), 4–5.

Kuehn, D. P., & Henne, L. J. (2003). Speech evaluation and treatment of patients with cleft palate. *American Journal of Speech-Language Pathology, 12,* 103–109.

Mossey, P. A., Shaw, W. C., Munger, R. G., Murray, J. C., Murthy, J., & Little, J. (2011). Global oral health inequalities: Challenges in the prevention and management of orofacial clefts and potential solutions. *Advances in Dental Research, 23*(2), 247–258.

Noordhoff, M. S. (2009). Establishing a craniofacial center in a developing country. *Journal of Craniofacial Surgery, 20*(Suppl. 2), 1655–1656.

Operation Smile. (n.d.). Retrieved from https://www.operationsmile.org/.

Persing, S., Patel, A., Clune, J. E., Steinbacher, D. M., & Persing, J. A. (2015). The repair of international clefts in the current surgical landscape. *Journal of Craniofacial Surgery, 26*(4), 1126–1128.

Prathanee, B., Dechongkit, S., & Manochiopinig, S. (2006). Development of community-based speech therapy model: For children with cleft lip/palate in northeast Thailand. *Journal of the Medical Association of Thailand, 89*(4), 500–508.

RSF-EARTHSPEAK. (n.d.). Retrieved from http://rsf-earthspeak.org

Ruiz-Razura, A., Cronin, E. D., & Navarro, C. E. (2000). Creating long-term benefits in cleft lip and palate volunteer missions. *Plastic and Reconstructive Surgery, 105*(1), 195–201.

Saboye, J., Chancholle, A. R., Tournier, J. J., & Maurette, I. (2004). Palatovelopharyngoplastie en un temps. Notre experience aux Philippines. *Annales de Chirurgie Plastique et Esthetique, 49*(3), 261–264.

Shrime, M. G., Sleemi, A., & Ravilla, T. D. (2015). Charitable platforms in global surgery: A systematic review of their effectiveness, cost-effectiveness, sustainability, and role training. *World Journal of Surgery, 39*(1), 10–20.

Silver, L. (2000). Creating long-term benefits in cleft lip and palate volunteer missions. *Plastic and Reconstructive Surgery, 106*(2), 516–517.

Smile Train. (n.d.). Beyond the smile: A story of lasting change. Retrieved from https://www.smiletrain.org/lp/beyond-the-smile-a-story-of-lasting-change

Weatherley-White, R. C., Eiserman, W., Beddoe, M., & Vanderberg, R. (2005). Perceptions, expectations, and reactions to cleft lip and palate surgery in native populations: A pilot study in rural India. *The Cleft Palate–Craniofacial Journal, 42*(5), 560–564.

Whitehead, E., Dorfman, V., Tremper, G., Kramer, A., Sigler, A., & Gosman, A. (2012). Telemedicine as a means of effective speech evaluation for patients with cleft palate. *Annals of Plastic Surgery, 68*(4), 415–417.

Yeow, V. K., Lee, S. T., Lambrecht, T. J., Barnett, J., Gorney, M., Hardjowasito, W., . . . Wilson, L. (2002). International Task Force on Volunteer Cleft Missions. *The Journal of Craniofacial Surgery, 13*(1), 18–25.

CREDITS

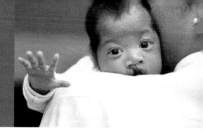
ablative surgery Surgery that involves removal of a part, such as a portion of the hard palate, due to a malignancy.

acrocentric When the centromere of a chromosome is very close to one end of the chromosome.

active speech characteristics Articulation productions that are abnormal in placement because of the individual's response to abnormal structure, such as velopharyngeal insufficiency or dental malocclusion, or abnormal neurophysiology, such as velopharyngeal incompetence; also known as *compensatory errors.*

acute otitis media Bacterial infection of the middle ear.

adenoid A mass of lymphoid tissue that is found on the posterior pharyngeal wall of the nasopharynx on the skull base; also called the *pharyngeal tonsil, adenoid pad*, or *adenoids.*

adenoid facies Facial characteristics caused by airway obstruction secondary to adenoid enlargement; characteristics include an open-mouth posture, anterior tongue position, the mandible in a forward or downward position, facial elongation, suborbital coloring and puffy eyes, and the appearance of pinched nostrils.

adenoid pad A mass of lymphoid tissue that is found on the posterior pharyngeal wall of the nasopharynx on the skull base; also called the *pharyngeal tonsil, adenoid*, or *adenoids.*

adipose Fat tissue.

affricate phonemes Pressure-sensitive consonants that require a buildup of intraoral air pressure and then slow release through a narrow opening; they are produced as a combination of a plosive and fricative and include /ʧ/ and /ʤ/.

ala nasi (pl. alae) Latin for "wing"; the outside curved part of the nostril.

alar base The area where the ala meets the upper lip.

alar rim The outside curved edge of each nostril.

allele The alternative form or variation of a given gene that is found at the same locus on a homologous chromosome.

allograft bone Bone that is obtained from a donor.

alveolar bone grafting A surgical procedure of grafting bone, often from the iliac crest (hip), to bridge the gap between the bony segments of the cleft alveolus; this helps to repair the alveolar ridge, serves as the missing nasal floor and pyriform (nasal) rim, and provides bone for eruption of teeth.

alveolar ridge The portion of the maxilla and mandible that form the base and the bony support for the teeth.

amnion Membrane surrounding the embryo and fetus.

amniotic bands Strands of tissue from the amnion that have ruptured and float in the amniotic cavity; these strands can attach to limbs, the head, or other body parts where they act as tourniquets, cutting off blood supply to developing structures, which results in amputations of limbs and digits, cleft lip, and encephalocele if the cranium is involved.

aneuploidy The presence of an abnormal number of chromosomes in a cell (e.g., a human cell with 45 or 47 chromosomes instead of the usual 46).

Angle's Classification System Differentiates normal occlusion and three types of malocclusion.

ankyloglossia A condition where the lingual frenulum is short or has an anterior attachment, resulting in restricted movement of the tongue tip; typically diagnosed if the patient cannot elevate the tongue tip sufficiently to touch the roof of the mouth with the mouth open and cannot protrude the tongue tip past the mandibular gingival ridge or incisors; also known as *tongue-tie.*

anotia Absence of the external auditory canal.

anterior crossbite A condition where a maxillary tooth or teeth are inside the mandibular arch; may involve any or all of the anterior teeth, such as the central incisors, lateral incisors, or canines; commonly seen in patients with dental or skeletal Class III malocclusion; also called *linguoversion* or *underjet*.

anterior fontanelle A soft spot on an infant's skull, located at the junction of the frontal, sagittal, and the coronal sutures.

anterior nasal spine The anterior point of the maxilla that corresponds to the base of the columella.

anterior–posterior (AP) view An X-ray view that allows the examiner to visualize the lateral pharyngeal walls at rest and during speech; the orientation of this view is as if one is looking straight through the nose; also called the *frontal view* or simply the *AP view*.

anticipation In genetics, the tendency for a disorder to have earlier age of onset or more severe manifestations.

apraxia of speech (adj. apraxic) Characterized by difficulty executing volitional oral movements and sequencing oral movements for connected speech; can result in an inability to adequately coordinate velopharyngeal movement with the other subsystems of speech (respiration, phonation, and articulation); also called *verbal apraxia*. When it occurs in children and affects speech development, it is called *childhood apraxia of speech (CAS)*.

articulators The oral structures that move to modify the airstream during speech; they include the lips, jaws (including the teeth), tongue, and velum.

aspiration Entry of material into the airway; often occurs with swallowing if there is a lack of adequate synchrony of breathing and swallowing.

association In genetics, when two or more abnormalities appear together frequently but have not yet been classified together as a syndrome.

attention deficit-hyperactivity disorder (ADHD) A cluster of behavioral characteristics involving impaired attention, distractibility, impulsivity, and hyperactivity; there appears to be a genetic basis to this disorder that affects the biochemical function in the brain.

attenuation The combined absorption and scattering of radiation proton particles by the tissues.

audible nasal emission Nasal emission through a medium-sized opening; there is some resistance to the flow so that it causes a friction-type sound.

auditory atresia Congenital closure or absence of the auditory canal that usually results in a conductive hearing loss; also called *aural atresia*.

auditory cortex Part of the brain that provides an awareness of sound.

auditory tube The tube that connects the middle ear with the nasopharynx; usually closed at the pharyngeal end at rest but opens with swallowing and yawning as a result of the action of the tensor veli palatini muscle; allows ventilation of the middle ear, equalization of air pressure on both sides of the tympanic membrane, and drainage of fluids; also known as the *eustachian tube*.

aural atresia Congenital closure or absence of the auditory canal that usually results in a conductive hearing loss; also called *auditory atresia*.

autogenous Produced by the individual; self-generating.

autosomal recessive Traits that are manifest only when they are present in both copies of a gene.

autosomes (adj. autosomal) Any chromosomes that are not sex chromosomes.

backing A compensatory articulation strategy characterized by the production of most phonemes with the back of the tongue and with the velum or the posterior pharyngeal wall.

base view X-ray view that allows the examiner to see the entire velopharyngeal sphincter during connected speech, as if looking up through the port; the relative contributions of the velum, the lateral pharyngeal walls, and posterior pharyngeal wall to closure can be determined; also called an *en face view*.

Bell's palsy A temporary facial paralysis caused by damage or trauma to facial nerves.

bilabial incompetence The inability to close the lips naturally at rest.

biofeedback A technique for making unconscious or autonomic physiological processes perceptible to the senses to manipulate them by conscious mental control; techniques are based on the learning principle that a desired response can be learned when it is determined that a specific thought process can produce the desired physiological response.

brachycephaly A short skull.

brachydactyly Abnormally short digits (fingers or toes).

breathiness A vocal quality where the vocal cords are held farther apart so that a larger volume of air escapes between them.

Brodie crossbite Occurs when the lingual cusps of all the maxillary posterior teeth are buccal to the mandibular teeth.

buccal (adj.) For the buccinator muscle of the cheeks; pertaining to, in the direction of, or adjacent to the cheek; the part of the dental arch that is posterior to the canine teeth and on the side of the teeth.

buccal crossbite Occurs when one or more maxillary teeth are positioned buccally such that the maxillary lingual cusps reside buccal to the mandibular cusps.

buccal pads Encapsulated fat masses inside the cheeks.

buccal sulcus (pl. sulci) The area between the cheeks and teeth.

café au lait macules Pigmented spots the color of "coffee with milk"; characteristic finding of neurofibromatosis 1.

canthus (pl. canthi) The angle or corner of the eye.

carriers Individuals who have one abnormal copy of a gene and are without detectable abnormalities.

central fossa (pl. fossae) The valley between the buccal cusp and the lingual cusp of a tooth.

centromere The area of constriction of a chromosome that divides the chromosome into two pairs of arms.

cephalogram A standardized lateral skull film used to measure the jaw relationship and the soft tissue profile of the forehead, nose, lips, and chin; often used in orthodontic and orthognathic surgery planning; often referred to as a *cephalometric radiograph*.

cephalometric radiograph A standardized lateral skull film used to measure the jaw relationship and the soft tissue profile of the forehead, nose, lips, and chin; often used in orthodontic and orthognathic surgery planning; often referred to as a *cephalogram*.

cheilorraphy Cleft lip repair.

childhood apraxia of speech (CAS) A motor speech disorder, usually of unclear etiology, that affects the child's ability to develop speech; it causes difficulty with the production and sequencing of motor movements for speech; speech is usually characterized by inconsistent errors that increase with utterance length or complexity; also called *developmental apraxia*, *verbal apraxia*, or just *apraxia*.

choana (pl. choanae) The opening on each side of the posterior part of the vomer that leads from the nasal cavity into the nasopharynx.

choanal atresia Congenital closure of the choana.

choanal stenosis A narrowing of the choana.

chromosome A strand of DNA in the nucleus that is encoded with genes. In most cells, humans have 22 pairs of *chromosomes* plus the two sex *chromosomes* (XX in females and XY in males) for a total of 46.

cineradiography Radiography of an organ in motion; an old method for evaluating velopharyngeal function by recording multiple views on motion picture film to observe several dimensions; often referred to as a *cine study*.

cine study Radiography of an organ in motion; an old method for evaluating velopharyngeal function by recording multiple views on motion picture film to observe several dimensions; often referred to as *cineradiography*.

circular pattern Pattern of velopharyngeal closure that occurs when all the velopharyngeal structures contribute equally and the closure pattern resembles a true sphincter.

circumvallate papilla A line of prominent taste buds that makes an inverted V on the posterior tongue.

Class I occlusion Normal dental arch relationship, although the teeth may be misaligned; the mesiobuccal (front outside) cusp of the first maxillary molar fits in the buccal (outside) groove of the first mandibular molar.

Class II malocclusion Abnormal dental arch relationship where the mesiobuccal (front outside) cusp of the first maxillary molar is anterior to the buccal (outside) groove of the first mandibular molar; the mandibular arch is too far behind the maxillary arch, often because of micrognathia.

Class III malocclusion Abnormal dental arch relationship where the mesiobuccal (front outside) cusp of the first maxillary molar is posterior to the buccal (outside) groove of the first mandibular molar; the mandibular arch is too far in front of the maxillary arch because of either maxillary retrusion or mandibular prognathism.

cleft An abnormal opening or a fissure in an anatomical structure that is normally closed.

cleft lip A congenital malformation that occurs in utero during the first trimester of pregnancy and involves a fissure of the lip and sometimes alveolus.

cleft muscle of Veau Refers to abnormal velar muscle insertion from a cleft palate; the levator veli palatini muscle does not interdigitate in the midline, and both this paired muscle and the palatopharyngeus muscles are inserted abnormally onto the posterior border of the hard palate, rendering them essentially nonfunctional.

cleft palate A congenital malformation that occurs in utero during the first trimester of pregnancy and involves a fissure in the soft palate and sometimes the hard palate.

cleft palate team (CPT) A team of professionals that consists of a surgeon, an orthodontist, a speech-language pathologist, and one additional specialist, according to the requirements of the American Cleft Palate–Craniofacial Association; other team members may include an audiologist, a dentist, a geneticist (dysmorphologist), a nurse, an oral surgeon (maxillofacial surgeon), and others.

clinodactyly Deflection or curvature of the digits (fingers or toes).

co-articulated When a consonant is characterized by one manner of production with simultaneous valving at two places of production.

cochlea A part of the inner ear that is composed of a bony spiral tube that is shaped like a snail's shell and is responsible for hearing.

cognition (adj. cognitive) Refers to the individual's ability to engage in conscious intellectual activities, such as thinking, reasoning, imagining, or learning.

colobomas Congenital defects, especially of the eye, which often involve a notch of the eyelid margin; usually affects the lower lid.

columella The "little column" at the lower portion of the nose that separates the nostrils; cartilage and mucosa that are located under the nasal tip and at the lower end of the nasal septum.

compensatory errors Articulation productions that are abnormal in placement because of the individual's response to abnormal structure, such as velopharyngeal insufficiency or dental malocclusion, or abnormal neurophysiology, such as velopharyngeal incompetence; also known as *active speech characteristics*.

complete cleft A cleft of the lip or palate that follows the embryological suture line(s) and extends all the way to the incisive foramen; a complete cleft lip involves the entire lip through the nostril sill(s) and the alveolus (or dental arch) and extends all the way to the area of the incisive foramen; a complete cleft palate involves the uvula, velum, and hard palate all the way to the incisive foramen.

complete crossbite When the maxilla is very narrow and as a result the entire maxillary arch is inside the mandibular arch during occlusion.

conductive hearing loss A type of hearing loss caused by a blockage or problem with sound conduction to the inner ear.

condyle The rounded articular surface of the bone, such as in the jaw joint.

congenital A disease or deformity that is present at birth; may be the result of an inherited (genetic or chromosomal) condition or may be caused by something that occurred during the pregnancy (exogenous factors).

conotruncal defects Major abnormalities of the heart's chambers or blood vessels; include truncus arteriosus, transposition of the great arteries, double outlet of the right ventricle, and tetralogy of Fallot.

consanguinity Mating between related individuals.

consulting team A team of professionals whose members provide opinions regarding the total care of the patient; the opinions and recommendations are forwarded to the treating professionals for follow-up.

contiguous gene syndromes Syndromes caused by deletions large enough to contain several genes but too small to be seen on routine cytogenetic analysis.

continuous positive airway pressure (CPAP) An instrument that delivers continuous airway pressure to the nasopharynx by means of a hose and nasal mask; used primarily in the treatment of obstructive sleep apnea to prevent pharyngeal collapse; has also been used to provide resistance training to strengthen the velopharyngeal musculature when there is velopharyngeal incompetence.

coronal pattern A pattern of velopharyngeal closure that is accomplished primarily by the posterior movement of the velum against a broad area of the posterior pharyngeal wall and the possible anterior movement of the posterior pharyngeal wall; there is less contribution of the lateral pharyngeal walls during closure with this pattern.

coronal suture The transverse suture in the skull separating the frontal bone from the parietal bones.

corpus callosum Nerve fibers that allow communication between the left and right cerebral hemispheres. Consists mostly of contralateral axon projections. It appears as a wide, flat region just ventral to (below) the cortex.

corticotomy A partial cut in the bone.

coupling Sharing acoustic energy.

craniofacial team (CFT) A team of professionals that consists of a craniofacial surgeon, an orthodontist, a mental health professional, and a speech-language pathologist, according to the requirements of the American Cleft Palate–Craniofacial Association; other members may include a neurosurgeon, an ophthalmologist, and others.

craniosynostosis Abnormal development of the cranial skeleton from premature ossification of one or more cranial sutures, resulting in malformation of the skull with growth; the shape of the skull depends on the sutures that are involved; can cause raised intracranial pressure (ICP) and mental retardation if not treated; can be syndromal from genetic factors or nonsyndromal.

crossbite A type of dental malocclusion where a maxillary tooth or teeth are inside the mandibular teeth; when the normal overlap of the upper teeth to the lower teeth is reversed so that the lower teeth overlap the upper teeth buccally; can be anterior or lateral.

cryptorchidism Undescended testes.

crypts Small tubular glands, pits, or recesses.

cul-de-sac resonance Abnormal resonance during speech, which occurs when the transmission of acoustic energy is trapped in a blind pouch in the vocal tract with only one outlet; the speech is perceived as muffled because the sound is contained in a cavity with no direct means of escape.

Cupid's bow The shape of the top of the upper lip, which includes a rounded configuration with an indentation in the middle.

cusps The points on the teeth.

cyanosis Bluish skin color resulting from poor circulation or inadequate oxygenation of the blood.

cytogenetics The branch of genetics that is concerned with the structure and function of the chromosomes within the cell; literally means "cell genetics."

damping To slow or stop the vibration or decrease the amplitude of an oscillating system.

deciduous teeth Primary, or "baby," teeth.

deep bite When the upper teeth overlap more than 25% of the lower teeth; the lower incisors may be in contact with the alveolar ridge of the palate.

deformation Birth defect that arises as a result of abnormal mechanical or physical forces in the fetal environment on an otherwise normal structure; usually results in the abnormal shape or form of a completely formed organ or structure, such as clubfoot; also known as *deformity*.

deformity Birth defect that arises as a result of abnormal mechanical or physical forces in the fetal environment on an otherwise normal structure; usually results in the abnormal shape or form of a completely formed organ or structure, such as clubfoot; also known as *deformation*.

dehisce To pull apart.

dehiscence A breakdown of a surgical repair or an unwanted opening in an area that has been surgically closed.

denasality Abnormal resonance from a lack of vibration of the sound energy in the nasal cavity; total nasal airway obstruction and the resultant effect on resonance.

dental implants Cylindrically shaped pieces of titanium that can take the place of a missing tooth's root and are able to support crowns and prosthetic devices.

dental occlusion The manner in which the maxillary teeth and mandibular teeth fit together, or the bite; in normal occlusion, the upper arch overlaps the lower arch.

dentures Removable prosthetic teeth that replace an entire dental arch.

deoxyribonucleic acid (DNA) A nucleic acid made up of building blocks called nucleotides; contained in the nuclei of animal and vegetable cells, it is the component of chromosomes; each DNA molecule contains many genes, which contain hereditary information; DNA consists of two strands that wrap around each other in the shape of a twisted ladder or double helix.

dermatoglyphics Creases on the hands or changes in the fingerprints that can give clues to early developmental problems.

diadochokinetic exercises Rapid production of syllables in different combinations with the /p/, /t/, and /k/ sounds (e.g., *pata pata pata* or *taka taka taka*, or *pataka pataka pataka pataka*); used to test for oral-motor dysfunction (e.g., apraxia of speech).

diastasis A separation between two normally joined structures, as in separation of the levator veli palatini muscles when there is a submucous cleft palate.

diastema A space or opening between the teeth, usually the upper central incisors.

direct instrumental procedures Instrumental procedures that allow the examiner to visualize the structures of the velopharyngeal valve during speech (and swallowing) and observe abnormalities of velopharyngeal structure or function; include the use of videofluoros-copy and nasopharyngoscopy.

disruption A morphologic defect resulting from an extrinsic breakdown or interference with a normal developmental process.

distal (adj.) Away from the center, midline, or point of origin.

distally (adv.) Away from the center, midline, or point of origin.

distraction osteogenesis A method for increasing bone length that involves making a corticotomy in the middle of a bone and then slowly pulling the cut ends apart (distracting) with a mechanical device; new bone is able to regenerate between the cut ends, obviating the need for bone grafts; can be used for maxillary or mandibular advancement.

dolichocephaly Long, narrow skull seen with prematurity.

dorsum The top surface, as on the tongue.

dose In speech therapy, refers to the number of learning opportunities experienced by the child, not to the number of therapy sessions or the length of a practice session.

double helix Coiled ladder of a DNA molecule that consists of two polymers of nucleotides.

dysarthria A motor speech disorder that affects the oral articulators and is characterized by abnormalities of muscular strength, range of motion, speed, accuracy, and tonicity from a neurological injury or insult; speech is very slow and characterized by inaccurate movement of the articulators.

dysmorphogenesis The process of abnormal tissue formation, resulting in abnormally formed features.

dysmorphologist Another term for a geneticist.

dysmorphology (adj. dysmorphic) The study of abnormal shape or form.

dysphonia (adj. dysphonic) Refers to voice disorder that results in an alteration in the normal phonatory quality of the voice; characterized by breathiness, hoarseness, low intensity, and glottal fry.

dysplasia An abnormal organization of cells into tissues and the outcome of the process.

eardrum Thin tissue that separates the outer ear from the middle ear; transmits sound energy through the ossicles to the inner ear; also called the *tympanic membrane*.

ectopic tooth A normal tooth that erupts in an abnormal position.

edema An excessive amount of fluid in cells and tissues, causing swelling.

encephalocele A congenital gap in the skull with herniation of brain tissue into the nose or palate.

endogenous A factor from within the organism rather than from the environment, such as the genetic makeup of the organism.

endoscope A specialized flexible fiberoptic instrument that consists of an eyepiece at the end of a long tube or scope; used for examination of an internal canal or organ; can be used for evaluation of the velopharyngeal mechanism, pharynx, or larynx; a type of endoscope is a *nasopharyngoscope*.

endoscopy A procedure that allows the visualization of the interior of a canal or hollow organ by means of a special instrument usually called an *endoscope*.

en face view X-ray view that allows the examiner to see the entire velopharyngeal sphincter during connected speech as if looking up through the port; the relative contributions of the velum, the lateral pharyngeal walls, and posterior pharyngeal wall to closure can be determined; also called a *base view*.

epibulbar lipodermoids Fatty cysts on the eyeball.

epicanthal folds Folds of tissue that extend from the upper eyelid to the lower part of the orbit at the inner canthus or corner of the eye.

epistaxis A nosebleed.

eustachian tube The tube that connects the middle ear with the nasopharynx; usually closed at the pharyngeal end at rest but opens with swallowing and yawning as a result of the action of the tensor veli palatini muscle; allows ventilation of the middle ear, equalization of air pressure on both sides of the tympanic membrane, and drainage of fluids; also known as the *auditory tube*.

exogenous A factor that is outside an organism and is not indigenous to that organism, such as drugs or smoke.

exophthalmos Protrusion of one or both globes of the eye beyond the socket from either congenital or pathological factors that provide pressure behind the eye; often associated with craniosynostosis involving the coronal suture.

external auditory canal A skin-lined canal of the external ear that leads to the eardrum.

external ear Part of the ear that comprises the pinna and the external auditory canal.

face mask A device used to advance the maxilla and improve an anterior crossbite; also called *reverse pull headgear*.

facial cleft A collective term that includes not only clefts of the lip and palate but also other less common types of clefts of the face, including those that involve the forehead, eyes, ears, nose, cheeks, mouth, and jaws.

faucial pillars Bilateral curtain-like structures in the posterior portion of the oral cavity; the anterior faucial pillar is formed as the velum curves downward toward the tongue, and the posterior faucial pillar is just behind the anterior pillar.

feeding obturator An obturator is a prosthesis that totally occludes an opening, such as an oronasal fistula or velopharyngeal opening. This type of prosthetic appliance can be used in the first few months of life to assist the infant with cleft palate in feeding; it keeps the tongue from resting inside the cleft and provides a solid surface so that the tongue can achieve compression of the nipple; no longer felt to be needed by most cleft centers.

fiberoptic endoscopic evaluation of swallowing (FEES) A procedure where a flexible endoscope is used in the evaluation of swallowing disorders; involves the transnasal passage of an endoscope for viewing of the pharyngeal and laryngeal structures to study the integrity of airway protection during swallowing.

fistula (pl. fistulae or fistulas) An abnormal hole or passage between two epithelialized organs that do not normally connect; examples include an oronasal (palatal) fistula or tracheoesophageal fistula.

fixed bridge Permanently placed prosthetic teeth typically used to replace dental segments.

fluorescence in situ hybridization (FISH) A procedure used in a cytogenetics laboratory that involves the use of a nucleic acid probe labeled with a fluorescent dye to localize a specified submicroscopic segment of DNA; used to determine deletion of parts of chromosomes, as in the diagnosis of velocardiofacial/22q11.2 deletion syndrome.

foramen (pl. foramina) A normal hole or opening in a bony structure or membranous structure; often serves as a passageway to allow blood vessels and nerves to pass through to the area on the other side.

forme fruste A partial or arrested form of a cleft lip where the overlying skin is intact, but the underlying muscle, nasal cartilage, and oral sphincter function usually are significantly affected; also called *microform cleft*.

founder effect When a relatively small number of original ancestors has led to a high frequency of carriers for certain disorders in a population.

foveae palati (sing. fovea palati) The bilateral midline depressions at the junction of the hard and soft palate that are the openings to minor salivary glands.

frenula (sing. frenulum) A connecting fold of membrane serving to support or restrain a part, such as the tongue.

fricative phonemes Pressure-sensitive sounds that require a gradual release of air pressure through a small opening, including /f/, /v/, /s/, /z/, /ʃ/, /ʒ/, /Θ/, /ð/.

frontal bones Bones that cover the frontal part of the skull.

frontal bossing A prominent, protruding forehead.

frontal view An X-ray view that allows the examiner to visualize the lateral pharyngeal walls at rest and during speech; the orientation of this view is as if one is looking straight through the nose; also called the *anterior–posterior view* or simply the *AP view*.

fundamental frequency The lowest frequency of a periodic waveform.

gamete A sex cell, either an ovum or a sperm cell.

gastrostomy tube (G-tube) A tube that is placed directly into the stomach through an opening that is surgically created to provide parenteral feeding.

gene (adj. genetic) A functional unit of heredity that is submicroscopic, resides at a specific location or locus on a chromosome, and is capable of reproducing itself with each cell division; consists of a sequence of nucleotide bases in a molecule of deoxyribonucleic acid (DNA).

genome Consists of chromosomes and DNA and contains a complete set of instructions for cell replication and differentiation for an organism.

genomics The branch of molecular biology concerned with the structure, function, evolution, and mapping of genomes.

gingivoperiosteoplasty A procedure to close the cleft of the alveolus with raised gingival flaps and the underlying periosteum on each edge of the cleft; raw surfaces are advanced and sewn together to allow the bone progenitor cells to lay down bone as the patient grows.

glossectomy Surgical removal of part of or all of the tongue.

glossoptosis The posterior displacement of the tongue in the pharynx; can cause airway obstruction.

glottal fricative A speech sound, /h/, produced by the friction of the airstream as it passes through the glottal opening.

glottal plosive A compensatory articulation production characterized by adduction (closure) of the vocal folds, a buildup of air pressure under the glottis, and then sudden opening of the vocal folds, resulting in a grunt-type sound; also called *glottal stop*.

glottal stop A compensatory articulation production characterized by adduction (closure) of the vocal folds. A buildup of air pressure, and then a sudden opening of the vocal folds, resulting in a grunt-type sound; also called *glottal plosive*.

glottis Space between the vocal cords.

greater segment Palatal segment on the noncleft side.

hair cells Sensory cells, as in the organ of hearing, that have hair-like properties.

hard palate A bony structure that serves as the roof of the mouth and floor of the nasal cavity and separates the oral cavity from the nasal cavity.

harmonics Component frequencies of a signal that are whole number multiples of the fundamental frequency; also called *overtones*.

hemangioma A congenital anomaly in which a proliferation of blood vessels results in a large mass.

hepatoblastoma A malignant liver tumor; a risk for individuals with Beckwith–Wiedemann syndrome.

heterogeneous A characteristic where more than one gene can cause the same clinical features.

heterozygous Having two different copies or alleles of a gene at the same locus on a pair of homologous chromosomes.

holoprosencephaly Failure of the forebrain to divide into the two hemispheres; often accompanied by a midline deficit in facial development or a midfacial cleft.

homozygotes Persons with two identical copies of a gene.

homozygous When genes have two similar alleles.

horizontal plates of the palatine bones Paired plates of the palatine bones located just behind the transverse palatine suture line; form the posterior portion of the hard palate, ending with the protrusive posterior nasal spine.

hydrocephalus A condition where fluid accumulates in the brain and, if untreated, can enlarge the head and cause brain damage.

hypernasality (adj. hypernasal) A resonance disorder that occurs when there is abnormal nasal resonance during the production of oral sounds caused by abnormal coupling of the oral and nasal cavities during speech; the perceptual quality of speech is often described as just "nasal," muffled, or characterized by mumbling; it is particularly perceptible on vowels.

hypertelorism Excessive distance between two paired organs, such as the eyes.

hypertrophy (adj. hypertrophic) Abnormal enlargement of a part of the body caused by enlargement of its constituent cells.

hyponasality A type of abnormal resonance that occurs when there is a reduction in nasal resonance during speech from a blockage in the nasopharynx or in the entrance to the nasal cavity; particularly affects the production of the nasal consonants (/m/, /n/, and /ŋ/).

hypopharynx Part of the pharynx, or throat, that is below the oral cavity and extends from the epiglottis inferiorly to the esophagus.

hypoplasia Underdevelopment or defective formation of a tissue (i.e., bone, muscles, and nerves) or an organ, usually because of a decrease in the normal number of cells.

hypoplastic Underdeveloped or defective formation of a tissue or an organ.

hypospadias Where the orifice of the penis is proximal to its normal location.

hypotelorism Narrow-spaced eyes.

hypotonia (adj. hypotonic) A state of low muscle tonicity and sometimes reduced muscle strength; caused by different diseases and disorders of the brain that affect the motor nerve control or muscle strength.

ideogram A schematic drawing of the banding pattern of a chromosome.

iliac crest The superior border of the wing of the ilium of the greater pelvis.

imprinting When some genes function differently, depending on whether they were inherited maternally or paternally.

inaudible nasal emission Nasal emission caused by a relatively large opening; is inaudible because there is very little resistance to the flow and hypernasality masks the sound.

incidence In epidemiological terms, refers to the number of new cases of a disease or disorder in a given population, such as the number of persons becoming ill with a certain disease.

incisive foramen A hole in the bone that is located in the alveolar ridge area of the maxillary arch, just behind the central incisors, and forms the tip of the premaxilla.

incisive papilla The slight elevation of the mucosa at the anterior end of the raphe of the palate.

incomplete cleft A cleft of the lip or palate that does not extend all the way to the incisive foramen.

incomplete penetrance The lack of a recognizable phenotype in an individual who carries a mutation that may cause an autosomal dominant trait or condition.

incus One of the ossicles in the middle ear; articulates with the malleus and the stapes.

indirect instrumental procedures Provide object data regarding the results of velopharyngeal function, such as airflow, air pressure, or acoustic output, but do not allow visualization of the structures; include the use of aerodynamic instrumentation or the Nasometer.

infant oral orthopedics A method used to align the alveolar segments in both unilateral and bilateral clefts of the palate prior to surgical correction; also known as *palatal orthopedics* and *premaxillary orthopedics*.

inner ear Part of the ear that consists of the cochlea and semicircular canals.

intentional fistula A nasolabial fistula that is deliberately left in the alveolus (under the lip) at the time of the primary palatoplasty to allow unrestricted facial growth; it is closed with a bone graft at a later time.

interdisciplinary team A group of professionals from various disciplines who work together to coordinate the care of a patient through collaboration, interaction, communication, and cooperation.

intermaxillary suture line Embryological suture line that begins at the incisive foramen and ends at the posterior nasal spine; separates the paired palatine processes of the maxilla and the horizontal plates of the palatine bones; also known as *palatine suture line* and *median palatine suture line*.

intonation Refers to the frequent changes in pitch throughout an utterance, as controlled by subtle changes in vocal fold length and mass and pharyngeal cavity size; variation of pitch is used for emphasis, to express feelings, ask a question, and for many other functions.

intravelar veloplasty A surgical reconstruction of the levator veli palatini sling during palatoplasty for correction of a cleft of the velum.

karyotype A gross chromosome analysis that is done by drawing blood, growing the cells in a culture, analyzing the white blood cells, photographing the chromosomes, and then arranging the chromosomes in pairs for display and assessment; a visual profile of an individual's chromosomes.

keloids Excessive scar tissue formed during healing.

labial (adj.) Relating to the lip; the outer part of the dental arch that touches the lip.

labial sulcus The furrow between the lip and gum.

labial tubercle The prominent projection on the inferior border, or free edge, of the midsection of the upper lip.

lambdoid suture The junction of the parietal bones, temporal, and the occipital bones of the skull.

laminography Use of a radiograph to measure distances and angles between landmarks.

laryngeal web A congenital anomaly that consists of a band of tissue between the vocal folds, usually in the anterior portion of the larynx, that can cause respiratory stridor.

laryngoesophageal cleft An opening between the larynx and the esophagus that can cause aspiration of food or liquids.

laryngomalacia Abnormally soft cartilage in the epiglottis and aryepiglottic folds at birth, resulting in loud inspiratory stridor that is particularly pronounced when the infant cries or breathes deeply.

lateral cephalometric X-rays Still radiographs of the head taken in the sagittal plane.

lateral crossbite Any of the maxillary teeth distal (posterior) to the canines are positioned inside the mandibular teeth; usually occurs because the maxilla is too narrow; also known as *posterior crossbite*.

lateral pharyngeal walls The side walls of the throat.

lateral view An X-ray view that shows the velum and posterior pharyngeal wall in a midsagittal plane; the orientation of the lateral view is as if we were able to look through the side of the head to view these structures.

lesser segment Palatal segment on the cleft side.

levator sling The levator veli palatini muscles from each side interdigitate and blend together to form a muscle sling.

levator veli palatini Paired muscle that forms the main muscle mass of the velum, primarily responsible for velar elevation.

lingual (adj.) Related to the tongue; also the inner part of the upper and lower dental arch that is in contact with the tongue.

lingual tonsil A mass of lymphoid tissue located at the base of the tongue and extending to the epiglottis.

linguoversion Malposition of an anterior tooth from the normal line of occlusion toward the tongue; also known as *anterior crossbite* or *underjet*.

lip adhesion A simple, straight-line surgical procedure to temporarily repair a cleft lip; this procedure is performed so that subsequent lip pressure draws the segments together, making the final repair more successful.

lip pits Depressions in the bottom lip that are usually bilateral and are associated with Van der Woude syndrome with cleft palate.

lobulated tongue The tongue appears to have multiple lobes, with fissures between each lobe.

lower esophageal sphincter (LES) Sphincter at the base of the esophagus that relaxes to allow a bolus to enter the stomach.

macroglossia Large tongue.

macrostomia A large mouth opening, often caused by failure of fusion between the maxillary and mandibular process of the embryonic development of the face.

magnetic resonance imaging (MRI) A noninvasive method to produce a very clear and detailed view of internal body structures using a magnetic field and radio waves.

malar bone The bone of the skull that forms the prominence of the cheek and articulates with the frontal, sphenoid, temporal, and maxillary bones. It is also known as the *zygomatic bone*.

malar eminence Related to the cheekbone.

malformation Defect in basic embryological plan caused by chromosomal or genetic factors.

malleus One of the ossicles in the middle ear and is firmly attached to the tympanic membrane and articulates with the incus.

malocclusion Abnormal dental or skeletal relationship of the maxillary and mandibular teeth so that the arches do not close together normally during biting.

mandible The bone that forms the lower jaw.

mastoid cavity A section of the temporal bone that is porous and located just behind the ear.

mastoiditis Inflammation or infection in any part of the mastoid process.

maxilla The bone that forms the upper jaw.

maxillary protrusion Characterized by a maxilla that is large and projects farther than normal.

maxillary retrusion Characterized by a small upper jaw (maxilla) relative to the lower jaw (mandible); a common anomaly, especially in individuals with repaired cleft lip and palate secondary to the inherent deficiency in the maxilla caused by the cleft and the possible restriction in maxillary growth with the surgical repair; also known as *midface deficiency*.

mean nasalance score Represents the relative amount of nasal acoustic energy in the person's speech as determined by the Nasometer; the ratio of nasal acoustic energy over total (oral plus nasal) acoustic energy during speech as determined through the use of the Nasometer. The score represents the mean of the percentage points that are calculated for an entire speech passage; also called *nasalance score*.

median palatine suture line Embryological suture line that begins at the incisive foramen and ends at the posterior nasal spine; separates the paired palatine processes of the maxilla and the horizontal plates of the palatine bones; also known as *intermaxillary suture line*.

meiosis The process of cell division.

mesial (adj.) The direction toward the midline, following the curvature of the dental arch.

mesiobuccal cusp Front outside cusp of a molar.

metacentric Chromosomes with a centrally located centromere.

metopic suture The junction between the frontal bones of the skull.

microcephaly Small head circumference in comparison to age-matched peers.

microform cleft A partial or arrested form of a cleft lip where the overlying skin is intact, but the underlying muscle, nasal cartilage, and oral sphincter function usually are significantly affected; also called *forme fruste*.

microglossia Small tongue.

micrognathia (adj. micrognathic) A small or hypoplastic mandible.

micropenis Small penis.

microphthalmia Small eyes.

microstomia A small mouth opening.

microtia Hypoplasia or absence of the external ear (pinna or auricle); often accompanied by aural atresia (a blind or absent external auditory meatus).

middle ear A hollow space within the temporal bone.

middle ear effusion Collection of fluids within the middle ear space caused by eustachian tube dysfunction.

mid-dorsum palatal stop An abnormal articulation production that is often compensatory for anterior oral cavity crowding; produced as a stop consonant that is articulated with the middle of the dorsum against the middle of the hard palate; is usually substituted for the lingual-alveolar sounds (/t/ and /d/), the velar sounds (/k/ and /g/), and in some cases, the sibilant sounds (/s/, /z/, /ʃ/, /ʒ/, /tʃ/, /dʒ/); also called a *palatal–dorsal plosive*.

midface deficiency Characterized by a small upper jaw (maxilla) relative to the lower jaw (mandible); a common anomaly, especially in individuals with repaired cleft lip and palate secondary to the inherent deficiency in the maxilla caused by the cleft and the possible restriction in maxillary growth with the surgical repair; also known as *maxillary retrusion*.

mixed dentition Presence of both primary and secondary teeth.

mixed resonance A combination of hypernasality, hyponasality, or cul-de-sac resonance during connected speech.

modified barium swallow (MBS) A radiographic procedure that allows an overall view of the oral, pharyngeal, and esophageal phases of swallowing as well as the interactions between the phases; also referred to as a *videofluoroscopic swallowing study (VFSS)*.

monosomy Absence of an entire chromosome of a pair of homologous chromosomes.

morphogenesis The process of embryonic tissue formation.

motor learning The acquisition of new motor skills to be able to execute complex motor movements and motor sequences; is necessary for the individual to perform all complicated motor movements and sequences without conscious thought; the key component of motor learning is feedback.

motor memory What develops the automaticity of newly learned motor movement and makes the new learning relatively permanent, although it can degrade with lack of use; the key component of motor learning is practice.

mucoperiosteum Tissue that covers the hard palate, consisting of a mucous membrane and periosteum.

mucosa Epithelial tissue that lines many body cavities (including the nasal cavity, oral cavity, and pharynx) and secretes mucus. Also known as *mucous membrane*.

mucous membrane (adj. mucosal) Epithelial tissue that lines many body cavities (including the nasal cavity, oral cavity, and pharynx) and secretes mucus. Also known as *mucosa*.

mucus A clear, viscid secretion from the mucous membranes for protection.

multidisciplinary team A group of professionals from various disciplines who work independently in evaluating and treating patients with complex medical needs; members of this type of team have well-defined roles and cooperate with each other, but there is little communication and interaction among the team members.

multifactorial inheritance A characteristic in the phenotype that is the result of a combination of many genes at different loci and/or factors from the environment; the combination of genes and other factors all have a small added effect to form the characteristic in the phenotype.

musculus uvulae A paired muscle that creates a bulge on the posterior nasal surface of the velum during phonation; during contraction, this bulge provides additional bulk and stiffness to the nasal side of the velum and helps to fill in the area between the velum and posterior pharyngeal wall, contributing to a firm velopharyngeal seal.

mutation A change in the sequence of base pairs in the DNA molecule that is reflected in subsequent divisions of the cell; a change in the chemistry of the gene that is reflected in the subsequent genotype and phenotype; can be as small as a substitution of a single base pair or as large as the deletion of an entire chromosome.

myopia Nearsightedness.

myringotomy A surgical puncture of the tympanic membrane so that fluid can be drained or suctioned out of the middle ear.

naris (pl. nares) Nostril.

nasal alveolar molding (NAM) A method of repositioning the nasal septum and ala in the infant prior to cleft lip repair; usually involves an intraoral/nasal appliance combined with taping.

nasalance distance The range between the maximum and minimum nasalance.

nasalance ratio The minimum nasalance divided by the maximum nasalance.

nasalance score Represents the relative amount of nasal acoustic energy in the person's speech as determined by the Nasometer; the ratio of nasal acoustic energy over total (oral plus nasal) acoustic energy during speech as determined through the use of the Nasometer. The score represents the mean of the percentage points that are calculated for an entire speech passage; also called *mean nasalance score.*

nasal bridge A saddle-shaped area that includes the nasal root and the lateral aspects of the nose.

nasal concha (pl. nasal conchae) A structure that is comparable to a shell in shape, such as the auricle or pinna of the ear or the turbinated bone within the nose.

nasal cul-de-sac resonance Resonance disorder that occurs when sound is partially blocked from exiting the nasal cavity during speech; most noticeable when there is a combination of VPI (which would otherwise cause hypernasality) and a blockage in the anterior part of the nose.

nasal endoscopy A minimally invasive endoscopic procedure that allows visual observation and analysis of the velopharyngeal mechanism or larynx during speech, phonation, or swallowing; commonly used in the evaluation of swallowing, upper airway obstruction, and the structure and function of the larynx and vocal cords; also called *nasopharyngoscopy, nasendoscopy,* or *video nasendoscopy.*

nasal grimace A muscle contraction during speech that is typically noted either above the nasal bridge (in the area between the eyes) or around the nares; occurs as an overflow muscle reaction when there is an attempt to achieve velopharyngeal closure; usually accompanied by nasal emission.

nasalization of oral phonemes An obligatory distortion from an open velopharyngeal valve; as a result, oral consonants sound more like their nasal cognates (e.g., m/b, n/d, and ŋ).

nasal meatuses (sing. meatus) The three passages in the nasal cavity that lie directly under a nasal concha.

nasal regurgitation Reflux of fluids into the nasopharynx and nasal cavity during drinking or vomiting.

nasal root The most depressed, superior part of the nose along the nasal ridge and at the level of the eyes.

nasal rustle A fricative sound that occurs as air is forced through a small velopharyngeal opening; airstream is released on the nasal side with pressure,

resulting in bubbling of nasal secretions; also called *nasal turbulence.*

nasal septum A wall separating the nasal cavity into two halves; consists of the vomer bone, the perpendicular plate of the ethmoid, and the quadrangular cartilage and is covered with mucous membrane.

nasal sill The base of the nostril opening.

nasal sniff An uncommon compensatory articulation production that is produced by a forcible inspiration through the nose; usually substituted for sibilant sounds, particularly the /s/, and typically occurs in the final word position.

nasal snort A burst of nasal emission that is produced by a forcible emission of air pressure through the nares during consonant production, resulting in a noisy, sneeze-like sound.

nasal turbinates Bony structures in the nose that are covered with mucosa; the superior and middle turbinates are parts of the ethmoid bone, and the inferior turbinate, which is the largest, is its own unique bone.

nasal turbulence A fricative sound that occurs as air is forced through a small velopharyngeal opening; airstream is released on the nasal side with pressure, resulting in bubbling of nasal secretions; also called *nasal rustle.*

nasal twang Increased nasality on vowels, as noted in some dialects.

nasal vestibule The most anterior part of the nasal cavity; it is enclosed by the cartilages of the nose.

nasendoscopy A minimally invasive endoscopic procedure that allows visual observation and analysis of the velopharyngeal mechanism or larynx during speech, phonation, or swallowing; commonly used in the evaluation of swallowing, upper airway obstruction, and the structure and function of the larynx and vocal cords; also called *nasopharyngoscopy, video nasendoscopy,* or *nasal endoscopy.*

nasion The midline point just superior to the nasal root and overlying the nasofrontal suture.

nasogastric tube (NG tube) A tube placed through the nose and down to the stomach that is used for feeding.

nasogram A contour display on a computer screen that represents the nasalance results of the spoken passage on the Nasometer.

nasolabial fistula A fistula in the alveolus (under the lip) that is often deliberately left by the surgeon during the initial repair to allow for maxillary growth. It is later closed by a bone graft; also known as an *intentional fistula.*

Nasometer A computer-based instrument (PENTAX Medical, Montvale, NJ) that measures the relative amount of nasal acoustic energy in a patient's speech.

nasometry A method of measuring the acoustic correlates of resonance and velopharyngeal function through a computer-based instrument.

nasopharyngeal airway tube A tube that is used to improve the airway of infants, such as those with Pierre Robin sequence; the tube is placed in the nose of the infant in such a way that one end sticks out of the nose and the other end extends to below the region of tongue obstruction.

nasopharyngoscope A type of endoscope that is used for examination of the pharynx, larynx, and velopharyngeal mechanism.

nasopharyngoscopy A minimally invasive endoscopic procedure that allows visual observation and analysis of the velopharyngeal mechanism or larynx during speech, phonation, or swallowing; commonly used in the evaluation of swallowing, upper airway obstruction, and the structure and function of the larynx and vocal cords; also called *nasendoscopy, nasal endoscopy,* or *video nasendoscopy.*

nasopharynx The part of the pharynx, or throat, that lies above the soft palate and just behind the nasal cavity.

necrosis Abnormal death of cellular tissue from toxins, infection, or trauma.

neurofibromas Large nerve sheath tumors.

nonpneumatic activities As they relate to the velopharyngeal valve: swallowing, gagging, and vomiting.

nosocomial infections Infections that are acquired while in the hospital.

nucleolus A structure within the nucleus of each cell in which genes are actively transcribed.

nucleotides Building blocks of DNA that consist of a 5-carbon sugar chemically bonded to a phosphate group and a nitrogenous base.

nucleus A part of a cell that contains genetic material that serves as instructions for cell and tissue functions; it is separated from the rest of the cell by a lipid membrane with specialized proteins.

obligatory distortions When the articulation placement (the function) of speech is normal, but an abnormality of the structure (i.e., dental malocclusion, velopharyngeal insufficiency, or an oronasal fistula) causes distortion of speech; include hypernasality, nasal emission, weak consonants, and short utterance length; also known as *passive speech characteristics.*

oblique view X-ray view that allows the examiner to see the lateral pharyngeal walls and velum during connected speech; used primarily if the base view cannot be obtained because of enlarged adenoids or the inability to hyperextend the neck.

obstructive sleep apnea (OSA) A period during sleep when the individual is exerting muscular forces to inspire but is unsuccessful in moving air into the lungs because of a blockage in the pharynx; often caused by enlarged tonsils, enlarged adenoids, or pharyngeal hypotonia during sleep.

obturator A prosthesis that totally occludes an opening, such as an oronasal fistula or velopharyngeal opening.

occipital bone The bone that forms the back of the skull.

occlusal cant A sloping transverse occlusal plane caused by inadequate vertical maxillary growth on one side, which is compensated by vertical alveolar growth in the mandible on the same side; common in patients with unilateral cleft lip/palate and those with hemifacial microsomia.

occlusion The way the maxillary and mandibular teeth fit together when the jaws are closed, as when biting.

occult submucous cleft A defect in the velum that is under the mucous membrane and not visible on the oral surface; this defect can usually be viewed on the nasal surface of the velum through nasopharyngoscopy.

open bite Occurs when one or more maxillary teeth fail to occlude with the opposing mandibular teeth; primarily affects the anterior dentition (anterior open bite) and less commonly the posterior dentition (lateral open bite).

oral cul-de-sac resonance Resonance disorder that occurs when sound is partially blocked from exiting the oral cavity during speech; can occur from microstomia; sounds like mumbling or speaking without opening the mouth normally.

oral gavage A means to deliver breast milk or formula directly to the stomach through a nasogastric (NG) tube.

orbicularis oris A complex of four independent quadrant muscles in the lips that encircle the mouth and are responsible for pursing and puckering of the lips.

organelles Internal structures in a cell that perform specific functions, such as metabolizing energy, building complex molecules such as proteins, and breaking down waste products.

organ of Corti The part of the inner ear where the mechanical energy introduced into the cochlea is converted into electrical stimulation.

orogastric tube A tube placed through the mouth and down to the stomach that is used for feeding.

oronasal fistula A hole or an opening in the palate that goes all the way through to the nasal cavity; usually the result of failure of the palate to heal after a palatoplasty; also known as a *palatal fistula*.

oropharyngeal isthmus The opening from the oral cavity to the pharynx; bordered superiorly by the velum, laterally by the faucial pillars, and inferiorly by the base of the tongue.

oropharynx The part of the pharynx, or throat, that lies below the soft palate at the level of the oral cavity or just posterior to the mouth.

orthognathic surgery Surgery that involves the bones of the upper jaw (the maxilla) and the lower jaw (the mandible).

Orticochea sphincteroplasty A type of pharyngoplasty to create a sphincter that encircles the velopharyngeal port; also known as *sphincter pharyngoplasty*.

osseointegrated implants Implants that are inserted in the bone; used for retention of bridges and prosthetic devices.

osseointegration (adj. osseointegrated) Creation of a connection between an implant and the bone.

ossicles (adj. ossicular) Three small bones in the middle ear, the malleus, incus, and stapes, that conduct sound energy from the tympanic membrane to the cochlea.

osteogenesis Creation of new bone.

osteotomy Surgical cut in a bone so the bone can be placed in a more functional and appropriate position.

ostium (pl. ostia) Small opening between a paranasal sinus and the nasal cavity.

overbite The vertical overlap of the upper and lower incisors; can be measured in millimeters but is often reported as a percentage of coverage of the lower incisors by the upper incisors; normal overbite is approximately 2 mm, or about 25%; greater amounts are called either deep overbite or *deep bite*.

overjet The horizontal relationship between the upper and lower incisors; typically measured in millimeters from the labial surface of the lower incisor to the labial surface of the upper incisor with the teeth in occlusion; a normal amount of overjet is about 2 mm with upper incisors and lower incisors in light contact; excessive overjet is when the maxillary incisors are labioverted or stick out toward the lips.

overlay dentures Dentures that fit over the existing teeth and usually provide more vertical dimension than with the existing teeth.

overtones Component frequencies of a signal that are whole number multiples of the fundamental frequency; also called *harmonics*.

overt submucous cleft A submucous cleft that can be identified on the nasal surface of the velum based on features such as a zona pellucida (thin zone); bifid or hypoplastic uvula; or apparent diastasis of the levator muscle, which is particularly apparent during phonation.

palatal (adj.) The inner part of the upper and lower arch that is in proximity to the surface of the hard palate.

palatal–dorsal fricative An abnormal articulation production that is often compensatory for anterior oral cavity crowding; produced as a fricative consonant that is articulated with the middle of the dorsum under the middle of the hard palate; is usually substituted for sibilant sounds (/s/, /z/, /ʃ/, /ʒ/, /ʧ/, /ʤ/).

palatal–dorsal plosive An abnormal articulation production that is often compensatory for anterior oral cavity crowding; produced as a stop consonant that is articulated with the middle of the dorsum against the middle of the hard palate; is usually substituted for the lingual-alveolar sounds (/t/ and /d/), the velar sounds (/k/ and /g/), and in some cases, the sibilant sounds (/s/, /z/, /ʃ/, /ʒ/, /ʧ/, /ʤ/); also called a *mid-dorsum palatal stop*.

palatal fistula A hole or an opening in the palate that goes all the way through to the nasal cavity; usually the result of failure of the palate to heal after a palatoplasty; also known as an *oronasal fistula*.

palatal lift A prosthetic appliance that can be used to raise the velum for speech in cases where the velum is long enough to achieve velopharyngeal closure but does not move well, often from neurological impairment.

palatal obturator A prosthetic appliance that can be used to cover an open palatal defect, such as an unrepaired cleft palate or a palatal fistula; this device can be used to improve an infant's ability to achieve compression of the nipple for suction or to close a palatal defect for speech.

palatal orthopedics A method used to align the alveolar segments in both unilateral and bilateral clefts of the palate prior to surgical correction; also known as *premaxillary orthopedics* or *infant oral orthopedics.*

palatal section (of a prosthesis) The body portion of a prosthetic appliance that fits over the palate.

palatal vault The rounded dome on the upper part of the oral cavity.

palatine aponeurosis A sheet of fibrous tissue located just below the nasal surface of the velum and extending about 1 cm posteriorly from its attachment on the posterior border of the hard palate; consists of periosteum, fibrous connective tissue, and fibers from the tensor veli palatini tendon; provides an anchoring point for the velopharyngeal muscles and adds stiffness to that portion of the velum; also called *velar aponeurosis.*

palatine processes of the maxilla Paired bones of the maxilla that are just behind the incisive suture lines and form the anterior three-quarters of the maxilla.

palatine raphe The thin white line that can often be seen running longitudinally down the middle of the hard palate and velum; an embryological suture line of the hard palate and velum.

palatine tonsils Masses of lymphoid tissue between the anterior and posterior faucial pillars on both sides of the oral cavity; also called simply the *tonsils.*

palatine torus A normal variation, not an abnormality, that consists of a prominent longitudinal ridge, or exostosis, on the oral surface of the hard palate in the area of the median palatine suture line; found most often in Caucasians, particularly those of northern European descent, and reportedly common in the northern Native American and Eskimo populations; also known as *torus palatinus.*

palatoglossus Paired muscles that act antagonistically to the levator veli palatini to depress the velum or elevate the tongue; these muscles contribute to lowering the velum for the production of nasal speech sounds.

palatomaxillary suture line An embryological suture line that separates the paired palatine processes of the maxilla, which form the anterior three-quarters of the

maxilla, and the paired horizontal plates of the palatine bones; also known as the *transverse palatine suture line.*

palatopharyngeus Paired muscle of the pharynx; the horizontal fibers are thought to be associated with the sphincteric action of the velopharyngeal valve, assisting with velopharyngeal closure by pulling the lateral pharyngeal walls medially to narrow the pharynx.

palatoplasty Palate repair.

palpebral fissures Openings between the eyelids.

panendoscope An older illuminated instrument that included an optical tube that is placed in the mouth and turned upward for visualization of the velopharyngeal sphincter; no longer used.

paranasal sinuses Four pairs of air-filled spaces, including the frontal sinuses (in the forehead area), maxillary sinuses (under the cheeks), ethmoid sinuses (between the eyes), and sphenoid sinuses (deep in the skull).

paresis (adj. paretic) Weakness of muscle movement; partial or incomplete paralysis or loss of movement.

parietal bones The bones that form the sides and top of the skull.

Passavant's ridge A shelf-like ridge that projects from the posterior pharyngeal wall into the pharynx during speech; occurs as a result of contraction of specific fibers of the superior pharyngeal constrictor muscles; found in normal speakers and speakers with velopharyngeal dysfunction.

passive speech characteristics When the articulation placement (the function) of speech is normal, but an abnormality of the structure (i.e., dental malocclusion, velopharyngeal insufficiency, or an oronasal fistula) causes distortion of speech; include hypernasality, nasal emission, weak consonants, and short utterance length; also known as *obligatory distortions.*

pedodontist A term sometimes used for a pediatric dentist.

periosteum A thick, fibrous membrane that covers the surface of bone.

perpendicular plate of the ethmoid The bone that projects down to join the vomer and lies between the vomer and the quadrangular cartilage; forms part of the nasal septum.

pharyngeal cul-de-sac resonance A resonance disorder that occurs when most of the sound remains in the oropharynx during speech; typically caused by large tonsils that block the exit of the oropharynx and thus the entrance to the oral cavity.

pharyngeal flap A type of pharyngoplasty designed to be a passive soft-tissue obturator of the middle of the velopharyngeal sphincter to improve or correct velopharyngeal function.

pharyngeal fricative A compensatory articulation production that is produced when the tongue is retracted so that the base of the tongue approximates, but does not touch, the pharyngeal wall; a friction sound occurs as the air pressure is forced through the narrow opening that is created between the base of the tongue and pharyngeal wall.

pharyngeal plexus A network of nerves that lies along the posterior wall of the pharynx and consists of the pharyngeal branches of the glossopharyngeal and vagus nerves, which provide motor innervation for the velar muscles that contribute to velopharyngeal closure.

pharyngeal plosive A compensatory articulation production that is produced with the back of the tongue articulating against the pharyngeal wall; also called *pharyngeal stop.*

pharyngeal stop A compensatory articulation production that is produced with the back of the tongue articulating against the pharyngeal wall; also called *pharyngeal plosive.*

pharyngeal tonsil A mass of lymphoid tissue that is found on the posterior pharyngeal wall of the nasopharynx on the skull base; also called the *adenoid, adenoid pad,* or *adenoids.*

pharyngeal wall augmentation An implant that is surgically placed or injected in the posterior pharyngeal wall or a rolled flap on the pharyngeal wall; placed in the area of the velopharyngeal opening to correct velopharyngeal dysfunction.

pharyngoplasty A surgical procedure of the pharynx that is designed to correct velopharyngeal dysfunction.

pharynx (adj. pharyngeal) The walls of the throat between the nasal cavity and the esophagus.

phenotype The manifestations of a genotype; range of characteristics associated with a genetic syndrome.

philtral ridges The raised lines on either side of the philtrum, which are embryological suture lines that are formed as the segments of the upper lip fuse.

philtrum (adj. philtral) A long dimple or indentation that courses from the columella down to the upper lip and is bordered by the philtral ridges on each side.

phonation The production of sound by vibration of the vocal cords; also called *voicing.*

phoneme-specific hypernasality Occurs when the individual has learned to consistently substitute a nasal sound for an oral sound, despite normal velopharyngeal anatomy and physiology.

phoneme-specific nasal emission (PSNE) Occurs when the individual has learned to produce pressure-sensitive consonants in the pharynx instead of the oral cavity, despite normal velopharyngeal anatomy and physiology; the airflow is released through the velopharyngeal valve as nasal emission that occurs only on those misarticulated phonemes; usually occurs on sibilant sounds, particularly s/z.

Pierre Robin sequence A congenital condition that consists of micrognathia, glossoptosis, and cleft palate; there is often upper airway obstruction for several months after birth.

pinna The delicate cartilaginous framework of the external ear; functions to direct sound energy into the external auditory canal.

plagiocephaly Asymmetric or abnormal skull shape.

pleiotropy The phenomenon where a single gene can affect multiple unrelated systems.

plosive phonemes Pressure-sensitive consonants that require a buildup of intraoral pressure prior to a sudden release (/p/, /b/, /t/, /d/, /k/, /g/).

pneumotachograph A device that determines the rate of airflow through the use of a flowmeter and a differential pressure transducer; one of the components of aerodynamic instrumentation to measure velopharyngeal orifice area or nasal resistance.

pneumatic activities As they relate to the velopharyngeal valve: blowing, whistling, sucking, and speech.

polydactyly Extra fingers and/or toes.

polymers Large molecules (macromolecules) composed of repeating structural units.

polymorphism Variability in genes that contributes to the uniqueness of individuals.

polysomnography A diagnostic test in which a number of physiologic variables are recorded during an overnight sleep study.

posterior crossbite Any of the maxillary teeth distal (posterior) to the canines are positioned inside the mandibular teeth; usually occurs because the maxilla is too narrow; also known as *lateral crossbite.*

posterior nasal fricative An abnormal articulation production that is produced with the velum somewhat down so that air pressure goes through a velopharyngeal opening, creating a friction sound with audible nasal emission; typically used as a substitution for sibilant sounds, particularly s/z; associated with phoneme-specific nasal emission (PSNE).

posterior nasal spine A midline bony protrusion from the posterior border of the hard palate.

posterior pharyngeal wall Back wall of the throat.

premaxilla A triangular-shaped bone that is bordered on either side by the incisive suture lines; this bony segment normally contains the central and lateral maxillary incisors.

premaxillary orthopedics A method used to align the alveolar segments in both unilateral and bilateral clefts of the palate prior to surgical correction; also known as *palatal orthopedics* or *infant oral orthopedics*.

pressure-equalizing (PE) tubes Small tubes that are surgically inserted in the eardrum to provide an alternate route for air to enter the middle ear for ventilation if the eustachian tube is nonfunctional; also called *ventilation tubes*.

pressure-flow technique Procedure using aerodynamic instrumentation to evaluate the dynamics of the velopharyngeal mechanism during speech; also used to evaluate nasal respiration and to quantify upper airway obstruction through measurements of nasal airway resistance.

pressure-sensitive phonemes Speech sounds that require oral air pressure for production; include plosives, fricatives, and affricates.

prevalence In epidemiological terms, refers to a measure of existing cases of a disorder in a given population.

primary palate The lip and palate anterior to the incisive foramen; includes the lip and alveolus.

prognathia (adj. prognathic) Protrusive mandible caused by mandibular hyperplasia.

prognathism A condition where the mandible is bigger than the maxilla.

prolabium The tissue that normally makes up the central portion of the upper lip between the philtral columns but is isolated when there is a bilateral cleft lip.

proptosis (adj. proptotic) Protrusion of the eyeball.

proptotic globes Relative protrusion of the eyes.

prosody Refers to the stress, intonation, and rhythm of speech.

prosthesis (adj. prosthetic) A fabricated substitute for a body part that is missing or malformed; also called a *prosthetic device*.

prosthetic device A fabricated substitute for a body part that is missing or malformed; also called a *prosthesis*.

prosthodontist A dental professional who deals with the restoration of teeth and the development of appliances to replace or improve the appearance of oral and facial structures or to assist with feeding and velopharyngeal closure.

provisionally unique syndrome Pattern of multiple anomalies in what appears to be an underlying syndrome, although a diagnosis cannot be made because the pattern is not one that has been previously described or reported.

pterygoid hamulus A hook-like structure at the lower end of the medial pterygoid plate of the sphenoid bone; the tensor veli palatini glides around it.

pterygoid process A part of the sphenoid bone that contains the medial pterygoid plate, the lateral pterygoid plate, and the pterygoid hamulus, all of which provide attachments for muscles in the velopharyngeal complex.

ptosis Drooping of the eyelids.

Punnett square A tabular summary of possible combinations of maternal and paternal alleles to predict the probability of an offspring having a particular genotype based on the rules of Mendelian inherittance.

purines Nitrogenous bases of nucleotides in a DNA molecule that consist of adenine and guanine.

pyriform aperture Literally means "pear-shaped opening"; the opening to the bony inside of the nose, sometimes spelled *piriform*.

pyrimidines Nitrogenous bases of nucleotides in a DNA molecule that consist of thymine and cytosine.

quad helix A palatal expansion device that consists of bands on the most posterior molars and frequently the primary canines, which are connected by a palatal spring that has two posterior and two anterior loops.

quadrangular cartilage The cartilage that forms the anterior nasal septum and projects anteriorly to the columella.

radiography The use of roentgen rays (X-rays) to image internal body parts.

rapid palatal expander (RPE) A palatal expansion device that consists of two or four molar bands and a jackscrew connecting them in the middle of the palate; turning the screw creates the necessary force to widen the dental arches.

reduction therapy A form of speech therapy where a prosthetic device is used to stimulate the movement of the velopharyngeal structures to avoid the need for surgery or reduce the extent of the surgery needed.

replication The process of making two identical DNA molecules from one, resulting in two double strands, each containing one original and one complementary newly synthesized strand of DNA.

resection Surgical removal of an organ or piece of a body part.

resonance As it relates to voiced speech, the modification of the sound that is generated by the vocal cords through selective enhancement of certain frequencies as it travels through the vocal tract (pharynx, oral cavity, and nasal cavity). The frequencies that are enhanced are determined by the size and shape of those cavities.

resonance disorder A disorder of the acoustics of speech due to abnormal transmission of sound energy through the oral, nasal, and/or pharyngeal cavities of the vocal tract during speech production.

retrognathia (adj. retrognathic) When one or both jaws is located posterior to its normal position; usually used in reference to a retrusive mandible; associated with micrognathia (mandibular hypoplasia).

reverse pull headgear A device used to advance the maxilla and improve an anterior crossbite; also called *face mask*.

rhythm With respect to speech, it refers to the alteration of stressed and unstressed syllables and the relative timing of each.

rugae Folds, ridges, or creases in a structure; the transverse ridges in the mucosal covering of the hard palate.

rule of 10s A guideline for the appropriate time for a cleft lip repair, which says that the infant must be at least 10 weeks of age and 10 pounds and have a hemoglobin of 10 gm prior to the lip repair.

saccule A sensory organ within the inner ear that provides a sensation of acceleration.

sagittal pattern The least common pattern of velopharyngeal closure; the lateral pharyngeal walls move medially to meet in midline to effect closure; the velum may move to close against the lateral pharyngeal walls rather than against the posterior pharyngeal wall.

sagittal suture The vertical division between the two parietal bones of the skull.

salpingopharyngeal folds Folds that originate from the torus tubarius at the opening to the eustachian tube on both sides of the pharynx and then course downward to the lateral pharyngeal wall; consist of glandular and connective tissue.

salpingopharyngeus Paired muscle that arises from the inferior border of the torus tubarius and courses vertically along the lateral pharyngeal wall and under the salpingopharyngeal fold; is not felt to have a significant role in achieving velopharyngeal closure given its size and location.

sclera (pl. sclerae) White portion of the eyeball.

secondary palate Structures that are posterior to the incisive foramen, including the hard palate (excluding the premaxilla) and the velum.

semicircular canals The loop-shaped tubular parts of the inner ear that provide a sense of spatial orientation; the loops are oriented in three planes at right angles to each other.

sensitivity The extent to which a test is able to correctly identify positive results; proportion of true positive results as intended to be revealed by a test.

sensorineural hearing loss A type of hearing loss caused by a problem with the creation of nerve impulses within the inner ear or the transmission of the nerve impulses through the brainstem to the auditory cortex.

sequence The occurrence of a pattern of multiple anomalies within an individual that arise from a single known or presumed prior anomaly or mechanical factor; where one anomaly leads to the development of the other anomalies, as in Pierre Robin sequence.

sex chromosomes The 23rd pair of chromosomes (X and Y), which function in determining gender.

sialorrhea Drooling.

sibilant phonemes Speech sounds that are produced by the friction of air pressure as it is emitted anteriorly through the incisors (i.e., /s/, /z/, ʃ/, /ʒ/, /ʧ/, /dʒ/)

Simonart's band A band of tissue that bridges a cleft lip that may result from partial fusion that has separated.

single-tooth crossbite A crossbite that involves only one upper and one lower tooth.

skeletal relationship The way the jaws (maxilla and mandible) come together during biting.

soft palate The part of the palate that is located in the back of the mouth and consists of muscles that are covered by the same mucous membrane as the hard palate; also known as the *velum*.

source–filter model Interaction between phonation and resonance where the vocal folds are the source and the vocal tract is the filter.

specificity The extent to which a test correctly identifies true negative results; the proportion of individuals with negative test results for what the test is intended to reveal.

speech aerodynamics A procedure to measure the aerodynamic properties of airflow and air pressure during speech production.

speech aid appliance A prosthetic device that can be considered when the velum is too short to close completely against the posterior pharyngeal wall; this device consists of a retaining appliance and a bulb (usually of acrylic) that fills in the pharyngeal space for speech; also known as a *speech bulb obturator*.

speech bulb obturator A prosthetic device that can be considered when the velum is too short to close completely against the posterior pharyngeal wall; this device consists of a retaining appliance and a bulb (usually of acrylic) that fills in the pharyngeal space for speech; also known as a *speech aid appliance*.

sphenoid bone An unpaired bone located at the base of the skull.

sphincter pharyngoplasty A type of pharyngoplasty to create a dynamic sphincter that encircles the velopharyngeal port; also known as the *Orticochea sphincteroplasty*.

Standard Precautions Recommended procedures, published by the Centers for Disease Control and Prevention, that are designed to protect the patient, the professional, and all others in a healthcare environment from the spread of infection.

stapes One of the ossicles in the middle ear; acts as a piston to create pressure waves within the fluid-filled cochlea.

stenosis An abnormal narrowing or stricture of a canal (e.g., choanal stenosis, pharyngeal stenosis, pyriform aperture stenosis, or subglottic stenosis).

stertorous A heavy snoring sound in respiration.

stigma A factor that is different from cultural standards and results in discrediting an individual's social acceptability.

stimulability The ability to correct an abnormal speech sound production when given minimal cues.

stoma An opening into a hollow organ, such as the mouth; can be surgically created, as in the stoma of the trachea following a tracheostomy.

stress Related to increased muscular effort and subglottic pressure during the production of a syllable; stressed syllables are produced with greater articulatory precision, are longer in duration, and are higher in pitch and intensity than unstressed syllables.

stridor A high-pitched, wheezing sound during breathing.

submetacentric When the centromere of a chromosome is closer to one end than the other.

submucous cleft palate A congenital defect that affects the underlying structures of the palate, whereas the structures on the oral surface are intact; can involve the muscles of the velum and those of the bony structure of the hard palate.

suborbital coloring Darkness under the eyes usually from lack of sleep; often called "black eyes."

succedaneous teeth Secondary or permanent teeth.

suckling An early form of sucking characterized by extension–retraction movements of the tongue.

superior constrictor Paired muscle of the pharynx; the upper fibers are responsible for the medial displacement of the lateral pharyngeal walls to effectively narrow the velopharyngeal port; also called *superior pharyngeal constrictor*.

superior pharyngeal constrictor Paired muscle of the pharynx; the upper fibers are responsible for the medial displacement of the lateral pharyngeal walls to effectively narrow the velopharyngeal port; also called *superior constrictor*.

supernumerary tooth Extra tooth; usually erupts in the line of the cleft.

syndactyly Fusion or webbing of the digits (fingers and/or toes).

syndrome A pattern of multiple anomalies or malformations that regularly occur together, are pathogenically related, and therefore have a common known or suspected cause; craniofacial syndromes (involving the head and face) cause affected individuals to look alike, even when there is no family relationship (e.g., Down syndrome).

tailpiece (of a prosthetic device) The part of a palatal lift or speech bulb appliance that extends posteriorly to either raise the velum or close the nasopharynx behind the velum.

temporal bones Located at the sides and base of the skull.

tensor veli palatini muscles Paired muscles that are believed to be responsible for opening the eustachian tubes to enhance middle ear aeration and drainage.

teratogens External chemical or physical agents, such as cigarette smoke, drugs, viruses, or radiation, that can interfere with normal embryological development and result in congenital malformations.

tongue-tie A condition where the lingual frenulum is short or has an anterior attachment, resulting in restricted movement of the tongue tip; typically diagnosed if the patient cannot elevate the tongue tip sufficiently to touch the roof of the mouth with the mouth open and cannot protrude the tongue tip past the mandibular gingival ridge or incisors; also known as *ankyloglossia*.

tonsillar fossa Space within the faucial pillars.

tonsillitis An infection of the tonsils.

tonsils Common name for the lymphoid tissue that is located on either side of the mouth between the anterior and posterior faucial pillars; also referred to as *palatine tonsils*. Note that there is the *lingual tonsil* at the base of the tongue and the *pharyngeal tonsil*, which is also referred to as the *adenoids*.

torus A slow-growing nodular protuberance of bone that can occur in either the hard palate or mandible.

torus palatinus A normal variation, not an abnormality, that consists of a prominent longitudinal ridge, or exostosis, on the oral surface of the hard palate in the area of the median palatine suture line; found most often in Caucasians, particularly those of northern European descent, and reportedly common in the northern Native American and Eskimo populations; also known as *palatine torus*.

torus tubarius A ridge in the nasopharyngeal wall, posterior to the opening of the eustachian tube, caused by the projection of the cartilaginous portion of this tube.

Towne's view A radiographic view that is sometimes used as an alternative to the base view because it also provides an en face orientation and allows the examiner to look down into the port.

tracheostomy A surgical procedure that involves placement of a tube directly in the trachea; done to relieve upper airway obstruction, which can be life threatening.

transdisciplinary team An interdisciplinary team where members understand the other disciplines and how they relate to the total care of the patient; this understanding of the various disciplines allows them to be able to see the "big picture" in the care of the patient.

transducers Used to convert the detected air pressure or flow into electrical signals for further processing as part of aerodynamic instrumentation.

translocation The result of a transfer of genetic material between two or more chromosomes; may not be associated with any abnormalities in the individual because the total amount of genetic material may be unchanged.

transverse palatine suture line Separates the anterior two-thirds of the maxilla (which consists of the paired palatine processes) from the posterior portion of the hard palate (which consists of the paired horizontal plates of the palatine bones); also known as the *palato-maxillary suture line*.

treating team Team members who provide a consultation regarding the total care of the patient and also offer treatment.

trisomy A condition where there is an extra chromosome in a homologous pair of chromosomes; for example, trisomy 21 or Down syndrome in humans is a condition where the cell contains 47 rather than 46 chromosomes.

tympanic membrane Thin tissue that separates the outer ear from the middle ear; transmits sound energy through the ossicles to the inner ear; also called the *eardrum*.

underbite The abnormal vertical overlap of the lower incisors over the upper incisors.

underjet A reversal of the normal incisor position, with the maxillary incisors linguoverted, or facing inward toward the tongue; also called *linguoversion* or *anterior crossbite*.

upper esophageal sphincter (UES) The upper end of the esophagus that normally is closed but stretches open as the bolus travels through the hypopharynx and into the esophagus.

utricle A sensory organ within the inner ear that provide the sensation of acceleration.

uvula A teardrop-shaped structure that is typically long and slender and hangs freely from the back or free edge of the velum; it has no known function.

uvulopalatopharyngoplasty (UPPP) A surgical procedure for the treatment of obstructive sleep apnea in adults; involves the excision of the remaining tonsil and resection of the free margin of the soft palate and uvula; the anterior and posterior tonsillar pillars are sewn together to open the oropharyngeal inlet.

variable expressivity Variability in the clinical presentation (phenotype) of patients with a particular genetic disorder; a gene can result in variations in the phenotype from a very pronounced effect in one individual to a barely noticeable effect in another.

velar aponeurosis A sheet of fibrous tissue located just below the nasal surface of the velum and extending about 1 cm posteriorly from its attachment on the posterior border of the hard palate; consists of periosteum, fibrous connective tissue, and fibers from the tensor veli palatini tendon; provides an anchoring point for the velopharyngeal muscles and adds stiffness to that portion of the velum; also called *palatine aponeurosis*.

velar dimple The area on the oral side of the velum where it bends during phonation or velopharyngeal closure as a result of the action of the levator veli palatini muscle; can be noted through an intraoral examination.

velar eminence A bulge on the nasal surface of the velum during phonation, which comes from the musculus uvulae muscles; can be seen through nasopharyngoscopy.

velar fricative Compensatory articulation production that is produced with the back of the tongue in the same position as for the production of a /j/ (as in "yellow") sound so that a small space is created between the back of the tongue and the velum; a fricative sound is produced as air is forced through that small opening.

velar plosive Speech sound that is produced with the back of the tongue against the velum; air pressure is built up behind the tongue and then released suddenly, including /k/ and /g/.

velar stretch The process where the velum elongates as it elevates to achieve velopharyngeal closure.

velopharyngeal dysfunction (VPD) One of the generic terms that is used to describe abnormal velopharyngeal function, regardless of the cause.

velopharyngeal impairment One of the generic terms that is used to describe abnormal velopharyngeal function, regardless of the cause.

velopharyngeal inadequacy One of the generic terms that is used to describe abnormal velopharyngeal function, regardless of the cause.

velopharyngeal incompetence A neuromotor or physiological disorder that results in poor movement of the velopharyngeal structures.

velopharyngeal insufficiency An anatomical or structural defect that precludes adequate velopharyngeal closure by causing the velum to be short relative to the posterior pharyngeal wall.

velopharyngeal mislearning Inadequate velopharyngeal closure from faulty learning of appropriate articulation patterns.

velum The part of the palate that is located in the back of the mouth and consists of muscles that are covered by the same mucous membrane as the hard palate; frequently referred to as the *soft palate*.

ventilation tubes Small tubes that are surgically inserted in the eardrum to provide an alternate route for air to enter the middle ear for ventilation if the eustachian tube is nonfunctional; also called *pressure-equalizing (PE) tubes*.

ventricular septal defect (VSD) A congenital hole in the wall that separates the lower chambers of the heart.

ventrum (adj. ventral) The underneath surface of the tongue.

vermilion The red pigmented portion of the upper and lower lips.

videofluoroscopic speech study An evaluation of the velopharyngeal mechanism during speech using videofluoroscopy.

videofluoroscopic swallowing study (VFSS) A radiographic procedure that allows an overall view of the oral, pharyngeal, and esophageal phases of swallowing as well as the interactions between the phases; also referred to as a *modified barium swallow (MBS)*.

videofluoroscopy An imaging technique used to obtain real-time moving images of internal structures; done through the use of a fluoroscope, which consists of an X-ray source and fluorescent screen; can be used for evaluation of velopharyngeal function or swallowing.

video nasendoscopy A minimally invasive endoscopic procedure that allows visual observation and analysis of the velopharyngeal mechanism or larynx during speech, phonation, or swallowing; commonly used in the evaluation of swallowing, upper airway obstruction, and the structure and function of the larynx and vocal cords; also called *nasopharyngoscopy*, *nasal endoscopy*, or *nasendoscopy*.

vocal fold paralysis The absence of movement of one or both vocal folds caused by dysfunction of the motor nerve supply to the larynx.

vocal nodules Small callus-like masses that typically occur symmetrically on both vocal cords and are caused by chronic abuse, misuse, or overuse of the cords.

voice The sound that results from vocal cord vibration, which is then emitted through the mouth or nose during speech and singing.

voicing The production of sound by vibration of the vocal cords; also called *phonation*.

vomer A flat bone of trapezoidal shape that is positioned so that it is perpendicular to the palate; the inferior border meets the nasal surface of the maxilla in midline and forms the inferior and posterior portion of the nasal septum.

Waldeyer's ring A complex of lymphoid tissue, including the adenoids (pharyngeal tonsil), palatine tonsils, and lingual tonsil, which encircles the pharynx and plays a role in the immune system.

W-arch A variation of the quad helix palatal expansion device.

white roll The white border tissue that surrounds the red tissue, or vermilion, of the upper and lower lips.

Wilms tumor A malignant tumor of the kidney; a risk for individuals with Beckwith–Wiedemann syndrome.

X-linked inheritance A condition caused by mutations in genes on the X chromosome.

zona pellucida A bluish area in the middle of the velum that is the result of abnormal insertion of the levator veli palatini muscles, effectively causing the velum to be thin and almost transparent in appearance.

Z-plasty A plastic surgery technique that is used to lengthen tissue.

zygomatic bone The bone of the skull that forms the prominence of the cheek and articulates with the frontal, sphenoid, temporal, and maxillary bones. It is also known as the *malar bone*.

CREDITS

Glossary opener photo: © PeopleImages/Getty Images

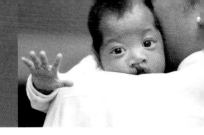

INDEX

Note: Page numbers followed by "*f*" and "*t*" indicate figures and tables respectively.

605